Handbook
of
Amyotrophic
Lateral
Sclerosis

NEUROLOGICAL DISEASE AND THERAPY

Series Editor

WILLIAM C. KOLLER

Department of Neurology
University of Kansas Medical Center
Kansas City, Missouri

1. Handbook of Parkinson's Disease, *edited by William C. Koller*
2. Medical Therapy of Acute Stroke, *edited by Mark Fisher*
3. Familial Alzheimer's Disease: Molecular Genetics and Clinical Perspectives, *edited by Gary D. Miner, Ralph W. Richter, John P. Blass, Jimmie L. Valentine, and Linda A. Winters-Miner*
4. Alzheimer's Disease: Treatment and Long-Term Management, *edited by Jeffrey L. Cummings and Bruce L. Miller*
5. Therapy of Parkinson's Disease, *edited by William C. Koller and George Paulson*
6. Handbook of Sleep Disorders, *edited by Michael J. Thorpy*
7. Epilepsy and Sudden Death, *edited by Claire M. Lathers and Paul L. Schraeder*
8. Handbook of Multiple Sclerosis, *edited by Stuart D. Cook*
9. Memory Disorders: Research and Clinical Practice, *edited by Takehiko Yanagihara and Ronald C. Petersen*
10. The Medical Treatment of Epilepsy, *edited by Stanley R. Resor, Jr., and Henn Kutt*
11. Cognitive Disorders: Pathophysiology and Treatment, *edited by Leon J. Thal, Walter H. Moos, and Elkan R. Gamzu*
12. Handbook of Amyotrophic Lateral Sclerosis, *edited by Richard Alan Smith*

Additional Volumes in Preparation

Handbook of Parkinson's Disease: Second Edition, Revised and Expanded, *edited by William C. Koller*

Handbook of Pediatric Epilepsy, *edited by Fereydoun Dehkharghani and Jerome Murphy*

Handbook
of
Amyotrophic
Lateral
Sclerosis

edited by
Richard Alan Smith
Center for Neurologic Study
San Diego, California

Marcel Dekker, Inc.   **New York • Basel • Hong Kong**

Library of Congress Cataloging-in-Publication Data

Handbook of amyotrophic lateral sclerosis / edited by Richard Alan Smith.
      p.   cm. -- (Neurological disease and therapy ; v. 12)
    Includes bibliographical references and index.
    ISBN 0-8247-8610-6 (alk. paper)
    1. Amyotrophic lateral sclerosis.   I. Smith, Richard Alan.
    II. Series.
    [DNLM: 1. Amyotrophic Lateral Sclerosis. W1 NE33LD v. 12 /
WE 550 H236]
RC406.A24H35   1992
616.8'3--dc20
DNLM/DLC
for Library of Congress   92-4386
                                                    CIP

This book is printed on acid-free paper.

MARCEL DEKKER, INC.
270 Madison Avenue, New York, New York 10016

Current printing (last digit):
10 9 8 7 6 5 4 3 2 1

PRINTED IN THE UNITED STATES OF AMERICA

Series Introduction

In the *Handbook of Amyotrophic Lateral Sclerosis*, Dr. Smith and his collaborators sum up what is currently known about amyotrophic lateral sclerosis (ALS). The clinical disorder is described, including genetic and epidemiological aspects. The pathology of this disorder is described in rich detail and both the neurophysiological and neuroimaging aspects of ALS are also thoroughly discussed. The treatment of the ALS patient is discussed in terms of providing total care to meet all the needs of the patient and his/her family. The second half of the book deals with research strategies. This is truly the exciting aspect of the battle against ALS. As our knowledge of neurodegenerative diseases has increased tremendously, it is likely that we will find the cause of these disorders in the near future and surely have better therapy to offer individuals afflicted with these devastating diseases. The experimental approaches discussed truly offer hope for the future. Contributors to the book clearly provide state-of-the-art knowledge on investigational strategies. It is the hope, and probably the reality, that in future editions of this book, many of the experimental therapies discussed will have become established therapies.

William C. Koller

Preface

Over the period that this book has been in preparation there has been a surge of public interest in the neurological sciences. The Congress of the United States has declared the 1990s to be the "Decade of the Brain" and numerous brain science companies have been founded. As this book goes to press, the gene location for familial amyotrophic lateral sclerosis (ALS) is in the news. This may mark a major milestone in the history of research into the cause of ALS, which has eluded discovery since its description in the last century. This is not the first time that a research result has generated great enthusiasm, leading to prediction of an imminent cure. In planning this book, it was decided to give balanced treatment to competing ideas, despite the temptation to give more attention to subjects that momentarily enjoy prominence. At one time or another, most of the etiological considerations included in the book have been in fashion. For example, in the 1960s it seemed almost certain that a viral cause for ALS would be discovered. More recently, the concept of an environmental cause of ALS has been resurrected after having been proposed some 40 years ago as an explanation for the high incidence of ALS on Guam. All these ideas are presented herein—in most instances by the people who have closely associated themselves with these subjects.

In the tradition of the Neurological Disease and Therapy series, this volume provides the reader with an overview, starting with an account of the clinical features of ALS. As of late, there has been renewed interest in this subject as more disorders mimicking ALS have been described. As chronicled by Norris, confusion about the diagnostic features of ALS has a long history, dating to the early 1800s. Then, as now, the problem is to sort out the cases of ALS from a myriad of other entities (see particularly the chapter by Thomas and Latov). Hopefully, practicing neurologists will find this exercise easier after review of the chapters dealing with the clinical description of ALS. For example, Stålberg and Sanders thoroughly review the electromyographic features that distinguish ALS from other disorders, and Hoffman and his colleagues discuss the radiological findings in ALS, including their results with positron emission tomography scanning. The clinical researcher will be interested in discussions of the quantitative methods employed to chronicle the course of ALS, including the possible use of single-fiber and macroelectromyography and the use of a quantitative neuromuscular examination as first introduced by Munsat. His studies reveal that deterioration in ALS is generally linear, although elsewhere Norris draws attention to cases of "benign" ALS. This concept emerges from a study of some 800 patients who were personally followed over the course of about 15 years. In a similar clinical tradition, Chou and Hirano and Kato elucidate the pathological findings in ALS, which suggest that there is a pathological continuum that is first represented by chromatolysis and later by progressive degeneration marked by loss of dendrites, pigmentary atrophy, axonal swelling, and dying back of the distal neuron. Furthermore, Chou offers an explanation for the occurrence of long-tract degeneration in ALS, which has not been easily explained. This is consonant with contemporary anatomical views about the origins of the pyramidal tract.

New ideas have not only invigorated our understanding of the clinical entity of ALS, but new technology has had a great impact on the care of ALS patients. It is odd that a treatment for ALS has eluded modern medicine, considering the therapeutic achievements of the time, but symptomatic treatment of ALS is highly developed. As discussed by Goldblatt, the care of ALS patients makes considerable demands on the physician. Not only is there a demand on one's technical skill, but one must also find the wisdom to guide patients along the difficult course that characterizes the disease. Along the way, patients with ALS encounter numerous difficulties, many of which are amenable to symptomatic treatment. The impact of technology on patient care is particularly evident in three areas: ventilatory and nutritional support and communication. The great strides made in the latter field are reviewed by Sutter, who provides insight into the theory that underlies communication technology utilized on behalf of the handicapped. In addition, he reports on his experience with the development of a communication system based on the use of evoked visual potentials. This would have seemed like pure science fiction a few years ago.

Although a number of legal and ethical issues impinge on patient care, little attention has been given in the ALS literature to the ethical aspects of experimental treatment. When this has been discussed, it has usually been in the context of protecting the patient from overzealous experimentation. Feenberg argues that some of these attitudes have resulted in a paternalism that does not always serve the needs of the patient. For a number of reasons, beyond the obvious one of personal benefit, patients with ALS are often highly motivated to participate in experimental treatment. Another aspect of this issue is the need to conduct rigorous clinical trials with the idea that both the patient and the research community deserve to know whether a putative treatment exhibits a therapeutic effect. To illuminate this subject various aspects of trial design are reviewed.

Although it is difficult to be certain where the clue to ALS will originate, it is likely that advances in the basic sciences will ultimately be the wellspring from which ALS is solved. In the instance of ALS, the brunt of the pathological process seems to focus on the motor neuron. Study of this cellular element is hampered by a number of factors, not the least of which is the inability to culture isolated adult human motor neurons. Strategies for dealing with this problem are reviewed by Cashman, who discusses the techniques of motor neuron purification using cell-sorting technology and the hybrid cell lines that can be immortalized. Furthermore, properties of the motor neuron include the role of the extracellular matrix, which may influence not only cell-to-cell contact within the central nervous system, but the properties of the neuromuscular junction. Perturbations of this system are suggested as a possible place to look for the cause of ALS. A novel proposal, long advocated by Festoff, is that ALS might actually start in the periphery owing to a disorder of the neuromuscular junction. Approaching the issue of neuron degeneration from a theoretical basis, Kuether and Lipinski developed computer simulations of the degenerative process, which leads to a better conceptual understanding of factors that ultimately influence the course of the disease process. Separate chapters dealing with epidemiology, immunology, virology, the cytoskeleton, growth factors, free radicals, neurotransmitters, and neurotoxicology focus on specific etiological considerations that have been explored in the instance of ALS. Although each of these ideas is treated separately, it is tempting to invoke a unitary hypothesis as to the cause of ALS, drawing on diverse disciplines. Considering the studies reported by Glasberg and Wiley and Salazar-Grueso and Roos, it can be seen, for example, that there are novel ways that a virus can bring about a disease. In transgenic mice, insertion of several retroviral genes has been associated with myositis and, in a recent experiment, with severe neuronal degeneration. Since some viral gene products appear to be growth factors, it does not stretch the imagination to suggest that a retrovirus, acting indirectly, could account for ALS on the basis of a unique pathology, possibly through an autoimmune mechanism. Obviously there is no shortage of such explanations. Idle hypotheses are not particularly helpful, but there are ways to approach such questions experimentally. One approach that comes to mind involves the search for ubiquinated proteins. Recently ubiquitin inclusions have been found in the motor neurons of patients dying of ALS (see Messer's chapter). Ubiquitin marks proteins scheduled for proteolysis. An unknown viral gene product might be detected by its association with this housekeeping protein.

Nowhere have human studies received more attention than on Guam, which could be considered a veritable neurological Rosetta stone. As reviewed by Kurland and his colleagues, the falling incidence of ALS in this island community seems to be giving way to an increased incidence of other neurodegenerative diseases. This could be accounted for on the basis of exposure to an environmental toxin, as elaborated on by Spencer and Kisby, who postulate the occurrence of "slow neurotoxins" as a cause of chronic, neurodegenerative disease. Although each research consideration discussed is promising, the genetic linkage studies reported by Figlewicz and her colleagues offer immediate promise for identifying a gene defect and, by extension, a specific protein that may be defective in ALS. The localization of the gene defect to chromosome 21, at least in some families, heightens the search for the gene that may prove to be the cause of ALS. This single finding could lead directly to a treatment for ALS if the problem turns out to be straightforward.

Looking ahead, Brown and Horvitz predict the future opportunities for ALS research. They suggest that the study of animal models for motor neuron disease could considerably enhance the search for the gene(s) responsible for motor neuron diseases and could serve as excellent models for experimental treatment. Calling on Horvitz's seminal studies with programmed cell death, they discuss the critical role that may be played by growth factors (also reviewed by Henderson) and the impact of possible "killer genes" in the instance of neurodegeneration. A future volume will no doubt be required to put these ideas in perspective.

Those who are familiar with the field will note that some subjects have not been included. Some were purposely omitted. In a few instances these seem to have been promoted beyond the facts, dying of their own weight. They will not be missed in this book or others. Only time will tell about the rest. Undoubtedly, there are some omissions that would have benefitted the reader. Where this is the case there are several explanations, the most embarrassing of which is ignorance. More permissible is the excuse that the pace of discovery and complexity of the subject constitute constraints on the editorial process. Almost any aspect of biology may well become germane in the instance of a disease, like ALS, that is characterized by the inexplicable degeneration of a rather select group of neurons. Almost weekly, the scientific literature is filled with mind-boggling reports that could point toward a new research direction. The wealth of information is comparable to the flowering of the arts that characterized the Renaissance. Hopefully, what was missed here will soon be given proper attention elsewhere.

Although it occurred to me to one day edit a book about ALS, having worked most of my professional life with this problem in mind, the idea for this book originated with the publisher. I must admit to some satisfaction in having been chosen to undertake this probject, although something of this sort unavoidably takes time that might be put to other use. With this task behind me and with the realization that there are fewer years ahead, I hope to devote more of my time to pursuing the ideas given life on these pages. To do so will require the continued faith of my patients, my family, and my numerous benefactors. It is to them and my colleagues who have given their time and effort to this endeavor that I dedicate this book.

ACKNOWLEDGMENTS

I am grateful to: colleagues Paul Marangos, Chris Mirabelli, Robert Fildes, Martin Nash, and Johnathan Licht; teachers Sherif Shafey, Paul Altrocchi, and Walter Dandlikker; patients Fred Clark, William Doro, Warren Irwin, John Stockton, Curtis Roberts, and Jim Waldal; friends Joan Thagard, Sandy and Bram Dykstra, David Gelles, Kevin McLean, Dee Norris, Henry Wineman, Jack and Mary Ann Olson, Ted Steffens, Rolly Koran, Steve Hoffman, Janice Roccio, Marcia Rosselini, and Jana Tognoli; supporters Arlene and George Hecht, Robert Curtis, Jr., Arlene Doro, Betty Bordner, Milton Fillius, and Ruth and William Frank; staff Shyla Hernandez, John Moon, Kristen Valderhaug, Teri Kataoka, and Fredric Storch; and family Norma Cohen, Gerri London, and Daryl and Tania Smith. Each of these people has reinforced my sense of purpose and well-being, but no person has done more to keep me working than George Thagard, Jr., to whom I will forever be indebted.

Richard Alan Smith

Contents

Contributors

Carmel Armon, M.D. Department of Neurology, Loma Linda University Medical School and Medical Center, and Jerry L. Pettis Memorial Veterans Affairs Medical Center, Loma Linda, California

Mark B. Atkinson, M.D. Department of Brain and Vascular Research, The Cleveland Clinic Foundation, Cleveland, Ohio

Orest B. Boyko, M.D., Ph.D. Department of Radiology, Duke University Medical Center, Durham, North Carolina

Anthony C. Breuer, M.D.* Departments of Neurology and Brain and Vascular Research, The Cleveland Clinic Foundation, Cleveland, Ohio

Benjamin Rix Brooks, M.D. ALS Clinical Research Center, University of Wisconsin—Madison, School of Medicine and Neurology Service, William S. Middleton Memorial Veterans Affairs Hospital, Madison, Wisconsin

Robert H. Brown, Jr., M.D., D.Phil. Department of Neurology, Massachusetts General Hospital, Boston, Massachusetts

---

*Present affiliation: Department of Neurology, Baptist Hospital, Nashville, Tennessee.

Neil R. Cashman, M.D.   Department of Neurology and Neurosurgery, McGill University, and Montreal Neurological Institute, Montreal, Quebec, Canada

Samuel M. Chou, M.D., Ph.D.   ALS Research Foundation, California Pacific Medical Center, San Francisco, California

Valerie A. Cwik, M.D.   Department of Neurology, University of Alberta, Edmonton, Alberta, Canada

W. Kent Davis, M.D.   Department of Radiology, Rex Hospital, Raleigh, North Carolina

Andrew Feenberg, Ph.D.   Department of Philosophy, San Diego State University, San Diego, California

Barry W. Festoff, M.D.   Neurobiology Research Laboratory, Veterans Affairs Medical Center, Kansas City, Missouri, and Department of Neurology, University of Kansas Medical Center, Kansas City, Kansas

Denise A. Figlewicz, Ph.D.   Department of Neurology, Montreal General Hospital, and Centre for Research in Neuroscience, McGill University, Montreal, Quebec, Canada

Mark R. Gilbert, M.D.*   Department of Neurology, The Johns Hopkins University School of Medicine, Baltimore, Maryland

Mark R. Glasberg, M.D.[†]   Department of Neurology, Henry Ford Hospital, Detroit, Michigan

David Goldblatt, M.D.   Department of Neurology, University of Rochester School of Medicine and Dentistry, Rochester, New York

James F. Gusella, Ph.D.   Molecular Neurogenetics Laboratory, Massachusetts General Hospital, Charlestown, Massachusetts, and Department of Genetics, Harvard Medical School, Boston, Massachusetts

Kenneth E. M. Hastings, Ph.D.   Montreal Neurological Institute and Departments of Neurology/Neurosurgery and Biology, McGill University, Montreal, Quebec, Canada

---

**Present affiliation:* University of Pittsburgh School of Medicine, Pittsburgh, Pennsylvania.
[†]*Present affiliation:* Neuroscience Center, Riverside Methodist Hospital, Columbus, Ohio.

Joseph M. Healey, Jr., J.D. Department of Community Medicine and Health Care, University of Connecticut School of Medicine, Farmington, Connecticut

Christopher E. Henderson, Ph.D. Centre de Recherche de Biochimie Macromoléculaire, CNRS-INSERM, Montpellier, France

Asao Hirano, M.D. Division of Neuropathology, Department of Pathology, Montefiore Medical Center, and Departments of Pathology and Neuroscience, Albert Einstein College of Medicine, Bronx, New York

John M. Hoffman, M.D. Department of Radiology, Duke University Medical Center, Durham, North Carolina

H. Robert Horvitz, Ph.D. Department of Biology, Massachusetts Institute of Technology and Howard Hughes Medical Institute, Cambridge, Massachusetts

Malcolm J. Jackson, Ph.D., M.R.C. Path. Department of Medicine, University of Liverpool, Liverpool, England

Edward J. Kasarskis, M.D., Ph.D. Departments of Neurology, Toxicology, and Nutrition, University of Kentucky and Veterans Affairs Medical Center, Lexington, Kentucky

Shuichi Kato, M.D. Division of Neuropathology, Department of Pathology, Montefiore Medical Center and Departments of Pathology and Neuroscience, Albert Einstein College of Medicine, Bronx, New York

Glen Kisby, Ph.D. Center for Research on Occupational and Environmental Toxicology, Oregon Health Sciences University, Portland, Oregon

Gerald Kuether, M.D. Neurological Clinic, Technical University, Munich, Germany

Leonard T. Kurland, M.D., Dr.Ph. Section of Clinical Epidemiology, Department of Health Sciences Research, Mayo Clinic and Mayo Foundation, Rochester, Minnesota

Norman Latov, M.D., Ph.D. Department of Neurology, College of Physicians and Surgeons, Columbia University, Neurological Institute, and Columbia-Presbyterian Medical Center, New York, New York

Hans Gerd Lipinski, Ph.D. MEDIS Institute, Munich, Germany

Robert L. Margolis, Ph.D.   Department of Basic Sciences, The Fred Hutchinson Cancer Research Center, Seattle, Washington

Anne Messer, Ph.D.   Wadsworth Center for Laboratories and Research, New York State Department of Health, and Department of Biomedical Sciences, State University of New York at Albany, Albany, New York

John Douglas Mitchell, M.D., F.R.C.P.   Department of Neurology, Royal Preston Hospital, Preston, England

Hiroshi Mitsumoto, M.D.   Neuromuscular Program, Department of Neurology, The Cleveland Clinic Foundation, Cleveland, Ohio

Nancy A. Muma, Ph.D.   Department of Pathology, The Johns Hopkins University School of Medicine, Baltimore, Maryland

Theodore L. Munsat, M.D.   Neuromuscular Research Unit, New England Medical Center, and Tufts University School of Medicine, Boston, Massachusetts

Forbes H. Norris, M.D.   ALS and Neuromuscular Research Foundation, California Pacific Medical Center, San Francisco, California

Raymond P. Roos, M.D.   Division of the Biological Sciences, Department of Neurology, Pritzker School of Medicine, The University of Chicago, Chicago, Illinois

Guy A. Rouleau, M.D., Ph.D.   Department of Neurology, Montreal General Hospital, and Centre for Research in Neuroscience, McGill University, Montreal, Quebec, Canada

Edgar F. Salazar-Grueso, M.D.   Division of the Biological Sciences, Department of Neurology, Pritzker School of Medicine, The University of Chicago, Chicago, Illinois

Donald B. Sanders, M.D.   Division of Neurology, Department of Medicine, Duke University, Durham, North Carolina

Glenn E. Smith, Ph.D.   Section of Clinical Epidemiology, Department of Health Sciences Research and Department of Psychiatry and Psychology, Mayo Clinic and Mayo Foundation, Rochester, Minnesota

Richard Alan Smith, M.D. Center for Neurologic Study, San Diego, California

Peter S. Spencer, Ph.D., M.R.C.Path. Center for Research on Occupational and Environmental Toxicology, Oregon Health Sciences University, Portland, Oregon

Erik V. Stålberg, Ph.D., M.D. Department of Clinical Neurophysiology, University Hospital, Uppsala, Sweden

John C. Steele, M.D., F.A.C.P., F.R.C.P.(C), M.Sc. (London) Micronesian Health Study, University of Guam, Mangilao, and Guam Memorial Hospital, Tamuning, Guam

Erich E. Sutter, Ph.D. Smith-Kettlewell Eye Research Institute, San Francisco, California

Florian Patrick Thomas, M.D. Montreal Neurological Institute, McGill University, Montreal, Quebec, Canada

Juan Cavieres Troncoso, M.D. Departments of Pathology and Neurology, The Johns Hopkins University School of Medicine, Baltimore, Maryland

Clayton A. Wiley, M.D., Ph.D. Departments of Pathology and Neurosciences, University of California—San Diego, La Jolla, California

D. B. Williams, M.B., B.S., Ph.D. Department of Neurology, John Hunter Hospital, Newcastle, New South Wales, Australia

Prologue

Stephen W. Hawking, C.B.E., F.R.S.

Lucasian Professor of Mathematics, Department of Applied Mathematics and Theoretical Physics, Cambridge University, Cambridge, England

I have had motor neuron disease for practically all my adult life. Yet it has not prevented me from having a very attractive family and being successful in my work. This is thanks to the help I have received from my wife, my children, and a large number of other people and organizations. I have been lucky, because my condition has progressed more slowly than is often the case. It shows that one need not lose hope.

I was born on January 8, 1942, exactly 300 years after the death of Gallileo. However, I estimate that about 200,000 other babies were also born that day. I don't know whether any of them was later interested in astronomy. I was born in Oxford, even though my parents were living in London. This was because Oxford was a good place to be born during the war: the Germans had an agreement that they would not bomb Oxford and Cambridge, in return for the British not bombing Heidelberg and Göttingen. It is a pity that this civilized sort of arrangement couldn't have been extended to more cities.

My father came from Yorkshire. His grandfather had been a wealthy farmer who had bought too many farms and gone bankrupt in the agricultural depression at the beginning of this century. This left my father's parents badly off, but they managed to send him to Oxford, where he studied medicine. He then went into research of tropical medicine. He went to east Africa in 1935. When the War began, he made an overland journey across Africa, to get a ship back to England, where he volunteered for military service. He was told, however, that he was more valuable in medical research.

My mother was born in Glasgow, Scotland, the daughter of a family doctor. The family moved south to Devon when she was 12. Like my father's family, they were not well off. Nevertheless, they managed to send my mother to Oxford. After Oxford, she had various jobs, including that of Inspector of Taxes, which she did not like. She gave that up to become a secretary. That was how she met my father, in the early years of the War.

We lived in Highgate, north of London. Our house was damaged by a V-2 rocket that landed a few doors away. Fortunately, we were not there at the time. In 1950, we moved to the cathedral city of Saint Albans, 20 miles north of London. My father wanted me to go to Westminster School, one of the main "public"—that is to say, private—schools. He himself had gone to a minor public school. He felt that this, and his parents' poverty, had led to his being passed over in favor of people with less ability, but more social graces. However, I was ill at the time of the scholarship exam, and so I did not go to Westminster. Instead, I went to the local school, Saint Albans School, where I got an education that was as good as, if not better than, what I would have had at Westminster. I have never found that my lack of social graces has been a hindrance.

I was a fairly normal small boy: slow to learn to read and very interested in how things worked. I was never more than about halfway up the class at school and never well coordinated. I was not good at ballgames and my handwriting was the despair of my teachers. Maybe for this reason, I didn't care much for sport or physical activities. When I was 12, one of my friends bet another friend a bag of sweets that I would never come to anything. I don't know if this bet was ever settled and, if so, which way it was decided.

My father would have liked me to study medicine. However, I felt that biology was too descriptive and not sufficiently fundamental. Maybe I would have felt differently if I had been aware of molecular biology, but that was not generally known about at the time. Instead, I wanted to study mathematics and physics. My father felt, however, that there would not be any jobs in mathematics, apart from teaching. He therefore made me study chemistry, physics, and only a small amount of mathematics. Another reason against mathematics was that he wanted me to go to his old college, University College, Oxford, and they did not teach mathematics at that time. I duly went to University College in 1959 to study physics, which was the subject that interested me most, since it governs how the universe behaves. To me, mathematics is just a tool with which to study physics.

Most of the other students in my year had done military service and were a lot older. I felt rather lonely during my first year and part of the second. It was only in my third year that I really felt happy at Oxford. The prevailing attitude at that time was very antiwork. You were supposed to either be brilliant without effort or accept your limitations and get a fourth-class degree. To work hard to get a better class of degree was regarded as the mark of a "gray man," the worst epithet in the Oxford vocabulary.

At that time, the physics course was arranged in a way that made it particularly easy to avoid work. I took one exam before I went up and then had 3 years at Oxford, with just the final exams at the end. I once calculated that I studied for about 1,000 hours of work in the three years I was at Oxford, an average of an hour a day. I'm not proud of this lack of work, I'm just describing my attitude at the time, which I shared with most of my fellow students: an attitude of complete boredom and feeling that nothing was worth making an effort for. One result of my illness has been to change all that: when faced with the possibility of an early death, it makes you realize that life is worth living, and that there are lots of things you want to do.

I had planned to get through the final exam by solving problems in theoretical physics, avoiding any questions that required factual knowledge. However, because of nervous tension, I didn't do very well. I was on the borderline between a first- and second-class degree, and I had to be interviewed by the examiners to determine which I should get. When they asked me about my future plans, I replied I wanted to do research. If they gave me a first, I would go to Cambridge. If I got only a second, I would stay at Oxford. They gave me a first.

I felt that there were two posible areas of theoretical physics that were fundamental and in which I might do research. One was cosmology, the study of the very large. The other was elementary particles, the study of the very small. I thought that elementary particles were less attractive, because, although lots of new particles were being found, there was no proper theory of elementary particles. All that could be done was to arrange the particles in families, as in botany. In cosmology, on the other hand, there was a well-defined theory, Einstein's General Theory of Relativity.

In my third year at Oxford, I seemed to be getting more clumsy, and I fell over once or twice for no apparent reason. But it was not until I was at Cambridge, in the following year, that I saw a specialist, and shortly after my 21st birthday, I went into the hospital for tests. I was in for two weeks, during which I had a wide variety of tests. The doctors took a muscle sample from my arm, stuck electrodes into me, and injected some radiopaque fluid into my spine and watched it going up and down with X-rays, as they tilted the bed. After all that, they didn't tell me what I had, except that it was not multiple sclerosis, and that I was an atypical case. I gathered, however, that they expected my condition to continue to get worse, and that there was nothing they could do, except give me vitamins. I could see that they didn't expect the vitamins to have much effect. I didn't feel like asking for more details, because they were obviously bad.

The realization that I had an incurable disease that was likely to kill me in a few years was a bit of a shock. How could something like that happen to me? Why should I be cut off like this? However, while I was in the hospital, I had seen a boy I vaguely knew die of leukemia, in the bed opposite me. It had not been a pretty sight. Clearly there were people who were worse off than I. At least my condition didn't make me feel sick. Whenever I feel inclined to be sorry for myself, I remember that boy.

Not knowing what was going to happen to me, or how rapidly the disease would progress, I was at loose ends. The doctors told me to go back to Cambridge and carry on with the research I had just started, in general relativity and cosmology. But I was not making much progress, because I didn't have much mathematical background. And, anyway, I might not live long enough to finish my Ph.D. I felt somewhat of a tragic character. I took to listening to Wagner, but reports in magazine articles that I drank heavily are an exaggeration. The trouble is, once one article said it, other articles copied it, because it made a good story. People believe that anything that has appeared in print so many times must be true.

My dreams at that time were rather disturbed. Before my condition was diagnosed, I had been very bored with life. There had not seemed to be anything worth doing. But shortly after I came out of the hospital, I dreamt that I was going to be executed. I suddenly realized that there were a lot of worthwhile things I could do, if I were reprieved. Another dream that I had several times was that I would sacrifice my life to save others. After all, if I were going to die anyway, it might as well do some good.

But I didn't die. In fact, although there was a cloud hanging over my future, I found, to my surprise, that I was enjoying life in the present more than before. I began to make progress with my research, and I got engaged to a girl named Jane Wilde, whom I had met just about the time my condition was diagnosed. That engagement changed my life. It gave me something to live for. But it also meant that I had to get a job, if we were to get married. To my great surprise, I got a research fellowship at Cambridge, and we got married a few months later.

I was lucky to have chosen to work in theoretical physics, because that was one of the few areas in which my condition would not be a serious handicap. And I was fortunate that my scientific reputation increased, at the same time that my disability got worse. This meant that people were prepared to offer me a sequence of positions in which I only had to do research, without having to lecture.

We were also fortunate in housing. When we were married, Jane was still an undergraduate, so she had to be away during the week. This meant that we had to find a place I could manage on my own, which was central, because I could not walk far. I asked the College if they could help, but was told that it was policy not to help Fellows find housing. We sublet a small house 100 yards from my university department and then we rented another house in the same road. After we had lived there for a few years, we wanted to buy the house, so we asked my College for a mortgage. However, the College did a survey and decided it was not a good risk. In the end, we got a mortgage from a building society, and my parents gave us the money to fix it up. We lived there until it became too difficult for me to manage the stairs. By this time, the College appreciated me rather more, and they offered us a ground-floor flat in a house they owned. This suits me very well, because it has large rooms and wide doors. It is sufficiently central that I can get to my university department, or the College, in my electric wheelchair. It is also nice for our three children, because it is surrounded by a garden, which is looked after by the College gardeners.

My research up to 1970 was in cosmology, the study of the universe on a large scale. My most important work in this period was on singularities. Observation of distant galaxies indicates that they are moving away from us: the universe is expanding. This implies that the galaxies must have been closer together in the past. The question then arises: was there a time in the past when all the galaxies were on top of one another, and the density of the universe was infinite? Or was there a previous contracting phase, in which the galaxies managed to avoid hitting one another? Maybe they flew past and started to move away from one another. To answer this question required new mathematical techniques. These were developed between 1965 and 1970, mainly by Roger Penrose and myself. We used these techniques to show that there must have been a state of infinite density in the past, if the General Theory of Relativity was correct.

This state of infinite density is called the Big Bang singularity. It would be the beginning of the universe. All the known laws of science would break down at a singularity. This would mean that science would not be able to predict how the universe would begin, if General Relativity is correct. However, my more recent work indicates that it is possible to predict how the universe began if one takes into account the theory of quantum mechanics, the theory of the very small.

General Relativity also predicts that massive stars will collapse in on themselves when they have exhausted their nuclear fuel. The work that Penrose and I had done showed that they would continue to collapse until they reached a singularity of infinite density. This singularity would be an end of time, at least for the star and anything on it. The gravitational field of the singularity would be so strong that light could not escape from a region around it, but would be dragged back by the gravitational field. The region from which it is not possible to escape is called a black hole, and its boundary is called the event horizon. Anything, or anyone, who falls into the black hole through the event horizon will come to an end of time at the singularity.

I was thinking about black holes as I got into bed one night in 1970, shortly after the birth of my daughter, Lucy. Suddenly, I realized that many of the techniques that Penrose and I had developed to prove singularities could be applied to black holes. In particular, the area of the event horizon, the boundary of the black hole, could not decrease with time.

From 1970 to 1974, I worked mainly on black holes. But in 1974, I made perhaps my most surprising discovery: black holes are not completely black!

When one takes the small-scale behavior of matter into account, particles and radiation can leak out of a black hole. The black hole emits radiation as if it were a hot body.

Since 1974, I have been working on combining general relativity and quantum mechanics into a consistent theory. One result was a proposal I made in 1983 with Jim Hartle, of Santa Barbara: that both space and time are finite in extent, but they don't have any boundary or edge. They would be like the surface of the earth, but with two dimensions. The Earth's surface is finite in area, but it doesn't have any boundary. In all my travels, I have not managed to fall off the edge of the world.

If this proposal is correct, there would be no singularities, and the laws of science would hold everywhere, including at the beginning of the universe. The way the universe began would be determined by the laws of science. I would have succeeded in my ambition to discover how the universe began. But I still don't know *why* it began.

Up to 1974, I was able to feed myself and get in and out of bed. Jane managed to help me and bring up two children, without outside help. However, things were getting more difficult, so we took to having one of my research students living with us. In return for free accommodation and a lot of my attention, they helped me get up and go to bed. In 1980, we changed to a system of community and private nurses, who came in for an hour or two in the morning and evening. This lasted until I caught pneumonia in 1985 and had to have a tracheostomy. After this, I had to have 24-hour nursing care. This was made possible by grants from several foundations.

Before the operation, my speech had been getting more slurred; only a few people who know me well could understand me. But at least I could communicate. I wrote scientific papers by dictating to a secretary, and I gave seminars through an interpreter, who repeated my words more clearly. However, the tracheostomy removed my ability to speak altogether. For a time, the only way I could communicate was to spell out words letter by letter, by raising my eyebrows when someone pointed to the right letter on a spelling card. It is pretty difficult to carry on a conversation like that, let alone write a scientific paper. However, a computer expert in California, Walt Woltosz, heard of my plight. He sent me a computer program he had written, called Equalizer. This allowed me to select words from a series of menus on the screen, by pressing a switch in my hand. The program can also be controlled by a switch operated by head or eye movement. When I have built up what I want to say, I can send it to a speech synthesizer. At first, I just ran the Equalizer program on a desktop computer. However, David Mason, of Cambridge Adaptive Communications, fitted a small portable computer and a speech synthesizer to my wheelchair. This system allows me to communicate much better than I could before. I can manage up to 15 words a minute. I can either speak what I have written or save it on disk. I can then print out or call it back and speak it sentence by sentence. Using this system, I have written a book and a dozen scientific papers. I have also given a number of scientific and popular talks. They have been well received. I think that is in large part due to the quality of the speech synthesizer, which is made by Speech Plus. One's voice is very important. If you have a slurred voice, people are likely to treat you as mentally deficient. This synthesizer is by far the best I have heard, because it varies the intonation and doesn't speak like a Dalek. The only trouble is that it gives me an American accent. However, the company is working on a British version.

In this summary of my experience in living with ALS, I have described just a few of the many problems faced by patients with this disease, and I have described how I coped with them.

DIAGNOSIS AND MANAGEMENT

1

Amyotrophic Lateral Sclerosis: The Clinical Disorder

Forbes H. Norris

*ALS and Neuromuscular Research Foundation, California Pacific Medical Center
San Francisco, California*

INTRODUCTION

Diseases causing progressive paralysis through systemic motor neuron degeneration are the *primary* motor neuron disorders (MNDs). The most common of these is amyotrophic lateral sclerosis (ALS), a progressive, usually fatal paralysis of adults, which is easily diagnosed in moderate to advanced cases, in which the clinical features are readily described. The onset, however, is variable and progression early in the illness is often insidious; indeed an old synonym is "creeping paralysis." There is considerable clinical variability from case to case, reminiscent to older clinicians of acute poliomyelitis (though in a greatly slowed time frame).

In some ALS cases, fascicular twitching of the muscles precedes by months, even years, any muscular weakness; in others, frequent, painful muscle cramps herald the creeping paralysis. Both these onsets are difficult to identify with certainty because everyone can experience a painful cramp or fascicular twitching, especially during or after vigorous exercise. (In this regard, the tendency of cramps to occur also during sound sleep as "night cramps" is a paradox.) Other ALS sufferers notice first an unusual fatigue, again (as with cramps and fasciculation) an exaggeration of a normal occurrence. As in normals and myasthenics, the fatigue syndrome usually responds to brief rest periods. Rarely there is slow, but steady progression of this fatigue syndrome, so that eventually even prolonged rest fails to restore the previous level of strength; every exertion seems to cause more weakness.

Some other ALS patients (or their families) first notice emotional lability, usually toward easier weeping but sometimes toward ready laughter ("the giggles"), even approaching an alarming hilarity. Particularly when the latter continues more than a minute and alarms the onlookers, or resists the patient's effort at control, there may be transition to frustrated weeping, and again this may not be controlled. Even trivial stimuli may provoke this emotional hyper-reflexia and lead to psychiatric attention, particularly in the self-conscious, affluent, modern societies when other signs and symptoms have not developed. Fatigue of the lower cranial nerve-supplied muscles can produce early symptoms of aspiration of saliva (manifest by a dry cough, rarely by aspiration pneumonitis even before other symptoms occur) and dysarthria, with or without emotional liability, and again these are changes we all notice occasionally, especially in times of great stress or emotional excitement, so that dating the onset of ALS from such symptoms can be very uncertain, nor do such symptoms necessarily indicate ALS.

Sooner or later in ALS there is chronic weakness with atrophy of affected muscles, and then the average patient seeks medical attention. Still, complaint of weakness has hundreds of causes, including the psychological, and until moderate muscle atrophy develops, the presence of so grave an illness as ALS may not be suspected by the physician even in the presence of quite abundant fasciculation, including similar twitching in normal muscles. All familiar with ALS will immediately recognize the ominous significance of such widespread fasciculation.

The weakness may be acute, though "creeping paralysis" is the rule. One patient, a banker, experienced sudden difficulty in pronunciation during an important business conference. He believed he was having a stroke and noted the time as 1014 hours on his conference pad. His physician diagnosed a cerebral thrombosis after appropriate workup disclosed no other cause of the symptom. It did not improve, however, as is typical of most strokes, and after 3–4 months the patient began to aspirate and after another month was found to have slight tongue atrophy with fasciculation. A neurological evaluation revealed generalized fasciculation with hyperreflexia at the knees, so ALS was suspected. An electromyogram (EMG) showed mild but diffuse denervation in the pattern characteristic of ALS. The typical progression then occured. But in the great majority of ALS patients, "creeping paralysis" makes it difficult to date the onset for scientific purposes.

The weakness can be in any body part, ranging from the bulbar-supplied muscles to the toes, so that one patient may present with toe weakness, another breathing problems, another finger clumsiness, another dysarthria, and another with apparent emotional disorder. Moreover, the difficulty can reflect either upper or lower motor neuron impairment, or a combination of upper and lower motor neuron lesions. For example, the emotional lability already noted is due to emotional reflex hyperactivity, a "pseudobulbar" manifestation, so nearly all those patients (even in the absence of other involvement) have hyperactive, sometimes clonic jaw jerks in the neurological examination. Owing to the characteristic mixture of upper and lower motor neuron lesions in ALS, such a patient (when becoming symptomatic enough to seek medical attention) also usually shows at least slight tongue atrophy with fasciculation and fibrillation. The gag reflex may also be hyperactive and spread to the larynx, causing temporary (but very distressing) upper airway obstruction from laryngospasm. The emotional reflexes are far more complex, however, so another patient may have a flaccid pharynx, no gag reflex, and no jaw jerk.

Another patient may present because of stumbling, catching one foot when walking or climbing stairs, and show no atrophy but have increased knee and ankle muscle stretch reflexes evidencing an upper motor dysfunction. At this point such patients usually do not manifest Babinski's sign in the examination, a valuable point in considering demyelinating and mass lesions in the differential diagnosis (1). Another patient with an identical history may have no ankle jerk, a reduced knee jerk, and anterior-compartment muscle atrophy, indicating lower motor neuron involvement at that time.

Most common of all at the time of diagnosis, however, is a generalized syndrome of progressive muscular weakness, painless except for cramps, sparing some muscles and moderately to severely affecting other muscles. Antecedent fatigue, cramps, fasciculation, emotional lability, and so forth, as discussed above, may have been absent but typically have been a problem for months or even years. ALS is further characterized by normal mental faculties, including preservation of the premorbid personality type (2), sparing of eye movements, the common and special senses, and bowel-bladder control. (Exceptions are infrequent and will be discussed below.) As recounted elsewhere in this volume, other (mimicking) conditions have been excluded by appropriate testing; the EMG shows not only diffuse denervation, but the giant or unstable motor units characteristic of ALS, with normal peripheral nerve conduction velocities.

From that time, the majority of patients experience steady progression of the weakness, though at varying rates; one patient progressed from no symptoms to death in 3 months, another in 4 months, though Professor Stephen Hawking has had ALS for 27 years and another patient is entering the 38th year of symptoms, 33 years after the diagnosis by an esteemed neurologist. Both these patients apparently had rather typical onsets and rates of progression early in the illness, which then slowed and later stabilized to result in continued major, but nonprogressive disability many years later.

TYPES OF PRIMARY MIND

That there are MND subtypes has been recognized for over a century; controversy has existed whether the less malignant, more restricted subtypes reflect
ALS in a patient having some resistance to the full disease process or truly a
different disease with partial or overlapping symptomatology. A familiar analogy
is liver disease caused by several etiologies (e.g., toxic-nutritional, viral, etc.)
but having similar, or even identical, clinical manifestations through ultimate
failure of a single target cell. The recognized subtypes of MND (Table 1) are as
follows:

Progressive muscular atrophy (PMA) is the lower motor and spinal MND
having earlier age of onset and sparing bulbar functions until very late in the
illness, which typically extends over decades, i.e., slower progression than ALS.
The onset is usually in the arms and hands with fasciculation. From lack of upper
motor involvement, the clinical picture is entirely amyotrophic with hypo- to
areflexia and great muscular atrophy, sometimes evolving before weakness is
noted.

Primary lateral sclerosis (PLS) is the mainly upper motor MND having onset
in spastic leg-foot muscles and then ascending paraparesis over many years,
usually decades, again a much slower progression than in ALS and again with
bulbar sparing. Late in the illness, the forearm and intrinsic hand muscles may

Table 1   Clinical Differentiation of Adult Idiopathic Motor Neuron Diseases (MNDs)

MND type	Sex	Usual onset	Atrophy	Muscle reflexes	Bulbar	Course
PMA	Male	Arms	Marked	Decr. to absent	Late	Decades
PLS	Either	Legs	Rare	Incr. to clonic	Late	Decades
PBP	Either	Bulbar	Mod. to marked	Incr. to clonic	Constant	Months–years
ALS	Either	Any	Mod. to marked	Absent to clonic	Usual	Months–years
GuamALS	Either	Arms	Mod. to marked	Absent to clonic	Usual	Years–decades
BenALS	Male	Arms or legs	Mod. to marked	Absent to clonic	Spared	Decades
PBspMA	Male	Girdles + bulbar	Mod. to marked	Variable	Constant	Decades
CMT II	Either	Legs	Marked	Absent	Late	Decades
WKW	Either	Girdles	Moderate	Absent	Late	Decades

develop atrophy, but fasciculation is rare. One patient developed this syndrome in 1953; respiratory compromise led to tracheostomy 35 years later, in 1988, when he also showed temporalis and masseter muscular atrophy as well as distal arm and hand muscle atrophy but still no fasciculation (which, as a physician, he confirmed). Death occurred in 1989 at age 78 years from myocardial infarction; PLS was confirmed by the necropsy. Rosenberg (3) is correct to emphasize that several other diseases, such as multiple sclerosis (MS) and high cord tumor, produce identical illnesses in some cases, but he is wrong to state that PLS is "a nondiagnosis."

Progressive bulbar palsy (PBP) is a bulbar motor neuron syndrome that is nearly always the early onset of ALS in the bulbar-supplied muscles (see below). The presentation may be either lower ("bulbar palsy") or upper motor neuron ("pseudobulbar palsy") or (commonly) a mixture of these syndromes. By strict definition (*bulbar*), there should be no weakness of neck flexion and extension, or of respiration, but in practice it seems that most neurologists accept such weakness to a mild degree if the major signs and symptoms are bulbar.

ALS as already described, is the occurence of both lower (hence, PMA-like) and upper (PLS-like) signs with rapid extension, including the bulbar functions (PBP-like) if spared early in the illness, though the onset may be bulbar and thus mimic PBP in the first weeks or months. The course to death from respiratory paralysis or aspiration pneumonitis is months to years. *Sporadic ALS* (Spor ALS) is ALS in a patient with no near relative having the disorder. *Familial ALS* (FamALS) is ALS in a patient having a near relative with the same illness. The clinical picture is identical to Spor ALS; despite the occurrence of dorsal column demyelination, FamALS patients usually show no clinical disturbance in sensation. If there is only one other affected relative, then it remains possible that the disease is SporALS striking the same family twice by coincidence. On the other hand, absence of such family history may merely indicate the family's lack of information about their relatives. An example is the orphan who develops ALS. Were there really no relatives with ALS or is the history merely silent on this point? Why was the patient given to the orphanage or put up for adoption? Unlike myotonic dystrophy, where the family often denies familial disease, in FamALS the relatives are often aware and readily inform their physicians. A positive history of FamALS is probably always accurate; a negative history in SporALS should be reviewed repeatedly with as many relatives as possible before concluding that it is really negative.

Guam ALS is very rare beyond the island except for the U.S. West Coast, where some Chamorro natives of Guam have immigrated. This subtype is also identical to SporALS, except that there is a much longer course in many Guam cases (4, 5), and also there are major differences in the pathology (6).

Benign ALS (BenALS) is a descriptive label for patients who developed typical SporALS, but after months or years, and after reaching a certain level of disability, were gratified to notice that the progression had become very slow or stopped altogether (7). These patients are also characterized by bulbar and respiratory muscle sparing and having an "ALS score" (8, 9) > 50 (normal = 98–100) with annual losses of 2 points or less in the score after relative stabilization. One such patient had the onset in 1953 and was diagnosed elsewhere in 1957 (so the early course was somewhat slower than usual); she has lost only 5 points on the ALS score in the past 20 years. It should be emphasized, however, that "benign" is not a satisfactory permanent designation for these patients; they all suffer major disabilities. On the other hand, Professor Hawking would not receive this diagnosis because of the severity and generalization of his paralysis, even though he has been nearly stable for some years.

Other idiopathic MND are much less frequent and readily differentiated from these adult disorders; for example, infantile-childhood *spinal muscular atrophy* (Werdnig-Hoffmann disease) usually runs a rapid course, but some patients live into early adult life and of course might present as new cases to a different MND clinic. That is more likely to happen in *Wohlfart-Kugelberg-Welander (WKW) disease*, a familial, proximal neurogenic atrophy having clinical onset later in childhood or adolescence and very slow progression, causing little or no reduction in life expectancy. It differs from PMA in the age of onset, the near absence of fasiculation, and the clear genetic background. Hausmanowa-Petrusewicz (10) has provided a good review. *Neuronal Charcot-Marie-Tooth* (CMT II) disease was originally differentiated from onion-bulb peripheral neuropathy (CMT I) on the basis of electrographic studies by Dyck and Lambert (11): a small percentage of apparent CMT sufferers have normal peripheral nerve conduction measurements, hence ventral horn cell or root origin of the denervation. They also tend to have a later onset age and even later development of the typical CMT sensory loss, and thus might also mimic PMA. *Progressive bulbospinal muscular atrophy (PBspMA)* is also a familial and relatively benign amyotrophy of the bulbar-supplied muscles and of proximal shoulder and arms, hip and thigh muscles with marked fasciculation, especially in the lower face and tongue muscles, described by Magee (12) and then by Tsukagoshi (13) and Kennedy and colleagues (14,14a). Despite the rather alarming bulbar involvement, and the adult onset, two patients at this center are remarkably functional in the seventh and ninth decades, respectively. Only one has a known affected family member. Asians seem more susceptible to this MND (15). Also seen more often in Asians is benign juvenile, distal, segmental upper extremity, neurogenic atrophy in adolescents and young adults, predominantly males with no family involvement (16). The onset is usually unilateral, but bilateral atrophy occurs and at least some cases manifest segmental cord atrophy (17, 18), which differentiates this MND from PMA, as does the strong tendency to stabilization after several years, without extension to other body parts.

CLASSIFICATION AND SEMANTIC PROBLEMS

The outline in Table 1 reveals the potential for diagnostic confusion and subsequent statistical error. Suppose a patient presents early in ALS with an entirely lower motor syndrome. Particularly if he is a vague historian and supposes such symptoms have been present for many years, the consulting neurologist may hopefully suggest a diagnosis of PMA, a label that can remain although clear upper motor signs evolve within a month and death occurs that year. As will be seen below, PBP is the most misused label; most accounts of MND treat it as a separate disease having a quarter to a third the incidence of ALS. When such patients are followed, however, it soon becomes apparent that the bulbar signs merely indicate the location of the onset of ALS, as is true for most cases initially diagnosed as PMA or PLS. Whether BenALS is arrested ALS or a different disease, subject to recrudescence at any future time, remains open, but thus far, by requiring relatively mild involvement (ALS score > 50) and objective evidence of very slow or no progression over at least 5 years, this subtype has remained "pure."

The main points to be made here are that the diagnosis of ALS and the other MND subtypes requires confirmation by time. Single examinations are usually not adequate [for contrary opinions, see Jablecki and Donnenfeld et al. (19,20)]; death certificates alone are not adequate; family histories must be scrutinized and reviewed critically. Finally, the remediable (or potentially remediable) disorders mimicking the primary or idiopathic MND must be well excluded.

HISTORY

In 1847, F.-A. Aran was appointed physician to the public hospitals of Paris and about this time he also began a "Clinical Review" in the new journal *l'Union Médicale*. One of these reviews, on Nov. 25, 1848, described a new syndrome, progressive forearm and hand muscle weakness and atrophy in a workman, Bernard, whose legs were also weak but seemed normal in appearance (21). This "terrible illness" was drawn to Aran's attention while on rounds with Professor Rayer at la Charité (22). It is of interest that Rayer also had a role in influencing Charcot toward study of neurology (23).

Aran's reviews were suspended on Feb. 22, 1849, due to illness (there was a cholera epidemic in Paris), and he only reappeared in the journal on Oct. 19, 1850, shortly after publication of his major work of lasting importance, "Récherches sur une maladie non encore décrite du système musculaire (atrophie musculaire progressive)" (22). Evidently Aran used his convalescence to seek out additional cases of the new syndrome and was able to add nine others plus one recently described by Dubois. Summaries in English have been published (24), and some features of these cases are presented in Table 2, where it can be

Table 2 Summary of Cases Presented by F.-A. Aran (22) in 1850

Case	Onset age	Sex	Suggested modern Dx
1	16	M	?Polymyositis
2	47	M	SporALS (?luetic amyotrophy)
3	38	M	SporALS
4	33	M	PMA
5	28	F	PMA
6	13	M	?PMA[a]
7	43	M	FamALS
8	33	M	SporALS[b]
9	45	F	?Postpolio
10	36	M	???
11	37	M	Lead toxicity

[a]With necropsy study.
[b]Necropsy reported later by Cruveilhier (29).

seen that, from the modern viewpoint and the understanding that muscle stretch and plantar reflexes were not then part of the clinical art, Aran was very likely describing SporALS in his cases 2, 3, and 8, and FamALS in case 7. Aran did not believe that his cases 9, 10, and 11 typified the new syndrome; he added them to demonstrate the previously unsuspected frequency of amyotrophic problems and to show variation in the clinical pattern seen in cases 2–8. He also introduced the possibility of an etiology, since in case 11 we would now suspect lead toxicity. Case 6 died of smallpox; the necropsy revealed no apparent central nervous system (CNS) lesion; in the muscles, there was patchy atrophy to the point of "gray connective tissue" in parts but not all of the affected muscles. (Today, can we imagine the courage of those physicians to autopsy an acute smallpox victim?)

Aran (22) emphasized that the intellectual functions and memory were preserved in all respects. The ordinary and special senses, including taste and smell, were also spared by the disease. The patient's general state of good health and usual lack of previous illness contrasted with the severity and gravity of the progressive paralysis. It was differentiated from the atrophy that can follow cerebral palsy and paralytic lesions at the medullary level. Plumbism was excluded because of its tendency in adults to affect mainly the extensor muscles of the wrist, although one of his cases (case 11) was surely lead intoxication, and in his discussion, Aran cited another case, seen by Duchenne, where occult lead poisoning was suspected as the cause of extensive muscular atrophy. Aran differentiated peripheral nerve lesions by pointing out that they customarily produce more rapid and severe atrophy confined to the muscles supplied by the damaged nerve. Galvanism seemed helpful in distinguishing the atrophy of progressive muscular atrophy from nonspecific wasting, for example that due to chronic rheumatism.

In some, but not all, cases there appeared to be a clear relationship between prolonged, vigorous use of certain muscles and the onset of the muscular atrophy. Aran was curious why some types of work could lead to the virtual disappearance of a muscle, as in progressive musuclar atrophy, but in other types of prolonged muscular usage there would be other phenomena, such as writer's cramp. Galvanic treatment by Duchenne seemed to give some immediate benefit, but when the patients were seen a few months later, they had progressed to a more serious state. Aran concluded that the muscular system could be the site of a nutritional atrophy independent of any circulatory disturbance; this atrophy could be partial, localized, or general but tended to affect certain muscles and spare others in the same limb; the disorder usually began as weakness followed by wasting in the upper extremities with cramps and twitching in the affected muscles. The last stage of the disease was the complete destruction of the affected muscles and their transformation into gray connective tissue. The disease could occur spontaneously but sometimes followed prolonged overuse of certain muscles. It tended to affect mainly young, robust, healthy individuals and cause severe disability. The duration of the disease was generally long, the progression slow. The disorder rarely remained in the muscles originally affected; more often it spread in the same part of the body or to the opposite limb; the affected muscle fibers showed electrical excitability up to the stage of degeneration, and this characteristic provided a useful diagnostic test. When the transformation of the muscular tissue became complete, no treatment could restore its integrity; before this stage, one might hope to arrest the disease by galvanic excitation of the affected muscles. It was possible to demonstrate at least weak galvanic contractions in some muscles that clinically seemed totally paralyzed.

An ironic commentary is provided by comparing Aran's (21) first thoughts about the etiology: "There is a disorder of the nervous system in some parts of the body, so the muscular system atrophies little by little and may even disappear completely." In the second report, Aran (22) opened his discussion of the etiology by stating that a spinal (or neural) origin should not be excluded, and he specifically compared the abundant fasciculations in one patient to those seen so commonly in spinal cord disorders (25). The striking muscular alterations in the case studied by necropsy (case 6) probably combined with the formidable opinion of Duchenne to sway Aran toward a muscular origin.

Another irony of medical history is the division of Aran's credit with Duchenne. The referral of some patients and the trials of galvanism by Duchenne were acknowledged in the reports by Aran (21,22), but Duchenne soon claimed all priority. He insisted that he had described progressive muscular atrophy to the

Académie des Sciences in either 1848 or 1849, while dating Aran's report as no earlier than 1851 (26–28). Duchenne was an impressive figure and the contemporary neurologists probably gave his claim credence, especially after it had been published several times and Aran had developed new interests. In fact, not only was Aran's first report published in 1848, but Duchenne only presented papers on electrical stimulation to the Academy in 1848–1850. In none of the Academy's abstracts for those years is there any mention of progressive muscular atrophy. Duchenne illustrated his presentations with clinical examples and might have included the results of galvanism in patients suffering from Aran's new disease; if so, he did not judge it worthy of inclusion in the published abstracts ("prepared by the author"). Moreover, though Aran grasped early the possibility of a neural lesion, Duchenne refused as late as 1859 to accept this basis of the muscular atrophy.

MOTOR NEURON DEGENERATION

The role of neuronal degeneration was not clarified for some years. The second recorded necropsy in the new disease occurred in 1853 after the death of Lecomte [Aran's case 8 (22)]. In a detailed necropsy, Cruveilhier (29) provided one of the more critical (and less quoted) articles which should have clearly indicated a neural etiology of MND.

Before presenting the necropsy result in the case of Lecomte, Cruveilhier (29) cited a similar case seen in 1832. The clinical features were similar and he had diagnosed a spinal cord disease, but was "stupefied" at the autopsy to find no CNS lesion. He decided that the discrepancy lay not in a lack of pathological anatomy but in his ability to find it. This experience was duplicated in 1849 [Aran's case 6 (22)]. The same muscular transformation was present but completely spared some muscles while totally involving others; some fascicles were normal and others affected within the same muscle. This was puzzling, but nevertheless Cruveilhier remained convinced of a spinal cord disorder and took special precautions when Lecomte was found dead in bed one morning in 1853.

The body was removed to Cruveilhier's laboratory and perfused with fixative. The only incidental finding, bronchopneumonia, was not surprising in view of the patient's bulbar palsy and intermittent lung symptoms in the last month of life. The muscles revealed the same changes found in the previous cases, again to variable degree and tending to a fascicular pattern of intramuscular atrophy. Some muscles were totally involved, others had been clinically weak but showed no pathology, and still other muscles had intermediate degrees of clinicopathological involvement. The gross examination of the CNS was notable only for marked atrophy of the motor roots, particularly the hypoglossal and the lower cervical ventral roots. Cruveilhier noted that the hierarchy of function from nerve to muscle would implicate the ventral root lesion as primary; he cited a case in which Dupuytren had correctly diagnosed a lesion at the hypoglossal foramen to account for hemiatrophy of the tongue; the motor nerve has a nutritive effect on the muscle it supplies. As for the etiology of the spinal cord disease that presumably led to the ventral root atrophy, Cruveilhier could only call for further studies, pointing out that the ultimate origins of the spinal roots were then unknown. He was clearly suspicious of a myelopathy even though no known cord disease provided an analogy. He proposed changing Aran's term from progressive muscular atrophy to progressive muscular paralysis with secondary atrophy. A further point from this little-known article: a treatment, to be successful, must occur before the development of severe neural and muscular atrophy, since the end-stage atrophy with tissue degeneration in this case was probably irreversible (29).

Additional instances of similar clinical features with ventral root atrophy were reported by Fromann (30) and Duménil de Rouen (31). Both cases were probably instances of ALS because of prominent, early bulbar symptoms and rapid progression. Fromann (30) clearly described cord and peduncular lesions.

The same year, Duchenne (28) distinguished "generalized spinal paralysis" from Aran's progressive muscular atrophy on the grounds that in the former the lesion "can be in no other part of the neural apparatus than the spinal cord," whereas in PMA the muscular alterations were prominent in the necropsies of three new cases but the ventral root atrophy was inconstant. Duchenne (32) differentiated PBP from the muscular atrophy of Aran only by the degree and rapidity of bulbar involvement and concluded that one patient had both diseases. In 1860 Luys (33) reported ventral horn cell degeneration in PMA, and later, Charcot's expositions of ALS (34,35) further shifted attention from the muscles to the spinal cord.

It is also ironic that the oft-cited 1869 paper by Charcot and Joffroy (36), describing ALS, was actually entitled "Deux cas d'atrophie musculaire progressive," although Charcot took care to differentiate his cases from Aran's muscular atrophy because of the shorter course, early bulbar involvement, and presence of rigidity (spasticity). He also noted that more men than women were afflicted by muscular atrophy (admitting, however, the feminine bias at his hospital, la Salpetrière) and that some familial cases of muscular atrophy contrasted with the negative family histories of his ALS patients (24). On this last point, he had evidently missed Aran's case 7 (Table 2). The only neuropathological difference was the lack of corticospinal tract pathology in muscular atrophy in contrast to the prominent tract lesion in ALS. Charcot believed that the latter could lead to ventral horn cell degeneration and so he further differentiated PMA, the protopathic disease, from ALS, a deuteropathic disease (34,35).

Despite the lively and sometimes vitriolic differences of opinion (32,34,37) in the nineteenth century among investigators handicapped by inadequate understanding or total ignorance of many normal functions, lacking tests deemed elementary today, using simple pathology techniques, the clinical picture of adult MND was recognized and the main neuropathology defined; the acute disorders, such as Landry's paralysis and poliomyelitis, were separated from the chronic progressive types, while in the latter a certain unity was appreciated (35). By 1882, Bramwell (38) could write that "the paralysis presents all the characteristic features which result from a lesion of the anterior horn."

A final irony is that Aran's great paper (22) has not only been omitted from most histories of ALS, but his credit for PMA has been half-apportioned to Duchenne ("Aran-Duchenne disease" = PMA). We can attribute this partly to Duchenne's own machinations as noted above, and partly to the tendency of reviewers to read titles or abstracts and not texts. As mentioned earlier, the reflexes were not part of the clinical art at that time, so is it not likely that in Aran's case 2 (Table 2), Bernard's normal-appearing, but progressively weaker legs reflected upper motor disorder? One fascinating aspect of Aran's (22) report is the description of fasciculation. He emphasized that it occurred in both clinically normal and affected muscles during relaxation but that fatiguing contractions tended to increase it. Fasciculation occurred mostly in the arms or thighs, rarely in the hands and face, but was also seen in the tongue in two cases.

Although the early reports emphasizes inevitable progression and the likelihood of a fatal outcome, especially in ALS-like cases, stabilization at any point in the illness, followed by chronic disability but no further progression, was noted by Gowers (39) and reemphasized by Potts (40). Such cases might be examples of what is here called "benign" ALS (BenALS).

Another historical article of great importance was the lecture on *abiotrophy* by Gowers (41). Aran (22) noted the active life-styles of his patients and how MND tended to become symptomatic first in those muscles most used. Hammond (42) speculated that vigorous muscular exercise leads to significant nutritional change in ventral horn cells. Gowers (39) was very aware of this association, and PMA (and, by extension, ALS) was the model he used to illustrate *abiotrophy*. The concept is simple, and based on probably thousands of years of folklore. Gowers theorized that every cell or tissue is endowed at birth with a certain "life energy," to be carefully husbanded throughout life to permit survival and good function of that tissue into old age. Careless or other overuse of this life energy would cause the cell or tissue to expire prematurely. Thus, the cause of PMA (and ALS) was overactivity in early years; the corollary (still recommended today by many physicians) is that the MND patient should go home, take to bed, and "conserve the remaining strength." Gowers (41) made no effort to reconcile the inevitability of abiotrophy with his earlier observation on stabilization in some cases (39).

WORKUP FOR MND

The occasional mimicry of ALS by another disease remains a rare occurrence. Of course, from the viewpoint of the patient concerned, such a diagnostic correction is potentially lifesaving and well worth the discomfort or pain, time, and expense involved in making the discovery of a different condition. Standard practice is to see a thorough general physical examination by a consulting internist, with a standard blood chemistry panel, urinalysis, and a quantitive pulmonary function test [in view of the frequent abnormalities found by Fallat et al. (43) even in early ALS cases]. As noted above, the EMG must show diffuse denervation with loss of motor units, including proximal segments and the paraspinal muscles, and unstable motor unit action potentials, but normal peripheral nerve motor and sensory conduction velocities. Further laboratory tests are for the parathormone level, the thyroid hormone level, the Lyme disease titer and a battery of autoimmune tests, including the specific levels of IgA, IgM, and IgG. Patients with predominantly lower motor signs and Jewish ancestry should be checked for hexoseaminidase deficiency and patients with PLS for antibodies to HTLV-1 virus. In all PLS patients a magnetic resonance (MR) image of the entire spinal cord should also be obtained, plus myelography if indicated, and this should also be done for at least the cervical segments in all ALS patients, with head scans also in search of atypical MS, syringomyelia, high cord cyst or tumor, etc. The actual cerebrospinal fluid should also be examined for cells, protein, VDRL (or equivalent) reaction, and the presence of oligoclonal bands. Two patients have only deteriorated slowly over 10 years and their cervical MR scans show several small "bright spots" suggestive of MS. It is not clear whether these patients suffer from MS with atypically severe anterior horn compromise or from ALS plus MS (44). Two other patients, with proven ALS, also showed such cord lesions in the MR image.

It is wise to consider muscle biopsy and perhaps nerve biopsy in all exclusively lower motor neuron syndromes, to aid in exclusion of atypical polymyositis and dysimmune polyneuritis. One patient had a 3-month history of progressive and generalized paralysis to the point of respiratory insufficiency; tracheostomy and ventilator support seemed imminent. A creatine kinase (CK) determination had been normal. There were no upper motor signs, but the diagnosis of PMA seemed unlikely from the ALS-like course. In desperation, plasma exchange with immunosuppression was tried; the patient improved! Repeat CKs were elevated and a biopsy showed myositis, so this treatment was continued. There was further improvement, but death occurred from pulmonary embolism. The necropsy was reported to show inflammation in many nerves but no primary muscle involvement, as though the original autoimmune pathophysiology had transferred from muscle to nerve.

There is great current interest in multifocal peripheral nerve conduction blocks causing an ALS-like syndrome. Specific immunoglobulin dyscrasias have been detected in many of these cases (45,46) and some have stabilized or improved with vigorous immunosuppression. Most of these cases have, however, been lower motor syndromes, thus PMA-like and not ALS-like. Shy (47) and Younger (48) and colleagues report a few patients with suspicious hyperreflexia (i.e., more ALS-like) and even autopsy proof of corticospinal tract involvement in a few cases. The resulting interest in immunosuppression has been heightened by Engelhardt and colleagues' (49) description of an experimental MND induced by autoimmunity.

In ALS renal biospy tissue, Oldstone and associates (50) found immune complex deposition in renal glomeruli and mesangia in patients having the most rapid courses. Immunosuppression treatment was begun, without detectable benefit. This approach to the treatment of ALS was intensified over several years to reach the following treatment protocol:

1. High-dosage, intravenous methylprednisolone for 1 week, during which
2. Oral cyclophosphamide administration was begun to lower the WBC to $\sim$2500 leukocytes/mm^3, meantime
3. 2–3-liter plasma exchange was performed every other day for 2 weeks, then twice weekly until 6 weeks from the start of treatment; the cyclophosphamide medication was continued until 3 months, when
4. It was replaced by azathioprine for an additional 3 months.

Some of the patients seemed to improve early in this final trial, but a placebo effect now seems likely because further vigorous treatment was only associated with typical neuromuscular deterioration. Thus, it does not seem reasonable to recommend further such trials of treatment in ALS, but Drachman and Kuncl (51) propose that in the pathology of ALS there might be an unconventional dysimmune process, resistant to standard treatment, thus opening a potential therapeutic door for patients willing to undergo the risks of even more intensive immunosuppression. Whatever the uncertainties of this treatment approach, all can agree on the necessity of careful investigation in each ALS patient for any evidence of a dysimmune process.

OTHER SPECIFIC EXCLUSIONS

Amyotrophic Spondylotic Myeloradiculopathy

The typical case of symptomatic cervical/lumbar spondylosis can be distinguished from primary MND by the presence of sensory symptoms or findings and by absence on examination of the usual extensive findings in MND, especially ALS. In other words, the patient with ALS usually has more extensive findings than the symptoms may indicate and, with rare exceptions, these are entirely motor findings. The presence of clearly positive bulbar and pseudobulbar motor neuron lesions strongly suggests that problems related to spondylosis are coincidental and that the postoperative course most likely will be downhill, so this problem in differentiation usually arises in cases with only spinal involvement. The problem that is best known in this regard is cervical spondylosis, but lumbar spondylosis can also be a problem, and sometimes both conditions afflict the same patient. Difficulties arise in atypical cases, particularly cases of spondylosis with long-standing neural encroachment at multiple levels but with minimal or no sensory changes. Differentiation can be remarkably difficult, and the physician should stress to the patient before any surgery that the final diagnosis depends in large part on the postoperative course. Needless to say, such a discussion will not increase the patient's interest in surgery, and the consulting surgeon may also lose interest.

The most satisfactory diagnostic test for amyotrophic spondylotic myeloradiculopathy is the myelogram. In one case, even though the patient refused lumbar puncture, a computerized tomogram of the cervical canal demonstrated significant narrowing in the anteroposterior diameter at several levels that corresponded to disc spaces; at one point in the sagittal plane, the diameter was only 5 mm. There were extensive changes in the plain x-rays suggesting a process of long duration, with heavy calcification of the lesions. The computerized tomogram may be less reliable than the myelogram for patients with softer lesions and shorter courses. While offering increasing and valuable application to this problem, the MR image of calcified lesions can also be misleadingly benign. Many cases of combined cervical and lumbar spondylosis have not yet yielded to rational preoperative analysis. When the ALS-like findings are mild and the spondylosis severe, it seems reasonable to proceed with posterior decompressive surgery if the patient consents after considering the anesthesia-surgery risks and the underlying concern about ALS. All such cases of compressive myeloradiculopathy have shown marked encroachment at the time of decompressive surgery; the lesions corresponded to those described previously by other authors (52). There is no explanation for the clinical sparing of sensory functions in these patients.

The patients in this group show no consistent abnormalities in spinal fluid that are not also seen in patients with idiopathic MND. Because simple lumbar puncture sometimes produces alterations that make subsequent myelography difficult or temporarily impossible, the lumbar puncture should be deferred until a complete set of spinal x-rays or scans has been obtained and the decision has been made for or against myelography.

Heavy-Metal Toxicity

Since the time of Aran (22), occasional cases of exposure to heavy metals have been reported in patients with MND (53). For MND patients with clear histories of exposure to a heavy metal, an open-bone biopsy is recommended (53) to permit mass spectrographic quantitation of the particular element in a dehydrated specimen of cortical bone. The biopsy is best done by an orthopedic surgeon using extensive local anesthesia to obtain a piece of bone from the iliac crest. In appropriate cases, a segment of rib cortex can be obtained during a muscle biopsy of the chest wall, conducted for other purposes (54).

Patients with elevated levels of metal in the cortical bone should be treated with the standard chelation therapy, intravenous calcium disodium edetate (EDTA), during 24-hr urine collections for measurement of other heavy metals as well as the one in question. The urine should be collected at least once before EDTA is administered and then every 24 hr during the treatment. Excretion of the metal more than threefold above the control level on 3 or more days during the 5 days of intravenous treatment may indicate significant mobilization of metal. Review suggests, however, that the optimal schedule for administration and dosage of EDTA, and the criteria for abnormality of metal excretion in the urine, have never been fully determined (53). Periodic follow-up evaluations are of major diagnostic assistance in assessment of abnormal levels of metal in the body. Some degree of sustained recovery may be viewed as evidence that the amount of metal in the body was elevated and that the administration of EDTA was of benefit. The development of prolonged neuromuscular stability may be gratifying but is not convincing scientific evidence of successful treatment as opposed to spontaneous stabilization of idiopathic MND (see above, benign ALS).

Such cases of apparent metal toxicity are extremely rare. In one series (53), none of the patients showed other signs of lead toxicity; even the excretion of lead during the 24 hr before treatment was within the normal range. Despite the rarity of exposure to heavy metals and the difficulty of establishing the diagnosis, MND patients should routinely be interviewed for this condition. Screening of urine for heavy metals should be abandoned in favor of the bone biopsy when the history clearly reveals undue exposure to a heavy metal.

MISCELLANEOUS DIFFERENTIATIONS

Hyperparathyroidism

At this center we have seen two cases of severe MND apparently caused by hyperparathyroidism; both patients are improving slowly after parathyroidectomy, one from .ventilator dependence. The notable feature in both cases was normal serum calcium measurements on one of three tests in one patient and two of four tests in the other. Neither patient had marked hypercalcemia at any time, as noted by Patten et al. (55). Possibly an increase of parathyroid hormone has some unappreciated neurotoxic effect on motor neurons (56). Hypophosphatemic osteomalacia may also mimic MND except for reversibility on administration of neutral phosphate (57).

Lyme Disease

Lyme disease has been associated with ALS in several cases, but in a large ALS series, Mandell and associates (58) showed no difference in Lyme titers compared to controls. Since the FTA-abs test also reacts with Lyme antibodies, the present series contains over 500 negatives by that test. One patient was positive, however, and positive also for specific Lyme IgG, so a course of antibiotic was administered for 2 months, during which the ALS signs and symptoms advanced at the previous rate. She had surely been exposed to the Lyme (*Borrelia*) spirochete in the past, but equally surely, that exposure was incidental to the current problem, ALS. Nevertheless, the neurological complications of Lyme disease are only now being described (59), so caution is necessary in neglecting positive tests in new patients.

Diabetic Amyotrophy

It is important to differentiate primary MND from diabetic amyotrophy, due to polyradiculopathy, which offers the chance for substantial recovery after appropriate treatment of the diabetes (60). Nearly all the patients described thus far have had severe, poorly regulated diabetes or were undiagnosed and thus untreated. Diabetic amyotrophy is notable for painful weakness in proximal leg muscles, with atrophy and reduced or absent muscle reflexes. Thus, these symptoms are more likely to mimic early polymyositis or perhaps PMA rather than ALS. The frequency of this complication of diabetes is unknown. Bruyn and Garland (61) found only about 200 cases of diabetic amyotrophy in the world literature up to 1969, but practicing clinicians probably see more cases than are reported. Asbury (62) suggested that both the clinical and pathological spectra of diabetic amyotrophy are broader than suspected.

Arteriosclerotic Myelopathy

Only brief note will be given arteriosclerotic myelopathy, chiefly because of its rarity as a *progressive* condition. At this center, two patients thought to have had this complication of arteriosclerosis, in association with severe diabetes mellitus, suffered steadily progressive paralysis, died, and at necropsy were found to have lesions typical of ALS, not arteriosclerotic myelopathy.

Postpoliomyelitic Amyotrophy ("Postpolio Syndrome", "Progressive Postpolio Muscular Atrophy" = PPMA)

Several surveys show an increased incidence of a history of paralytic poliomyelitis in patients who develop ALS (24). Some of these patients seem to have symptoms typical of ALS, including rapid deterioration with a fatal outcome. In others, however, the less malignant, PPMA course has been observed. Campbell (63) and then Mulder and colleagues (64) drew attention to this subgroup of patients with MND: Focal paralysis results from a febrile illness (presumably poliomyelitis) many years before; relative stability follows recovery from the illness; in later years, further weakness develops, with a corresponding increase in atrophy in the part of the body that previously was paretic; the illness subsequently extends to other parts of the body but runs a much slower course than ALS, and there are no corticospinal signs and symptoms.

Chronic Inflammatory Polyradiculopathy

Dyck and associates (65) described a series of patients in whom chronic inflammatory disease had greatest impact on the spinal nerve roots and the peripheral nerves. Administration of corticosteroids appeared to be of benefit in some of these cases. Many cases in that series are readily distinguishable from idiopathic MND in that some exhibited sensory loss; some had involvement of the special senses, impotence, or impaired bowel or bladder control. But lower motor neuron involvement could be the predominant feature, thus raising PMA as a differential diagnosis.

Among new patients with motor neuron disease sent for evaluation, fewer than 0.1% have displayed spinal fluid findings consistent with inflammatory disease. All such patients had been investigated previously by experienced neurologists, who diagnosed either PMA or ALS by discounting abnormal spinal fluid findings or failing to perform a lumbar puncture. The possibility of luetic amyotrophy (66) mandates that the spinal fluid be examined at least once in every patient diagnosed as having MND. In PLS suspects, the HTLV-1 virus antibody level is also imperative in view of the many cases of "tropical spastic paraparesis" (67,68) now associated with that infection.

Myasthenic States

The electrographic study (EMG and nerve conduction measurements) should include assessment of neuromuscular transmission in several nerve-muscle pairs. This caution is not so much for myasthenia gravis (which is unlikely with the typical atrophy and reflex changes usually seen in ALS), but for the Lambert-Eaton myasthenic myopathy, which was actually found by this test in one patient after this author had examined him and agreed with the referral diagnosis of

PMA, possibly early ALS. Several months after the Lambert-Eaton syndrome was detected, a rapidly enlarging axillary lymph node showed small-cell (oat-cell) carcinoma. (Follow-up note: No other masses were detected in 1975, but a course of mediastinal and axillary radiation was administered. The myasthenic syndrome remitted, and despite recent coronary artery disease the patient continues in his profession of public school administration, 16 years later!) Again, this single case is of little significance for nearly all MND cases except the next one to present in this fashion with the Lambert-Eaton syndrome.

THE CLINICAL PICTURE AND COURSE IN ALS FROM POPULATION-BASED STUDY

Introduction

A digression is necessary at this point in order to illustrate a "population-based study," though neurologists are becoming increasingly aware of its importance in ALS, mainly from the work of Leonard Kurland and his associates at the Mayo Clinic. Two scenarios may illustrate the problem created by "referral patients" (or series) in comparison to the population-based study. An otherwise healthy young businessman, diagnosed as having ALS, may well become dissatisfied with his local physicians and undertake a lengthy, expensive trip to obtain an opinion elsewhere. He plays golf with a heart surgeon and cannot believe that, in this modern era of heart transplantation, he has not only an incurable disease, but one whose cause is unknown and that he should retire from his work, go home, and stay in bed to conserve his strength. On the other hand, an elderly woman, perhaps already disabled from arteriosclerotic heart disease, is much more apt to acquiesce in the verdict of her local physician and not undertake a much shorter trip to the consultant.

In an uncommon disorder such as ALS, the practice of the distant consultant will therefore contain a disproportionate number of active, younger (and wealthier) males over their natural occurrence in the whole disease population. Most of the patients will be seen only once, so the course of the disease in an individual patient will not be seen. Because the disease is uncommon, the local physicians never see more than a few cases and are therefore unable to see the true picture of the disease as it affects various ages, races, and sexes, and may not see the typical progression of the disease. Possible risk factors, such as past trauma or exposure to polio, will also differ between the two groups, so none of these physicians obtains an accurate picture of the disease.

In ALS, the reports of Kondo (69–71) on the Japanese experience, Li and colleagues (72) in England, Hudson and colleagues (73) in Ontario, Angelini (74) and Schiffer and associates (75) in northern Italy, Jokelainen (76,77) in Finland, Murray and colleagues in Nova Scotia (78), and Gunnarsson and associates (79) in Sweden provide the best information to date because of the large number of cases in relatively stable populations having medical care and data collection of good quality. A problem affecting all these studies, however, is uncertainty about such factors as mode of onset, date of onset, and so forth, because the patients were examined by a variety of physicians, who surely had variable interest in and expertise with neuromuscular disorders, and usually the analyzed data was only that found on death certificates. The Rochester, Minnesota, population-based study being carried out at the Mayo Clinic (80) is probably the most complete of all such studies, but the total number of ALS patients thus far is less than 50, from which it is not feasible to draw firm conclusions about such basic matters as age and sex patterns.

The following data about ALS are, unless stated otherwise, from a defined area of northern California, begun in 1967. Because large percentages of ALS, ALS-suspect, and other MND patients were not seen immediately, the series being cited now was begun on Jan. 1, 1970. To provide adequate follow-up, the study was closed on Dec. 31, 1989, so the minimum follow-up time is now over 4 years. This study is being reported in detail elsewhere (81), so only summary data will be given in this chapter. It should be noted, however, that the series is large enough to provide a sound statistical base: 870 patients were collected during that time; of these, 761 cases were considered to show typical adult MND, with follow-up in 756. The advantages of such a study are that it was prospective and population-based; all patients within the area of the study were accepted; a single physician interviewed all the patients; and the major physical findings were checked personally by this physician.

Methods

The patients were accrued because of MND, diagnosed by another neurologist, from Jan. 1, 1970, through Dec. 31, 1986, with a minimum follow-up of 4 years or to death or to respirator dependence (when the patient would have died in the natural course of the disease). The patients lived within 1-hr travel time of clinics in northern California. Patients unable to travel were seen at home, and patients becoming progressively more disabled and unable to visit a clinic were followed at home later in the illness.

The routine EMG study included finding the characteristic pattern of denervation with giant potentials in three or more muscles of at least three major body parts, including the paraspinal musculature. There was preservation of normal peripheral nerve motor conduction velocity in at least two major peripheral nerves, including one affected limb (plus two normal sensory nerve conduction studies after 1975). In each case without clear upper motor involvement on admission, two muscle biopsies showed only neurogenic atrophy characteristic of ALS, including type grouping and isolated small fibers. In all types except PMA, significant hyperreflexia developed during the course of the illness if it was not present on admission; definite lower motor involvement in at least two major body parts was manifest by muscular atrophy with fasciculation. Although many patients reported sensory disturbances, particularly early in the illness (see below, "Atypical Symptoms"), the admission sensory examination was normal or showed only minor abnormality attributable to other causes, and the special senses were entirely preserved. Bowel and bladder control were intact. No evidence was found for any other disorder that could be causing such a picture; normal or negative blood tests included vitamin B_{12} and folic acid, electrolytes including calcium, thyroid hormone, erythrocyte sedimentation rate, antinuclear antibodies, serum protein electrophoresis (and, since 1980, IgG, IgA, and IgM specifically), VDRL (FTA-abs since 1977), parathormone since 1984, and the Lyme titer since 1987. Any other indicated tests were always carried out in every case, such as myelography in patients with both ALS and spondylosis.

Definitions

The *onset* of the illness was the date of definite weakness in any body part, admitting that in some cases there were antecedent periods of months to years in which abnormal fatigue, painful muscle cramps, or fasciculation activity was present (see above). *Survival months* are months to death, or to intubation and artificial ventilation, or to Dec. 31, 1990. Patients who died of other causes are omitted from this calculation. *Survivership* is the percentage of patients alive without ventilator support at a given time from the onset. *Trauma* is any fracture, or concussion, or dislocation of any major joint within the 5 years prior to the onset of MND.

Results

A total of 870 cases of MND were obtained from the specified area during 1970–1986. There were 761 cases of idiopathic adult MND disease with better than 99% follow-up; the various subgroups are shown in Table 3. There were 167 necropsy studies, which confirmed the diagnosis in each such case. Though begun as a population-based study, Support Group and memorial donation records suggest that only 80–85% of the cases in the defined area were actually seen, so the following data may be skewed in unknown ways.

There were no cases of PBP. All patients who presented with bulbar palsy developed rather rapid extension to other body parts, from which the correct diagnosis of ALS soon became apparent. This paucity of PBP cases does not mean that it does not exist, only that PBP is very rare.

Table 4 presents the male-female ratios for the various idiopathic MNDs. BenALS and PMA are predominantly male disorders; contrary to common teaching, SporALS is not. Table 5 compares the age in years at onset and the survival months by sex. Although SporALS tends to occur earlier in men than women, it carries the same prognosis. There is no such age difference in FamALS, but

Table 3 Frequency of Idiopathic MND Cases[a] in Population-Based Study (81)

Dx	Number	%	No. lost	Follow-up %
SporALS	626	82	2	>99
FamALS	56	7	0	100
GuamALS	5	1	0	100
BenALS	29	4	1	97
PMA	17	2	2	88
PLS	27	4	0	100
PBP	0	0	—	—
All types	761	100	5	>99

[a]Excluding the several cases of CMT II, WKW, and PBspMA.

Table 4 Sex Differences in MNDs

Dx	Male	Female	Total	M/F
SporALS	356	270	626	1.3
FamALS	30	26	56	1.2
BenALS	24	5	29	4.8
PMA	15	2	17	7.5
PLS	14	13	27	1.1

Source: From Northern California study by Norris et al. (81).

survival months are significantly increased in males with FamALS. In the onset of symptoms, only bulbar onset in 26 and 23%, respectively, differentiated SporALS and FamALS from BenALS, which had only 4% bulbar onsets. Onset in arms or legs and the presence of Babinski signs were not different. The only other major point of difference was frequent, coarse fasciculation activity in 59 and 62% of SporALS and FamALS cases, respectively, versus 41% in BenALS when first examined. Regarding the course, arm versus leg onset had little or no difference, but a bulbar onset reduced the survival months to 33 in SporALS and 27 in FamALS.

The age of onset was clearly a major factor in the prognosis (Table 6). The survival months fell steadily to age 65, then stabilized, and was not shorter in patients over age 80 at the onset. The Asian patients had an earlier age of onset but the same survival time; black and Caucasian patients did not differ in age of onset or survival months.

The ALS conference in Tokyo, in 1978, introduced the concept of *ALS cachexia* (7), although surely many clinicians and pathologists had previously seen in ALS patients the characteristic disproportionate loss of body weight,

Table 5 Role of Sex on Age and Survival

MND	Onset age[a]			Survival months[a]		
	Male		Female	Male		Female
SporALS	57 ± 1	$p < 0.01$	60 ± 1	44 ± 2		43 ± 2
FamALS	50 ± 2		52 ± 3	74 ± 12	$p < 0.003$	43 ± 10
	$p < 0.001$		$p < 0.005$	$p < 0.006$		
BenALS	48 ± 3		54 ± 10	160 ± 15		209 ± 48
	$p < 0.002$			*		$p < 0.0003$
PMA	45 ± 3		(61)	190 ± 31		(89)
	$p < 0.0003$			*		
PLS	52 ± 3		46 ± 3	180 ± 23	$p < 0.003$	279 ± 3
				*		*

[a]Mean ± SE, p values *below* the mean ± SE give significance of difference from SporALS in that column.
*$p < 0.0001$.
Results in parentheses from too few cases for statistical analysis.
Source: From Northern California study by Norris et al. (81).

Table 6 Age at Onset of SporALS in Relation to Survival Months and Age of the Total Population

Onset age	Survival months (mean ± SE)	% ALS patients	% total population[a]	Age
<35	71 ± 8	4.4	54.2	<35
35–44	57 ± 4	7.5	14.8	35–44
45–54	49 ± 4	21.0	11.1	45–54
55–64	42 ± 2	33.6	9.3	55–64
65–74	36 ± 2	27.2	6.2	65–74
≥75	33 ± 3[b]	6.4	4.2	≥75

[a]1980 census data calculated from County and City Data Book 1988, U.S. Census Bureau, Government Printing Office, Washington, DC.
[b]For 12 patients (1.9%) over age 80, the mean survival was 40 ± 9 months.
Source: From Northern California population study by Norris et al. (81).

including loss of subcutaneous and peritoneal fat first reported by Gowers (39). For this study, ALS cachexia was defined as unexplained body weight loss exceeding 20% early in the illness (± 6 months from onset of weakness). At the time, ALS cachexia seemed to herald death within months, but in subsequent experience ALS cachexia has not dramatically shortened the course although

Table 7 Risk Factors in Past Illness/Exposure and Family History

	Number of cases						
	SporALS	FamALS	BenALS	PMA	PLS	All MND	%
Illness or exposure							
Neoplasm	21	0	1	1	0	23	3.0
Trauma	51	4	5	1	2	63	8.2
Heavy metal	18	3	0	0	0	21	2.7
Other toxin	1	0	0	0	1	2	—
Polio	6	1	3	0	0	10	1.3
Family history							
Parkinson	33	3	0	2	1	39	5.1
Alzheimer	9	1	0	0	0	10	1.3
Total cases	626	56	27	17	27	761	100

Source: From Northern California study by Norris et al. (81).

such patients are slightly older. Table 7 presents the occurrence of other putative risk factors. The trauma incidence of about 8% in this series is remarkably less than the 30–43% found by Kondo and Tsubaki (70) and the 19% by Angelini and colleagues (74). The other risk factors seem too low to be of any etiological significance. Despite the link on Guam between ALS, Parkinsonism, and dementia, this northern California population showed no evidence of such an association (Table 7).

ATYPICAL SYMPTOMS

Dementia

A major unresolved issue in ALS is the occurrence of dementia. Cognitive defects of varying severity may be seen (82). The best-known association of frank dementia with ALS occurs on Guam, in the ALS-Parkinsonism-dementia complex, but there the ALS patients are not demented although the Parkinsonism-dementia patients suffer slight-to-moderate amyotrophy (83). Elsewhere, dementia rarely complicates ALS, although as bulbar/pseudobulbar palsy advances, the patients become very difficult to test. Even when there does seem to be a cognitive problem, differentiation from the pseudodementia of severe reactive (situational) depression is rarely addressed. Clear-cut dementia ("organic psychosis") just antecedent to ALS, in which bulbar symptoms and depression could be excluded as causes of the mental changes, was first described by

Weschler and Davison (84). Mitsuyama and Takamiya (85) suggested that dementia with ALS is a disease entity, possibly more frequent in Japan, since Mitsuyama (86) was able to report 26 cases by 1984, more than the total cases available for the reviews by Hudson (87) and Horoupian and associates (88). French students of the problem, dealing however with only a small number of Caucasian cases, proposed that dementia with ALS be designated a subtype of ALS (89).

It seems clear, whatever the ultimate resolution, that such very rare cases as the Dutch children with hereditary ALS and dementia reported by Staal and associates (90,91) probably manifest a different disease, perhaps a common toxic exposure in the seven children who lived on a barge (90). Similarly, Burnstein's (92) family with schizophrenia, dementia, and ALS is difficult to relate to the average case of ALS.

When dementia does complicate ALS, it usually develops a year or two before the outset of bulbar symptoms or sometimes during the course of an ALS illness notable for severe bulbar involvement (87,88,93). In the northern California ALS series, dementia occurred in 13 patients, 11 of the 626 SporALS (1.8%) and 2 of the 56 FamALS cases (3.6%), none with demented near relatives. The onset of ALS was bulbar in 10 of the 13, and nine of the 13 were men. Their onset ages were not different from the nondemented patients, and survival was the same in SporALS, but the two FamALS patients, both men, died after just 10 and 43 months, respectively (cf. Table 5). Wikstrom and colleagues (93) emphasized severe cachexia in each of their three patients, but the California series contains only two cases of "ALS cachexia" as strictly defined (see above and Ref. 7).

Improved case finding might alter this picture of ALS dementia, since, as noted, the bulbar patients become progressively less testable and no special efforts were made to detect dementia late in the illness; an earlier study (2) in these California patients did not approach this issue. Gallassi and associates (94) found significant cognitive impairment in 6 of 22 (27%) consecutive patients free of depression and systemic disorders apt to affect mentation. While Poloni and co-workers (95) could not substantiate that high percentage, they noted a puzzling lack of correlation with cerebral atrophy as seen in computerized tomograms. In this older population, the significance of slight or even moderate cerebral atrophy is another topic for future research. Hudson's review (87) found dementia in 15% of FamALS case, far more than the 3–4% in the California population.

Horoupian and associates (88) advanced an interesting hypothesis, that the frontal lobe neuronal disease not only causes the dementia but, by denervating pyramidal cells, leads to the corticospinal tract disease as well.

Sensory Symptoms

Many reliable, nonneurotic MND patients, usually with ALS, report abnormal sensibility in the illness, usually early and sometimes as the first symptom. These are usually irritative symptoms, i.e., heightened sensitivity (usually to just one or two somatic modalities, rarely taste or smell, very rarely visual or auditory stimuli), and on examination the physician finds nothing (96). These histories are usually discounted (96), but sensory involvement is not surprising, indeed is predictable in view of the recognized pathology affecting sensory pathways both centrally and peripherally in ALS (97,98).

In the present MND population, the patients were evaluated for sensory dysfunction at 3-month intervals throughout their illnesses and probably 20% (the data are not yet tabulated) were found to have sensory involvement at one stage or another of the illness. In agreement with Mulder (96), these were usually irritative or positive symptoms early in the illness, without objective findings at that time. Jamal and associates (99) found a thermal sensory abnormality in up to 80% of ALS cases; Radtke and colleagues (100) found abnormal brain-evoked sensory potentials in 47% of their patients. Tashiro and associates (101) found reduced perception of vibration in 43%.

In some patients, the occurrence of specific neuralgias highlights clinical sensory symptoms as a probable consequence of the neural disease. For example, patient M.B. was a man who noted the first ALS symptoms in 1976 at age 65 and died of respiratory problems and complicating myocardial infarction in 1982. The main clinical features were spinal upper motor neuron involvement until late in the course, when both lower motor and pulmonary problems appeared. In 1978, for 3 months, he also endured typical trigeminal neuralgia. In 1980, he suffered 6 months from identical pain, readily controlled by carbamazepine, on the other side. This was worrisome and the relevant diagnostic studies were repeated, negatively. Later that same year, he developed typical lateral femoral cutaneous neuralgia for 2 months. Then, in 1981, a year before death, he again suffered from trigeminal neuralgia for 1 month (it might have troubled him longer but for continuing carbamazepine treatment).

Patient D.O. was a man who had the onset of ALS in 1977 at age 25 and died in 1988 from respiratory paralysis. His signs and symptoms were classic but for the appearance of bulbar and respiratory problems only in the last year of the illness. In 1981, he also suffered from lateral femoral cutaneous neuralgia for 5 months. In 1982, the other nerve manifested identical symptoms; both responded to carbamazepine but the latter only with toxic doses, so surgical neurectomy was performed to terminate this neuralgia. In 1983, he was afflicted 1 month with trigeminal neuralgia, responsive to carbamazepine. In 1987, and until death 6 months later, he again suffered from the femoral neuralgia on the original side.

Bowel/Bladder Continence

Some MND and particularly ALS patients also suffer from "urgency incontinence" of urine in the absence of dementia, and sometimes a fecal control problem, in the absence of bladder/rectal sensory or urethral/anal sphincter disturbances. All such cases should, of course, have urological/gynecological evaluations, especially for outflow (prostate) obstruction in men and "pelvic floor" problems in women. Other investigations have not been pursued since finding that the administration of oxybutynin provides relief.

Pseudoincontinence of feces is common in advanced ALS, due to partial impaction from severe, chronic constipation (obstipation) and dehydration. Careful attention to the diet and laxatives is the solution to this problem (102), which arises simply from the requirement for daily physical activity to promote normal bowel contractility. In advanced paralysis (from any cause) this normal bowel stimulus is reduced or absent. As bulbar involvement increases, many patients reduce their fluid intake in order to reduce aspiration. Another explanation may be the autonomic dysfunction dicussed below.

Several nondemented patients became truly incontinent of both bowel and bladder but after developing far-advanced generalized paralysis, at which time neither dementia nor severe depression causing pseudodementia is possible to determine. Perhaps in such tragic circumstances some patients become psychotic, a state that might also interfere with continence. Two patients had patulous anal sphincters, but certainly the average patient and family can be reassured that this is a very rare complication of ALS.

Autonomic Involvement

Cold, swollen, cyanotic feet and toes, made worse by dependency, are quite common in ALS and PLS. Elevation of the legs may not reverse these symptoms completely, and another indication of dysautonomia is the occasional development of similar alterations in the hands and fingers. One patient had it in first one and later the other forearm, resembling the old comic-book character Popeye. This dysfunction may also contribute to the bowel and continence symptoms just described as well as the marked increase of salivation seen sometimes in ALS as the initial bulbar symptom. In other, rare cases there is reduction of tears and oropharyngeal secretions, and then, of course, the workup for autoimmune disorders should be repeated. The cold sensitivity reported by many ALS patients may also indicate autonomic involvement in ALS, for which the studies reported by Daube's group (103) lend support.

Fatigability

The increased muscular fatigue of most ALS patients is so severe in some patients that a "myasthenic state" exists, which can be confirmed objectively by electrographic testing (104,105). Some of these patients obtain at least transient benefit from anticholinesterase medication although rarely as satisfactorily as patients with myasthenia gravis. Many complaints of fatigue in ALS may be due to mental factors in a depressing illness.

Eye Movements

Nearly every account of ALS cites normal eye movements, although on careful inspection and particularly with electronic measurement (electronystagmography) (ENG), there are frequent abnormalities in ALS (106). There is a bewildering range of ENG abnormalities in all the MND (106), most commonly irregular pursuit movements, which may be seen at the bedside (107). Several patients have also developed gaze palsies although gaze impersistence is more frequent. The two patients mentioned above with sphincter paralysis had also lost all eye movement and even blinking.

DISCUSSION

One perennial problem has been whether FamALS and SporALS are the same disease. FamALS could occur more often in families having genetically determined increase of sensitivity or common exposure to the causative agent, or SporALS could occur infrequently in families possessing genetically determined resistance or lack of much exposure to the agent, to name a few possibilities. The results in Table 5 are not compatible with such possibilities. ALS has a slight male dominance (Table 4), which is consistent with the significantly earlier male onset age in SporALS, but the earlier onset in FamALS is not different for men and women (Table 5), and the longer male survivorship in FamALS (Table 5) cannot be explained by such a male factor.

Similarly, it has been questioned whether BenALS and PMA are SporALS in patients having ''resistance'' to the full disease (108). The marked male dominance in BenALS and PMA (Table 4) makes it impossible to reconcile those entities with SporALS in view of their much better prognoses (Table 5).

Lilienfeld and colleagues (109) and Gunnarsson and colleagues (79) report data showing that ALS is increasing in incidence; Buncher and colleagues (110) report similar data. One can question improved diagnoses by increasing numbers of graduates of neurology training programs. Again, criticism must be directed at studies based necessarily on potentially inaccurate death certificates. A neat form of control, not so far reported, would be to examine the incidences of the more benign MND in those populations with apparently increasing ALS. Similar increases in the other MND would strongly suggest improved diagnosis rather than a real increase in SporALS.

Finally, controversy continues over the role of age in ALS. Kurtzke (111) found that the incidence of ALS peaks in the seventh decade and then declines; all subsequent reports, including the California population study (Table 6), support that conclusion, but Hudson and associates (73) found the age-adjusted incidence to level off in extreme old age, and the Mayo Clinic–Hennepin County series is showing the increasing incidence with aging (personal communications) reported by Yoshida and colleagues (80).

This point is vital in consideration of the etiology of ALS. For example, if ALS is clearly related to age (as found by the Mayo investigators), then future research should delve heavily into the effects of aging on motor neurons, whereas that approach might be wasted if age is only a secondary risk factor. The results in Table 6 do not support *age alone* as a major risk factor, since the course stabilizes over the onset age of 65. The subsequent fall in new cases (Table 6) raises other etiological possibilities, such as the possibility that a motor neuron toxin came into the population in past years but before the oldest citizens were at a susceptible age or before they would have the necessary long-term exposure. Other possibilities come to mind, but in such scenarios age is only a cofactor or even secondary in the risk factors. A marker for neuronal aging is lipofuscin accumulation. Measurements of lipofuscin in single neurons show that in ALS there is no excess (112).

At the other extreme, childhood or *juvenile ALS* remains very much an enigma, mainly because of the rarity of such cases. The literature even fails to define the cutoff age satisfactorily; for example, BenHamida and Hentati (113) accept as "juvenile" any case having the onset before age 30. They emphasize slower courses in these younger patients, whereas Hudson's review (87) suggests unusually rapid courses. Neuronal RNA-rich inclusions may indicate some essential difference in the pathophysiology or even the etiology (114). As suggested above, the Dutch children with dementia plus widespread brain lesions (90,91) seem to manifest a very special kind of encephalomyelopathy.

Finally, lest some important points have been neglected or wrongly interpreted herein, other recent reviews are provided by Mulder (115), Tandan and Bradley (116), Festoff (117), and Mitsumoto and associates (118). Rowland (119) reviews current research, and several recent symposium volumes have been published (120–123).

ACKNOWLEDGMENT

This work was supported by the Shelly Byers Chapter of the ALS and Neuromuscular Research Foundation. Dr. Eric Denys aided greatly by criticizing the manuscript. Many members of the San Francisco Neurological Society referred cases. Linda Elias, R.N., and Dolores Holden, R.N., aided the follow-up.

Holten Norris provided the computer program for the California study. Marge Dodge and Janet Owen prepared the typescript.

REFERENCES

1. Norris FH, Denys EH, U KS. Differential diagnosis of adult motor neuron disease. In: Mulder DW, ed. The diagnosis and treatment of amyotrophic lateral sclerosis. Boston: Houghton-Mifflin, 1980:53–78.
2. Houpt JL, Gould BS, Norris FH. Psychological characteristics of patients with amyotrophic lateral sclerosis (ALS). Psychosom Med 1977;39:299–303.
3. Rosenberg RN. Inherited, congenital and idiopathic degenerative diseases of the nervous system. In: Wyngaarden JB, Smith LH, eds. Cecil textbook of medicine. Philadelphia; Saunders, 1982:2036–2044.
4. Mulder DW, Espinosa RE. Amyotrophic lateral sclerosis: Comparison of the clinical syndrome in Guam and the United States. In: Norris FH, Kurland LT, eds. Motor neuron diseases. New York, London: Grune & Stratton, 1969:12–19.
5. Mukai E, The prognosis of amyotrophic lateral sclerosis in Guam and Japan. Clin Neurol (Jpn) 1982;22:139–144.
6. Tan N, Kakulas BA, Masters CL, et al. Observation on the clinical presentations and the neuropathological findings of amyotrophic lateral sclerosis in Australia and Guam. Ann Acad Med (Aust) 1986;15:62–66.
7. Norris FH, Denys EH, U KS. Old and new clinical problems in ALS. In: Tsubaki T, Toyokura Y, eds. Amyotrophic lateral sclerosis. Tokyo: University of Tokyo Press, 1979:3–26.
8. Norris FH, Calanchini PR, Fallat RJ, et al. The administration of guanidine in amyotrophic lateral sclerosis. Neurology 1974;24:721–728.
9. Norris FH. Charting the course in amyotrophic lateral sclerosis. In: Rose FC, ed. Amyotrophic lateral sclerosis. New York: Demos, 1990:83–92.
10. Hausmanowa-Petrusewicz I. Spinal muscular atrophy. Springfield, VA: US Dept of Commerce, 1978.
11. Dyck PJ, Lambert EH. Lower motor and primary sensory neuron diseases with peroneal muscular atrophy, II. Arch Neurol 1968;18:619–625.
12. Magee KR. Familial progressive bulbar-spinal muscular atrophy. Neurology 1960;10:295–305.
13. Tsukagoshi H, Nakanishi T, Kondo K, et al. Hereditary proximal neurogenic muscular atrophy in adult. Arch Neurol 1965;12:597–603.
14. Barkhaus PE, Kennedy WR, Stern LZ, Harrington RB. Hereditary proximal spinal and bulbar motor neuron disease of late onset. Arch Neurol 1982;39:112–116.
14a. Kennedy WR, Alter M, Sung JH. Progressive proximal spinal and bulbar muscular atrophy of late onset. Neurology 1968;18:671–680.
15. Mukai E. Clinical features of bulbo-spinal muscular atrophy. Clin Neurol (Jpn) 1980;20:255–263.
16. Sobue I, Saito N, Isida M, Andro K. Juvenile type of distal and segmental muscular atrophy of upper extremities. Ann Neurol 1978;3:429–432.

amyotrophic lateral sclerosis and their relationship with CT scan–assessed cerebral atrophy. Acta Neurol Scand 1986;74:257–260.

96. Mulder DW. Clinical limits of amyotrophic lateral sclerosis. In: Rowland LP, ed. Human motor neuron diseases. New York; Raven Press, 1982:15–22.

97. Averback P, Crocker P. Regular involvement of Clarke's neurons in sporadic motor neuron disease. Arch Neurol 1982;39:155–156.

98. Bradley WG, Good P, Rasool CG, Adelman LS. Morphometric and biochemical studies of peripheral nerves in amyotrophic lateral sclerosis. Ann Neurol 1983;14: 267–277.

99. Jamal GA, Weir AL, Hansen S, Ballantyne JP. Sensory involvement in motor neuron disease: Further evidence from automated thermal threshold determinations. J Neurol Neurosurg Psychiatry 1985;48:906–910.

100. Radtke R, Erwin A, Erwin C. Abnormal sensory evoked potentials in amyotrophic lateral sclerosis. Neurology 1986;36:796–801.

101. Tashiro K, Moriwaka F, Matsuura T, et al. Sensory findings in amyotrophic lateral sclerosis. In: Tsubaki T, Yase Y, eds. Amyotrophic lateral sclerosis: Recent advances in research and treatment. Amsterdam: Excerpta Medica, ICS 769, 1988: 183–188.

102. Norris FH, Smith RA, Denys EH. Motor neurone disease: Towards better care. Br Med J 1985;291:259–262.

103. Daube JR, Litchy WJ, Low PA, Windebank AJ. Classification of ALS by autonomic abnormalities. In: Tsubaki T, Yase Y, eds. Amyotrophic lateral sclerosis; recent advances in research and treatment. Amsterdam: Excerpta Medica, ICS 769, 1988:189–191.

104. Mulder DW, Lambert EH, Eaton LM. Myasthenic syndrome in patients with amyotrophic lateral sclerosis. Neurology 1959;9:627–631.

105. Denys EH, Norris FH. Amyotrophic lateral sclerosis: impairment of neuromuscular transmission. Arch Neurol 1979;36:74–80.

106. Lebo CP, Norris FH, Steinmetz EF. Electronystagmography in amyotrophic lateral sclerosis. 72. Arch Neurol 1983;40:525–526.

107. Jacobs L, Bozian D, Heffner RR, Barron SA. An eye movement disorder in amyotrophic lateral sclerosis. Neurology 1981;31:1282–1287.

108. Mulder DW, Howard FH. Patient resistance and prognosis in amyotrophic lateral sclerosis. Mayo Clin Proc 1976;51:537–541.

109. Lilienfeld DE, Chan E, Ehland J. Rising mortality in motoneuron disease in the USA, 1962–84. Lancet 1989;1:710–713.

110. Buncher CR, White M, Moomaw CJ. ALS mortality rates in Ohio, 1960–1986. In: Rose FC, Norris FH, eds. Amyotrophic lateral sclerosis: Recent advances in toxicology and epidemiology. London: Smith-Gordon, 1990:7–10.

111. Kurtzke JF. Epidemiology of amyotrophic lateral sclerosis. In: Rowland LP, ed. Human motor neuron diseases. New York: Raven Press, 1982:281–301.

112. McHolm GB, Aguilar MJ, Norris FH. Lipofuscin in amyotrophic lateral sclerosis. Arch Neurol 1984;41:1187–1188.

113. BenHamida M, Hentati F. Maladie de Charcot et sclérose laterale amyotrophique juvenile. Rev Neurol (Par) 1984;140:202–206.

114. Nelson JS, Prensky AL. Sporadic juvenile amyotrophic lateral sclerosis. Arch Neurol 1972;27:300–306.
115. Mulder DM, Amytrophic lateral sclerosis: the clinical syndrome. In: Chen KM, Yase Y, eds. Amyotrophic lateral sclerosis in Asia and Oceania. Taiwan: Shyan-Fu Chou, 1984:3–18.
116. Tandan R, Bradley WG. Amyotrophic lateral sclerosis. Ann Neurol 1985;18: 271–280.
117. Festoff BW. Amyotrophic lateral sclerosis. In: Davidoff RA, ed. Handbook of the spinal cord. New York, Basel: Marcel Dekker, 1987:607–664.
118. Mitsumoto H, Hanson MR, Chad DA. Amyotrophic lateral sclerosis, recent advances in pathogenesis and therapeutic trials. Arch Neurol 1988;45:189–202.
119. Rowland LP. Research progress in motor neuron diseases. Rev Neurol (Par) 1988;144:623–629.
120. Cosi V, Kato AC, Parlette W, et al, eds. Amyotrophic lateral sclerosis: Therapeutic, psychological and research aspects. New York: Plenum Press, 1987.
121. Tsubaki T, Yase Y, eds. Amyotrophic lateral sclerosis: Recent advances in research and treatment. Amsterdam: Excerpta Med, ICS 769, 1988.
122. Rose FC, Norris FH, eds. Amyotrophic lateral sclerosis: Recent advances in toxicology and epidemiology. London: Smith-Gordon, 1990.
123. Rowland LP. Motor neuron research. New York: Raven Press, 1991.

2

Familial Amyotrophic Lateral Sclerosis
The Relationship Between Age-Dependent Gene Expression and Patterns of Familial Aggregation

D. B. Williams

John Hunter Hospital
Newcastle, New South Wales, Australia

INTRODUCTION

As long ago as 1850, Aran explicitly described familial aggregation of amyotrophic lateral sclerosis (ALS) (1). This was in the first report of the condition he termed "progressive muscular atrophy." Despite the subsequent publication of several reports concerning similar familial conditions (reviewed in Refs. 2 and 3), it was not for another 100 years that familial aggregation of ALS became widely recognized (3). Kurland and Mulder, impressed by the familial occurrence of ALS in Guam (Marianas Islands), were the first to systematically elicit a family history of the disease from a series of ALS patients. At the Mayo Clinic, 6% of unselected ALS patients reported that at least one additional family member had suffered from a similar condition (4). The familial aggregations initially studied and reported were interpreted as being consistent with autosomal dominant inheritance (3). Subsequent clinical (5,6) and pathological (7) investigation of familial ALS cases suggested that these were different from sporadic cases in several ways, which implied to some the existence of two diseases with different etiologies.

Although this conceptualization of familial ALS as a separate disease with a unique etiology has the appeal of clarity and simplicity, it is challenged by a variety of recent data, which do not yet permit unambiguous interpretation (8–10). Many familial aggregations are not consistent with unmodified autosomal dominant inheritance. The etiology of these aggregations is moot—some may be due to autosomal dominant inheritance modified by late age of onset, or modified by other genes, and some may be due to other genetic mechanisms, such as recessive inheritance, mitochondrial inheritance, or more complex gene-environment interactions. The clinical characteristics of familial disease are variable, and there is a continuum from familial through sporadic disease. This continuum is the basis for the belief that understanding the etiology of familial aggregation will also help in determining the etiology of many cases of sporadic disease (6).

CLINICAL VARIATION AND ETIOLOGICAL HETEROGENEITY

Familial aggregation does not necessarily imply a specific pathogenesis or etiology. Genetically determined disease, infectious disease (including "vertical transmission" of an infectious agent), and common exposure to an environmental agent may all produce familial aggregation (9,11). Therefore, although most evidence can be interpreted as suggesting that there are important genetic determinants in familial ALS (3,5,11), no incontrovertible data support such an interpretation. This precludes dismissing any etiological hypothesis and, as a corollary, should caution against assuming that one pathogenetic mechanism or etiology accounts for all familial aggregations.

Familial ALS, in different families, may be associated with Parkinsonism, dementia, or other neurological abnormalities (12–14). However, even if discussion is restricted to familial ALS unassociated with other neurological disturbances, there is a broad spectrum of clinical variation. Sensitive tests may sometimes detect additional subclinical variation (15,16). Kurland and Mulder (3) emphasized that there is both intrafamilial and interfamilial variation in such features as age at onset and disease duration. In spite of the intrafamilial variation, when sufficient numbers of affected family members can be studied, there often appear to be features that distinguish one family from another (5). These can include a preponderance of bulbar onset (17) or tendency to short (18), or long survival (19). Statistically, the interfamilial variation in age at onset and disease duration is reported to be greater than the corresponding intrafamilial variation. In the context of previous observations, this latter finding suggests that there may be fundamental differences between families (8).

A significant consequence of developments in molecular genetics has been the demonstration that clinical heterogeneity is not necessarily due to underlying genetic heterogeneity. Allelic variation at the disease locus or the action of unlinked modifying genes may produce marked phenotypic variation, as is postulated in Huntington's disease (20). Conversely, clinical homogeneity is no guarantee that the same genetic defects are responsible in different familial aggregations (21). Nonetheless, despite the inexact correlation of clinical features with etiological determinants, it is suspected that the wide spectrum of clinical variation in familial ALS is at least partly due to underlying etiological, probably genetically determined, heterogeneity.

PATTERNS OF FAMILIAL AGGREGATION

In the absence of pathophysiological and etiological correlation, any classification must be considered temporary, but for the purposes of discussion and analysis, I divide familial aggregations of ALS into three groups. The first group consists of families in which the disease appears to be dominantly inherited; the second group consists of families in which dominant inheritance is possible, but diminished penetrance, or some other mechanism, must be postulated; and the third group consists of aggregations for which many different etiological hypotheses are equally plausible.

In many of the original reports of familial ALS, and most literature reports of single families, the pattern of aggregation is consistent with segregation of a single, autosomal dominant disease gene (3,7,18,22). An example of such a family is shown in Figure 1. Affected individuals can be traced through successive generations, males and females appear equally likely to be affected,* male-male transmission of the disease trait can be confirmed, and the ratio of affected to unaffected adults in "at-risk" sibships approaches 50%. Individuals who must have carried the postulated disease gene but failed to develop the disease [H-II(1) and H-III(1)] are found to have died before passing the known risk period for the disease (Fig. 2). It may be postulated that they would have developed the disease had they lived longer.

In the second group are families in which the pattern of familial aggregation is not consistent with unmodified transmission of a single autosomal disease gene (23,24). Figure 3 illustrates such a family. Because ALS is a rare disease (responsible for approximately 1 in 800 deaths), chance alone cannot account for the observed aggregation in this and similar families. However, the pattern of aggregation is not consistent with unmodified transmission of a single autosomal disease gene, because a number of individuals, such as I(1), I(2), II(2), II(5), II(6), II(11), II(13), were not known to develop the disease although they must have carried the disease gene if one assumes autosomal dominant inheritance. In addition, the ratio of affected to unaffected individuals in affected sibships is much less than 50%. Unlike the family in Figure 1, unaffected (assumed) gene carriers had lived through most of the known risk period for the disease in this

---

*In the family shown in Figure 1. there were more affected females than males, but the observed sex-specific risk is not statistically significantly different from expected because more adult females were at risk for the disease.

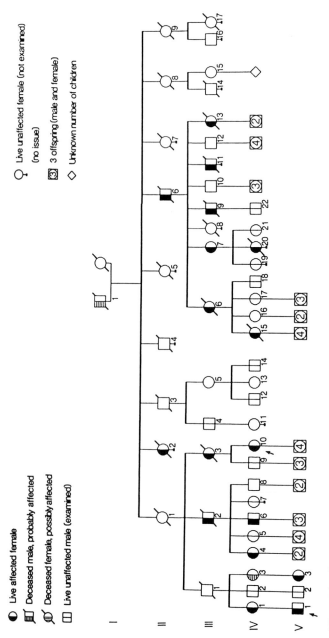

Figure 1 Occurrence of ALS in the H family suggests autosomal dominant transmission of a disease gene. In generation II, unaffected individuals without descendants all died as children, and many of the descendants in generations IV and V were quite young adults when the family was ascertained. (Reproduced from Ref. 25.)

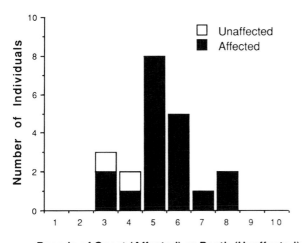

Decade of Onset (Affected) or Death (Unaffected)

Figure 2   Solid bars represent the distribution of ages of onset of affected individuals in the H family illustrated in Figure 1. The open bars, representing the ages at death of II-1 and III-1, show that these two individuals failed to live through the majority of the known risk period for the disease in this family. (Reproduced from Ref. 25.)

family (Fig. 4), and the majority of affected individuals were initially diagnosed as having sporadic rather than familial ALS (24).

Trivial explanations for the difference between the familial aggregation illustrated in Figure 3 and that depicted in Figure 1 seem unlikely. One person (this author) pursued the family history, pertinent medical records, and death certificates in the two families with equal vigor, and no difference in the social circumstances of the two families suggested that disparity in access to medical care was responsible for the contrasting patterns of aggregation.

In neither of the families described above was there any known consanguinity, and individuals were affected in successive generations, so recessive inheritance is highly unlikely. Affected individuals came from widely different geographical regions of Australia and died at different times over several decades, and no spouses were affected, so common exposure to an environmental neurotoxin is an inadequate explanation of the observations. The possible modifying effect of late age of onset or other potential mechanisms besides autosomal dominant inheritance are considered in the next section.

The third group of familial aggregation forms the majority of cases in some series (9,25). These consist of families in which only two or three individuals are known to have been affected. The affected individuals may be siblings, first-degree relatives in consecutive generations, or more distantly related individuals.

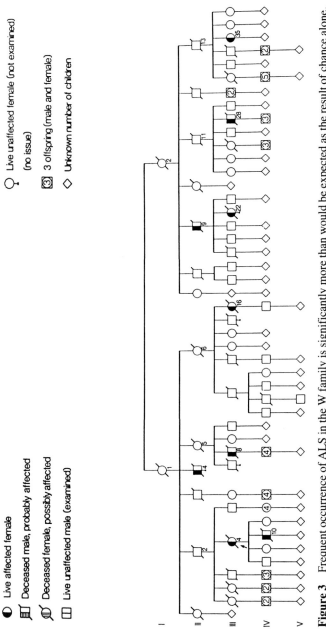

Figure 3 Frequent occurrence of ALS in the W family is significantly more than would be expected as the result of chance alone, but simple autosomal dominant inheritance is an inadequate explanation of the familial aggregation. [Reproduced from Ref. 25. Family first reported by Selby (24).]

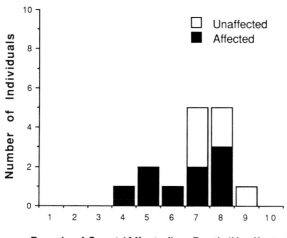

Figure 4 Solid bars represent the distribution of ages of onset of affected individuals in the W family illustrated in Figure 3. In contrast to the H family (Figs. 1 and 3), the disease in the W family tends to develop at a later age, and unaffected individuals who must have transmitted any postulated disease gene had passed all, or the majority, of the known risk period for the disease in this family. (Reproduced from Ref. 25.)

In some of these aggregations, lack of information about preceding generations may allow the supposition, sometimes confirmed by additional research, that the affected individuals are part of a larger familial aggregation of the type shown in Figure 1. In other cases, such as that shown in Figure 5, diligent genealogical research demonstrates that the few known affected individuals are members of a larger aggregation, more reminiscent of that illustrated in Figure 3. Then it seems likely that the affliction of two first-degree relatives brought an otherwise un-recognized aggregation to attention. As there are considerable practical problems in identifying aggregations such as these, the absence of evidence for additional affected relatives in any specific family cannot be taken as evidence that they do not exist. Therefore, we do not yet know how frequently apparently sporadic ALS patients, or aggregations of two or three affected individuals, closely re-lated, are actually part of a larger family grouping similar to those illustrated in Figures 1, 3, and 5.

Undoubtedly, it is possible that some of these small aggregations may also be due to chance aggregation of sporadic ALS, or common environmental expo-sure. However, small aggregations cannot simply be dismissed as being due to that mechanism. With current knowledge there is no way to determine whether it is more likely that most aggregations of two or three affected individuals are

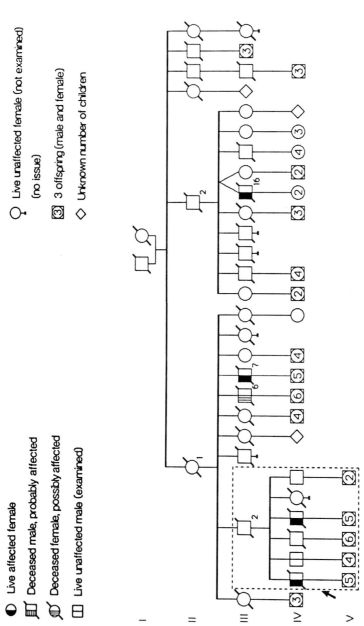

- ● Live affected female
- ▥ Deceased male, probably affected
- ⬗ Deceased female, possibly affected
- ☐ Live unaffected male (examined)

- ○ Live unaffected female (not examined)
  (no issue)
- ③ 3 offspring (male and female)
- ◇ Unknown number of children

Figure 5 An initial family history may be misleading because of insufficient information. At first, in the family illustrated here, only two siblings were known to be affected. Reliable information was confined to the family group outlined by the dotted rectangle. Subsequent research over several months revealed other individuals definitely affected by ALS, and at least one additional individual suspected of being affected.

coincidental associations of sporadic disease, or that many apparently sporadic ALS patients (like those in Figures 3 and 5) are actually members of larger, commonly unrecognized familial groups.

FAMILIAL ALS—ETIOLOGICAL HYPOTHESES

The hypothesis of autosomal dominant inheritance would be strongly supported by the detection of a genetic marker, such as a protein or cDNA sequence, linked to the postulated disease gene. Such cDNA sequences are being sought by several investigators, and some negative data have been published that exclude specific chromosomal regions from linkage with the postulated disease gene (25,26). Discussion of alternative etiological hypotheses, or potential modifiers of autosomal dominant inheritance, is currently believed to concern mainly families in the second and third groups described above.

There are a variety of potential explanations for the second and third types of familial aggregation, including modified autosomal dominant inheritance (diminished penetrance), other modes of inheritance (multigenic, recessive, mitochondrial), gene-environment interactions, and common environmental exposure. These are discussed in general, and the effect of the distribution of ages of onset on aggregation is discussed in detail.

Phenotypic variability in disease determined at one genetic locus may result from allelic variation at that locus or the modifying action of other, nonlinked autosomal genes. This has been postulated to be responsible for the clinical heterogeneity of Huntington's disease. The existence of that disease is determined at one genetic locus, but the form in which it is expressed may be determined by the specific allele present at the disease locus or the effect of other, nonlinked, autosomal genes (20). A similar mechanism could be responsible for the large variation in clinical features observed in familial ALS.

As outlined above, recessive inheritance is unlikely in families with affected individuals in multiple generations, especially in the absence of consanguineous unions. Few convincing reports of recessive inheritance of typical ALS exist in the medical literature (19,27–29). Lack of confirmatory evidence and the variety of possible alternative explanations leave this question unresolved. A recessive syndrome indistinguishable from classical ALS, apart from consistently longer disease duration, exists in Tunisia (Dr. R. Brown, personal communication), but has yet to be reported in other communities.

With improved understanding of mitochondrial disorders has come increasing awareness of the genetic complexity and phenotypic variability of these diseases. Mitochondrial proteins are encoded by both nuclear and mitochondrial DNA, so mitochondrial genetic abnormalities may be inherited in either an autosomal or maternal pattern. In addition, mitochondrial DNA has a faster mutation rate than nuclear DNA and lacks DNA repair enzymes, a combination of circumstances that might lead to relatively frequent metabolic disturbance (30,31). Mitochondrial diseases have mainly been recognized as disorders of cells with high metabolic rates, such as muscle. However, tissue-specific, heteroplasmic expression of abnormal mitochondrial DNA has recently been reported in mitochondrial myopathy (32) and pancytopenia (33). Therefore, although there is currently no evidence that neuron-specific mitochondrial disease occurs, or that it produces an ALS-like syndrome, there are at least theoretical reasons to consider this possibility in some cases (30).

Gene-environment interactions can potentially explain all the variation in all diseases. Therefore, in the absence of specific hypotheses, this explanation can never be disproven. However, some specific hypotheses of this general type can now be tested. An example is the recent report that in both motor neuron disease (ALS) and Parkinson's disease, affected individuals are deficient in the ability to sulfate and sulfoxidate several xenobiotic test compounds when compared with the ability of control subjects (34,35). This suggests that either or both of these neurodegenerative disorders could be the result of idiosyncratic metabolism of an agent that is readily detoxified by most people, or of excessive production of a toxic intermediary metabolite. There is good evidence for the latter mechanism causing parkinsonism following N-methyl-4-phenyl-1,2,3,6-tetrahydropyridine (MPTP) exposure (36,37). The enzymes determining the functional capacities of metabolic detoxification pathways are at least partly under genetic control (38,39), so this is one potential means by which both genetic and environmental factors could determine familial aggregation. The causes of the reported abnormal glutamate metabolism in ALS (40) are not yet known, and a similar defect has not been shown in familial cases, but this mechanism could potentially link cases of familial and sporadic ALS. A similar mechanism might underlie the current, unresolved debate concerning the possible etiological role of β-N-methylamino-L-alanine (BMAA) in ALS-Parkinsonism-dementia complex of Guam (41–43). It can be postulated that among the Chamorro people prone to develop the neurodegenerative complex, genetically determined susceptibility to specific environmental agents has arisen from geographical isolation.

One factor that has been proposed as modifying the pattern of aggregation of familial ALS is interfamilial variation in the age of onset of the disease (10). The hypothesis is that in families with a later average age of disease onset, proportionally more family members who possess the disease gene will die of other causes before the disease becomes clinically manifest.

In several families with individual family members who were not known to be affected but must have carried any postulated disease gene (assuming autosomal dominant inheritance), different authors have suggested that those individuals may have developed the disease if they had lived longer (3,6,19,44). However, the suggestion has not previously been extended as a general explanation of interfamilial variability or been subjected to rigorous examination.

Table 1 Patterns of Aggregation in Familial ALS

	Av. onset age ($\pm$ SD)	Sex ratio
Author's families		
Strong agg.	47.5 $\pm$ 12.9 years (n = 43)	0.9:1
Weak agg.	59.1 $\pm$ 12.3 years (n = 29)	1.4:1
Small fam.	56.5 $\pm$ 11.5 years (n = 33)	1.1:1
Literature analysis		
Strong agg.	42.9 $\pm$ 12.0 years (n = 170)	1.2:1
Weak agg.	51.4 $\pm$ 9.3 years (n = 44)	1.2:1
Small fam.	50.9 $\pm$ 11.7 years (n = 90)	1.4:1

Av. = average; SD = standard deviation; agg. = aggregation; fam. = families.
Source: Reproduced from Ref. 25.

The hypothesis can be tested by separating families into "strong" and "weak" aggregation groups and comparing the ages of onset in the respective groups. Families with only two or three known affected individuals are analyzed separately. Such an analysis was performed on 21 Australian families ascertained by the author and 73 families reported in the scientific literature (25). The results are shown in Table 1. The families were separated into strong and weak aggregation groups using two different criteria,* but the assignment of specific families remained essentially unaltered, so only the results of the first analysis are given. The significant result is that the average age of onset in the weak aggregation group is significantly higher than in the strong aggregation group. This is consistent with the hypothesis that in the strong aggregation families the lower average age of disease onset results in most disease gene carriers developing symptomatic disease before they succumb to another condition, while in the

---

*(a) Aggregation was regarded as strong if each affected individual had an affected parent (unless the parent died under the age of 60 years). If a family otherwise had strong aggregation, but no information was available concerning the parents of one affected individual, the categorization was unchanged.

(b) For each family, the ratio of affected individuals with an affected parent to all affected individuals was calculated. Strong aggregation families were defined as those with a ratio > 0.5.

The division of Australian families into two groups was the same regardless of which definition was used.

weak aggregation families later age of disease onset exposes carriers of the disease gene to the increasing risk of succumbing to one of the many more common conditions associated with aging before they develop symptomatic ALS. If this hypothesis is correct, the true difference between strong and weak aggregation families must be even greater than the observed difference, because the observed distribution of risk arises only from consideration of those individuals who developed the disease at a relatively young age for that particular family. This conclusion is implied by the histogram in Figure 4.

The average age of onset in the group of families with only two or three known affected individuals is also significantly higher than in the strong aggregation families and not significantly different from the average for the weak aggregation families. This would be consistent with these smaller families being "fragments" of larger families with an aggregation similar to the weak aggregation families (as shown in Figures 3 and 5), but most other etiological explanations discussed above are also equally plausible explanations for these aggregations.

This evidence supports the contention that later average age of onset of ALS in a family is a modifying factor that could account for some of the observed variation in familial aggregation. A critical test of the hypothesis is the prediction that those who are recognized by their relationship to other affected family members to carry the postulated disease gene should develop the disease if they live sufficiently long. Of the six individuals representing such occurrences known to this author, the prediction was fulfilled in two patients aged 84 and 82, respectively [O-II(3) in Ref. 25; III-3 of family B in Ref. 7; L. T. Kurland, personal communication). In addition, one 80-year-old patient had upper motor neuron signs and assymetrical wasting and weakness attributed to two other disease processes by her local physician (D. B. Williams, unpublished data), one patient had signs compatible with early motor system disease at age 90 [O-II(1) in Ref. 10), and two others had no clinical signs of motor system disease on the one occasion each was examined at age 38 and 94, respectively (D. B. Williams, unpublished data). In each of these cases the patient was a woman, and disease onset or the identification of abnormal neurological signs occurred during the 9th decade of life, well beyond the age range considered "typical" for the onset of familial ALS (5,11), but in an age group now known to be at high risk for developing ALS in general (45–47). This is not to suggest that these individuals coincidentally had sporadic ALS, but to emphasize that the age-specific risk of developing familial ALS is unknown and may not conform with previous assumptions.

LATE DISEASE ONSET AND ITS IMPLICATIONS

If, as suggested by the analysis above, some families have a significant risk of developing familial ALS in the 7th, 8th, and 9th decades, there are several important consequences. First, some family members who carry the disease gene will die before they manifest the clinical features of ALS. Second, others who develop the disease will do so at such a late age that there is a diminished likelihood that it will be correctly diagnosed. Because of these two phenomena, fewer first-degree relatives will be affected, and the chances of the disease being recognized as familial will be diminished.

As the average lifespan in the population increases, and neurological diagnosis and the provision of medical care to the elderly improves, this hypothesis predicts that more older people will be diagnosed as having ALS, and familial aggregation will be increasingly recognized. No formal test of these consequences has yet been reported, but it is this author's impression that both phenomena are occurring. A corollary of the hypothesis is that familial aggregation is likely to be underestimated.

THE FREQUENCY OF FAMILIAL AGGREGATION

Accepted estimates of the frequency of familial ALS range between 5% and 10% (48). However, the comparative rarity, late onset, and short duration of ALS mitigate against recognition of familial aggregation, and there are no clinical features that allow one to reliably distinguish between the familial and sporadic forms of ALS. Therefore, a negative family history must always be regarded as provisional, and it seems likely that the frequency of familial aggregation is underestimated.

The three reasons a familial aggregation may not be recognized are that other family members with the disease gene do not develop the disease, that they develop the disease but it is not diagnosed, or that despite an accurate diagnosis other family members are unaware of it.

An individual may have apparently sporadic disease either because no other predisposed or susceptible family member lived sufficiently long to develop the late-onset disease or the follow-up period was too short. As follow-up for two generations may be required in some cases to detect familial disease (cf. Figs. 3 and 5), very few patients with apparently sporadic disease can be regarded as having had familial disease definitely excluded.

An individual may appear to have sporadic disease because other family members with the disease were not correctly diagnosed. This may occur for many different reasons, but is more likely to occur in the elderly (49–51). Patients with MND/ALS do not feel ill, but present because they can no longer undertake certain activities that they expect themselves to be capable of performing. Consequently, if the patients are senile, or the progressive weakness they experience is consistent with their expectation of the effects of aging, they will effectively be asymptomatic. The high prevalence of cognitive impairment among the elderly (52) suggests that it is very likely that some elderly individuals with ALS fail to bring their neuromuscular symptoms to attention or have them diagnosed (53). Family practitioners are reported to be aware of less than 60% of their elderly patients' disabilities (54). Even if an elderly patient reports progressive weakness, MND/ALS may only be diagnosed by exclusion. Therefore, if the patient suffers from neoplastic disease, chronic heart or lung disease, or arthritis, the symptoms may readily be ascribed to the coexisting condition without further investigation. Even if an additional diagnosis is suspected, complicated investigations may be avoided because the patient is considered unlikely to benefit from precise diagnosis. False negative diagnosis of MND/ALS is correspondingly more likely.

Finally, an individual may appear to have sporadic disease if the patient is ignorant of other affected relatives. ALS is a rare condition, often unfamiliar to the lay public, and it has been referred to by a variety of pseudonyms and euphemisms in the recent past (e.g., creeping paralysis, progressive muscular atrophy, motor neuron disease, amyotrophic lateral sclerosis, motor degenerative disorder, and Lou Gehrig's disease). In addition, the phenotypic variation of the disease may be misleading to a lay observer. Many families in the last two generations have been disrupted by war, migration, divorce, or adoption, which can severely limit the available family history at the initial presentation. Even in the absence of these phenomena, few individuals can confidently describe the cause of death of all their grandparents or elderly aunts, uncles, and cousins. In some cases the medical practitioner may be responsible for perfunctory questioning concerning affected relatives.

Two recent studies critically examined the question of familial aggregation in ALS. In the first study (25), 50 consecutive patients at an ALS clinic at the University of Sydney had a standard family history elicited as part of the routine neurological assessment. Subsequently, additional family history was obtained from other family members and validated by examination of death certificates and medical records. At the initial assessment, 4/50 (8%) gave a history consistent with familial ALS. However, following the additional investigation, 7/50 (14%) had a definitively positive family history, and an additional 2/50 (4%) patients had what the author regarded as a probable family history of the same disease. In the second study, a case-control comparison of sporadic ALS patients diagnosed at the Mayo Clinic, ALS patients were 2 to 3 times more likely than matched controls to report having had an elderly relative with an undiagnosed history of painless, progressive weakness and wasting (C. Armon, personal communication).

Both these studies suggest that familial ALS is underestimated. The first study confirms that lack of knowledge concerning other family members who did have ALS diagnosed, or the limitation of short-term follow-up, is an important reason for underestimation of familial aggregation, and both the first and second studies suggest that underdiagnosis of ALS at the extremity of life may be an additional important factor.

THE RELATIONSHIP BETWEEN FAMILIAL AND SPORADIC DISEASE

Some authorities have been impressed not by the differences, but by the similarities between familial and sporadic ALS (6). Indeed, in the absence of a family history it is impossible to determine by any other means whether a patient has familial rather than sporadic disease. Some biological evidence suggests a link between familial and sporadic ALS. In a recent report, all six patients dying of sporadic ALS had heterotopic spinal cord neurons on neuropathological examination (55). The generation, migration, and differentiation of spinal cord neurons are all very early developmental events. Therefore, if heterotopy in ALS is confirmed, it implies that either genetic or intrauterine developmental factors are essential etiological determinants in apparently sporadic disease. Reports of ALS in dizygotic twins have been interpreted as evidence both for (29) and against (56) the hypothesis of intrauterine etiological determinants.

It is possible to estimate the relative contribution of hereditary and environmental factors from careful twin studies comparing monozygotic and dizygotic twins (57). Unfortunately, no systematic study has yet addressed this question in ALS, and the few case reports may be used to support contradictory interpretations. It should, however, be noted that if ALS has multigenic determinants, concordance rates in monozygotic twins may be predicted to be low because of the low ALS population frequency (57,58). In addition, monozygotic twins have been reported to be discordant for familial ALS for more than 10 years before the surviving cotwin developed the disease (25). Therefore, variable age of onset should also be considered a potential confounding factor in the interpretation of ALS twin studies.

Despite the fact that individual cases of familial and sporadic ALS are clinically indistinguishable, some characteristics of familial ALS have been proposed to differentiate these patients (as a group) from sporadic ALS. The features that have been held to distinguish them are: earlier age at onset, a tendency to develop the disease first in the lower limbs, and an equal sex ratio. In addition, the distinctive pathological involvement of the spinal cord dorsal columns and other areas outside the area of clinically evident motor degeneration has been proposed as a further distinguishing characteristic. Critical evaluation of the available clinical data suggests that features which appear to distinguish familial from sporadic ALS may be artifacts of selective recognition of familial disease. In addition, the existence of marked intrafamilial neuropathological variation should caution against ascribing etiological significance to neuropathological differences between families and between familial and sporadic ALS.

The characteristics of the strong aggregation families are summarized in Tables 1 and 2. As described above, they have a significantly lower average age of disease onset than that found in the weak aggregation families and in families

Table 2 Clinical Features of Familial and Sporadic ALS

	Familial (SA) ($n = 30$)	Familial (ALL) ($n = 105$)	Sporadic ($n = 106$)
Ratio M:F	0.87:1	1.06:1	1.21:1
Onset age (years)	47.5 ± 12.9	53.5 ± 13.1	59.2 ± 10.8
Onset site			
UL	26.7%	45.0%	27.2%
LL	56.7%	31.0%	43.7%
Bulbar	16.7%	19.0%	29.1%
Respiratory	0.0%	5.0%	1.9%
Av. dur.	3.4 ± 2.3	2.6 ± 1.7	2.7 ± 2.1
(Years)	($n = 24$)	($n = 69$)	($n = 76$)

SA = Strong aggregation; UL = upper limb; LL = lower limb; Dur. = duration.
Source: Reproduced from Ref. 25.

with only two or three known affected individuals. The age of onset in these latter familial cases was close to that reported in most clinical series of sporadic ALS (6,59) and in the comparison group in Table 2. In addition, although there is a slight female preponderance in the strong aggregation families, the sex ratio is not significantly different from 1:1, and there is a strong tendency for the disease to develop in the lower limbs. By contrast, in both the weak aggregation families and the families with only two or three known affected individuals, there is a male preponderance. This male preponderance is statistically significant in the latter group of families ascertained from the medical literature. If one takes all familial cases together, the apparent tendency to develop the disease first in the lower limbs is lost.

Li and associates compared sporadic and familial ALS using hospital records (9). The majority of their families had only two or three known affected individuals. Although there was a tendency for the familial cases to have a younger age of onset, the difference was small and could not be tested statistically. In addition, there was no statistically significant difference between the sex ratio for affected sporadic and familial cases. Finally, they did not find that there was a greater tendency for familial cases to develop the disease in the lower limbs first compared with sporadic cases.

Taken together, the foregoing evidence suggests that the characteristics that have been proposed as distinguishing features of familial ALS are the characteristics of strong aggregation families. These families are most impressive when encountered, the family history is well known to family members, and these families are much more likely to have been previously recognized and reported.

Until recently, aggregations of two or three individuals had been reported only infrequently, which suggests that the distinguishing facts of familial ALS are the result of selective recognition and reporting of familial disease.

In 1959 Engel and colleagues reported familial disease clinically indistinguishable from ALS, in which neuropathological examination of affected individuals showed severe degeneration in the "middle root zones" of the posterior columns (7). Subsequently, although additional, similar families have been reported (14,22,60–62), it is now known that posterior column involvement is seen in only a minority of familial ALS cases. The majority have pathological findings indistinguishable from sporadic disease (1,5,60). Conversely, it has been known for some time that apparently sporadic cases of ALS do demonstrate involvement of structures outside the motor pathways (63–66), including the posterior columns and spinocerebellar pathways. Loss of cells in Clarke's nucleus may only be detectable using quantitative methods (67).

There are relatively few reports concerning the neuropathological features of more than one affected individual in each family. In some, the neuropathological features are very similar in different affected family members (3,7). However, in other families there is significant intrafamilial neuropathological variation (18,25,44,68–70). In some cases the variation is simply in the degree to which certain structures are affected, or in the presence or absence of descending motor pathway involvement (18). However, in other cases the degree of variation is more marked. In those families one or more affected family members showed pathological changes in the posterior columns (25,69), spinocerebellar pathways (25,44,70), or other central nervous system structures (62,68), while other affected family members failed to show the same changes. These observations suggest that there exists wide intrafamilial neuropathological variation and caution against uncritically assuming that neuropathological heterogeneity in ALS is necessarily the consequence of differing etiological factors. The observations also emphasize the absence of any sensitive, specific markers that differentiate familial from sporadic ALS.

MOLECULAR GENETICS AND FAMILIAL ALS

The search for genetically determined disease markers and understanding of genetic diseases have both changed radically since the discovery of restriction endonucleases, which cleave at specific DNA base sequences, and the development of DNA electrophoresis and the Southern blotting technique. Theoretically, all genetically determined disorders may now be identified by determination of the aberrant DNA sequences that are their cause. As a preliminary step, polymorphic DNA segments may be used as linkage markers in regions close to the disease gene (71). These techniques have recently proven successful in both Duchenne muscular dystrophy (72) and cystic fibrosis (73–75). However, the potential of molecular genetic techniques can be maximized only by detailed clinical knowledge—benefit from the interaction between laboratory and clinical research commonly proves to be mutual. Familial ALS is one of the most difficult (presumed) genetic diseases to study, and molecular biology techniques will prove most useful when accurate clinical understanding allows appropriate interpretation of laboratory findings.

The major requirements for linkage analysis using log-odds (LOD) analysis include a well-characterized phenotype, a "sufficient" number of informative meioses,* and polymorphic markers "close" to the chromosomal location of the disease gene. Unfortunately, the first two conditions (a well-characterized phenotype and sufficient informative meioses) may be difficult to fulfill in familial ALS, and there are few clues as to the chromosomal region most likely to harbor a familial ALS gene.

Large pedigrees in which one might find sufficient informative meioses are rare, and because familial ALS has late onset and a short duration, the majority of known affected individuals are dead. DNA from the surviving spouse and offspring of an affected individual may permit reconstruction of that individual's genotype, but in these cases the accuracy of the original diagnosis may remain questionable. In order to obtain the benefit of additional meioses in an analysis, LOD scores from different families may be added together. However, this procedure presupposes that the same genetic defect is responsible in each family, and as has been emphasized, there is reason to suspect genetic if not other forms of etiological heterogeneity in familial ALS. Linkage can still be obtained using LOD scores from heterogeneous disorders, but it requires considerably more data to do so (76).

There have been few studies of linkage markers in familial ALS, although some studies have compared the frequency of specific genetically determined markers in sporadic ALS and control patients. In sporadic ALS Haberlandt (77) reported that among 100 patients with ALS or progressive bulbar palsy (PBP) there was no significant perturbation in the frequency of ABO, MN, or Rh blood groups, or in the ability to taste phenylthiocarbamide (a genetically determined trait) compared with the general German population. There were fewer than expected cases of color-blindness in the study population, but the difference was not statistically significant. Subsequently there have been reports of an increased frequency of blood group B (79) and the HLA-A3 allele (78), but these results were not confirmed in more extensive studies (80,81).

---

*An informative meiosis is one in which an affected individual, heterozygous for the polymorphic marker under investigation, has an offspring of known phenotype in which the specific allele conferred by the affected parent can be identified.

Until recently, few studies of potential linkage markers had been performed in familial ALS. Poser and colleagues reported that serum arginine concentrations were depressed in some patients with familial ALS (82). Recently, exclusion mapping detected no significant evidence of linkage for ABO, Fy, ACP_1, $APOC_2$, PGMQ, ESD, Rh, and two X-chromosome markers, and linkage at $\theta \leq 0.05$ was excluded for the MNS system (26). In addition to confirming the results for ABO, Fy, Rh, and the MNS system, tight linkage has also been excluded for the β-NGF gene, the β-globin gene 3' linkage group, the γ-crystallin pseudogene, the D14S21 region, the Kidd system, the insulin hypervariable region, and the PTH and alpha-fetoprotein genes (25).

A variety of strategies have been adopted in the search for genetic markers and etiological determinants in familial ALS. Increased numbers of informative meioses may be obtained through identification of new familial aggregations of ALS and careful follow-up of known families. However, additional clinical, electrophysiological, biochemical, and neuropathological study of familial ALS is still required to identify reliable phenotypic discriminators that will permit accurate subclassification for genetic analysis. Genealogical research that links otherwise unrelated families can provide strong evidence for identical etiological determinants.

DNA from all individuals known to be affected by familial ALS should be preserved, preferably as an immortalized cell line in a centralized cell banking facility. Because a patient may not be recognized as suffering from familial disease at the initial presentation, and ALS is commonly fatal in a short time, there is an argument for preserving DNA from all ALS patients. However, this strategy is dependent on the cost and availability of appropriate storage facilities.

Any clue to the chromosomal location of the disease gene in familial ALS, or the specific cellular pathophysiology in the disease, would greatly decrease the quantity of work required to establish linkage. In familial Alzheimer's disease, clinical clues to the location of a disease gene on chromosome 21 (83) included the occurrence of pathological changes indistinguishable from those of Alzheimer's disease in relatively young adults with trisomy 21 (84) and the reports of an excessive number of patients with trisomy 21 among the relatives of those affected by Alzheimer's disease (85,86).

In familial ALS, no associations with localizable chromosomal abnormalities have been recognized, but are being sought. As information concerning specific abnormalities of axonal transport, transmitters, or other cellular function becomes available in ALS, or the understanding of normal cellular events (such as programmed cell death during neuronal development) suggests possible mechanisms for the development of ALS, relevant candidate genes can be examined to determine possible etiological relationships with the postulated genetic defect.

CONCLUSIONS

1. In some, but not all, families, familial ALS occurs in a pattern consistent with autosomal dominant inheritance. In these families the sex ratio of affected individuals is approximately 1:1, and there is a tendency for the disease to develop among younger individuals than other forms of ALS, and to commence first in the lower limbs.

2. In some families deviations from the expected pattern of autosomal dominant inheritance may be due to late expression of the disease gene. However, the true age-specific risk of developing the disease in these families is unknown, so alternative explanations of the familial aggregation remain possible.

3. Aggregations of two or three known affected individuals are sometimes found to be members of families such as those in (1) and (2) above, but many are not. The proportion of these families and the number of apparently sporadic ALS cases who have genetically determined disease depend on the true age-specific risk of developing the disease in each family, and these data remain to be determined.

4. Clinical features that appear to distinguish groups of familial ALS cases from groups of sporadic ALS may be artifacts of selective recognition and analysis of familial ALS cases.

5. Neuropathological differences between families and between familial and sporadic ALS should not be accepted as unequivocal evidence of different etiology.

6. Many practical difficulties are associated with current strategies for studying cDNA markers in familial ALS.

REFERENCES

1. Aran FA. Récherches sur une maladie non encore décrite du système musculaire (atrophie musculaire progressive). Arch Gen Med 1850;24:15–35, 172–214.
2. Brown MR. "Wetherbee Ail": The inheritance of progressive muscular atrophy as a dominant trait in two New England families. N Engl J Med 1951;245:645.
3. Kurland LT, Mulder DW. Epidemiologic investigations of amyotrophic lateral sclerosis. 2. Familial aggregation indicative of dominant inheritance. Neurology 1955;5:182–196, 249–268.
4. Mulder DW. The clinical syndrome of amyotrophic lateral sclerosis. Mayo Clin Proc 1957;32:427–436.
5. Bonduelle M. Amyotrophic lateral sclerosis. In: Vinken PJ, Bruyn GW, eds. Handbook of clinical neurology. Amsterdam: North-Holland, 1975;22:281–347.
6. Mulder DW, Kurland LT, Offord KP, Beard CM. Familial adult motor neuron disease: Amyotrophic lateral sclerosis. Neurology 1986;36:511–517.
7. Engel WK, Kurland LT, Klatzo I. An inherited disease similar to amyotrophic

lateral sclerosis with a pattern of posterior column involvement. An intermediate form? Brain 1959;82:203–220.

8. Chio A, Brignolio F, Meineri P, Schiffer D. Phenotypic and genotypic heterogeneity of dominantly inherited amyotrophic lateral sclerosis. Acta Neurol Scand 1987;75:277–282.

9. Li T-M, Alberman E, Swash M. Comparison of sporadic and familial disease amongst 580 cases of motor neuron disease. J Neurol Neurosurg Psychiatry 1988;51:778–784.

10. Williams DB, Floate DA, Leicester J. Familial motor neuron disease: Differing penetrance in large pedigrees. J Neurol Sci 1988;86:215–230.

11. Emery EH, Holloway S. Familial motor neuron diseases. In: Rowland LP, ed. Human motor neuron diseases. New York: Raven Press, 1982:139–147.

12. Hudson AJ. Amyotrophic lateral sclerosis and its association with dementia, Parkinsonism and other neurological disorders: A review. Brain 1981;104:217–247.

13. Schmitt HP, Emser W, Heimes C. Familial occurrence of amyotrophic lateral sclerosis, parkinsonism, and dementia. Ann Neurol 1984;16:642–648, 1984.

14. Kurent JE, Hirano A, Foley JM. Familial amyotrophic lateral sclerosis with spino-cerebellar degeneration and peripheral neuropathy. J Neuropathol Exp Neurol 1975;34:110.

15. Daube JR, Litchy WJ, Low PA, Windebank AJ. Classification of ALS by autonomic abnormalities. In: Tsubaki T, Yase Y, eds. Amyotrophic lateral sclerosis. Amsterdam: Elsevier, 1988:189–191.

16. Mulder DW, Bushek W, Spring E, Karnes J, Dyck PJ. Motor neuron disease (ALS): Evaluation of detection thresholds of cutaneous sensation. Neurology 1983;33: 1625–1627.

17. Wolfenden WH, Calvert AF, Hirst E, Evans W, McLeod JG. Familial amyotrophic lateral sclerosis. Clin Exp Neurol 1973;9:51–55.

18. Hawkes CH, Cavanagh JB, Mowbray S, Paul EA. Familial motor neurone disease: Report of a family with five post-mortem studies. In: Rose FC, ed. Research progress in motor neurone disease. London: Pitman, 1984:70–98.

19. Horton WA, Roswell E, Brody JA. Familial motor neuron disease. Neurology 1976;26:460–465.

20. Sax DS, Bird ED, Gusella JF, Myers RH. Phenotypic variation in 2 Huntington's disease families with linkage to chromosome 4. Neurology 1989;39:1332–1336.

21. Rowland LP. Molecular genetics, pseudogenetics, and clinical neurology. Neurology 1983;33:1179–1195.

22. Metcalf CW, Hirano A. Amyotrophic lateral sclerosis. Clinicopathological studies of a family. Arch Neurol 1971;24:518–523.

23. Husquinet H, Franck G. Hereditary amyotrophic lateral sclerosis transmitted for five generations. Clin Genet 1980;18:109–115.

24. Selby G. Hereditary motor neuron disease. Clin Exp Neurol 1987;24:145–151.

25. Williams DB. Genetic factors in motor neuron disease. Ph.D. Thesis, University of Sydney, 1989.

26. Siddique T, Pericak-Vance MA, Brooks BR, Roos RP, Hung W-Y, Antel JP,

Munsat TL, et al. Linkage analysis in familial amyotrophic lateral sclerosis. Neurology 1989;39:919–925.

27. Dumon J, Macken J, de Barsy TH. Concordance for amyotrophic lateral sclerosis in a pair of dizygous twins of consanguineous parents. J Med Genet 1971;8:113–115.

28. Magee KR. Familial progressive bulbar-spinal muscular atrophy. Neurology 1960;10:295–305.

29. Estrin WJ. Amyotrophic lateral sclerosis in dizygotic twins. Neurology 1977;27: 692–694.

30. Linnane AW, Marzuki S, Ozawa T, Tanaka M. Mitochondrial DNA mutations as an important contributor to ageing and degenerative diseases. Lancet 1989;1:642–645.

31. Zeviani M, Bonilla E, DeVito DC, DiMauro S. Mitochondrial diseases. Neurol Clin 1989;7:123–156.

32. Holt IJ, Harding AE, Morgan-Hughes JA. Deletions of muscle mitochondrial DNA in patients with mitochondrial myopathies. Nature 1988;331:717–719.

33. Rotig A, Colonna M, Blanche S, Fischer A, Le Deist F, Frezal J, Saudubray J-M, Munnich A. Deletion of blood mitochondrial DNA in pancytopenia. Lancet 1988;2: 567–568.

34. Steventon GB, Heafield MTE, Waring RH, Williams AC. Xenobiotic metabolism in Parkinson's disease. Neurology 1989;39:883–887.

35. Steventon G, Williams AC, Waring R, Pall HS, Adams D. Xenobiotic metabolism in motor neurone disease. Lancet 1988;2:644–647.

36. Burns RS, Chiueh CC, Markey SP, Ebert MH, Jacobowitz DM, Kopin IJ. A primate model of Parkinsonism: Selective destruction of dopaminergic neurons in the pars compacta of the substantia nigra by *N*-methyl-4-phenyl-1,2,3,6-tetrahydropyridine. Proc Natl Acad Sci USA 1983;80:4546–4550.

37. Davis GC, Williams AC, Markey SP, et al. Chronic Parkinsonism secondary to intravenous injection of meperidine analogues. Psychiatry Res 1979;1:249–253.

38. Weinshilboum R. Methyltransferase pharmacogenetics. Pharmacol Ther 1989;43: 77–90.

39. Weinshilboum R. Sulfotransferase pharmacogenetics. Pharmacol Ther 1989 (in press).

40. Plaitakis A, Caroscio JT. Abnormal glutamate metabolism in amyotrophic lateral sclerosis. Ann Neurol 1987;22:575–579.

41. Spencer PS, Nunn PB, Hugon J, Ludolph AC, Ross SM, Dwijendra NR, Robertson RC: Guam amyotrophic lateral sclerosis–Parkinsonism dementia linked to a plant excitant neurotoxin. Science 1987;237:517–522.

42. Duncan MW, Kopin IJ, Garruto RM, Lavine L, Markey SP. 2-Amino-3(methylamino)-propionic acid in cycad-derived foods is an unlikely cause of amyotrophic lateral sclerosis/Parkinsonism. Lancet 1988;2:631.

43. Garruto RM, Yanagihara R, Gajdusek DC. Cycads and amyotrophic lateral sclerosis/Parkinsonism dementia. Lancet 1988;2:1079.

44. Gardner JH, Feldmahn A. Hereditary adult motor neuron disease. Trans Am Neurol Assoc 1966;91:239–241.

45. Juergens SM, Kurland LT, Okazaki H, Mulder DW. ALS in Rochester, Minnesota, 1925–1977. Neurology 1980;30:463–470.
46. Yoshida S, Mulder DW, Kurland LT, Chu C-P, Okazaki H. Follow-up study on amyotrophic lateral sclerosis in Rochester, Minn., 1925 through 1984. Neuroepidemiology 1986;5:61–70.
47. Lilienfeld DE, Chan E, Ehland J, Godbold J, Landrigan PJ, Marsh G, Perl DP. Rising mortality from motoneuron disease in the USA, 1962–84. Lancet 1989;2: 710–712.
48. Tandan R, Bradley WG. Amyotrophic lateral sclerosis. Part 1. Clinical features, pathology, and ethical issues in management. Ann Neurol 1985;18:271–280.
49. Bradley WG. Recent views on amyotrophic lateral sclerosis with emphasis on electrophysiological studies. Muscle Nerve 1987;10:490–502.
50. Buckley J, Warlow C, Smith P, Hilton-Jones D, Irvine S, Tew JR. Motor neuron disease in England and Wales 1959–1979. J Neurol Neurosurg Psychiatry 1983;46: 197–205.
51. Mulder DW. Clinical limits of amyotrophic lateral sclerosis. In: Rowland LP, ed. Human motor neuron diseases. Raven Press: New York, 1982:15–22.
52. Evans DA, Funkenstein HH, Albert MS, Scherr PA, Cook NR, Chown MJ, Hebert LE, Hennekens CH, Taylor JO. Prevalence of Alzheimer's disease in a community population of older persons: Higher than previously reported. JAMA 1989;262: 2551–2556.
53. Larson EB, Reifler BV, Featherstone HJ, English DR. Dementia in elderly outpatients: A prospective study. Ann Intern Med 1984;100:417–423.
54. Williamson J, Stokoe, IH, Gray S, Fisher M, Smith A, McGhee A, Stephenson E. Old people at home: Their unreported needs. Lancet 1964;1:1117.
55. Kozlowski MA, Williams C, Hinton DR, Miller CA. Heterotopic neurons in spinal cord of patients with ALS. Neurology 1989;39:644–648.
56. Jokelainen M, Palo J, Lokki J: Monozygous twins discordant for amyotrophic lateral sclerosis. Eur Neurol 1978;17:296–299.
57. Smith C. Heritability of liability and concordance in monozygous twins. Ann Hum Genet 1970;34:85–91.
58. Edwards JH. Familial predisposition in man. Br Med Bull 1969;25:58–63.
59. Vejjajiva A, Foster JB, Miller H. Motor neuron disease. A clinical study. J Neurol Sci 1967;4:229–314.
60. Hirano A, Kurland LT, Sayre GP. Familial amyotrophic lateral sclerosis. Arch Neurol 1967;16:232–243.
61. Takahashi K, Nakamura H, Okada E. Hereditary amyotrophic lateral sclerosis. Histochemical and electron microscopic study of hyaline inclusions in motor neurons. Arch Neurol 1972;27:292–299.
62. Tanaka J, Nakamura H, Tabuchi Y, Takahashi K. Familial amyotrophic lateral sclerosis: Features of multisystem degeneration. Acta Neuropathol (Berl) 1984;64: 22–29.
63. Brownell B, Oppenheimer DR, Hughes JT. The central nervous system in motor neurone disease. J Neurol Neurosurg Psychiatry 1970;33:338–357.

64. Davison C, Wechsler IS. Amyotrophic lateral sclerosis with involvement of posterior column and sensory disturbances. Arch Neurol Psychiatry 1936;35:229–239.
65. Hassin GB. Amyotrophic lateral sclerosis complicated by subacute combined degeneration of the cord. Arch Neurol Psychiatry 1933;29:125–138.
66. Lawyer T, Netsky MG. Amyotrophic lateral sclerosis: A clinicoanatomic study of fifty-three cases. Arch Neurol Psychiatry 1953;69:171–192.
67. Averback P, Crocker P. Regular involvement of Clarke's nucleus in sporadic amyotrophic lateral sclerosis. Arch Neurol 1982;39:155–156.
68. Alter M, Schaumann B. Hereditary amyotrophic lateral sclerosis. Eur Neurol 1976;14:250–256.
69. Farmer TW, Allen JN. Hereditary proximal amyotrophic lateral sclerosis. Trans Am Neurol Assoc 1969;94:140–144.
70. Igisu H, Ohta M, Yamashita Y, Kuroiwa Y. Familial motor neurone disease. Jpn J Hum Genet 1974;19:108–109.
71. Botstein D, White RL, Skolnick M, Davis, RW. Construction of a genetic linkage map in man using restriction fragment length polymorphisms. Am J Hum Genet 1980;32:314–331.
72. Koenig M, Monaco AP, Kunkel LM. The complete sequence of dystrophin predicts a rod-shaped cytoskeletal protein. Cell 1988;53:219–226.
73. Kerem B, Rommens JM, Buchanan JA, Markiewicz D, Cox TK, Chakravarti A, Buchwald M, Tsui L-C. Identification of the cystic fibrosis gene: Genetic analysis. Science 1989;245:1073–1080.
74. Riordan JR, Rommens JM, Kerem B, Alon N, Rozmahel R, Grzelczak, Zielenski J, Lok S, Plavsic N, et al. Identification of the cystic fibrosis gene: Cloning and characterization of complimentary DNA. Science 1989;245:1066–1073.
75. Rommens JM, Iannuzzi MC, Kerem B, Drumm ML, Melmer G, Dean M, Rozmahel R, Cole JL, Kennedy, D, Hidaka N, et al: Identification of the cystic fibrosis gene: Chromosome walking and jumping. Science 1989;245:1059–1065.
76. Ott J. Analysis of human genetic linkage. Baltimore, London: Johns Hopkins University Press, 1985:Chapter 5.
77. Haberlandt WF. Genetic aspects of amyotrophic lateral sclerosis and progressive bulbar paralysis. Acta Genet Med Gemell 1959;8:369–373.
78. Antel JP, Arnason BGW, Fuller TCS, Lehrich JR. Histocompatibility typing in amyotrophic lateral sclerosis. Arch Neurol 1976;33:423–425.
79. Vejjajiva A, Foster JB, Miller H: ABO blood-groups in motor-neurone disease. Lancet 1965;1:87.
80. Myrianthopoulos NC, Leyshon WC. The relation of blood groups and the secretor factor to amyotrophic lateral sclerosis. Am J Hum Genet 1967;19:607–616.
81. Norris FH, Terasaki PI, Henderson B. HLA typing in amyotrophic lateral sclerosis. Arch Neurol 1986;43:7 (letter).
82. Poser CM, Johnson M, Bunch LD. Familial amyotrophic lateral sclerosis. Dis Nerv Syst 1965;26:697–702.
83. St George-Hyslop PH, Tanzi RE, Polinsky RJ, Haines JL, Nee L, Watkins PC, Myers RH, et al. The genetic defect causing familial Alzheimer's disease maps on chromosome 21. Science 1987;235:885.

84. Burger PC, Vogel FS. The development of the pathologic changes of Alzheimer's disease and senile dementia in patients with Down's syndrome. Am J Pathol 1973;73:457–476.
85. Heston LL. Alzheimer's disease, trisomy 21, and myeloproliferative disorders: Associations suggesting a genetic diathesis. Science 1977;196:322.
86. Heyman LA, Wilkinson WE, Hurwitz BJ, Schmechel D, Sigmon AH, Weinberg T, Helms MJ, Swift M. Alzheimer's disease: Genetic aspects and associated clinical disorders. Ann Neurol 1983;14:507–515.

3

The Natural History of Amyotrophic Lateral Sclerosis

Theodore L. Munsat

New England Medical Center and Tufts University School of Medicine
Boston, Massachusetts

INTRODUCTION

A clearly defined natural history of a disease is of considerable importance. It provides the clinician with information about prognosis, allowing the family to adjust their life-style and future plans more appropriately. It can also provide useful clues into the etiology and pathogenesis of the disease. This type of analysis led to important insight into the etiology of McArdle's disease, the myoglobinuric myopathies, and the vasculitic neuropathies. In addition, accurate natural history information is essential for proper design of clinical trials.

Most "natural history" studies of amyotrophic lateral sclerosis (ALS) have been in great part anecdotal and descriptive, often relying on personal experience, second-hand information, or mail surveys. However, recently several groups have attempted to define ALS more precisely using better defined clinical criteria and more exact methods of measuring the disease. It is these studies that we will emphasize.

Disease Definition

Before attempting to delineate the natural history of ALS, it is necessary to carefully define the disorder. ALS is a true "system degeneration" which is essentially limited to the voluntary motor system. Although occasional patients may have sensory complaints and the pathological findings may extend beyond the classical voluntary motor system (especially in the familial and Guamanian forms), the true hallmark of ALS is its remarkable clinical sparing of other neurological systems. The process involves both the lower motor neurons (LMN) and upper motor neurons (UMN), typically in the same anatomical region. Although at the outset ALS may appear to be limited to UMN or LMN alone in some patients, with time, usually within a period of 2 years, both levels of the voluntary motor system will become affected.

In the past, disease of the LMN alone has been considered a form of ALS under the designation "progressive muscular atrophy" (PMA). However, these patients are indistinguishable from patients with late-onset spinal muscular atrophy by clinical, electrophysiological, and pathological criteria. Since the adult-onset spinal muscular atrophies have a much more favorable prognosis and much more benign course, which typically spares bulbar function, it led to the view that certain patients with "ALS" could have a favorable outlook. However, beginning with Norris' excellent clinical study in 1975 (1) in which he demonstrated that almost all patients diagnosed as having PMA, if followed long enough, evolved into true ALS with both UMN and LMN damage, the term has lost its nosological significance. In recent years death certificate analysis has revealed a decrease in the use of the term (2). In addition, with the pending definition of the gene for SMA, the diagnosis should be more easily established with greater certainty.

Patients with UMN deficit alone—primary lateral sclerosis—also have a slower evolution and a more favorable prognosis and were similarly previously considered to be part of the ALS spectrum. However, with the advent of newer diagnostic techniques, particularly magnetic resonance imaging, most of these patients were shown to have demyelinating disorders (3,4) indistinguishable from late-onset, slowly progressive multiple sclerosis.

These two types of motor neuron disease led to previous statements that certain patients with ALS may have a very benign course or may even spontaneously arrest. In the following analysis of the natural history of ALS we will exclude those patients with pure UMN or pure LMN disease, excluding a group with a more favorable prognosis. In addition, we will exclude those patients with a motor neuron disease associated with either a definable biochemical abnormality, such as hexoseaminidase deficiency (5), or a serum protein abnormality, such as plasma cell dyscrasia (6) or antineuronal antibody elevation (7). We will define ALS as a progressive disease limited to the voluntary motor system with clinical evidence of both UMN and LMN damage at more than one level of the neuraxis and without a specific associated biochemical abnormality.

The clinical manifestions of Guamanian ALS are similar to the "sporadic" disease occurring elsewhere in the world except for two features. "Overlap" syndromes occur with concurrent evidence of dementia and/or Parkinson's disease, and pathological examination may reveal neuronal damage outside the voluntary motor system similar to that seen in familial ALS. However, with the apparent disappearance of the high-incidence focus in this region, it seems unnecessary to consider these patients separately at the present time.

Techniques of Evaluating Natural History

At the present time a description of the natural history of ALS must be limited to those clinical features which can be assessed by clinical techniques. Unfortunately, there are currently no biochemical markers that can be used to assess progression or change in course. Although the serum creatine kinase is elevated in over half of ALS patients, these levels do not correlate with clinical change or rate of progression. Neither do purported elevations of anti-GM1 or GD1a antibodies correlate with disease severity (8). Central nervous system imaging reveals only nonspecific alterations of uncertain significance, and pathological descriptions are essentially limited to terminal disease and cannot be used to analyze historical features. Magnetic stimulation of the pyramidal tracts does not produce useful longitudinal information, and recent data suggest the procedure may be of little value in any context (9). Although muscle biopsy (10) and electrophysiological testing (11) can occasionally provide information that can be correlated with the stage of the disease, their main value is in establishing the diagnosis in uncertain cases. Bradley (12) recently reviewed in detail the utility and significance of electrophysiological studies in ALS. Thus, we must rely on clinical phenomena to provide the most useful information about natural history. The traditional bedside neurological examination is most useful in establishing the diagnosis and localizing a lesion. It is seriously deficient in assessing longitudinal change in deficit. More recent observers have thus utilized defined functional testing or quantitative instrumented strength measurement to define change in ALS.

PRECIPITATING EVENTS

Over the years a number of predisposing factors, epidemiological characteristics, or associated events have appeared in the literature with suggestions that one or more of these factors may play a role in the initiation of ALS. These have been reviewed recently by Mitsumoto et al. (13) and include the cycad nut and mineral soil alterations for Guamanian patients (clearly not a factor in non-Guamanians), exposure to animal skins, excessive milk intake, previous poliomyelitis, heavy physical activity, cancer, lead exposure, parathyroid dysfunction, or exposure to fertilizer. It is safe to say that none of these have supporting scientific data to presently consider them as established etiological factors.

MORTALITY DATA

The use of mortality statistics alone in defining the natural history of ALS has certain inherent problems. Although it provides a clear measurable end-point of disease progression, it may not be an accurate representation of the rate of motor unit loss or the aggressiveness of the disease process because of the prominant regional character of the disease. Thus, in certain patients, intercostal muscle weakness and particularly diaphragmatic impairment leading to respiratory insufficiency may be an early or even presenting feature. These patients may expire at a stage when limb function is reasonably normal if respiratory support is not provided. In addition, the time of death is often significantly influenced by associated intrinsic pulmonary disease such as emphysema, chronic bronchitis, or a history of smoking.

In the first analysis of ALS deaths due directly to the disease itself, Leone et al. (2) reported that age-specific mortality rates increased with age until the early 70s and then began to drop, although studies from the Mayo Clinic (14) suggest a more linear relationship between age and disease incidence.

Mulder (15) has observed that 50% of his referrals died within 3 years, 20% lived for 5 years, 10% for 10, and a few for as long as 20 years. Rosen (16) recorded a 39.4% 5-year survival in 668 patients evaluated by mail survey. Juergens et al. (14) reported a mean survival period of 22.5 months and noted that younger-onset patients had a better prognosis.

Jablecki et al. (17) recently devised a statistical technique to predict time of death. Using a modified Norris ALS score to define deficit at any point in time, historical information about the duration of weakness, and the age of the patient, they constructed a table which in their view gives an accurate assessment of time of death. For example, a patient with an average deterioration rate who is age 55 when examined would be informed that his expected longevity was a mean of 22 months. However, because the variances are so high (11–53 months for the 25th–75th percentile in the example cited), it would be difficult to use this approach for any single patient. In our experience, survival is most closely linked to change in respiratory status.

INITIAL COMPLAINTS, DISEASE ONSET

The presenting symptoms of a patient developing ALS depend on the region of onset as ALS is a disease with prominent regional characteristics. Patients with bulbar onset typically experience dysarthria at the outset followed by dysphagia. Quite commonly these complaints are interpreted as an otolaryngologic problem. If the disease begins in the arms, complaints are typically those of difficulty performing fine skilled tasks followed by weakness in carrying out heavier work. Regional onset in the legs is expressed by gait disturbances and, less frequently, difficulty negotiating stairs. Although ALS often begins asymmetrically, it soon becomes symmetrical and rates of deterioration in opposite limbs are similar.

Cramps are relatively uncommon as a spontaneous initial complaint but most patients will respond positively if questioned directly. Fasciculations usually accompany cramps and occasionally antedate weakness. Both cramps and fasciculations are most common in the early months of the disease and are less prominent as the weakness and functional disturbance increase. Although vague sensory symptoms occur in about 25%, these are rarely a significant presenting complaint.

Unexplained weight loss, apparently without reduction in food intake, is commonly observed in the early phases of ALS. It has been speculated that this may be a result of muscle mass loss, but this has not been substantiated.

REGION OF ONSET AND SUBSEQUENT HISTORY

On occasion, patients will present with respiratory impairment and may present a diagnostic dilemma. If these individuals are not provided with respiratory support, death will occur early. They die not because the disease process is particularly malignant or rapidly progressive, but because of the location of the damage. Conversely, if respiration is spared, patients may do extremely well for long periods of time.

Mulder (15) suggested that the course of ALS is similar regardless of region of onset except for respiratory onset. Recent observations support the fact that mortality and longevity may not be accurate indicators of the natural history, but rather reflect the regionality of the process. In this regard it has been noted that arm onset has a particularly poor prognosis (18), probably because of the proximity of respiratory motor cells to the arm muscles.

Recently Brooks (19) carried out a much needed, precise analysis of the sequence of progression in ALS. They observed that the region of onset correlated with subsequent disease progression. If the disease began in one arm or one leg, it probably spread to the contralateral limb next. Spread from the arm or leg to the other limb on the same side is faster than spread to a different limb on the other side. As expected, when onset was with dysarthria swallowing was affected next. Bulbar deficit was more likely the next area affected with arm onset compared to leg onset. All these observations suggest that ALS progresses in a patterned manner—not randomly—first spreading to adjacent homologous groups of motoneurons and then vertically to adjacent motoneuron pools. Spread is more likely to be contiguous than noncontiguous and random. This consistent with our own factor analysis studies showing regionality (20).

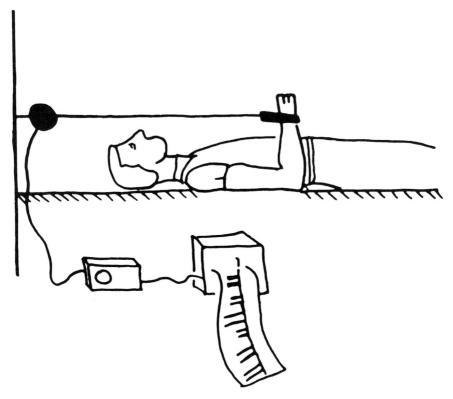

Figure 1 Modified examination table used for quantifying muscle strength includes a strain gauge tensiometer and direct writeout.

NATURAL HISTORY AS DETERMINED BY RATING SCALES

The first attempt to quantify neurological deficit in ALS was by Norris (21). His ALS score consisted of a series of functional ratings and reflex measurements, as well as assessment of fasciculations, wasting, emotionality, fatiguability, and tone. Most of the 34 functions tested were rated on a 0–3 scale for a theoretical normal sum of 100 points. However, the scale has several deficiencies. Pulmonary function was not measured. The values consisted of a mixture of signs, symptoms, and observations. There was no attempt to measure muscle strength directly. The items were not properly weighted, many had different designations, and reliability data were never published.

Appel (22) recently modified the Norris ALS scale to correct these deficiencies. The "Baylor" scale includes more individual test items, complete manual muscle testing, and pulmonary function studies. In addition, some of the more subjective test items of the ALS scale are omitted. Items are grouped into subscores for bulbar function, respiratory function, and upper and lower extremity function, which could then be assessed individually or summated into a total ALS score. Reliability studies produced a mean of 2.9% of the total score on test-retest, with subgroup correlations of greater than 0.96.

Utilizing this measurement instrument to assess natural history, it was observed that deterioration occurred in a linear fashion for all patients followed for at least 1 year. There was an approximate 20-fold difference in deterioration rates between the slowest and the most rapid courses. Deterioration rates based on total ALS scores were also used to predict demise.

QUANTITATIVE STRENGTH STUDIES

In our own studies of the natural history of ALS, we have elected to assess the rate and distribution of motor neuron loss by measurement of maximum voluntary isometric contraction (MVIC) utilizing a strain guage tensiometer (Fig. 1). Contrary to what one might intuitively expect, MVIC is both highly reliable (20) and very valid; i.e., it reflects the functional status of the motor unit pool (23,24). It also has the capability of assessing most body muscle groups and it provides interval data. It also is more sensitive to early loss, compared to manual muscle testing and rating scales (Fig. 2). Assessing patients longitudinally in this

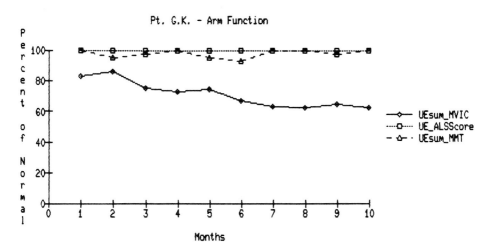

Figure 2 Monthly evaluation of ALS patient by maximum voluntary isometric contraction (MVIC), rating scale (ALS Score), and manual muscle testing (MMT). Note relative insensitivity of rating scale and MMT.

Table 1 Extracted Data from a Six-Factor Solution Rotated
Factor Analysis of 47 Data Items[a]

	Rotated factor loadings (pattern)			
	Factor 1	Factor 2	Factor 3	Factor 4
FVC		0.732		
MVV		0.712		
pa				−0.899
pata				−0.919
phoneR			0.689	
phoneL			0.539	
pegbdR			0.734	
pegbdL			0.501	
shdflexR		0.798		
shdflexL		0.867		
shdextR		0.798		
shdextL		0.878		
elbflexR		0.626		
elbflexL		0.808		
elbextR		0.713		
elbextL		0.820		
gripR		0.598		
gripL		0.615		
hipextR	0.570			
hipextL	0.552			
hipflexR	0.546			
hipflexL	0.608			
kneextR	0.588			
kneextL	0.623			
kneflexR	0.665			
knefledL	0.750			
dorsiflexR	0.721			
dorsiflexL	0.781			

[a]Only values above 0.5 are included.

manner, several new aspects of the disease were documented. Using a loaded
factor analysis program (Table 1), in which we assessed the commonality of
change in various muscle groups, we observed that muscle groups (motoneuron
groups) that were anatomically near each other shared the time of disease onset,
degree of weakness at any point in time, and similar rates of deterioration. This
confirmed existing clinical observations about the regional character of the disease—not only in area of onset, but in deterioration rate as well.

Table 2 Deterioration Rate of 50 Patients Expressed as Decline in Standard Deviation Units per Year

Megaslopes	Mean ± SD	Range
1	−1.000 ± 0.82	−0.080 to −4.033
2	−0.777 ± 0.58	−0.009 to −2.143
3	−1.073 ± 0.89	−0.020 to −4.176
4	−0.978 ± 0.66	−0.031 to −3.139
5	−0.829 ± 0.62	−0.230 to −3.770

Megaslope numbers refer to subgroup scores for different neuraxis levels. 1 = respiratory; 2 = bulbar; 3 = hand; 4 = arm; 5 = leg.

An understanding of the regionality of the disease process is particularly important in trial design as summed scores of regional deterioration rates may give a false impression of both the course of the disease and its response to therapeutic intervention.

We also observed (25) that bulbar function deteriorated more slowly than respiratory, arm, or leg function, although this could be due in part to the fact that the bulbar testing procedure is less sensitive to change. We observed no difference between age at onset and rate of deterioration or between region of onset and deterioration rate. No significant male-female differences were observed. Deterioration rates were similar between homologous muscle groups and between proximal and distal muscles.

In this study (25) considerable effort was taken to describe the actual course of motoneuron loss. Using several statistical criteria, it was found that during the active phase of motoneuron loss, the loss was remarkably linear with the exception of the early and very late phases. Plateaus may be seen prior to the onset of deterioration and late in the course, when a very small number of functioning moror units may remain for several months. Deterioration rates vary considerably among patients (Table 2), but intrapatient deterioration between different regions is more similar.

Although still incomplete, new data that more accurately characterize the natural history of ALS are accumulating. These data should be extremely useful for patient counseling as well as for basic and applied research.

REFERENCES

1. Norris FH. Adult spinal motor neuron disease. In: Vinken PJ, Bruyn BW, eds. Handbook of clinical neurology. Amsterdam: North-Holland, 1975:1–56.
2. Leone M, Chandra V, Schoenberg BS. Motor neuron disease in the United States, 1971 and 1973–1978. Neurology 1987; 37:1339–1343.

3. Younger DS, Chou S, Hays AP, Lange DJ, Emerson R, Brin M, Thompson H, Rowland LP. Primary lateral sclerosis. A clinical diagnosis reemerges. Neurology 1988; 45:1304–1307.

4. Miska RM, Pojunas W, McQuillen MP. Cranial magnetic resonance imaging in the evaluation of myelopathy of undermined etiology. Neurology 1987; 37:840–843.

5. Mitsumoto H, Sliman RJ, Kaufman SCS, Horwitz WA. Motor neuron disease and adult hexosaminidase A deficiency in two families: Evidence for multisystem degeneration. Ann Neurol 1985; 17:378–385.

6. Shy ME, Rowland LP, Smith T, Trojaborg W, Latov N, Sherman W, Pesce MA, Lovelace RE. Motor neuron disease and plasma cell dyscrasia. Neurology 1986; 36:1429–1436.

7. Pestronk A, Cornblath DR, and Ilyas AA. A treatable multifocal motor neuropathy with antibodies to GM1 ganglioside. Ann Neurol 1988; 24:73–78.

8. Pestronk A, Adams RN, Cornblath D, Kuncl RW, Drachman DB, Clawson L. Patterns of serum IgM antibodies to GM1 and GD1a gangliosides in amyotrophic lateral sclerosis. 1989; 25:98–102.

9. Eisen A, Shytbel W, Murphy K, Hoirch M. Cortical magnetic stimulation in amyotrophic lateral sclerosis. Muscle Nerve 1990; 13:146–151.

10. Wakata N, Brenner J, Adelman L, Kelly JJ, Munsat TL. Reinnervation in amyotrophic lateral sclerosis. Neurology 1986; 36:138.

11. Kelly Jr J, Thibodeau L, Andres PL, Finison LJ. Use of electrophysiologic tests to measure disease progression in ALS therapeutic trials. Muscle Nerve 1990 (in press).

12. Bradley WG. Recent views on amyotrophic lateral sclerosis with emphasis on electrophysiological studies. Muscle Nerve 1987; 10:490–502.

13. Mitsumoto H, Hanson M, Chad D. Amyotrophic lateral sclerosis Recent advances in pathology and therapeutic trials. Arch Neurol 1988; 45:189–202.

14. Juergens SM, Kurland LT, Okazaki H, Mulder DW. ALS in Rochester, Minnesota, 1925–1977. Neurology 1980; 30:463–470.

15. Mulder DW. Clinical limits of amyotrophic lateral sclerosis. In: Rowland LP, ed. Human motor neuron diseases. New York: Raven Press, 1982, pp 15–22.

16. Rosen AD. Amyotrophic lateral sclerosis. Clinical features and prognosis. Arch Neurol 1978; 35:638–642.

17. Jablecki CK, Berry C, Leach J: Survival prediction in amyotrophic lateral sclerosis. Muscle Nerve 1989; 12:833–841.

18. Festoff BW. Amyotrophic lateral sclerosis. In: Davidoff RA, ed. Handbook of the spinal cord. New York, Basel: Marcel Dekker, 1987, pp 607–664.

19. Brooks BR. Multicenter controlled trial: No effect of alternate-day 5 mg/kg subcutaneous thyrotropin releasing hormone (TRH) on isometric strength decrease in amyotrophic lateral sclerosis. Neurology 1989; 39:332.

20. Andres PL, Hedlund W, Finison L, Conlon T, Felmus M, Munsat TL. Quantitative motor assessment in amyotrophic lateral sclerosis. Neurology 1986; 36:937–941.

21. Norris FH, Calanchini PR, Fallat RJ, Panchari S, Jewett B. The administration of guanidine in amyotrophic lateral sclerosis. Neurology 1974; 24:721–728.

22. Appel SH, Stockton-Appel V, Stewart SS, Kerman RH. Amyotrophic lateral scle-

rosis. Associated clinical disorders and immunological evaluations. Arch Neurol 1986; 43(3):234–238.

23. Munsat TL. The use of quantitative techniques to define amyotrophic lateral sclerosis. In: Munsat TL, ed. Quantification of neurologic deficit. Stoneham: Butterworth, 1989.

24. Munsat TL, Andres PL, Skerry IM. Quantitative assessment of deficit in amyotrophic lateral sclerosis. In: Fowler W, ed. Physical medicine and rehabilitation: State of the art reviews. Philadelphia: Hanley & Belfus.

25. Munsat TL, Andres PL, Finison L, Conlon T, Thibodeau L. The natural history of motoneuron loss in ALS. Neurology 1988; 38:452–458.

4

Postpoliomyelitis Syndrome

Valerie A. Cwik

University of Alberta
Edmonton, Alberta, Canada

Hiroshi Mitsumoto

The Cleveland Clinic Foundation
Cleveland, Ohio

INTRODUCTION

According to the U.S. National Health Survey (1), poliomyelitis is estimated to be the second most prevalent cause of residual paralysis in America. Poliomyelitis, an acute motor neuron disease resulting from poliovirus infection, is sometimes associated with chronic progressive lower motor neuron disease in later life, known as "late sequelae of acute poliomyelitis" or "postpoliomyelitis syndrome" (PPS). That unique problems occur late in life in those who had acute poliomyelitis has been known for some time. However, concern has recently grown as those affected in the last epidemic, before the development of the Salk and Sabin vaccines in the early 1950s, are stricken with this difficult medical syndrome (2).

Poliomyelitis and PPS clearly differ from amyotrophic lateral sclerosis (ALS) in many respects, but they share similar features of progressive muscular atrophy (3). A thorough understanding of the pathogenesis of PPS can be invaluable to understanding that of ALS. Thus, we review here the historical, clinical, and laboratory features of PPS, its management, and its pathogenesis. We also discuss the relationship between poliomyelitis and ALS.

HISTORICAL ASPECTS

As early as the latter part of the 19th century, European researchers recognized that persons with poliomyelitis could develop "spinal" diseases in later life. In

77

1875, Raymond (4), with a contribution from Charcot, and Cornil and Lepine (5) independently described for the first time a progressive new weakness and muscular atrophy in patients with remote poliomyelitis. In 1899, Hirsch (6) reviewed the European literature regarding progressive muscular atrophy in patients with remote poliomyelitis and described the three patterns of its clinical presentation: (a) new muscular weakness in muscles unaffected by infantile paralysis; (b) new weakness in previously affected as well as unaffected muscles; and (c) new weakness limited to muscles previously affected by infantile paralysis. He also summarized the prevailing theories regarding the etiology of the new symptoms, none of which is yet proven or disproved: (a) the old lesion makes the spinal cord a ''locus minoris resistentiae'' susceptible to further disease; (b) a vulnerability in the anterior horn cells gives rise to acute poliomyelitis at one time and to progressive muscular atrophy at another; and (c) the old lesion, produced by the initial inflammation, is a latent, but permanent inflammatory focus that may reactivate and produce new symptoms (6).

Potts (7), in 1903, reviewed 36 cases of new spinal disease that developed in patients with a history of poliomyelitis. He attributed the majority (28 cases) to progressive muscular atrophy resulting from poliomyelitis, four cases to a second attack of poliomyelitis, two cases to ALS, and two cases to other causes. Salmon and Riley (8), in 1935, also recognized that a variety of disorders were related to remote poliomyelitis. Among the 60 cases of progressive muscle weakness they reviewed from the literature, the majority had new weakness and atrophy related to prior poliomyelitis, which the authors called ''chronic anterior poliomyelitis'' or ''progressive spinal muscular atrophy'' (8). They believed that inapparent viral infection could occur and that the dormant virus became active years later to produce chronic anterior poliomyelitis.

In 1962, Zilkha (9) investigated 137 of his own patients who had a benign course of motor neuron disease and noted that 11 had had poliomyelitis before the age of 6. He believed poliomyelitis and motor neuron disease to be closely related. Poskanzer et al. (10), in 1969, also believed there was an association between ALS and remote paralytic polio. Mulder and colleagues (11), in 1972, suggested that acute poliomyelitis may, many years later, give rise to a syndrome resembling, but not identical to, ALS that they called ''forme fruste ALS''; they could not completely exclude a causal relationship between the two disorders.

PPS AND PROGRESSIVE POSTPOLIOMYELITIS MUSCULAR ATROPHY

The definition of PPS has been somewhat confusing and controversial, depending on the criteria proposed. Mulder et al. (11) require the following criteria for the diagnosis of the syndrome of late progression of anterior poliomyelitis: (a) credible history of poliomyelitis; (b) a partial recovery of function; (c) a minimum of 10 years in stabilized recovery following acute poliomyelitis; and (d) the subsequent development of progressive muscular weakness. Cashman et al. (12) state that the stereotyped symptoms of weakness, fatigue, and pain occurring decades after acute poliomyelitis constitute a "post-polio-myelitis syndrome." PPS, as Dalakas (3) defines it, includes only the new neuromuscular symptoms that some patients develop 25–35 years after maximum recovery from acute poliomyelitis. The symptoms consists of: (a) musculoskeletal complaints resulting indirectly from the late effects of polio; (b) postpoliomyelitis progressive muscular atrophy (PPMA), which includes only those patients with progressive lower motor neuron disease and a history of polio infection; or (c) a combination of (a) and (b).

Precise epidemiological data regarding patients with remote polio are not available, but there may be 250,000–400,000 survivors of polio with residual weakness in the United States alone (2). In several recent surveys, up to 87% of patients with remote polio reported new health problems and new problems with activities of daily living (2,13,14). These new problems may have a significant impact on life-style, leading to changes in employment, recreation, and methods of transportation (15).

CLINICAL PRESENTATION

Many years after maximum recovery from the initial parlytic attack, postpolio patients may begin to notice fatigue and decreased endurance as well as new muscle weakness and atrophy. The severity of the acute poliomyelitis infection appears to be a factor in predicting the incidence of PPS. Those at greatest risk for developing PPS are those who required hospitalization for the original infection, needed ventilatory support, or developed quadriparesis (2,11,13). Several investigators have suggested that infection in early childhood, before 10 years of age, is a risk factor for the development of late weakness (9,11,15–17), whereas Speier et al. (2) and Halstead et al. (13) noted that acute infection after the age of 10 is associated with a higher risk of developing new problems. The reports on gender-related risk of PPS also differ: some reports indicate a male preponderance (8,11), while others find no such trend (2,13,14,18).

The new weakness tends to begin in previously affected muscles, but it may also affect muscles thought to have been spared by the initial acute infection. Patients may relate deterioration in health and function to a recent fall, minor trauma, or prolonged bed rest, or these changes may occur without provocation (13). One or more limbs deteriorate, generally asymmetrically, resulting in increased motor disability. Patients may experience frequent falls, with resultant long-bone fractures, and joint pain or instability resulting from the added stress on already overworked joints and muscles.

Fasciculations occur frequently in newly weakened muscles, but are also seen in muscles of unchanged strength. There are no sensory abnormalities. Reflexes generally are either normal or absent, although Babinski extensor plantar sign has been seen in some patients (3,11,16,19). This sign may actually be false and result from paralysis of the flexor hallucis longus tendon or from improper foot positioning in patients with footdrop (20). In acute poliomyelitis, brainstem lesions, particularly in the reticular formation, are thought to be responsible for spasticity; the precentral gyrus may be affected by poliovirus infection, but lesions in this area are not thought to be severe enough to cause spasticity (21). Whether brainstem lesions are responsible for Babinski sign in patients with PPS is unknown. In addition, spasticity and a positive Babinski sign can be the result of concomitant cervical spondylitic myelopathy.

New weakness can occur in bulbar and respiratory muscles, but is less frequently noted than in extremity muscles. Patients with prior or residual bulbar and respiratory weakness may be at higher risk for developing new dysarthria and respiratory difficulty. Pharyngeal and laryngeal muscle weakness may result in dysphagia, nasal reflux, and choking (22,23); dysphonia occurs as a result of vocal cord paralysis (23,24).

Respiratory problems may result from a variety of causes. Bulbar weakness may lead to the accumulation of secretions, aspiration, and airway obstruction (25). Hypoventilation, as the result of the weakness of respiratory muscles and dysfunction of medullary respiratory centers, may lead to hypoxia, atelectasis, and pneumonia; prolonged hypoxia may cause pulmonary hypertension and cor pulmonale (25). Previously nonprogressive scoliosis may resume, and spinal curvature may increase as a result of new muscle weakness, which can contribute to progressive immobility and respiratory deterioration (26).

The three main characteristics of late-onset respiratory dysfunction in PPS are: (a) fatigue, often accompanied by headaches, depression, and an inability to concentrate; (b) exertional dyspnea and greater susceptibility to respiratory tract infections; and (c) abnormal sensitivity to cold, especially of the extremities, with peripheral cyanosis, edema, or both, and a tendency to develop systemic hypertension (27). Nocturnal hypoventilation may cause headaches on waking, excessive daytime sleepiness, and disturbed sleep (25,26).

In addition to scoliosis, exaggerated lumbar lordosis and torsion deformities of the spine resulting from acute poliomyelitis may produce abnormal postures and excessive stress on muscles, tendons, ligaments, and joints. Patients may compensate well for many years, but new muscular weakness may overload these already overworked systems, leading to muscle strain, ligamentous sprain, and hip, back, and limb pain (25). Other orthopedic problems, not strictly part of PPS, that may contribute to functional deterioration in PPS patients include cervical spondylosis, osteoarthritis, and severe osteoporosis (26).

The diagnosis of PPS is made by exclusion; other causes of increased or new disability must be ruled out: These causes include entrapment neuropathy, radiculopathy, and myelopathy secondary to spondylosis, arthritis, or arthropathy, skeletal problems (such as scoliosis and postural problems from unequal limb length), and obesity. Other treatable systemic disorders, such as diabetes, connective tissue disorders, electrolyte imbalance, and intercurrent infections, must also be ruled out.

Weakness with PPS may progress steadily or in a stepwise fashion (18,25). Dalakas (18) estimated the progression of weakness, based on the Medical Research Council scale, to be 1% per year in 27 patients followed for an average of 8.2 years. Brown and Patten (29) followed seven patients for an average of 5.6 years and found the annual progression to be 7%, based on grip strength and the number of seconds that the leg or head could be raised against gravity.

LABORATORY FINDINGS

Routine blood chemistries are generally normal in PPS (16,18,28), although elevated serum creatine kinase (CK) is found in some patients (18,29). The cerebrospinal fluid (CSF) is also generally normal (16,18). Dalakas et al. (18,30) found weak oligoclonal bands in the CSF in up to 40% of their patients with PPS. However, the significance of these CSF changes in PPS has not been clarified.

To date, no consistent immunoregulatory abnormality has been found in PPS. High titers of poliovirus antibodies have been demonstrated in the sera of PPS patients (30), but there is no specific production of the antibody in the CSF (18,31). Ginsberg et al. (32) found the CD4 and CD8 subsets of T-cell lymphocytes to be depleted in patients with remote polio infection, but asymptomatic patients with remote polio and patients with PPS did not differ significantly in this respect.

ELECTROPHYSIOLOGICAL FINDINGS

Routine electromyographic (EMG) studies are useful in assessing patients with remote polio to confirm earlier disease of the anterior horn cells (33). Muscles known to have been affected by polio show chronic neurogenic changes: high-amplitude, long-duration, sometimes polyphasic motor unit potentials with a reduced interference pattern. However, muscles thought to have been previously spared demonstrate similar changes, indicating that the disease was actually more widespread than initially suspected or remembered (34–36).

Routine EMG studies do not differentiate between stable, remote polio and PPS (33). In addition to chronic neurogenic changes, fibrillation potentials may be seen in the muscles of polio patients who have no new weakness. Usually considered a sign of recent denervation, fibrillation potentials may persist for years in both stable and newly weakening muscles of remote polio patients and therefore do not reliably indicate progressive PPS (12,18,33,36).

New weakness may develop for reasons other than PPS in patients with remote polio. Routine EMG studies may help identify these other neuromuscular problems, such as entrapment neuropathies or peripheral polyneuropathies (33). The EMG study may be less useful in identifying a superimposed radiculopathy in a previously affected extremity that already demonstrates changes on needle electrode examination suggestive of chronic and active neurogenic disease.

Single-Fiber EMG

The single-fiber EMG shows increased fiber density in muscles affected by remote polio, both stable and newly weakening muscles, reflecting muscle-fiber type grouping that occurs by the process of continuous reinnervation (12,18, 34,37). Fiber density may be significantly higher in muscles with wasting and weakness than those of normal strength; however, fiber density does not differentiate between stable weakness and the new weakness of PPS (34). Increased jitter and blocking in the single-fiber EMG are found to the same degree in both stable and weakening muscles, suggesting terminal axon or axon terminal dysfunction with impaired neuromuscular transmission (12,18,37).

Macro-EMG

While routine and single-fiber EMGs are useful for confirming antecedent poliomyelitis, the macro-EMG may be more useful for identifying muscles newly weakened by PPS. In patients with remote polio, muscles of normal strength, as well as weak and atrophied muscles that have remained stable since the initial infection, have large-amplitude and often markedly increased macro-EMG signals (38). Newly weakening muscles of PPS show lower, and sometimes below-normal, macro-EMG amplitudes, and the amplitude may decrease as clinical weakness progresses (38).

MUSCLE BIOPSY

Muscle biopsies from remote polio patients reveal a spectrum of abnormalities, ranging from: (a) chronic denervation changes; (b) a combination of chronic and active denervation changes; (c) myopathic changes only; and (d) mixed neurogenic and myopathic changes; to (e) apparently normal findings (11,19,28,39). Changes are found in muscles both affected and spared by the initial infection. Furthermore, both stable and newly weakening muscles may show signs of chronic denervation and reinnervation, as well as ongoing denervation with scattered small angulated fibers (11,19,39). Muscle fibers immunoreactive for neural cell adhesion molecules, a marker for ongoing denervation, are also found in both stable and newly weakening muscles (11). As seen in EMG analyses, the histological data from PPS patients suggest that the denervating process is still active in apparently stable muscles.

In the series by Dalakas (39), biopsy specimens from 40% of PPS patients (13 of 27) with new weakness had mild perivascular or interstitial and predominantly lymphocytic inflammation; there was no evidence of vasculitis or immune complex disease. The significance of the inflammation is unknown, but inflammation is unrelated to phagocytosis and may represent an ongoing disease activity. In fact, biopsies from patients with no new weakness showed no inflammation (39). In acute poliomyelitis, transient leukocytic (both lymphocytic and neutrophilic) inflammation in areas of necrotic muscle fibers and mild perivascular lymphocytic inflammation may be observed (40,41). Similar changes are occasionally noted in muscles more than 1 year after the acute infection; it is not clear whether these inflammatory reactions are secondary to denervation or are a direct effect of the poliovirus on the muscle (40). How long the inflammation persists after acute polio infection is unclear, but inflammation found in newly weakening muscles in PPS patients suggests that it may persist in some muscles for long periods.

So-called "myopathic" changes, such as central nucleation, fiber degeneration with phagocytosis, endomysial fibrosis, fiber splitting, and muscle fiber regeneration, may be seen in muscles partially recovered from the acute paralysis, and in both stable and newly weakening muscles of PPS (28,39). These myopathic changes may appear alone, but they are frequently combined with typical neuropathic features. These features are thought to result from a loss of innervation in cases of long-standing partial denervation, and not from a primary myopathic process (28).

SPINAL CORD PATHOLOGY

Pezeshkpour and Dalakas (42) found neuronal loss and atrophy of some surviving motor neurons, active gliosis, and perivascular and parenchymal inflammation (primarily lymphocytes and plasma cells) in the spinal cords of patients with remote polio. Meningeal lymphocytic infiltration was present in almost every case. The changes were similar both in stable patients and in those with new weakness, suggesting that slow disease activity continues for many years in the spinal cords of PPS patients.

The spinal cord pathology of vaccine-related chronic progressive poliomyelitis in immunodeficient patients is similar to that of other patients, in that it includes neuronal loss, astrogliosis, and infiltration by mononuclear cells and microglia (43,44). However, the clinical course of immunodeficient patients is different from that of other postpolio patients, in that it steadily progresses to death within a few months; thus it may not represent an analogous condition.

In acute poliomyelitis, predominantly lymphocytic infiltration occurs in the affected gray matter, often forming perivascular cuffing and inflammatory nodules (41). Active neuronophagia usually fades after several weeks, but patchy meningeal inflammatory cells can persist for weeks or months. As with the inflammation found in muscles from patients with acute poliomyelitis, how long the inflammation persists in the spinal cord is not known. However, the inflammation may persist for years after acute polio infection and may lead to new muscle weakness and atrophy in PPS.

TREATMENT AND MANAGEMENT

Management of PPS patients begins with identification and treatment of other disorders that can cause increased or new disability, as mentioned. Treatment is then aimed at symptomatic intervention of new problems directly related to the new weakness of PPS.

While intensive exercise programs are generally not advisable, nonfatiguing strengthening exercises may stabilize or even improve newly weakening muscles in PPS (13,45). Recently, low-impact aerobic training has been advocated for improving the general neuromuscular function of PPS patients (46). Resumption of or additional bracing or the use of crutches and wheelchairs may be necessary to improve patients' daily activity (13,15). Patients with new respiratory complaints may benefit from IPPB treatments or assisted ventilation (27). Tracheostomy may prevent airway obstruction (24). If dysphagia and choking episodes are severe, dietary changes or tube feeding by percutaneous endoscopic gastrostomy may be necessary (23,24).

PATHOGENESIS

As discussed earlier, several hypotheses have been proposed for the pathogenesis of PPS. They include increased susceptibility of the spinal cord to further disease after polio infection, a specific vulnerability of anterior horn cells to poliovirus infection, a permanent inflammatory focus causing new weakness, or a reactivation of latent viral infection (6,8,16). Mulder et al. (11) suggested that acute anterior poliomyelitis made anterior horn cells vulnerable to further injury by the aging process and other illnesses of later life.

While earlier pathogenetic theories of PPS focused on a "central" cause at the spinal cord (6,11,16,17), recent theories focus on a "peripheral" cause. In these latter theories, degeneration or dysfunction of individual axon terminals in the motor unit, rather than degeneration of the anterior horn cell, is thought to be responsible for the new weakness (18). Motor units are thought to undergo continual remodeling and repair throughout life by the outgrowth or sprouting of axons, but in healthy persons the actual number of motor units remains fairly constant until approximately age 60 (47,48). Beyond age 60 a striking and progressive loss of motor neuron function takes place and causes muscle denervation, which is probably part of the normal aging process (48). This may be the result of as yet unknown, age-dependent changes in the capacity of nerves to sprout and regenerate (47–49). The axon and its terminal branches depend solely on the neuronal cell body for metabolic support, and any impairment with the metabolism of motor neurons (from, for example, toxins, metabolic derangements, trauma, or infection) could hasten normal aging (50,51).

In patients with PPS, motor units are no longer normal, even before age 60. From the acute infection, anterior horn cells have been lost, denervation and often widespread reinnervation has occurred, and motor units have been enlarged, sometimes to several times their normal size, all of which has increased the metabolic demands on individual motor neurons (3). As "normal" remodeling of motor units occurs throughout life, motor neurons already stressed to the limits of their capabilities may not be able to meet the demands of the motor unit; terminal axon branches may be deprived of essential nutrients or metabolites and become dysfunctional or degenerate. This deterioration, called "stress-induced exhaustion," may cause motor neurons to age faster than normal, resulting in premature denervation of muscle fibers (48,49). Hyperfunctioning motor neurons may not be able to reinnervate these muscle fibers, and if enough muscle fibers are denervated, new weakness appears (18,51,52). The concept of degeneration of the terminal axon branches is supported by the findings of scattered angulated fibers in biopsied muscles (18).

Oligoclonal bands in CSF and chronic inflammation in the muscles and spinal cord in some PPS patients suggest that immune mechanisms play a role in the pathogenesis of PPS (3,18,30,53). Further studies are certainly required because immunological abnormalities are not consistently found in these patients.

Relapse from a latent viral infection may occur, but the fact that the specific antibody to poliovirus is seldom found in PPS patients suggests that such a relapse is unlikely (53).

As already discussed, persistent poliovirus infection producing chronic progressive poliomyelitis occurs in immunodeficient individuals, but this infection is not clinically analogous to PPS (43,44). However, prolonged asymptomatic poliovirus infection can occur in laboratory animals. But, despite documented infection of brain homogenates by viral cultures, serum-neutralizing antibodies to poliovirus are not detected, and poliovirus RNA is detected in only half the animals with culture-proven infections (54). Another experiment, in which cyclophosphamide-pretreated mice were infected with poliovirus, showed that chronic polio infection can be induced (55). A higher dose of virus results in chronic polio with a shorter latency period, whereas infection with a lower dose results in a longer latency period before onset of the disease (55).

Such animal studies suggest that asymptomatic infection could eventually occur in the course of a latent viral infection in PPS. These studies also suggest that prolonged asymptomatic infection may occur and not be detected by routine serological tests or RNA detection techniques and that PPS might bear some relationship to chronic neurological diseases, such as ALS.

RELATIONSHIP BETWEEN ALS AND PPS

PPS, more specifically PPMA, after Dalakas (3), is not ALS, but ALS can occur in persons with remote polio (11,56). Clinically, the two diseases are superficially similar with progressive asymmetrical weakness and atrophy, diffuse fasciculations, and lack of sensory abnormalities. Except for an occasional Babinski sign, upper motor neuron signs are not a feature of PPS, but they are a requirement for the diagnosis of typical ALS (52). Perhaps the most compelling feature that distinguishes PPS from ALS, and which has tremendous prognostic implications, is the slow progression of PPS (3). ALS progresses more rapidly, leading to death in 2–5 years in the majority of patients (52). Therefore, it is crucial for consulting physicians to assure patients with PPS that PPS or PPMA is not ALS.

Laboratory data do not support the notion that poliovirus causes ALS (52). The virus has not been identified from cultures or immunofluorescence staining of brain, spinal cord, or muscle tissue from ALS patients at necropsy (57–59). A nucleic acid hybridization assay has been developed by Kohne et al. (60) to sensitively detect the presence of poliovirus RNA in the brain or spinal cord tissue. With this technique, poliovirus RNA has been identified in a control case and in 1 of 14 cases of ALS (60). Although these findings support the idea that picornaviruses may persist in the human nervous system, their significance remains a matter of speculation, in part because the study by McClure and Perrault (61) suggests that ribosomal RNA may contain sequences that are homologous to viral genomes, including polio (61). The presence of such sequences could result in a false-positive hybridization signal (62).

The negative results to identify poliovirus, however, could not discount a viral etiology for ALS because: (a) viral activity may be so low that the tests cannot detect the virus; (b) the virus may be present early in the illness and not later or at necropsy; or (c) viral genetic information may be mutated so that genetic probes do not recognize the mutated genes (63). Bartfeld et al. (64), however, found a significantly increased in vitro, cell-mediated immune response to poliovirus in ALS tissue, suggesting that a specific sensitization to poliovirus takes place and that a resulting autoimmune process may be involved in ALS. Again, failure to identify poliovirus does not exclude the possibility that defective poliovirus is related to the pathogenesis of ALS (63,64).

Pietsch and Morris (65) found an association between HLA-A3 and HLA-A7 and paralytic poliomyelitis. They suggest that the presence of these histocompatibility antigens on neuronal cells might facilitate poliovirus infection of the nervous system. Alternatively, HLA-A3 and HLA-A7 may link to an immune response gene, so that the neuronal damage is not caused by direct viral infection but by the immune response activated by the viral infection (65). In PPS, such immune response could explain the inability to culture the virus from the CSF, brain, or spinal cord. Antel et al. (66) noted a link between HLA-A3 and ALS and suggested an infectious or autoallergic cause for ALS. In noting an increase in HLA-A3, both in patients with poliomyelitis and in those with ALS, they suggested that the association would be consistent with a causal link between the two diseases.

The reinnervation of denervated muscle fibers is the common feature in PPS (see above) and ALS (51,67,68), although reinnervation is much more prominent in PPS. A failure of the reinnervation may be the common process leading to progressive weaknes and atrophy in both conditions. In PPS, the terminal axonal degeneration may take place in the motor unit that has already reinnervated an enormous number of muscle fibers (3,18). On the other hand, in ALS, normal reinnervation may be impaired by a progressive neuronal or immunological disease (51,69). A better understanding of how and why the reinnervation process fails in PPS may provide an important clue for understanding of the pathogenesis of ALS (52).

CONCLUSION

Although an effective vaccine has controlled acute poliomyelitis in developed countries, PPS will remain a major health threat to large numbers of polio survivors of the last epidemic for at least several more decades. Even with widespread availability of the vaccine, acute poliomyelitis has not totally disappeared in developed countries (70,71). Worldwide poliomyelitis is still prevalent, which means that PPS will continue to be a significant medical problem for years to come. Although research continues (10,13), more vigorous investigations, including large-scale prospective follow-up studies of polio survivors, are required to understand PPS. This knowledge will not only help polio survivors, but also greatly expand our understanding of motor neuron diseases in general.

ACKNOWLEDGMENT

The authors thank Mr. Thomas Lang, Department of Scientific Publication, The Cleveland Clinic Foundation, who kindly reviewed the manuscript.

REFERENCES

1. Prevalence of Selective Impairments. National Health Survey Vital and Health Statistics series 10, 134. Washington, DC: National Center for Health Statistics, 1977.
2. Speier JL, Owen RR, Knapp M, Canine JK. Occurrence of postpolio sequelae in an epidemic population. Birth Defects 1987;23:39–48.
3. Dalakas MC. Post-poliomyelitis motor neuron disease: What did we learn in reference to amyotrophic lateral sclerosis? In: Hudson AJ, ed. Amyotrophic lateral sclerosis: Concepts in pathogenesis and etiology. Toronto: University of Toronto Press, 1990:326–357.
4. Raymond M. Paralysie essentialle de l'enfance atrophie musculaire consecutive. Gaz Med Par 1875;225.
5. Cornil, Lepine. Sur un cas de paralysie generale spinale anterieure subaigue, suivi d'autopsie. Gaz Med Par 1875;127.
6. Hirsch W. On the relations of infantile spinal paralysis to spinal diseases of later life. J Nerv Ment Dis 1899;26:269–286.
7. Potts CS. A case of progressive muscular atrophy occurring in a man who had had acute poliomyelitis nineteen years previously. Univ Pa Med Bull 1903;16:31–37.
8. Salmon LA, Riley HA. The relation between chronic anterior poliomyelitis or progressive spinal muscular atrophy and an antecedent attack of acute anterior poliomyelitis. Bull Neurol Inst NY 1935;4:35–63.
9. Zilkha KJ. Discussion on motor neuron disease. Proc R Soc Med 1962;55:1028–1029.
10. Poskanzer DC, Cantor HM, Kaplan GS. The frequency of preceding poliomyelitis in amyotrophic lateral sclerosis. In: Norris FH Jr, Kurland LT, eds. Motor neuron diseases: Research on amyotrophic lateral sclerosis and related disorders. New York: Grune & Stratton, 1969:286–290.
11. Mulder DW, Rosenbaum RA, Layton DD. Late progression of poliomyelitis or forme fruste amyotrophic lateral sclerosis? Mayo Clin Proc 1972;47:756–761.
12. Cashman NR, Maselli R, Wollmann RL, Roos R, Simon R, Antel JP. Late denervation in patients with antecedent paralytic poliomyelitis. N Engl J Med 1987;317:7–12.
13. Halstead LS, Wiechers DO, Rossi CD. Late effects of poliomyelitis. Part II. Results of a survey of 201 polio survivors. South Med J 1985;78:1281–1287.
14. Cosgrove JL, Alexander MA, Kitts EL, Swan BE, Klein MJ, Bauer RE. Late effects of poliomyelitis. Arch Phys Med Rehabil 1987;68:4–7.
15. Anderson AD, Levine SA, Gellert H. Loss of ambulatory ability in patients with old anterior poliomyelitis. Lancet 1972;2:1061–1063.
16. Campbell AMG, Williams ER, Pearce J. Late motor neuron degeneration following poliomyelitis. Neurology 1969;19:1101–1106.
17. Kayser-Gatchalian MC. Late muscular atrophy after poliomyelitis. Eur Neurol 1973;10:371–380.
18. Dalakas MC, Elder G, Hallett M, et al. A long-term follow-up study of patients with post-poliomyelitis neuromuscular symptoms. N Engl J Med 1986;314:959–963.

19. Palmucci L, Bertolotto A, Doriguzzi C, Mongini T, Schiffer D. Motor neuron disease following poliomyelitis. Eur Neurol 1980;19:414–418.
20. El-Sherbini KB. False Babinski sign in poliomyelitis. Arch Phys Med Rehabil 1971;52:130–132.
21. Bodian D. Histopathologic basis of clinical findings in poliomyelitis. Am J Med 1949;6:563–578.
22. Sonies B, Dalakas M. New bulbar symptoms in previously asymptomatic post-polio patients: A dynamic study of oral-motor dysfunction with video fluoroscopy. Neurology 1988;38(Suppl 1):425 (abstract).
23. Coehlo CA, Ferrante R. Dysphagia in post polio sequelae: Report of three cases. Arch Phys Med Rehabil 1988;69:634–636.
24. Cannon S, Ritter FN. Vocal cord paralysis in postpoliomyelitis syndrome. Laryngoscope 1987;97:981–983.
25. Frustace SJ. Poliomyelitis: Late and unusual sequelae. Am J Phys Med 1987;66: 328–337.
26. Howard RS, Wiles CM, Spencer GT. The late sequelae of poliomyelitis. Q J Med 1988;251:219–232.
27. Lane DJ, Hazleman B, Nichols PJR. Late onset respiratory failure in patients with previous poliomyelitis. Q J Med 1974; 172:551–568.
28. Drachman DB, Murphy SR, Nigam MP, Hills JR. "Myopathic" changes in chronically denervated muscle. Arch Neurol 1967;16:14–24.
29. Brown S, Patten BM. Post-polio syndrome and amyotrophic lateral sclerosis: A relationship more apparent than real. Birth Defects 1987;23:83–98.
30. Dalakas M, Elder G, Sever J. A 9-year follow-up study of patients with late post poliomyelitis muscular atrophy (PPMA). Neurology 1985;35(Suppl 1):108 (abstract).
31. Brooks BR, Kurent J, Madden D, Sever J, Engel WK. Cerebrospinal fluid antiviral antibody (Ab) titres in ALS and late post-poliomyelitis progressive muscular atrophy (LPPPMA). Neurology 1978;28:338 (Abstract).
32. Ginsberg AH, Gale MJ, Rose LM, Clark EA. T-cell alterations in late postpoliomyelitis. Arch Neurol 1989;46:497–501.
33. Block HS, Wilbourn AJ. Progressive post-polio atrophy: The EMG findings. Neurology 1986;36(Suppl 1):137 (Abstract).
34. Cruz Martinez A, Perez Conde MC, Ferrer MT. Chronic partial denervation is more widespread than is suspected clinically in paralytic poliomyelitis. Eur Neurol 1983;22:314–321.
35. Hayward M, Seaton D. Late sequelae of paralytic poliomyelitis: a clinical and electromyographic study. J Neurol Neurosurg Psychiatry 1979;42:117–122.
36. Ravits J, Hallett M, Baker M, Nilsson J, Dalakas M. Clinical and EMG studies of post poliomyelitis muscular atrophy. Neurology 1987;37(Suppl 1):161 (Abstract).
37. Wiechers DO, Hubbell SL. Late changes in the motor unit after acute poliomyelitis. Muscle Nerve 1981;4:524–528.
38. Lange DJ, Smith T, Lovelace RE. Postpolio muscular atrophy: Diagnostic utility of macroelectromyography. Arch Neurol 1989;46:502–506.

39. Dalakas MC. Morphologic changes in the muscles of patients with postpoliomyelitis neuromuscular symptoms. Neurology 1988;38:99–104.

40. Denst J, Neuberger KT. A histologic study of muscles and nerves in poliomyelitis. Am J Pathol 1950;28:863–875.

41. Leestma JE. Viral infections of the nervous system. In: Davis RL, Robertson DM, eds. Textbook of neuropathology. Baltimore: Williams & Wilkins, 1985:704–787.

42. Pezeshkpour GH, Dalakas MC. Long-term changes in the spinal cords of patients with old poliomyelitis. Arch Neurol 1988;45:505–508.

43. Feigen Rd, Guggenheim MA, Johnsen SD. Vaccine-related paralytic poliomyelitis in an immunodeficient child. J Pediatr 1971;79:642–647.

44. Davis LE, Bodian D, Price D, Butler IJ, Vickers JH. Chronic progressive poliomyelitis secondary to vaccination of an immuno deficient child. N Engl J Med 1977;297:241–245.

45. Feldman RM, Soskolne CL. The use of nonfatiguing strengthening exercises in post-polio syndrome. Birth Defects 1987;23:335–341.

46. Jones DR, Speier J, Canine K, Owen R, Stull GA. Cardiorespiratory responses to aerobic training by patients with postpoliomyelitis sequelae. JAMA 1989;261:3255–3258.

47. Pestronk A, Drachman DB, Griffin JW. Effects of aging on nerve sprouting and regeneration. Exp Neurol 1980; 70:65–82.

48. McComas AJ, Upton ARM, Sica REP. Motoneurone disease and ageing. Lancet 1973;2:1477–1480.

49. Brown WF. Functional compensation of human motor units in health and disease. J Neurol Sci 1973;20:199–209.

50. Grafstein B, McQuarrie IG. Role of the nerve cell body in axonal regeneration. In: Cotman CW, ed. Neuronal plasticity. New York: Raven Press, 1978:155–195.

51. Bradley WG. Recent views on amyotrophic lateral sclerosis with emphasis on electrophysiological studies. Muscle Nerve 1987;10:490–502.

52. Mitsumoto H, Hanson MR, Chad DA. Amyotrophic lateral sclerosis: Recent advances in pathogenesis and therapeutic trials. Arch Neurol 1988;45:189–202.

53. Dalakas MC, Sever JL, Madden DL, Papadoupoulos NM, Shekarchi IC, Albrecht P, Krezlewiez A. Late postpoliomyelitis muscular atrophy: Clinical, virologic and immunologic studies. Rev Infect Dis 1984;6:S562–S567.

54. Miller JR. Prolonged intracerebral infection with poliovirus in asymptomatic mice. Ann Neurol 1981;9:590.

55. Jubelt B, Meagher JB. Poliovirus infection of cyclophosphamide-treated mice results in persistence and late paralysis. I. Clinical, pathologic, and immunologic studies. Neurology 1984;34:486–493.

56. Roos RP, Viola MV, Wollmann R, Hatch MH, Antel JP. Amyotrophic lateral sclerosis with antecedent poliomyelitis. Arch Neurol 1980;37:312–313.

57. Weiner LP, Stohlman SA, Davis RL. Attempts to demonstrate virus in amyotrophic lateral sclerosis. Neurology 1980;30:1319–1322.

58. Oshiro LS, Cremer NE, Norris FH, Lennette EH. Viruslike particles in muscle from a patient with amyotrophic lateral sclerosis. Neurology 1976;26:57–60.

59. Cremer NE, Oshiro LS, Norris FH, Lennette EH. Cultures of tissues from patients with amyotrophic lateral sclerosis. Arch Neurol 1973;29:331–333.

60. Kohne DE, Gibbs CJ, White L, Tracy SM, Meinke W, Smith RA. Virus detection by nucleic acid hybridization: Examination of normal and ALS tissue for the presence of poliovirus. J Gen Virol 1891;56:223–233.

61. McClure MA, Perrault J. Poliovirus genome RNA hybridizes specifically to higher eukaryotic rRNA. Nucleic Acids Res 1985;13:6797–6897.

62. Smith RA. Treatment of amyotrophic lateral sclerosis with interferon. In: Smith RA, ed. Interferon treatment of neurologic disorders. New York: Marcel Dekker, 1988:265–276.

63. Viola MV, Myers JC, Gann KL, Gibbs JC, Roos RP. Failure to detect poliovirus genetic information in amyotrophic lateral sclerosis. Ann Neurol 1979;5:402–403.

64. Bartfeld H, Dham C, Donnenfeld H, et al. Immunological profile of amyotrophic lateral sclerosis patients and their cell-mediated immune responses to viral and CNS antigens. Clin Exp Immunol 1982;48:137–147.

65. Pietsch MC, Morris PJ. An association of HL-A3 and HL-A7 with paralytic poliomyelitis. Tissue Antigens, 1974;4:50–55.

66. Antel JP, Arnason BGW, Fuller TC, Lehrich JR. Histocompatibility typing in amyotrophic lateral sclerosis. Arch Neurol 1976;33:423–425.

67. Brown WF, Jaatoul N. Amyotrophic lateral sclerosis: Electrophysiologic study (number of motor units and rate of decay of motor units). Arch Neurol 1974;30: 242–248.

68. Stalberg E, Schwartz MS, Trontelj JV. Single fibre electromyography in various processes affecting the anterior horn cell. J Neurol Sci 1975;24:403–415.

69. Gurney ME, Belton AC, Cashman N, et al. Inhibition of terminal axonal sprouting by serum from patients with amyotrophic lateral sclerosis. N Engl J Med 1984;311: 933–939.

70. Morrison EG, Embil JA. Poliomyelitis in North America: The disease is not dead yet. Can Med Assoc J 1987;137:1085–1087.

71. Poliomyelitis—United States, 1975–1984. MMWR 1986;35:180–182.

5

Sporadic and Western Pacific Amyotrophic Lateral Sclerosis
Epidemiological Implications

Carmel Armon

Loma Linda University Medical School and Medical Center and Jerry L. Pettis Memorial Veterans Affairs Medical Center Loma Linda, California

Leonard T. Kurland and Glenn E. Smith

Mayo Clinic and Mayo Foundation Rochester, Minnesota

John C. Steele

University of Guam, Mangilao, and Guam Memorial Hospital Tamuning, Guam

This chapter provides a review of recent developments in the epidemiology of sporadic and Western Pacific amyotrophic lateral sclerosis (ALS); familial ALS is covered in another chapter of this volume. The etiological and pathogenetic implications of these recent developments will be emphasized in our effort to build on, rather than duplicate, previous recent reviews of the epidemiology of ALS (1–3).

GENERAL EPIDEMIOLOGICAL CONSIDERATIONS IN ALS

Potential Uses of Epidemiological Data and Methods

In general, descriptive or observational studies may serve to identify new diseases or phenotypic variants of known diseases and may delineate the natural history of those diseases. Such information may be used to infer prognosis for individual patients and for purposes of public health planning and resource allocation (4). Analytical or comparative studies can help identify temporal trends and geographic variations; within that framework, the discovery of geographic isolates (5) or clusters (6) offers a special research potential. The use of epidemiological data to generate or test hypotheses of causation or etiology is not a self-evident process. It is derived from a basic premise or axiom that disease does not occur randomly, but in patterns that reflect the operation of underlying causes (7). One particular reason why epidemiological data on ALS may be of particular importance in generating etiological hypotheses is the fact that animal models have failed to reproduce its features or to provide therapeutic leads (8,9).

General Methodological Issues in ALS

Major methodological issues as they relate to the epidemiology of ALS are: case definition, case ascertainment, and the use of reference populations or controls. An advantage of familiarity with the statistical and analytical procedures in descriptive and comparative studies of ALS is the ability to critique data derived from such studies.

Case Definition

Motor neuron disease (MND) is a group of system degeneration diseases that include ALS, progressive muscular atrophy (PMA), and progressive bulbar palsy (PBP) (10). Strictly speaking, the term (classic) ALS should be reserved for patients who have clinical involvement of both upper and lower motor neurons, the term PMA for patients with primary involvement of skeletal muscle innervated by lower motor neurons, and the term PBP for patients with primary involvement of bulbar-innervated muscles. Since ALS in its early stages may present as either PMA or PBP, the term ALS has been used interchangeably with motor neuron disease to describe all three clinical forms (11). The current emphasis on lower motor neuron syndromes, some of which may respond to treatment (12), has made the desirability of distinguishing ALS from ''motor neuron disease'' more than a matter of semantics. Recent studies have used the term ALS in the restrictive sense implying evidence of upper and lower motor neuron involvement (13–15). Attention to these methodological and terminological differences is necessary in comparing recent to earlier studies.

Case Ascertainment

In order for an individual with a particular disease to enter into a potential epidemiological database, several things must occur. First, a correct diagnosis needs to be made; second, that diagnosis should be entered into an archive where it will be found by future investigators. These processes, combined with the efforts of the investigators to identify cases, enable case ascertainment, upon which temporal and regional comparisons depend.

As it relates to ALS, underascertainment has undoubtedly occurred in the past in the elderly, in women, and in socially or racially disadvantaged populations. The tendency of families in the past to attribute 80-year-old grandma's progressive weakness to her "arthritis" is a case in point. Furthermore, a general practitioner can be expected to observe a new case of ALS only five or six times in a lifetime of service; it is not unreasonable to expect him to fail to recognize such a case, especially in the very elderly where other findings may support an alternative diagnosis. Also, the apparent futility of making a diagnosis for a condition for which there is no cure may have discouraged many general practitioners from looking further. We have attempted to estimate the potential size of these problems within a case-control study of sporadic ALS (15). On careful questioning of the controls in that study, a history of painless, progressive wasting and weakening illness in the last years or months of life was provided for at least one relative aged over 60 by 10% of the controls. Of 1881 relatives of controls, 23 (1.2%) had such a condition attributed to them by the control who was interviewed. On earlier or routine questioning, these relatives were described variously as having died of "old age," of an "unknown cause," or of an "unspecified cause." This number, 1.2%, is 12 times higher than the estimate of the U.S. death ratio for ALS: 1/1000 of those reaching adulthood. While we doubt that all the relatives for whom we elicited a history of painless, progressive wasting and weakening illness had ALS, we consider 1.2% of the relatives as a potential pool of individuals, some of whom may have died of undiagnosed motor neuron disease.

Furthermore, not all individuals diagnosed with ALS will have that diagnosis appear on their death certificates. It is thus inappropriate to equate the increased appearance of a diagnosis of motor neuron disease, ALS, or any other neurodegenerative disease on death certificates as representing true increases in mortality from these conditions (16–18), a point previously made by others (19,20). The fact that the rates, as determined from these death certificate data, fall short of the incidence rates for the Rochester, Minnesota, population (11), where no significant increase has been detected, gives additional impetus to interpret increased appearance of ALS on death certificates conservatively.

Another reason for an apparent increase is a shift in physicians' practice from reporting ALS as a secondary or contributing cause of death to that of the underlying cause. It was noted (21) that for the years 1971–1978 about 25% of motor neuron disease diagnoses were not reported as underlying cause, which would tend to underestimate the mortality and incidence rates. Listing ALS as the underlying cause, as recommended by the World Health Organization, would be expected to result in an apparent increase in the ALS mortality rate.

Improved diagnosis of ALS has resulted from increased public awareness of ALS, a relative increase in the number of neurologists, the increased availability of neurodiagnostic techniques, the increased awareness by the aging population that progressive weakness is not a normal part of aging, and enactment of the

Medicare Act in 1965 (which guaranteed improved access to health care for the elderly). These trends, coupled with improved reporting practices, including proper death certification, can be expected to result in further increases in the recognized mortality from ALS.

Choice of Controls

A major concern in any study of coexistent conditions in patients with ALS or in case-control studies of risk factors is the choice of controls. A case in point is the putative association of thyroid disease with ALS. Five anecdotal reports and a recent uncontrolled study claimed such an association existed (22). Subsequent series (23–25) and our own population-based case-control study (26) have revealed no excess association with thyroid disease. It remains a matter of speculation whether therapeutic trials with thyrotropin-releasing hormone (TRH) in patients with ALS (27,28), an agent that ultimately proved to be ineffective in this disease, were influenced by the earlier reports. Immunosuppressant treatments in ALS also appear to have been based on anecdotal evidence of immune dysfunction in conditions mimicking this disease or on nonspecific immune abnormalities which may be as much a response to the disease as its cause. They, too, have proved unsuccessful (29–32).

The choice of controls can seriously affect the results of case-control studies and the interpretation of pathological data from patients such as those on Guam and in other foci. These issues will be explored later in this chapter.

Types of ALS

On the basis of epidemiological and genetic features, three major types of ALS have been identified: (a) the classic and usually sporadic form, (b) the familial and presumably hereditary form, and (c) the Western Pacific (Mariana Islands) form, first described among the indigenous population (Chamorros) of Guam (33), often in association with another progressive and fatal disorder referred to as Parkinsonism-dementia complex (PDC). This same form of ALS (with PDC) was subsequently recognized in two villages on the Kii Peninsula of Japan (34,35) and among the Auyu and Jakai people of Irian Jaya (western New Guinea) (36).

Clinical and Pathological Features of ALS

The clinical and pathological features of the three major types of ALS are presented in Table 1; however, as pointed out in a recent review of ALS (37), in the last decade increasing attention has been directed to the fact that ALS may involve parts of the central and peripheral nervous systems outside the upper and lower motor neurons. Systems affected, albeit to a lesser extent than the motor system, include peripheral (38) and central (39–42) sensory nerves, sensory cortex (43), spinocerebellar neurons (44), and autonomic function (45,46); oc-

Table 1 Clinical and Pathological Features of Sporadic (Classic), Familial, and Western Pacific ALS

Type	Clinical features	Pathological features
Sporadic (classic)	90% of patients Cause of death in ≈1 of 800 men, 1 of 1200 women Male:female ratio 1.6:1 Mean age at onset 66 years (oldest group) Frequency of involvement of additional systems (sensory, autonomic, cognitive) now a subject of investigation	Degeneration of cortical Betz cells and anterior horn cells; demyelination of corticospinal tracts Involvement of additional systems recently identified
Familial	10% of patients Autosomal dominant inheritance Male:female ratio 1:1 Mean age at onset 45–50 years (intermediate age group) Three major genotypic/phenotypic variants, with greater variation between than within families Duration generally less than in sporadic form; rarely long	Degeneration of cortical Betz cells and anterior horn cells; demyelination of corticospinal tracts Demyelination of posterior columns, involvement of spinocerebellar tracts and columns of Clarke
Western Pacific	3 foci in Western Pacific Incidence rates originally 100 times those of continental U.S. Linked to cycad exposure Male:female ratio > 2:1 Mean age at onset 45 years (youngest group) Associated with Parkinsonism-dementia complex	Degeneration of cortical Betz cells and anterior horn cells; demyelination of corticospinal tracts Degeneration of substantia nigra and locus ceruleus Excess neurofibrillary tangles and intracytoplasmic inclusion (granulovacuolar) bodies widespread in the central nervous system, particularly in the hippocampus, substantia nigra, locus ceruleus, and cerebellum

ulomotor neuron involvement has been documented at autopsy in respirator-sustained patients (47).

Cognitive involvement in ALS may also be more frequent than previously suspected. Frank dementia has previously been reported in about 5% of sporadic and familial cases (37,48). Some cases of amyotrophy presenting with dementia pathologically resemble ALS more than Creutzfeldt-Jakob disease or other dementias (49,50). Also, there is a lack of transmissibility to nonhuman primates in almost all such cases tested (49). One of us (C.A.) recently suspected cognitive impairment in 21/61 (34%) of patients without articulatory or respiratory problems, based on their performance within a structured interview setting (15) compared to 25/199 (13%) of controls ($p < 0.0001$). Formal cognitive testing in 37 unselected patients with ALS revealed mild, but significant impairment in various measures of cognitive performance compared to matched controls (51).

The evidence for frequent involvement of nonmotor systems in what is otherwise typical sporadic ALS implies that such involvement should not be considered reason to discard the diagnosis in individual patients or to exclude them from studies of sporadic ALS, since it may transpire that with sufficiently sensitive testing the majority of patients with classic ALS may have evidence of involvement of additional nuclei or neuronal tracts. We do not favor calling such patients "ALS +," in distinction to the approach of designating patients with Parkinson's disease and findings of involvement of additional systems as "Parkinson's +." The diagnostic criteria for ALS should continue to be the core clinical findings of progressive upper and lower motor neuron abnormalities and electromyographic evidence of widespread muscle denervation.

Age at Onset of Symptoms and Age at Diagnosis

On average, about 12 months elapse between onset of the first clinical symptom of ALS and its diagnosis, according to several careful studies (11,13,15,26). There is the general belief that more persistent questioning may elicit an even earlier date of onset. Furthermore, the onset of first clinical symptoms must surely occur sometime after the disease has been biologically active. Since progression after onset to death averages 3 years, when 90% or so of the anterior horn cells at affected levels have degenerated, and if clinical disease can be recognized only when half the motor neurons are affected, it could be argued that the biological onset also predates clinical onset by as much as 3 years. Thus, the dates of biological and clinical onset of disease may be somewhat uncertain. There is usually less uncertainty about the date of diagnosis. Given these concerns, it is probably appropriate to provide survival data, both from age at onset of first recognized clinical symptom and from age at diagnosis.

Figure 1, modified from Mulder et al. (52), shows the cumulative percentage for age at onset of symptoms in five groups of patients with motor neuron disease. It demonstrates the following points: (a) curves are similar for all five groups, but shifted compared to each other; (b) mean and median ages at onset are lowest for the Mariana Islands type and increase, respectively, for the familial, referral, and population-based groups; and (c) the referral sample has a younger mean age at onset than the population-based group and is the only sample to achieve a plateau (flat line after age 65 years). The more recent Mayo

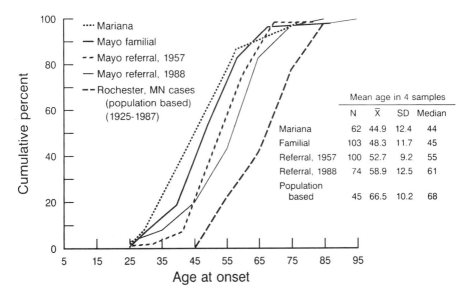

Figure 1 Cumulative percent for age at onset of symptoms in five data groups with motor neuron disease, Mayo Clinic, Rochester, Minnesota. [Modified from Mulder et al. (52).]

Clinic referral sample (15) had a mean age at onset of 58.9 years, reflecting increased referral of older people with ALS. This referral sample did not achieve a plateau at age 65 years because the oldest age at onset for this group of patients was 83 years. Thus, we now know that age-specific incidence rates increase with age (11,16) rather than peaking at 55–60 years, as shown in referral-based case series. This is significant because it means that ALS is more akin to other neurodegenerative disorders, such as Alzheimer's disease and Parkinson's disease, than might have been inferred from the earlier data (4).

The feature that distinguishes the Rochester, Minnesota, population-based cohort from referral series is the absence in the Rochester series of early-onset-aged patients, the youngest being 48 years, whereas 5–15% in the usual referral series is 45 years and under. Indeed, the mean age at onset of the subgroup of our recent referral series patients (15) who were 50 years and older was 63.8 years, which is comparable to the Rochester population-based series. The absence of younger individuals with motor neuron disease in the Rochester population-based series, in the context of adequate ascertainment in older age groups, if not due to chance, may reflect life-style and environmental factors unique to Rochester, Minnesota.

SPORADIC (CLASSIC) ALS

Descriptive Studies

Four major descriptive population-based parameters can be used to describe the frequency of disease. "Incidence rate" refers to the number of cases developing or being newly diagnosed with a disease during a stated interval of time, divided by the population at risk. "Prevalence rate" refers to the number of cases present at a given point in time, divided by the population at risk. "Mortality rate" is the number of deaths from the disease during a stated period of time, divided by the population at risk; and the "death ratio" is the proportion of deaths from a specific cause divided by all deaths in the population at risk during a given period of time.

As these definitions relate to motor neuron disease, there is some evident ambiguity in the definition of incidence rate, as one to several years may elapse between the time symptoms develop and the time the diagnosis is made. Thus, it is essential that this rate be specified as "symptomatic" (onset) or "diagnostic" incidence rate. As a corollary, prevalence rates will be underestimates to the extent that there are patients in whom the disease has begun but is not yet diagnosed. Mortality rates and death ratios are readily available, inexpensive to obtain, and unambiguous, but depend on the methods and accuracy of reporting the disease on the death certificate. Assignment of ALS as the primary or as a contributory cause can also affect the death rate and death ratio (53).

Some rounded figures approximating frequency values for the population of the United States follow. The incidence rate is about 2 per 100,000 per year and this should equal the mortality rate; however, underreporting on death certificates accounts for a lower reported rate, which in the 1980s was under 1.5 per 100,000 per year, for all ages combined. With an average duration of nearly 3 years, the prevalence should be three times the incidence rate, or about 6 per 100,000 population on a given date. The death ratio incorporates the concepts of a cumulative incidence of the probability of developing the disease during a lifetime. In the United States, the death ratio from ALS is about 1 in 1000 deaths for those reaching adulthood. Since the sex ratio of affected individuals is about 1.6 males per female, this translates into a death ratio of 1 in 800 men and 1 in 1200 women. Annegers et al. have computed the death ratio from the Rochester, Minnesota, incidence rates and find the ratio is approximately 1 in 300 for men and 1 in 600 for women (11; and J.F. Annegers, personal communication). Reports of annual incidence of motor neuron disease in other countries have ranged from 0.8 to 1.8 per 100,000 population. This variability may be due at least in part to different levels of ascertainment, although there may be true differences in incidence rates. Prevalence rates have been even more variable (4).

Based on death certificate data for motor neuron disease, the mortality rate per 100,000 population increased from 0.7 to 1.1 between 1944 and 1977 (4) and continued to rise through 1984 (16). This leads us to suspect that ascertainment of ALS as the cause of death has improved with time, because the increasing mortality rates have yet to match the incidence rates in the Rochester population. Furthermore, all the reported rise in mortality (16) has taken place in individuals aged 70 years and over regardless of gender or race. This feature also suggests that crude ascertainment, diagnosis, and documentation of cause of death in the elderly, rather than a true increase in incidence, accounts for these trends in reported mortality.

A critical approach to the interpretation of population-based data will be illustrated by reviewing several recent studies.

Review of the following studies demonstrates the potential pitfalls introduced by referral bias, ascertainment bias, and issues of diagnosis into the interpretation of epidemiological data (54–57). These studies relied on diagnoses in patients admitted to regional hospitals during the mid-1970s to mid-1980s. They reported annual incidence rates for ALS ranging from 0.44 to 0.78 per 100,000 inhabitants (54,55,57), and for MND, 1.01 per 100,000 (56). The degree of distinction between ALS and the other forms of MND in these studies is not always clear, because all the authors subdivide ALS further into conventional (atrophic, classic), bulbar, and pseudopolyneuritic forms, presumably according to site of clinical onset. Longest survival is reported with the pseudopolyneuritic form, next longest with the conventional form, and significantly shorter survival with the bulbar form.

Mean age at onset in the three studies of ALS ranged from 54.3 to 61.4 years; median age at onset was 60.5 in the study of MND. A higher mean age at onset was present in the studies with the higher incidence rates. Mean survival was shorter (27–28 months) in the two studies (55,56) that reported higher incidence rates of ALS or MND than in the other studies (34–42 months) (54,57). The correlation of higher mean age at onset and shorter survival with higher reported incidence rates suggests that referral bias leading to underascertainment in the elderly or in patients with a short course may account for the differences. These studies suggest that improved diagnosis may identify patients with a course shorter than the previously considered average of 3 years. Other studies have shown that, indeed, bulbar findings at diagnosis and age at onset of over 60 years may predispose to a shorter course (13,14).

Features suggesting more complete case ascertainment have emerged from national mortality data for MND from Sweden (58). These data showed an increase in average mortality for ALS/PBP from 1.4 per 100,000 in 1961–1969 to 2.0 per 100,000 in 1970–1977 and to 2.3 per 100,000 in 1978–1985. When directly age-adjusted to a standard European population, the rates were 1.3, 1.7, and 1.8, respectively. When age-standardized to the U.S. population of 1976, the 1978–1985 rate was 1.7. The male:female ratio was 1.2:1. When the data were analyzed by birth cohort, age-adjusted mortality rates continued to rise through age 85 +, except that the 1887–1900 male cohort peaked at 80–84 years of age.

High representation of the elderly and a male:female ratio approaching unity suggest that ascertainment in this study (58) was more complete than in those discussed previously (54–57), resulting in higher absolute rates. The rise in age-adjusted mortality rates shown is comparable to the rise in age-specific incidence rates in the Rochester, Minnesota, population-based data for 1925–1984 (11), which provides an additional feature suggesting that ascertainment in the elderly was less limited by referral bias in this (58) than in other studies. Nevertheless, the Rochester, Minnesota, average annual incidence rate for 1925–1984, adjusted to the 1970 U.S. population, was 2.4 per 100,000, higher than the 1.7 per 100,000 average adjusted Swedish mortality rate for 1978–1985, for a population that is genetically similar. This suggests some under-ascertainment in the Swedish mortality data, despite the other evidence for its completeness.

Racial differences in death rates from ALS in the United States were noted in 1959–1961 mortality data studies: the rates for whites exceeded those for non-whites by 1.7:1 (59). Subsequent studies of the rates for 1971 and 1973–1978 (53) and 1962–1984 (16) continued to show lower rates among nonwhites, particularly those older than 60 years, especially women. These differences (1.5:1 to 1.7:1 overall, unadjusted for age) have been considered "small" (53). We consider them evidence for continued underascertainment in this population. Of particular note is the fact that the rise of ascertainment of MND between 1962 and 1984 in individuals aged over 70 years, whites (men and women), and nonwhite men has not occurred among nonwhite women. In that group, the age-specific mortality pattern reported for 1980–1984 resembled that for 1962–1964 (16). A door-to-door survey, such as the Copiah County Study for the prevalence of major neurological disorders (60) undertaken in 1978, has not been reported for ALS. That study revealed, in one county, considerable underdiag-nosis (42%) of another neurodegenerative disease, Parkinson's disease, in both black and white populations (61). However, gender appeared to have been a greater risk factor for underdiagnosis than race; of 13 newly diagnosed patients, 10 were women (five black, five white) and three were men (two black, one white). Racial or gender differences in the age-adjusted prevalence rates of Parkinson's disease were not striking (61).

Given the potential confounding effect of underascertainment, we believe that no statement can be made regarding the effect of race on the true incidence of ALS. While we have illustrated this point with data from the United States, we believe it may apply to international comparisons. We further suspect that the long-standing observation of gender differences in the incidence of sporadic ALS may prove to have similarly resulted, at least in part, from selective underascertainment of ALS in women, particularly in the older age groups.

Analytical or Comparative Studies

Three major types of analytical studies may identify potential risk factors for disease: cross-sectional or prevalence studies, cohort (prospective or follow-up) studies, and case-control studies. Because of the relatively low incidence of ALS, cross-sectional surveys and cohort studies are generally impractical as a means of identifying risk factors (1).

This leaves the case-control study, where the affected are selectively included and the size of the group is limited only by the resources available and the perseverance of the investigator. This method is suitable for generating or confirming multiple hypotheses with regard to possible causative agents. The chief disadvantages are recall bias and the concern that by testing multiple hypotheses (a "fishing expedition") some may attain significance by chance alone. However, at the present time it is the only feasible epidemiological approach for comparative or analytical studies for an uncommon disease such as ALS. Hypotheses can then be the subject of further confirmatory studies if they appear to be biologically plausible and if the association is noted for a significant proportion of the affected.

Unfortunately, most case-control studies to date have not been rigorously designed. Furthermore, there is concern that publication bias whereby a positive finding is more likely to be published than the lack of such a finding favors the identification of spurious risk factors. As a result, case-control studies have implicated previous mechanical, chemical, and electrical trauma, surgery, exposure to heavy metals, occupations dealing with leather, solvent exposure, and physical (manual) labor (62–73). Poor study design and recall bias may account for some of the inconclusive or conflicting results.

Methodological Issues in Case-Control Studies of ALS
We present some methodological considerations in the design of case-control studies of ALS that hopefully will help readers in evaluating published studies and in designing their own studies.

Patient Homogeneity. Sporadic motor neuron disease is a heterogeneous group of disorders with more than a single clinical form, and possibly more than a single cause. It is therefore advantageous to study as homogeneous a group as can be determined on clinical grounds. This may be done by limiting the study to patients with the ALS form, i.e., requiring evidence of involvement of upper and lower motor neurons. Patients with progressive bulbar palsy may be included if there is additional evidence of extensive lower motor neuron involvement or if

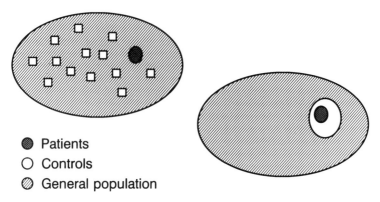

Figure 2   Matching and overmatching between cases and controls.

autopsy shows involvement of the corticospinal tracts. It is appropriate to deal separately with those patients with a positive family history and those who have resided in high-prevalence loci.

Choice of Controls.   Two conflicting influences affect the choice of controls. The first is the desire to have controls representative in some way of the general population in order to infer from the study how the cases differ from the general population (the external validity of the study). The second influence, which operates through the process of matching, tends to make the controls more like the patients than the general population. This process itself has a positive influence and prevents inappropriate comparisons, such as 70-year-old men and adolescent girls. However, the matching process may result in controls that are more similar to patients with respect to variables of interest than to the general population. Such a situation, termed "overmatching," is illustrated in Figure 2. Comparisons with such controls may not bring out true associations of disease with those particular variables, and in addition, from such comparisons it may be incorrect to make external inferences to the general population. It is often appropriate to select controls in more than a single way in an attempt to take into account the potential biases inherent in any particular way of selecting controls. For example, a spouse who may have shared many biographic experiences with the patient is predisposed to a different occupational history, yet will be overmatched for residence. By contrast, an age- and sex-matched social peer of the patient may be overmatched for activities.

Recall Bias.   It is recognized that people with a fatal disease may be more likely to recall those details of their past that they think may be associated with the disease. It is possible to attempt to control for this by at least three means. First, a sequential questionnaire/interview design may be used to standardize the information-gathering process (15). This provides two opportunities to prompt the patient's memory, an opportunity for the patient to ask questions about the questionnaire and so confirm that he/she understood them, and ascertainment by the interviewer of the completeness of the responses. Such a design is an improvement over that of previous studies, including our own (67). Unrelated questions may be included in the questionnaire to estimate the effect of recall bias and suggestibility. Second, it is appropriate to decide ahead of time to analyze separately (perhaps in a subsequent case-control study) information that is clearly a result of a unique research effort by an individual patient who has convinced himself that a specific risk factor is causative. For example, most individuals do not know the chemical composition of pesticides they use, but an individual patient may have gathered such information. Third, it is appropriate to ask patients if they have any specific hypotheses about the causation of their disease in order to see if such hypotheses might bias their recall. It should also be recognized that some patients might not share their hypotheses with the interviewer.

Quantification of Activities or Exposures. To the extent possible, it is helpful to quantify data, e.g., for residence, the number of years lived in a particular community; for occupational and recreational activities, the number of hours per week and the number of years spent at that activity. It is important to exclude events and activities that occurred after the onset for both the index case and the control.

Testing of Multiple Hypotheses. A major advantage of the case-control study is the ability to test for multiple possible risk factors. Exploitation of this advantage is constrained by two considerations. First, the chance of finding a spurious association increases with the number of hypotheses tested. On the average, when testing, at the 0.05 level of significance 100 potential associations where no association exists, up to five may be found "significant" by definition, owing to chance alone. Attempting to compensate for this by using more stringent acceptance criteria (e.g., Bonferroni's correction) may result in the rejection of true associations. Second, the more specific and detailed the information sought, the less likely it is to be available or remembered. Three approaches may be used to address this concern. The first is to make a distinction between those hypotheses for which the study should be considered confirmatory or hypothesis-confirming and those for which it should be considered exploratory or hypothesis-generating. Second, it is important to limit the number of hypotheses for which the study should be considered confirmatory; each should be entered on the basis of preexisting rationale. Third, it is important to recognize that looking for rare or infrequent antecedent events will lead, at best, to identification of associations of possible etiological significance in only a small minority of patients or to identification of multiple different antecedent events which, in turn, will lead to more and more hypotheses to be tested. It is, therefore, appropriate to ask about those activities or exposures that may be expected to be relatively common and that the majority of people might recall reliably. These considerations are demonstrated in the following analysis of specific risk factors.

Amyotrophic Lateral Sclerosis and Trauma

A number of reports (15,63,64,66,74–77) address the question of the association of trauma and ALS. Percentages of ALS patients reporting histories of trauma have ranged from 7.5% (66) to 58% (63). Risk ratios for these case-control studies have ranged from 1.78 to 2.68. Kondo (78) concluded that mechanical injuries are "known beyond doubt" to be a motor neuron disease risk factor. Because of the deficiencies in design and methodology in his and other studies to be reviewed, we take serious issue with this statement. The role of trauma in ALS remains controversial at best. Given the continuing need for rational, viable etiological models of ALS and the medicolegal implications of pronouncements such as Kondo's, careful attention to methodology and a cautious approach is essential before drawing conclusions.

Specific Methodological Considerations—Trauma and ALS. Applying the criteria outlined above, several features should receive careful attention in analyzing past (and future) studies:

1. The diagnostic criteria used for ALS should be defined and the method of documenting diagnosis should be explicit and sound. The criteria for establishing a diagnosis of ALS are presented elsewhere in this volume.

2. The nature of trauma (agent, anatomical site, and severity) should be clearly defined and the time of exposure specified.

3. The observed rates of exposure to trauma should be evaluated against baseline trauma rates, i.e., expected rates for a specific trauma during a specific exposure period. Trauma to the patient occurring at times other than the period just prior to onset should also be described in detail.

Table 2 lists the annual incidence in the United States for injuries as established by the National Center for Health Statistics' National Health Survey in 1980–1981 (79). The table reflects that in a given year approximately one-third of the U.S. population will experience trauma of some form. Overall rates for trauma are highest in the young and lessen with age.

The interview data obtained in the National Health Survey are in general accord with incidence data obtained from medical records data in the population of Olmsted County, Minnesota (80). For example, the 0.9% incidence rate for lower limb fractures reported by the National Health Survey compares with a 0.6% rate reported by Garraway et al. at Mayo Clinic (81). In general, the National Health Survey should reflect slightly higher incidence since it included injuries for which no medical treatment was sought.

Table 2 Annual Percentage of Traumatic Injuries by Type and Age Group in the United States: 1980–1981

Injury	All ages	<17 years	17–44 years	45–64 years	≥65 years
All injuries	33.2	38.7	38.3	22.6	19.5
Skull fractures and intracranial injuries	1.0	1.3	1.4	0.2	0.5
Lower limb fractures	0.9	0.5	1.0	1.1	1.2
Upper limb, neck, and trunk fractures	1.8	2.3	1.7	1.1	2.2
Open wounds	8.0	11.2	8.9	4.9	2.8
Sprains and strains	7.6	6.4	10.5	5.1	3.7
Contusions	5.2	6.9	5.2	3.4	4.6
All other injuries	8.7	10.1	9.6	6.8	4.5

Source: Adapted from National Center for Health Statistics (79).

As noted, Table 2 shows that in a given year 33% of the population will experience trauma sufficiently severe to be recalled at interview. Assuming that an individual's risk for trauma is independent of previous trauma, it follows that within 10 years 98% of people will have experienced such trauma ($0.98 = 1 - \{1 - 0.33\}^{10}$). It is clear that a reasonable assessment of ALS risk associated with trauma can occur only in conditions where types of injury and exposure windows are specific and/or narrow.

4. The method of establishing association must be valid. Methods of establishing association between trauma and ALS can be organized into a hierarchy, from least to most useful. These studies can be grouped into anecdotal reports/case studies, case series, case-control retrospective studies, and prospective studies. In addition to noting the differing validity of different methods in establishing an association, distinctions between association and causation should be maintained. If associations are found, these should be subjected to criteria that allow us to draw conclusions about causative relations. These criteria have been succinctly described by Sartwell and Last (82) and include strength of association, consistency, dose-response relationship, chronological relationship, specificity, and biological plausibility.

To summarize, each year 5000 persons in the United States will develop ALS while at least 83 million will suffer a significant injury; thus, the probability that there may be a chance association of the two in individual cases is high. In a 1-year interval, one-third of those with newly diagnosed ALS, or about 1667 cases, would also have had an injury purely by chance. For many, the injury may have been precipitated by the developing skeletal muscle weakness rather than the converse. Furthermore, true onset of ALS probably occurs 1–3 years prior to its clinical recognition. Thus, the establishment of a timely association is subject to even greater uncertainty with respect to recent trauma.

Analysis of Past Studies

Case Reports and Case Series: We recognize that case reports and case series are far more likely to be reported and published than are negative studies. Thus, there have been many anecdotal reports of an association between trauma and ALS (63,74). While anecdotal reports are useful sources of research hypotheses, they cannot be used to test an hypothesis because they are subject to nearly every bias (sampling, selection, response, and observer) found in epidemiological research. The same can be said of case series such as that of Bharucha (83). Case series may reduce some idiosyncracy of single case reports; however, case series are simply an aggregate of anecdotal reports and thus continue to suffer from all the biases of single case reports. Case studies and case series fail to meet methodological criteria that allow for tests of association and thus can lead to no conclusions.

Case-Control Studies: Retrospective case-control studies are at the first level of methodology that provides an actual opportunity for tests of association between exposure and disease. Several studies with this design have investigated trauma and ALS (15,63,66,76,77). However, problems of poor case definition, broad definitions of trauma, and selection and recall biases can be seen in a number of retrospective case-control studies. A recent study (63) may be used to demonstrate the effect of poor case selection and recall bias. It purports to examine ALS and trauma. In fact, the authors based subject selection on the broader diagnosis of motor neuron disease. Questionnaires were mailed to 135 ALS cases. Of those receiving the mailing, 37% belonged to an association whose newsletter frequently published anecdotal reports of trauma/ALS onset associations. Controls were drawn from a listing of patients belonging to a multiple sclerosis association. Seventy-eight ALS patients with prior mechanical trauma were identified; of these, 59 had head and neck injuries. This number was compared to the number of head and neck injuries in a control sample of multiple sclerosis patients selected *not for history of trauma*, but merely for their ability to return the questionnaires mailed to them. While using multiple sclerosis patients as controls should have reduced recall bias problems, any benefits from this choice were undone by the other sampling and selection biases.

Kondo and Tsubaki's retrospective case-control study of 712 cases of ALS in Japan (76) is among the most widely cited studies to support the notion that trauma is a risk factor for ALS. However, this study suffers from several significant shortcomings. The first pertains to defining the ALS sample. Although ALS was distinguished from other motor neuron diseases, death records in Japan for the years 1965 and 1966 were used to determine the diagnosis. An attempt was made to corroborate these death certificate diagnoses by contacting the certifying physician, but it is not specified how this was done. The average interval from death of the patient until interview of the respondents was not reported; however, the study was not published until 15 years after the target years for death certification. Also, the use of mortality data for case identification biases the sample by failing to include patients with ALS in the target years who survived and cases whose death certificates listed other causes of death (e.g., pneumonia, heart attack).

Controls for more than 50% of these cases were reporting spouses. Under these conditions, it was impossible for the interviewer to be blinded to the status of the interviewee. The interval from death of the case to interview of the family member was not reported. The difference in rates of reported trauma may reflect recall bias. This bias may be seen by considering that trauma was defined as mechanical injury of any type, provided it required physician attention (76). The data indicated that the mean time from injury to ALS onset was approximately 13 years. There was no maximum placed on the interval between injury and onset of ALS that could be allowed for establishing etiologically significant associations. Within this framework, the rate of trauma from mechanical injuries was 42.9% in cases compared to 19.7% in controls. It was noted above that in the United States in the 1980s, a 98% cumulative incidence for trauma could be expected in as little as a 10-year period. While the cumulative incidence rate of trauma in Japan in the 1950s and 1960s is uncertain, it is most unlikely that expected rates would have been only 20% for mechanical injury over a 40- to 60-year lifetime.

The most striking feature of these retrospective studies is that their rates of trauma for both cases and controls are less than expected, probably due to differential underrecall. The National Health Survey data are based on inquiries regarding injuries in the 2 weeks prior to the survey, rather than over long periods. Over longer periods of time, injuries, especially lesser ones, may be forgotten. The rates in these retrospective studies differ between cases and controls because of selective forgetting, i.e., recall bias. Recall of an injury may be solicited during the medical history-taking process or in the patients' own efforts to understand their disease. It is then likely to be rehearsed many times over in further medical history taking or contemplations by the patient. Thus, we cannot conclude that ALS patients are more likely to have had mechanical injury. We can only conclude that controls are more likely to forget the trauma they experienced.

The problem of recall bias is intrinsic to retrospective studies and may be illustrated further in a study by Deapen and Henderson (65), who observed an increased odds ratio for trauma with loss of consciousness in ALS cases compared to controls. However, they noted an inverse relationship when examining duration; controls reported longer periods of unconsciousness. Shorter episodes of unconsciousness are more likely to be forgotten than longer losses of consciousness, suggesting that some process is operating to enhance recall of brief episodes of unconsciousness in the ALS cases.

A study by Kurtzke and Beebe (66) attempted an innovative method to avoid the recall bias arising from retrospective reporting (i.e., reporting that follows disease detection). They utilized the military enlistment records of World War II servicemen who later developed ALS and reported rates of 7.5% injuries (occurring before service) in cases compared to rates of 3.2% injuries in controls. These differences were statistically significant. However, a different bias may have operated in that study: underreporting of prior injuries during physical examination of those entering the service in World War II. Table 2 suggests that the annual incidence rate for those in the age groups <17 years and 17–44 years is over 35% (79), significantly greater than the cumulative rates of 7.5% reported for cases and 3.2% for controls (66). While there is no basis to assume "bias" across cases and controls in these reports, inferential statistics based on such incomplete data should be viewed with caution.

The case-control study by Gresham et al. (77) may possess the soundest methodology. The objective diagnostic and eligibility criteria used to select ALS patients in their study were clearly defined. An active case identification approach was used, focusing only on fractures, as they could be expected to be well diagnosed and recalled. Cases and controls were matched for age and sex, and statistics appropriate to paired comparisons were used. There were no differences in the rate of fractures between cases and controls. In samples with an approximate mean age of 55, the cumulative incidence rates were 52% for cases and 55% for controls.

In a recent case-control study (15), Armon et al. also did not find an increased incidence of trauma in ALS patients; in fact, up to age 20 years the controls reported an increased incidence of trauma.

It appears that, as attention to methodological detail of case-control studies increases, support for an association of ALS and trauma disappears.

Prospective Studies: Prospective studies should follow cohorts of individuals who sustained trauma to determine whether the subsequent incidence of ALS exceeds that of the general population. If there is adequate sampling of trauma cases, response and observer bias are not problems, as the trauma (not ALS) is the index. However, adequate diagnosis of ALS must follow. Unfortunately, we could not find any published reports of prospective studies of the onset of ALS in patients diagnosed with trauma. We, therefore, recently embarked on such studies, using an existing data source describing a large cohort of patients with lumbar disc surgery and another cohort with head injury. The records of 942 Olmsted County, Minnesota, patients who underwent lumbar disc surgery between 1950 and 1979 for confirmed or suspected prolapse formed the first cohort. Disc surgery was related to a history of back injury in nearly all these cases. In this cohort, where the minimum follow-up interval was 11 years, no subsequent cases of ALS were observed. In a similar follow-up of 943 patients with traumatic head injuries sustained between 1935 and 1989, one patient developed ALS, which is consistent with expectations from age-specific incidence rates for ALS.

Applying the "Rules of Evidence." Applying Sartwell and Last's (82) criteria to the data on an association between ALS and trauma reinforces the conclusion that trauma is unlikely to contribute to etiology of ALS.

Strength of the Association: Trauma occurs so frequently (100%) in the absence of ALS that the strength of the association can never be high.

Consistency: Thus, as expected, methodologically sound investigations have not demonstrated the association of trauma and ALS reported in earlier studies.

"Dose-Response" Relationship: The study by Deapen and Henderson (65) reports an inverse dose-response relationship between ALS and degree of injury as indexed by length of loss of consciousness. This speaks against a causal relationship.

Chronological Relationship: Kondo and Tsubaki's (76) mean lag from injury to ALS of greater than 12 years, with a range of 0–45 years, fails to serve as a convincing proximate chronological relationship.

Specificity: Gresham et al. (77) show that when trauma is more specifically defined (e.g., fracture), an association to trauma is not observed.

Biological Plausibility: No theory currently exists that accounts for a process induced by trauma that affects motor neurons selectively. Bonduelle (84) points out that trauma generally involves focal injury while ALS is a system disease. Riggs (85) suggests that injury to motor neurons may take place at the time of a fracture. He conjectures that in the hypermetabolic state following neuronal injury, the lower motor neuron may become susceptible to other causes of ALS. However, the selective susceptibility of motor neurons is not discussed. Riggs notes that the data show a distribution of fractures that does not correspond to the site of initial weakness and amyotrophy. Thus, the same data that are interpreted to show a putative association between trauma and ALS also undermine that association.

Conclusions. The existence of an association between ALS and trauma is not supported by a review of the literature, with careful attention to methodological rigor. Prospective studies with long-term follow-up of very large samples of defined, clearly documented cases of trauma have been negative regarding subsequent excess ALS. This, we believe, is the most convincing evidence against an association of trauma and ALS.

Specific Risk Factors—Exposure to Lead and Others

In a recent case-control study of the Mayo referral population (15), five hypotheses were identified in advance as those for which the study was to be confirmatory. Of these, only greater exposure to lead in men was confirmed. As noted, there were no differences between patients and controls with regard to trauma or major surgery, nor were there differences in hard physical labor (men only), family history of neurodegenerative disease, or years lived in a rural community. Occupational and recreational data (physical labor and lead hypotheses) were analyzed only for the 47 male patients and the 47 matched controls, as data for women were insufficient. The other hypotheses were tested on all 74 patients with ALS and 201 controls. Exposure to lead was determined in 20 of 45 patient/control pairs. Of these, 16 were discordant for exposure to lead, with the ALS patient as the exposed member in 14 of these pairs ($p < 0.003$). The association remained significant when minimal exposures were excluded. Our data further indicated that men with ALS had worked more frequently at blue-collar jobs ($p = 0.1005$) and at welding or soldering ($p < 0.01$). We noted that the association with lead affected a significant minority of our population and was an extension of previous findings in a separate population of an association of ALS with exposure to heavy metals (67). We thus concluded that it probably was not due to chance alone. However, despite what we believe to have been a rigorous study design, we cautioned against inferring causation from this association and recommended testing the effect of inhaled lead vapor in laboratory models (15).

The Role of Geographic Clusters

Although theoretically promising, investigations of clusters of chronic disease identified in a community have an inconsistent track record as sources of epidemiologically useful information. The chief reasons (86) are that, on careful evaluation, the apparent cluster did not represent a true excess of the specified disease or that a plausible environmental explanation for the apparent cluster did not surface. Better case ascertainment is due to increased public awareness, better diagnostic capabilities, and specialist availability, especially for the elderly. The incidence rates from Olmsted County, Minnesota, where neurological case ascertainment is high, may serve as a better basis for comparison with the suspect cluster than historical national rates frequently used in reported clusters. The use of poorly defined denominators, inappropriate "expected" numbers, or the process whereby most community-generated clusters are identified (comparable to drawing the bull's eye after seeing where the bullet struck) all increase the likelihood that such clusters may be due to selective ascertainment or chance rather than the operation of some local etiological factor. The problem is similar to that of multiple comparisons (87,88). We have recently suggested that the threshold for significance be increased by a factor of 1.3–2.0, depending on the number of expected cases, and that field work and case ascertainment be reserved only for those clusters large enough to meet these modified criteria for potential significance (6).

Clusters identified by investigators using techniques that are not influenced by the findings (87) may potentially provide more fruitful ground for investigation. Taylor and Davis, in a recent study of clustering of ALS in Wisconsin (89), restated this point, but then proceeded to ignore their own advice and took part in a case-control study of an apparent cluster of six cases of ALS in a town located in one of the counties with a lower-than-average death rate from ALS (90).

With regard to chronic neurological diseases, even clusters identified by investigators, including the geographic isolates in the Western Pacific (vide infra), have not provided a convincing etiological explanation. To the extent that they do not relate to new forms of disease or to its appearance in unexpected age groups, most clusters of chronic neurological disease noted in a community or subgroup of the population (90,91) should not be expected to yield epidemiologically significant leads.

WESTERN PACIFIC ALS

Epidemiological Considerations

The Western Pacific form of ALS has aroused interest over the past 35 years, not only because of its distinctive characteristics, but because its incidence, prevalence, and mortality rates when first identified were 50–100 times those of the sporadic form in the continental United States. The male:female ratio approximated 2:1 and the median age at onset was 44 years. Furthermore, clusters of ALS have been noted in three distinct geographic isolates (92): the southern Mariana Islands, in two villages of the Kii Peninsula of Japan, and among the Auyu and Jakai people in a small area of Irian Jaya (western New Guinea) (Fig. 3). From the standpoint of epidemiological research, the distinction between these investigator-identified geographic isolates and community-identified clusters is important. Other than the way these foci were identified, two major differences from community-identified clusters are the extreme excess occurrence (100-fold rather than just a fewfold greater than the expected number) and especially the persistence of this excess over time. It is these differences that fuel the expectation that the study of Western Pacific ALS may demonstrate genetic or ecological associations that have not been observed or appreciated through the study of the sporadic form, and that these will provide clues to the etiology of the sporadic form. It is these considerations that also underlie the controversy whether Western Pacific ALS is declining in incidence or is persisting (vide

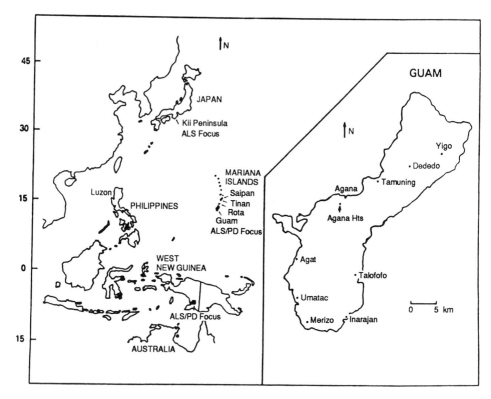

Figure 3 Map of the Pacific islands, showing the three foci of ALS/PDC that have been identified—the Kii Peninsula in Japan, Guam, and Irian Jaya (western New Guinea). The map of Guam (inset) indicates villages where ALS/PDC prevalence has been determined.

infra) and how the geographic pattern and trend relate to the various etiological hypotheses.

Pathology

The lower and upper motor neuron degeneration in Western Pacific ALS is similar to that of sporadic ALS, with the additional feature of an excess of neurofibrillary tangles and intracytoplasmic inclusion (granulovacuolar) bodies, particularly in the nerve cells of the hippocampus and other subcortical areas (93–95). The specificity of the neurofibrillary tangles in Western Pacific ALS and PDC is unclear because an excess of such tangles has also been found in a large proportion of Chamorros who died apparently free of these conditions [57% of people aged 40–59 and 95% of people aged ≥60 years (96)]. The neurofibrillary tangles occurring in Chamorros both with and without ALS/PDC have been shown to be similar to those of Alzheimer's disease by immunocytochemical characterization techniques (97). This is discussed in greater detail in other chapters of this volume.

Patterns of Distribution and Etiological Implications

Familial aggregation of ALS/PDC on Guam was recognized in the first published reports (98–100). This pattern has persisted to date, with the result that some families are considered ''afflicted'' and, possibly, their members may be perceived as less than ideal candidates for marriage. However, the pattern of putative inheritance within ''afflicted families'' has not followed simple Mendelian patterns. Questions of false paternity should be resolved with modern tissue-typing techniques. The possibility of mitochondrial inheritance of a predisposition to ALS/PDC is also being pursued. The prevalence of excessive neurofibrillary tangles in asymptomatic Chamorros, which may suggest a predisposition to neurodegenerative disorders, is also under intensive study. In the present study, asymptomatic Chamorros who have shown none of the features of ALS or PDC have been examined and will be reexamined periodically; autopsies on such well-documented asymptomatic individuals are expected to provide a much needed neuropathological reference, against which the findings in affected individuals can be compared.

The following factors suggest that genetics alone does not account for the high prevalence of ALS/PDC among Chamorros on Guam and in the other Western Pacific foci: (a) three apparently different populations are involved; (b) there appears to be an excess of ALS or PDC among Filipinos who settled in Guam as young adults (although little is known regarding ALS/PDC endemicity in the Illocos region of northwestern Luzon, the origin of most Filipino migrants to Guam (101); and (c) there has been a remarkable increase in age at onset of ALS and PDC in the southern villages of Guam over the past 30 years (102).

Thus, while strong consideration should be given to genetic predisposition as an important factor in the development of Western Pacific ALS/PDC, a genetic explanation alone does not account for its pattern of distribution.

Environmental Considerations

Two types of environmental hypotheses have been proposed to account for Western Pacific ALS/PDC. One is the presence of an exogenous toxin common to the three affected areas, and the other is the absence of essential minerals.

The leading candidate as the source of exogenous toxin has been the seed of the false sago palm, *Cycas circinalis*. *C. circinalis* is a member of the order Cycadeles, the palmlike evergreens that flourish in subtropical and tropical climates. The seeds of *C. circinalis* have been known to be highly toxic for humans since ancient times. Some populations learned how to process the seeds for food so that the acute toxicity could be avoided. Among the Chamorros of Guam a ritual of prolonged soaking developed, and during times of famine, especially following hurricanes and in times of conflict such as World War II, cycad became an important source of carbohydrate in the diet. The husk of the nut was sometimes used as a chew, and the freshly ground cycad seed was also used as a medicinal, particularly in the form of a poultice applied to ulcers and other lesions of the skin. The cycad seed was identified as a potential culprit within field studies by Margaret Whiting (103). The most immediately active toxin of *C. circinalis* is cycasin, a glycoside component in which hepatotoxic and carcinogenic properties predominate, with only minimal neurotoxic effects identified. This toxin is usually removed by the soaking process whereby cycad is prepared for consumption. The focus thus shifted from cycasin to other potential toxins in cycad.

A single animal experiment by Dastur in 1964 (104) described muscle weakness and degeneration of anterior horn cells in a young rhesus monkey fed washed cycad with no cycasin detected by the methods available at the time. Subsequently, after interest in cycad was revived, Dastur reported similar changes in pathological specimens of additional animals that had been fed cycad, but had not developed clinical changes (and therefore had not been studied at the time) (105). The initial finding was not pursued because it appeared to be an isolated response. When another toxin from the cycad seed, α-amino-β-methylaminopropionic acid or β-*N*-methylamino-L-alanine (BMAA), was isolated in the late 1960s (106,107), it was felt to have no etiological relevance to ALS because its only apparent acute effects were "convulsions and paralysis in mice when delivered in high doses." In the face of no supporting evidence from contemporary animal models, the cycad hypothesis was nevertheless kept alive by Kurland (108,109). A renewed impetus for the cycad hypothesis has been given by Spencer and colleagues, who suspected that there might be parallels between the toxin responsible for lathyrism, β-*N*-oxalylamino-L-alanine (BOAA) (110) and the BMAA from cycad. Both these chemicals have structures similar to that of glutamic acid (Fig. 4). The neurotoxicity of BOAA and of BMAA has been demonstrated when applied to cortex or cord explants (111,112). Using a purified L-isomer of BMAA, Spencer was able to produce in monkeys an illness with features of human ALS and possible Parkinson's disease (113,114). Spencer has further reported unwashed cycad use as a medicinal in both other foci of Western Pacific ALS, namely, the Irian Jaya focus in western New Guinea (as a poultice) and the Kii Peninsula of Japan (as a "tonic" made from dried seeds of *Cycas revoluta*) (115,116). The feeding experiment in monkeys by Spencer has not been replicated; others have made efforts to feed monkeys cycad, but have failed to reproduce Spencer's findings (117). However, these apparently negative findings raise questions of the potency of the cycad, since one would expect hepatic toxicity to cycasin if the monkeys had indeed

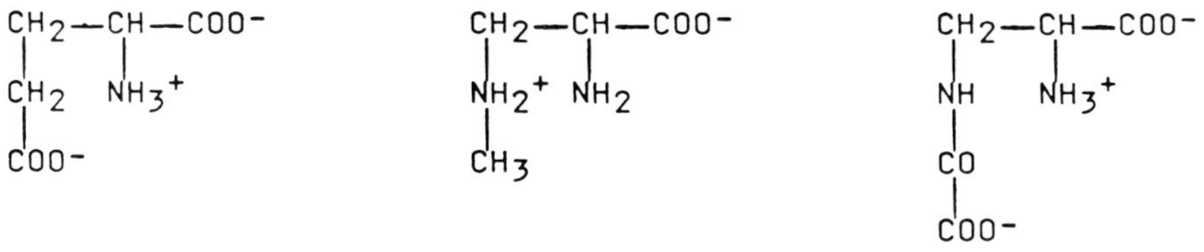

$$CH_2-CH-COO^-$$
$$| \quad\quad |$$
$$CH_2 \quad NH_3^+$$
$$|$$
$$COO^-$$

$$CH_2-CH-COO^-$$
$$| \quad\quad |$$
$$NH_2^+ \quad NH_2$$
$$|$$
$$CH_3$$

$$CH_2-CH-COO^-$$
$$| \quad\quad |$$
$$NH \quad NH_3^+$$
$$|$$
$$CO$$
$$|$$
$$COO^-$$

Glutamic
acid

β-N-methylamino-
L-alanine
(BMAA)

β-N-oxalylamino-
L-alanine
(BOAA)

Figure 4 Chemical structure of BOAA and BMAA, showing similarity to glutamic acid.

been fed fresh unwashed cycad. The absence of such a toxic response suggests that the cycad may have been modified by long storage or some handling procedure. Hence, it is unclear whether the monkeys who showed no apparent neurological disease were fed BMAA in quantities corresponding to Spencer's experiment. Seawright et al. recently reported a neurotoxic effect in the cerebellum with pathological confirmation in rats fed BMAA (118).

Recently, Kisby and Spencer (119) suggested that methylazoxymethanol, the aglycone of the cycad carcinogen cycasin, may react with naturally occurring amino acids to produce derivatives that have neurotoxic properties similar to those of the glutamate agonist *N*-methyl-D-aspartate (NMDA), as demonstrated in cortical organotypic cultures. A compound like BMAA was produced when monkey serum was incubated with methylazoxymethanol under physiological conditions (119).

An alternative hypothesis has been that the absence or excess of essential minerals is related to Western Pacific ALS. Low levels of calcium and magnesium in the soil and water have been proposed as culprits (120,121). However, recent studies on Guam have shown an adequate calcium and magnesium content of water and foods grown in the soil of areas such as Umatac where ALS and PDC are particularly prevalent (122 and D.R. McLachlan, personal communication). Garruto has demonstrated deposition of aluminum in affected neurons (123) and more recently has shown that a low-calcium, high-aluminum diet may induce motor neuron pathology in cynomolgus monkeys (124).

It remains to be seen whether either of these hypotheses, the exogenous toxin or the absence of essential minerals, can by itself explain the etiology of Western Pacific ALS/PDC. To one of us (L.T.K.), cycad remains the primary candidate; others believe that more than one mechanism may be acting on a genetically susceptible population. It is in the context of these competing hypotheses that the nature and quality of epidemiological data from Guam need to be reviewed.

The Epidemiological Data from Guam and the Mariana Islands

There is evidence for a high incidence of ALS among the Chamorro population of Guam as early as 1815 (125). Frequent reports of "lytico" and "paralytico" have been found in the earliest death certificates, dating back to the early 1900s. The clinical and pathological features were thought initially to be those of classic ALS. Early reports by Zimmerman (126), Arnold et al. (98), Koerner (99), and Tillema and Wijnberg (127) were confirmed in surveys by Kurland and Mulder (100,128), who showed that ALS was 50–100 times more prevalent among the Chamorros of Guam than in the population of the continental United States. ALS was also prevalent in the Chamorros on the nearby island of Rota and among those who had moved to California in the previous 40 years (102). It was less common among the Chamorros on Saipan, and there was some uncertainty about whether an atypical form of motor neuron disease characterized by paraparesis was occurring among the Carolinians on Saipan who had partly adopted Chamorro customs. In the Caroline Islands to the south, neither ALS nor PDC was found (100,128). On Guam the highest prevalence rate of ALS was in the southern village of Umatac (Fig. 3). A genetic explanation for the observed familial aggregation was initially proposed (125).

During the first surveys by Kurland and Mulder, patients were encountered with what was first regarded as postencephalitic Parkinsonism. Japanese B encephalitis had been reported on Guam in the 1940s. It became evident that this was in fact a new entity, referred to as Parkinsonism-dementia complex (PDC), which had been well recognized by the native population as "bodig" or "rayput," meaning slowness or laziness. The intensive clinical, pathological, and familial studies that were carried out suggested that PDC was a clinical variant of the local form of ALS, often coexisting with it (33,93,94). Cases of presenile dementia without Parkinsonism or ALS, which have become prevalent in recent years, were not described in the 1950–1960 surveys. It cannot be determined at this stage if there was indeed an absence of such patients or whether they were missed because they were overshadowed by the ALS/PDC patients with more striking pathology.

The unusual concentration of individuals with neurological disease on Guam led to the establishment of a National Institute of Neurologic Disease and Stroke (NINDS) research center registry, which recorded incident cases of neurodegenerative disease from 1945 to 1985. However, the reports based on review of that registry at 10-year intervals (130–132) showed a steady decline in the annual incidence of ALS, reportedly down to only two to three times the rate found on the mainland, so that, by 1982, it was concluded that the high incidence of

ALS/PDC on Guam had "disappeared" (133). It was this apparent disappearance of neurodegenerative disease from Guam that led to the reduction of staff in 1982 and, finally, the closure of the NINDS research center registry in 1985.

There was, however, reason to doubt the completeness of case ascertainment within the NINDS research center registry as compared to that attained with the earlier surveys by Mulder and Kurland. This difference was due not only to the methodological shortcomings of passive versus active surveillance, but also to the existence of financial disincentives for patients to be registered: the legislation providing for free care for ALS and PDC patients at the Guam Memorial Hospital was linked to revocation of the medical insurance entitling them to private care. This led to a disincentive for both patients and local practitioners to report cases.

A follow-up study by Reed et al. (134) of a cohort identified in 1968 showed that the ALS incidence rate was decreasing, but that of PDC continued to be high. Active ascertainment of neurodegenerative disease in three villages in Guam was therefore undertaken (102). These villages were chosen for survey because they had high prevalence rates of ALS in previous surveys and had maintained a traditional Chamorro culture. These surveys showed that the prevalence of ALS in these villages continued to be high, 50 times greater than that of Rochester, Minnesota, and for those over 55 years old, 70 times greater than in Rochester, Minnesota. Prevalence of Parkinsonism was five times that of Parkinson's disease in Rochester, Minnesota, and prevalence of dementia alone was three times greater, and for those aged 55 years and over, five times that of Alzheimer's disease in Rochester, Minnesota. In the continental United States, ALS, Parkinson's disease, and Alzheimer's disease tend to occur as single diseases in patients, although as many as one-third of those with Parkinson's disease will develop cognitive impairment. However, on Guam, a combination of two or all three of these disorders (ALS, Parkinsonism, and dementia) frequently occur in the same patient. When one, two, or all three conditions are considered and the number of persons affected is counted, the prevalence rate on Guam is 2.8 times greater than the corresponding rate in the population of Rochester, Minnesota; and for those aged 55 years and older, it is 3.8 times greater than that of Rochester, Minnesota. The reason for this dramatic difference in relative risks between the individual diseases and the number affected is that almost all patients on Guam have more than one component of the ALS/Parkinsonism dementia complex. Also, the lifetime risk for the mainland population aged 55 years and over differs greatly by disease—risk of ALS is about 1:500, risk of Parkinson's disease is 1:40, and risk of Alzheimer's disease is 1:10.

Furthermore, in the course of these surveys, supranuclear disturbances of ocular motility were noted in some of the patients (135), and, on occasion, a pathological picture suggestive of Pick's disease has also been noted. There is thus the suggestion that the spectrum of neurodegenerative disease on Guam is broader than previously suspected and includes features of ALS, Parkinson's disease, Alzheimer's disease, and progressive supranuclear palsy. Compared to the survey in 1953, the mean age at onset for ALS and PDC has increased by about 10 years; however, for all villages, the male:female ratio continues to be 2:1. In the southern villages, dementia alone or in association with Parkinsonism was noted predominantly in older women; this may reflect their selective survival.

Observations that at present are of uncertain significance are the collagen changes in the skin of patients with Guamanian ALS/PDC (136) as well as in patients in the continental United States with sporadic ALS but not spinal muscular atrophy (137,138). Another new discovery under investigation is the pigmentary retinopathy resembling posterior ophthalmomyiasis interna discovered in 26 of 49 Chamorros with ALS/PDC as well as in 6 of 37 clinically asymptomatic individuals from the southern villages of Guam. The pathology in these cases shows no evidence of a parasite. There is focal degeneration of the retinal pigmented epithelium similar to that described in two cases of olivopontocerebellar degeneration (139).

The persistence of high prevalence of neurodegenerative disease in some villages on Guam suggests the continued presence of an etiological mechanism. The changing spectrum may reflect improved case ascertainment or temporal differences between the interaction of environmental factors and susceptible individuals. One might consider a constant level of exposure to an environmental toxin that peaked during World War II and has declined but not disappeared. Individuals exposed to higher doses of that toxin might develop ALS at a relatively early age with or without associated PDC. Individuals exposed to a lesser dose might develop, at a later date, ALS with or without PDC, PDC alone, or dementia alone. Additional surveys on Guam in villages with historically lower incidence of neurodegenerative disease, careful review of the genetics of afflicted and nonafflicted individuals, and careful review of ecological and life-style factors within case-control studies may help identify the factor(s) responsible for the increased prevalence of neurodegenerative disease on Guam.

IMPLICATIONS FOR SPORADIC NEURODEGENERATIVE DISEASES

Two leading contemporary hypotheses with regard to ALS are that it is an unconventional autoimmune disease (140) and that it is due to glutamate dysfunction (141–144). Both hypotheses have generated therapeutic trials (29–32, 145–147). They are reviewed in detail elsewhere in this volume. The results of these clinical trials have not been encouraging, giving rise to the concern that the abnormal findings that generated these hypotheses are part of the disease rather than its direct cause. Alternative explanations might be that the treatments used have not affected or reached the target organ (brain and spinal cord) or that they have been of the right type but of insufficient intensity. The presence of lymphocytic infiltration in the pyramidal tract of patients with ALS, but not in those with pyramidal degeneration due to other causes, may, similarly, be a result of the unique changes in ALS rather than its cause (148). The affinity of this infiltrate to areas in which heterotopic neurons have been found in spinal cords of patients with ALS is intriguing (149). It is apparent that the intersection of the hypotheses generated by western Pacific ALS and the two previously mentioned hypotheses for sporadic ALS favors a neurotoxic etiology that is endogenous, exogenous, or derived from a combination of the two.

An outbreak of toxic encephalopathy caused by eating mussels contaminated with domoic acid (150) has provided, in humans, data on the long-term sequelae of acute intoxication with a glutamic acid analog similar to kainic acid. The chronic residua in these patients were memory dysfunction and a motor neuron-opathy or axonopathy. The acute findings on nerve conduction studies were "markedly diminished compound motor unit potentials with well preserved conduction velocities," and, on concentric needle electromyography, "9 of 10 had findings consistent with various degrees of acute denervation, such as spontaneous activity and unstable motor unit potentials." In seven patients who had a follow-up examination after 11–14 months, "the signs of acute denervation were partially resolved, whereas the compound motor unit potentials remained unchanged." Positron emission tomography in two severely affected patients showed decrease in glucose metabolism in amygdala and hippocampus, which correlated with the patients' memory scores.

Neuropathological studies in the four patients exposed to domoic acid who died acutely showed neuronal necrosis and loss predominantly in the hippocampus and amygdala, in a pattern similar to that observed experimentally in animals after the administration of kainic acid. However, pathological features of Alzheimer's disease (neurofibrillary tangles, granulovacuolar degeneration, and senile plaques) were not observed in these patients. Furthermore, there was no loss of motor neuron cells in the brainstem and spinal cord, and anterior horn axonal spheroids were not detected. The authors, therefore, emphasize the difference in the distribution and cytopathology of lesions in acute domoic acid intoxication from those described in the idiopathic neurodegenerative syndromes hypothesized to be mediated by glutaminergic mechanisms. This begs the issue of the appropriateness of comparing the neuropathological changes in acute intoxication to those which evolve in a more chronic form. This may be clarified if the survivors of domoic acid intoxication are eventually studied for long-term pathological effects. However, the electrophysiological findings showing only partial resolution of acute denervation and no change in the diminished amplitude of the compound muscle action potentials suggest a long-term effect of this acute intoxication, which at least is interfering with the expected pattern of recovery (151). Additional electrophysiological studies may enable the recovery of lower motor neurons to be monitored during life.

Conversely, it does not follow automatically that an agent producing, in high doses, acute neurotoxicity with chronic sequelae may necessarily be capable of producing chronic neurodegenerative disease with chronic exposure to low doses or many years after a single exposure to a high dose. In both in vivo and in vitro systems, the acute neuronotoxic action of L-BOAA is said to be mediated via quisqualate and/or kainate glutamate receptors, whereas L-BMAA action is attenuated in a dose-dependent manner by 2-amino-7-phosphonoheptanoic acid, a selective antagonist for the *N*-methyl-D-aspartate (NMDA) glutamate receptor (152).

A recent review of the excitatory amino acid hypothesis in ALS (142) cautions that ''although the hypothesis is intriguing, considerably more information needs to be gathered prior to concluding that excitatory amino acids plays a role in ALS,'' and ''if a generalized defect in glutamate metabolism does exist in ALS, perhaps it is a proximate cause of selective neuronal vulnerability but not the primary one.'' In concurrence with this viewpoint, we consider motor neuron disease as the final outcome of a chain of events which may be triggered at one or more points by endogenous or exogenous causes or a combination thereof.

The epidemiological similarities of the three neurodegenerative diseases (ALS, Parkinson's disease, and Alzheimer's dementia) are: a 5–15% familial pattern, increased incidence with increasing age, and a high incidence in the Western Pacific foci, often coexisting in a single individual. These similarities support a common underlying endogenous or environmental mechanism(s) for all three. They may represent an abiotrophic interaction between aging and environment (153) or they may be responses of genetically susceptible individuals to particular life-styles, life events, or environmental toxins. Even as case-control studies and therapeutic trials attempt to provide leads to the etiology of the sporadic forms of these diseases, intensive study of the familial forms and of the western Pacific forms may provide an added advantage through the ability to narrow the search to a limited number of genetic, life-style, or environmental possibilities.

ACKNOWLEDGMENT

The authors thank Mrs. Laura Long for editorial assistance and manuscript preparation. The research reported here has been supported in part by Grants NS17750, AG06786, and AG08802 from the National Institutes of Health, Bethesda, Maryland.

REFERENCES

1. Armon C, Kurland LT. Classic and Western Pacific amyotrophic lateral sclerosis: Epidemiologic comparisons. In: Hudson AJ, ed. Amyotrophic lateral sclerosis: Concepts in pathogenesis and etiology. Toronto: University of Toronto Press, 1989:144–165.
2. dePedro Cuesta J, Litvan I. Epidemiology of motor neuron disease. In: Anderson DW, ed. Neuroepidemiology: A tribute to Bruce Schoenberg. Boca Raton, FL: CRC Press, 1991:265–296.
3. Mitsumoto H, Hanson MR, Chad DA. Amyotrophic lateral sclerosis: Recent advances in pathogenesis and therapeutic trials. Arch Neurol 1988;45:189–202.
4. Kurtzke JF, Kurland LT. The epidemiology of neurologic disease. In: Baker AB, ed. Clinical neurology, Vol. IV, Chapter 66. Philadelphia: Harper & Row, 1983;1–143.
5. Kurland LT, Mulder DW. Recent epidemiologic developments in the context of earlier observations on ALS: Geographic isolates in the Marianas and other islands of the Western Pacific. In: Tsubaki T, Yase Y, eds. Amyotrophic lateral sclerosis: Recent advances in research and treatment. Amsterdam: Elsevier Science Publishers (Biomedical Division), 1988:3–9.
6. Armon C, Kurland LT. When is a cluster a true cluster? Ann Neurol 1989;26: 140–41 (Abstract).
7. Fox JP, Hall CE, Elveback LR. Epidemiology: Man and disease. London: Macmillan (Collier-Macmillan), 1970:185.
8. Sillevis Smitt PAE, deJong JMBV. Animal models of amyotrophic lateral sclerosis and the spinal muscular atrophies. J Neurol Sci 1989;91:231–258.
9. Cork LC, Kitt CA, Struble RG, Griffin JW, Price DL. Animal models of degenerative neurologic disease. Prog Clin Biol Res 1987;229:241–269.
10. Adams RD, Victor M. Principles of neurology, 4th ed. New York: McGraw-Hill, 1989;953–956.
11. Yoshida S, Mulder DW, Kurland LT, Chu C-P, Okazaki H. Follow-up study on amyotrophic lateral sclerosis in Rochester, Minnesota, 1925–1984. Neuroepidemiology 1986;5:61–70.
12. Pestronk A, Chaudhry V, Feldman EL, et al. Lower motor neuron syndromes defined by patterns of weakness, nerve conduction abnormalities and high titres of antiglycolipid antibodies. Ann Neurol 1990;27:316–326.
13. Christensen PD, Højer-Pedersen E, Jensen NB. Survival of patients with amyotrophic lateral sclerosis in two Danish counties. Neurology 1990;40:600–604.
14. Jablecki CK, Berry C, Leach J. Survival prediction in amyotrophic lateral sclerosis. Muscle Nerve 1989;12:833–841.
15. Armon C, Kurland LT, Daube JR, O'Brien PC. Epidemiologic correlates of sporadic amyotrophic lateral sclerosis. Neurology 1991;41:1077–1084.
16. Lilienfeld DE, Chan E, Ehland J, et al. Rising mortality from motoneuron disease in the USA, 1962–1984. Lancet 1989;1:710–713.
17. Martyn CN, Barker JP, Osmond C. Motoneuron disease and past poliomyleitis in England and Wales. Lancet 1988;1:1319–1322.

18. Kahana E, Zilber N. Changes in the incidence of amyotrophic lateral sclerosis in Israel. Arch Neurol 1984;41:157–160.

19. Kurtzke JF. Epidemiology of amyotrophic lateral sclerosis. In: Rowland LP, ed. Human motor neuron diseases. Advances in Neurology 36. New York: Raven Press, 1982:281–302.

20. Swash M, Schwartz MS, Lie T-M. Trends in mortality from motor neuron disease. Lancet 1989;1:958 (Letter).

21. Chandra V, Bharucha NE, Schoenberg BS. Mortality data for the U.S. for deaths due to and related to 20 neurologic diseases. Neuroepidemiology 1984;3:149–168.

22. Appel SH, Stockton-Appel V, Stewart SS, Kerman RH. Amyotrophic lateral sclerosis: Associated clinical disorders and immunological evaluations. Arch Neurol 1986;43:234–238.

23. Kiessling WR. Thyroid function in 44 patients with amyotrophic lateral sclerosis. Arch Neurol 1982;39:241–242.

24. Iwasaki Y, Kinoshita M. Normal thyroid function in 32 patients with amyotrophic lateral sclerosis. Jpn J Med 1989;28:309–311.

25. Malin JP, Kodding R, Fuhrmann H, von zur Muhlen A. T_4, T_3, and rT_3 levels in serum and cerebrospinal fluid of patients with amyotrophic lateral sclerosis. J Neurol 1989;236:57–59.

26. Armon C, Kurland LT, O'Brien PC, Mulder DW. Antecedent medical diseases in patients with amyotrophic lateral sclerosis: A population-based case-controlled study in Rochester, Minnesota, 1925–1987. Arch Neurol 1991;48:283–286.

27. Brooks BR, Sufit RL, Montgomery GK, Beaulieu DA, Erickson LM. Intravenous thyrotropin-releasing hormone in patients with amyotrophic lateral sclerosis: Dose-response and randomized concurrent placebo-controlled pilot studies. Neurol Clin 1987;5(1):143–58.

28. Munsat PL, Taft J, Kasdon D. Intrathecal thyrotropin releasing hormone in amyotrophic lateral sclerosis. Neurol Clin 1987;5(1):159–170.

29. Olarte MR, Schoenfeldt RS, McKiernan G, Rowland LP. Plasmapheresis in amyotrophic lateral sclerosis. Ann Neurol 1980;8:644–645.

30. Kelemen J, Hedlund W, Orlin JB, et al. Plasmapheresis with immunosuppression in amyotrophic lateral sclerosis. Arch Neurol 1983;40:752–753.

31. Brown RH, Hauser SL, Harrington H, Weiner HL. Failure of immunosuppression with a 10–14 day course of high-dose intravenous cyclophosphamide to alter the progression of amyotrophic lateral sclerosis. Arch Neurol 1986;43:383–384.

32. Appel SH, Stewart SS, Appel V, et al. A double-blind study of the effectiveness of cyclosporine in amyotrophic lateral sclerosis. Arch Neurol 1988;45:381–386.

33. Kurland LT, Choi NW, Sayre GP. Implications of incidence and geographic patterns on the classification of amyotrophic lateral sclerosis. In: Norris FH Jr, Kurland LT, eds. Motor neuron diseases: Research on amyotrophic lateral sclerosis and related disorders. New York: Grune & Stratton, 1969:28–50.

34. Kimura K, Yase Y, Higashi Y, et al. Epidemiological and geomedical studies on amyotrophic lateral sclerosis. Dis Nerv Syst 1963;24:155–159.

35. Shiraki H. The neuropathology of amyotrophic lateral sclerosis (ALS) in the Kii Peninsula and other areas of Japan. In: Norris FH Jr, Kurland LT, eds. Motor

neuron diseases: Research on amyotrophic lateral sclerosis and related disorders. New York: Grune & Stratton, 1969;80:84.

36. Gajdusek DC, Salazar AM. Amyotrophic lateral sclerosis and Parkinsonian syndromes in high incidence among the Auyu and Jakai people of West New Guinea. Neurology 1982;32:107–26.

37. Tandan R, Bradley WG. Amyotrophic lateral sclerosis. Part 1. Clinical features, pathology, and ethical issues in management. Ann Neurol 1985;18:271–280.

38. Ben Hamida M, Letaief F, Hentati F, Ben Hamida C. Morphometric study of the sensory nerve in classical (or Charcot disease) and juvenile amyotrophic lateral sclerosis. J Neurol Sci 1987;78:313–329.

39. Ghezzi A, Mazzalovo E, Locatelli C, et al. Multimodality evoked potentials in amyotrophic lateral sclerosis. Acta Neurol Scand 1989;79:353–356.

40. Radke RA, Erwin A, Erwin GW. Abnormal sensory evoked potentials in amyotrophic lateral sclerosis. Neurology 1986;36:796–801.

41. Zanette G, Polo A, Gasperini M, Bertolasi L, De Grandis D. Far-field and cortical somatosensory evoked potentials in motor neuron disease. Muscle Nerve 1990;13:47–55.

42. Fucco E, Micaglio G, Liviero MC, et al. Sensory motor conduction time in amyotrophic lateral sclerosis. Riv Neurol 1989;59:108–112.

43. Hatazawa J, Brooks RA, Dalakas MC, Mansi L, Di Chiro G. Cortical motor sensory hypometabolism in amyotrophic lateral sclerosis: A PET study. J CAT 1988;12:630–636.

44. Williams C, Koslowski MA, Hinton DR, Miller CA. Degeneration of spinocerebellar neurons in amyotrophic lateral sclerosis. Ann Neurol 1990;27:215–225.

45. Barron SA, Mazliah J, Bental E. Sympathetic cholinergic dysfunction in amyotrophic lateral sclerosis. Acta Neurol Scand 1987;75:62–63.

46. Chida K, Sakamaki S, Takasu T. Alteration in autonomic function and cardiovascular regulation in amyotrophic lateral sclerosis. J Neurol 1989;236:127–130.

47. Hayashi H, Kato S. Total manifestations of amyotrophic lateral sclerosis: ALS in the totally locked-in state. J Neurol Sci 1989;93:19–35.

48. Wikström J, Paetau A, Palo J, Sulkava R, Haltia M. Classic amyotrophic lateral sclerosis with dementia. Arch Neurol 1982;39:681–683.

49. Salazar AM, Masters CL, Gajdusek DC, et al. Syndromes of amyotrophic lateral sclerosis and dementia: Relation to transmissible Creutzfeldt-Jakob disease. Ann Neurol 1983;14:17–26.

50. Morita K, Kaiya H, Ikeda T, Namba M. Presenile dementia combined with amyotrophy: A review of 34 Japanese cases. Arch Gerontol Geriatr 1987;6:263–277.

51. Petersen RC, Ivnik RJ, Litchy WJ, Windebank AJ, Daube JR. Cognitive function in amyotrophic lateral sclerosis. Neurology 1990;40(Suppl. 1):315 (Abstract).

52. Mulder DW, Kurland KT, Offord KP, Beard CM. Familial adult motor neuron disease: amyotrophic lateral sclerosis. Neurology 1986;36:511–517.

53. Leone M, Chandra V, Schoenberg BS. Motor neuron disease in the United States, 1971 and 1973–1978: Patterns of mortality and associated conditions at the time of death. Neurology 1987;37:1339–1343.

54. DeDomenico P, Malara CE, Marabello L, et al. Amyotrophic lateral sclerosis: An

epidemiologic study in the province of Messina, Italy, 1976–1985. Neuroepidemiology 1988;7:152–158.

55. Scarpa M, Colombo A, Panzetti P, Sorgato P. Epidemiology of amyotrophic lateral sclerosis in the province of Modena, Italy. Influence of environmental exposure to lead. Acta Neurol Scand 1988;77:456–460.

56. López-Vega JM, Calleja J, Combarros O, Polo JM, Berciano J. Motor neuron disease in Cantabria. Acta Neurol Scand 1988;77:1–5.

57. Salemi G, Fierro B, Arcara A, et al. Amyotrophic lateral sclerosis in Palermo, Italy: An epidemiologic study. Ital J Neurol Sci 1989;10:505–509.

58. Gunnarsson L-G, Lindberg G, Söderfelt B, Axelson O. The mortality of motor neuron disease in Sweden. Arch Neurol 1990;47:42–46.

59. Kurland LT, Kurtzke JF, Goldberg ID, Choi NW. Amyotrophic lateral sclerosis and other motor neuron diseases. In: Kurland LT, Kurtzke JF, Goldberg ID. Epidemiology of neurologic and sense organ disorders (Vital and Health Statistics Monograph, American Public Health Association). Cambridge, MA: Harvard University Press, 1973:108–127.

60. Anderson DW, Schoenberg BS, Haerer AF. Racial differentials in the prevalence of major neurological disorders: Background and methods of the Copiah County study. Neuroepidemiology 1982;1:17–30.

61. Schoenberg BS, Anderson DW, Haerer AF. Prevalence of Parkinson's disease in the biracial population of Copiah County, Mississippi. Neurology 1985;35:841–845.

62. Tandan R, Bradley WG. Amyotrophic lateral sclerosis. Part 2. Etiopathogenesis. Ann Neurol 1985;18:419–431.

63. Gallagher JP, Sanders M. Trauma and amyotrophic lateral sclerosis: A report of 78 patients. Acta Neurol Scand 1987;75:145–150.

64. Gawel M, Zaiwalla Z, Rose FC. Antecedent events in motor neuron disease. J Neurol Neurosurg Psychiatry 1983;46:1041–1043.

65. Deapen DM, Henderson BE. A case-control study of amyotrophic lateral sclerosis. Am J Epidemiol 1986;123:790–799.

66. Kurtzke JF, Beebe GW. Epidemiology of amyotrophic lateral sclerosis. 1. A case-control comparison based on ALS deaths. Neurology 1980;30:453–462.

67. Roelofs-Iverson RA, Mulder DW, Elveback LR, et al. ALS and heavy metals: A pilot case-control study. Neurology 1984;34:393–395.

68. Plato CC, Garruto RM, Fox KM, Gajdusek DC. Amyotrophic lateral sclerosis and Parkinsonism-dementia on Guam: A 25-year prospective case-control study. Am J Epidemiol 1986;124:643–656.

69. Gresham LS, Molgaard CA, Golbeck AL, Smith R. Amyotrophic lateral sclerosis and occupational heavy metal exposure: A case-control study. Neuroepidemiology 1986;5:29–38.

70. Gunnarsson L-G, Palm R. Motor neuron disease and heavy manual labor: An epidemiological survey of Varmland County, Sweden. Neuroepidemiology 1984;3:195–206.

71. Pierce-Ruhland R, Patten BM. Repeat study of antecedent events in motor neuron disease. Ann Clin Res 1981;13:102–107.

72. Campbell AMG, Williams ER, Barltrop D. Motor neurone disease and exposure to lead. J Neurol Neurosurg Psychiatry 1970;33:877–885.
73. Hawkes CH, Cavanagh JB, Fox AJ. Motoneuron disease: A disorder secondary to solvent exposure? Lancet 1989;1:73–76.
74. Jelliffe SE. The amyotrophic lateral sclerosis syndrome and trauma. J Nerv Ment Dis 1935;82:415–435, 536–550.
75. Felmus MT, Patten BM, Swanke L. Antecedent events in amyotrophic lateral sclerosis. Neurology 1976;26:167–172.
76. Kondo K, Tsubaki T. Case-control studies of motor neuron disease. Arch Neurol 1981;38:220–226.
77. Gresham LS, Molgaard CA, Golbeck AL, Smith R. Amyotrophic lateral sclerosis and history of skeletal fracture: A case-control study. Neurology 1987;37:717–719.
78. Kondo K. Environmental factors in motor neurone disease. In: Gourie-Devi M, ed. Motor neurone disease. New Delhi: Oxford and IBH, 1987:53–60.
79. National Center for Health Statistics, J. G. Collins. Types of injuries and impairments due to injuries, United States. Vital Health Statistics. Series 10, No. 159. DHHS No. (PHS) 87-1587. Public Health Service. Washington, DC: US Government Printing Office, 1986:24.
80. Annegers JF, Grabow JD, Kurland LT, Laws ER. The incidence, causes and secular trends of head trauma in Olmsted County, Minnesota, 1935–1974. Neurology 1980;30:912–919.
81. Garraway WM, Stauffer RN, Kurland LT, O'Fallon WM. Limb fractures in a defined population. I. Frequency and distribution. Mayo Clin Proc 1979;54:701–707.
82. Sartwell PE, Last JM. Epidemiology. In: Last JM, ed. Maxcy-Rosenau public health and preventive medicine, 11th ed. New York: Appleton-Century-Crofts, 1980:9–86.
83. Bharucha NE. Motor neurone disease. J PostGrad Med 1973;19:51–62.
84. Bonduelle M. Amyotrophic lateral sclerosis. In: Vinken PJ, Bruyn GW, eds. Handbook of clinical neurology, Vol 22. Amsterdam: Elsevier North-Holland Biomedical, 1975;281–330.
85. Riggs JE. Trauma and amyotrophic lateral sclerosis. Arch Neurol 1985;42:205 (Letter).
86. Schulte PA, Ehrenberg RL, Singal M. Investigation of occupational cancer clusters: Theory and practice. Am J Public Health 1987;77:52–56.
87. Armitage P, Berry G. Statistical methods in medical research. Oxford: Blackwell Scientific Publications, 1987:478–483.
88. Taylor WF. Table 1. In: Kyle RA, Greipp PR. Multiple myeloma and the monoclonal gammopathies. In: Fairbanks VF, ed. Current hematology, Vol. 1. New York: Wiley, 1981:476–477.
89. Taylor JA, Davis JP. Evidence for clustering of amyotrophic lateral sclerosis in Wisconsin. J Clin Epidemiol 1989;42:569–575.
90. Sienko DG, Davis JP, Taylor JA, Brooks BR. Amyotrophic lateral sclerosis: A

case-control study following detection of a cluster in a small Wisconsin community. Arch Neurol 1990;47:38–41.

91. Hyser CL, Kissel JT, Mendell JR. Three cases of amyotrophic lateral sclerosis in a common occupational environment. J Neurol 1987;234:443–444.

92. Kurland LT. Geographic isolates: Their role in neuroepidemiology. In: Schoenberg BS, ed. Neurological epidemiology: Principles and clinical applications. New York: Raven Press, 1978;69–82.

93. Hirano A, Kurland LT, Krooth RS, Lessell S. Parkinsonism-dementia complex, an endemic disease on the island of Guam. I. Clinical features. Brain 1961;84:642–661.

94. Hirano A, Malamud N, Kurland LT. Parkinsonism-dementia complex, an endemic disease on the island of Guam. II. Pathological features. Brain 1961;84:662–679.

95. Malamud N, Hirano A, Kurland LT. Pathoanatomic changes in amyotrophic lateral sclerosis on Guam: Special reference to the occurrence of neurofibrillary changes. Arch Neurol 1961;5:401–415.

96. Chen L. Neurofibrillary change on Guam. Arch Neurol 1981;38:16–18.

97. Shankar SK, Yanagihara R, Garruto RM, et al. Immunocytochemical characterization of neurofibrillary tangles in amyotrophic lateral sclerosis and Parkinsonism-dementia of Guam. Ann Neurol 1989;25:146–151.

98. Arnold A, Edgren DC, Palladino VS. Amyotrophic lateral sclerosis: Fifty cases observed on Guam. J Nerv Ment Dis 1953;117:135–139.

99. Koerner DR. Amyotrophic lateral sclerosis on Guam: A clinical study and review of the literature. Ann Intern Med 1952;37:1204–1220.

100. Kurland LT, Mulder DW. Epidemiologic investigations of amyotrophic lateral sclerosis: 1. Preliminary report on geographic distribution, with special reference to the Mariana Islands, including clinical and pathologic observations. Neurology 1954;4:355–378.

101. Garruto RM, Gajdusek DC, Chen K-M. Amyotrophic lateral sclerosis and Parkinsonism-dementia among Filipino migrants to Guam. Ann Neurol 1981;10:341–350.

102. Lavine L, Steele JC, Wolfe N, Calne DB, O'Brien PC, Williams DB, Kurland LT, Schoenberg BS. Amyotrophic lateral sclerosis/Parkinsonism-dementia complex in southern Guam: Is it disappearing? In: Rowland LP, ed. Amyotrophic lateral sclerosis and other motor neuron diseases: Advances in Neurology, Vol. 56. New York: Raven Press, 1991:271–285.

103. Whiting MG. Toxicity of cycads. Econ Bot 1963;17:271–302.

104. Dastur DK. Cycad toxicity in monkeys: clinical, pathological, and biochemical aspects. Fed Proc 1964;23:1368–1369.

105. Dastur DK, Palekar RS, Manghani DK. Toxicity of various forms of cycas circinalis in rhesus monkeys: Pathology of brain, spinal cord and liver. In: Rose FC, Norris F, eds. ALS: New advances in toxicology and epidemiology, chapter 18. London: Smith, Gordon, 1990:129–141.

106. Polsky FI, Nunn PB, Bell EA. Distribution and toxicity of α-amino-β-methylaminopropionic acid. Fed Proc 1972;31:1473–1475.

107. Vega A, Bell EA. α-Amino-β-methylaminopropionic acid, a new amino acid from seeds of *Cycas circinalis*. Phytochemistry 1967;6:759.

108. Kurland LT, Molgaard CA. Guamanian ALS: Hereditary or acquired? In: Rowland LP, ed. Human motor neuron diseases. New York: Raven Press, 1982:165–171.
109. Kurland LT, Mulder DW. Overview of motor neurone disease. In: Gourie-Devi M, ed. Motor neurone disease: Global clinical patterns and international research. New Delhi: Oxford and IBH, 1987:31–44.
110. Spencer PS, Schaumburg HH. Lathyrism: A neurotoxic disease. Neurobehav Toxicol Teratol 1983;5:625–629.
111. Nunn PB, Seelig M, Zagoren JC, Spencer PS. Stereospecific acute neuronotoxicity of "uncommon" plant amino acids linked to human motor-system diseases. Brain Res 1987;410:375–379.
112. Weiss JH, Koh J-Y, Choi DW. Neurotoxicity of BMAA and BOAA on cultured cortical neurons. Brain Res 1989;497:64–71.
113. Spencer PS. Guam ALS/Parkinsonism-dementia: A long-latency neurotoxic disorder caused by "slow toxin(s)" in food? Can J Neurol Sci 1987;14:347–357.
114. Spencer PS, Nunn PB, Hugon J, et al. Motor neuron disease on Guam: Possible role of a food toxin. Lancet 1986;1:965.
115. Spencer PS, Palmer VS, Herman A, Asmedi A. Cycad use and motor neurone disease in Irian Jaya. Lancet 1987;2:1273–1274.
116. Spencer PS, Ohta M, Palmer VS. Cycad use and motor neurone disease in the Kii Peninsula of Japan. Lancet 1987;2:1462–1463.
117. Garruto RM, Yanagihara R, Gajdusek DC. Cycads and amyotrophic lateral sclerosis/parkinsonism dementia. Lancet 1988;2:1079 (Letter).
118. Seawright AA, Brown AW, Nolan CC, Cavanagh JB. Selective degeneration of cerebellar cortical neurons caused by cycad neurotoxin, L-β-methylaminoalanine (L-BMAA), in rats. Neuropath Appl Neurobiol 1990;16:153–169.
119. Kisby G, Spencer PS. Neurotoxic amino acids from the cycad carcinogen methylazoxymethanol. Int ALS·MND Update 1989;2Q89:27–28 (Abstract).
120. Gajdusek DC, Garruto RM, Salazar AM. Ecology of high incidence foci of motor neuron disease in Eastern Asia and Western Pacific and the frequent occurrence of other chronic degenerative neurological diseases in these foci. Tenth International Congress on Tropical Medicine and Malaria, Manila, Philippines, Nov 9–15, 1980:382.
121. Yase Y. The basic process of amyotrophic lateral sclerosis as reflected in Kii Peninsula and Guam. Excerp Med Int Cong Ser 1977;434:413–427.
122. Zolon WJ, Ellis-Neill L. University of Guam Technical Report No. 64, 1986.
123. Garruto RM. Neurotoxicity of trace and essential elements: Factors provoking the high incidence of motor neurone disease, Parkinsonism and dementia in the Western Pacific. In: Gourie-Devi M, ed. Motor neurone disease: Global clinical patterns and international research. New Delhi: Oxford and IBH, 1987:73–82.
124. Garruto RM, Shankar SK, Yanagihara R, Salazar AM, Amyx HL, Gajdusek DC. Low calcium, high aluminum diet-induced motor neuron pathology in cynomolgus monkeys. Acta Neuropathol 1989;78:210–219.
125. Kurland LT. Epidemiologic investigations of amyotrophic lateral sclerosis. 3. A genetic interpretation of incidence and geographic distribution. Proc Staff Meet Mayo Clin 1957;32:449–462.

126. Zimmerman HM. Monthly report to medical officer in command, U.S. Naval Medical Research Unit No. 2, June 1, 1945.

127. Tillema S, Wijnberg CJ. "Endemic" amyotrophic lateral sclerosis on Guam: Epidemiological data, preliminary report. Doc Med Geogr Trop (Amst) 1953;5: 366–370.

128. Mulder DW, Kurland LT. Amyotrophic lateral sclerosis in Micronesia. Proc Staff Meet Mayo Clin 1954;29:666–670.

129. Torres J, Iriarte LLG, Kurland LT. Amyotrophic lateral sclerosis among Guamanians in California. Calif Med 1957;86:385–388.

130. Reed D, Plato C, Elizan T, Kurland LT. The amyotrophic lateral sclerosis/Parkinsonism-dementia complex: A ten-year follow-up on Guam. I. Epidemiologic studies. Am J Epidemiol 1966;83:54–73.

131. Reed DM, Brody JA. Amyotrophic lateral sclerosis and Parkinsonism-dementia complex on Guam, 1945–1972. I. Descriptive epidemiology. Am J Epidemiol 1975;101:287–301.

132. Rodgers-Johnson P, Garruto RM, Yanagihara R, Chen KM, Gajdusek DC, Gibbs CJ. Amyotrophic lateral sclerosis and Parkinsonism-dementia on Guam: A 30-year evaluation of clinical and neuropathologic trends. Neurology 1986;36:7–13.

133. Garruto RM, Yanagihara R, Gajdusek DC. Disappearance of high-incidence amyotrophic lateral sclerosis and Parkinsonism-dementia on Guam. Neurology 1985;35:193–198.

134. Reed D, Labarthe D, Chen K-M, Stallones R. A cohort study of amyotrophic lateral sclerosis and Parkinsonism-dementia on Guam and Rota. Am J Epidemiol 1987;125:92–100.

135. Lepore FE, Steele JC, Cox TA, Tillson G, Calne DB, Duvoisin RC, Lavine L, McDarby JV. Supranuclear disturbances of ocular motility in lytico-bodig. Neurology 1988;38:1849–1853.

136. Fullmer HM, Siedler HD, Krooth RS, Kurland LT. A cutaneous disorder of connective tissue in amyotrophic lateral sclerosis: A histochemical study. Neurology 1960;10:717–724.

137. Ono S, Toyokura Y, Mannen T, Ishibashi Y. "Delayed return phenomenon" in amyotrophic lateral sclerosis. Acta Neurol Scand 1988;77:102–107.

138. Ono S, Mannen T, Toyokura Y. Differential diagnosis between amyotrophic lateral sclerosis and spinal muscular atrophy by skin involvement. J Neurol Sci 1989;91:301–310.

139. Cox TA, McDarby JV, Lavine L, Steele JC, Calne DB. A retinopathy on Guam with high prevalence in lytico-bodig. Ophthalmology 1989;96:1731–1735.

140. Drachman DB, Kuncl RW. Amyotrophic lateral sclerosis: An unconventional autoimmune disease. Ann Neurol 1989;26:269–274.

141. Plaitakis A. Glutamate dysfunction and selective motor neuron degeneration in amyotrophic lateral sclerosis: A hypothesis. Ann Neurol 1990;28:3–8.

142. Young AB. What's the excitement about excitatory amino acids in amyotrophic lateral sclerosis? Ann Neurol 1990;28:9–11 (Editorial).

143. Perry TL, Krieger C, Hansen S, Eisen A. Amyotrophic lateral sclerosis: Amino acid levels in plasma and cerebrospinal fluid. Ann Neurol 1990;28:12–17.

144. Rothstein JD, Tsai G, Kuncl RW, et al. Abnormal excitatory amino acid metabolism in amyotrophic lateral sclerosis. Ann Neurol 1990;28:18–25.

145. Baumann J. Results of treatment of certain diseases of the central nervous system with ACTH and corticosteroids. Acta Neurol Scand 1965;41(Suppl 13):453–461.

146. Norris FH, Denys EH, Mielke CH. Plasmapheresis in amyotrophic lateral sclerosis. In: Clark EC, Dau PC, eds. Plasmapheresis in the immunobiology of myasthenia gravis, Chapter 24. Boston: Houghton-Mifflin, 1979:258–264.

147. Plaitakis A, Smith J, Mandeli J, Yahr MV. Pilot trial of branched-chain amino acids in amyotrophic lateral sclerosis. Lancet 1988;1:1015–1018.

148. Troost D, van den Oord JJ, de Jong JMBV, Swaab DF. Lymphocytic infiltration in the spinal cord of patients with amyotrophic lateral sclerosis. Clin Neuropathol 1989;8:289–294.

149. Koslowsky MA, Williams C, Hinton DR, Miller CA. Heterotopic neurons in spinal cord of patients with ALS. Neurology 1989;39:644–648.

150. Perl TM, Bédard L, Kosatsky T, et al. An outbreak with toxic encephalopathy caused by eating mussels contaminated with domoic acid. N Engl J Med 1990;322:1775–1780.

151. Teitelbaum JS, Zatorre RJ, Carpenter S, et al. Neurologic sequelae of domoic acid intoxication due to the ingestion of contaminated mussel. N Engl J Med 1990;322:1781–1787.

152. Ross SM, Seelig M, Spencer PS. Specific antagonism of excitotoxic action of "uncommon" amino acids assayed in organotypic mouse cortical cultures. Brain Res 1987;425:120–127.

153. Calne DB, Eisen A, McGeer E, Spencer P. Alzheimer's disease, Parkinson's disease, and motoneurone disease: abiotrophic interaction between ageing and environment. Lancet 1986;2:1067–1070.

6

Pathology–Light Microscopy of Amyotrophic Lateral Sclerosis

Samuel M. Chou

ALS Research Foundation, California Pacific Medical Center
San Francisco, California

INTRODUCTION

Amyotrophic lateral sclerosis (ALS), the most common form of motor neuron disease (MND) in humans, occurs sporadically in middle or late adult life and can be divided into three clinical subtypes irrespective of bulbar or spinal predominance. This classification, which is not infallible, but is convenient for conceptualization of pathology germane to ALS, includes: (a) lower motor neuron type, or primary muscular atrophy (PMA) (Aran's disease) (1), (b) upper motor neuron type, or primary lateral sclerosis (PLS) (Erb's disease) (2), and (c) upper-lower motor neuron type, or classic ALS. On the basis of some 20 clinical and five autopsy cases, Charcot (3,4) coined the term ALS, recognizing that the disease started in the lateral columns of the spinal cord, hence "lateral sclerosis," propagated to the bulbar gray and anterior horns, and secondarily produced muscle atrophy, as connoted by the word "amyotrophic." Many atypical forms of ALS, all with a high familial incidence, have recently been added. They include: (a) familial ALS, (b) Guamanian ALS, (c) Kii Peninsula ALS in Japan, (d) ALS in Auyu and Jaki people of West New Guinea, and (e) familial juvenile ALS. Gowers (5) believed that the degeneration in both upper and lower motor neurons might occur simultaneously or independently; thus, pure lower motor

---

This work is dedicated to my mentor, Dr. Gabriele M. ZuRhein, in honor of her 70th birthday.

133

neuron diseases have become separated. With this notion, one is obligated to compare the pathology of ALS with that of other MNDs, such as Werdnig-Hoffmann disease, Fazio-Londe disease, Kugelberg-Welander disease, familial spastic paraplegia of Strümpell, and the neuronal type of Charcot-Marie-Tooth disease. Strümpell disease is chosen for comparison in this chapter. Through the years, a number of reviews have been published concerning the pathology of ALS or MND (6–11), and they serve as the guideline for the current reviews on the pathology of ALS.

PHYSIOLOGICAL ANATOMY OF THE MOTOR SYSTEM

Whether the disease process of ALS involves only the motor system remains to be seen; however, there is little doubt that the motor system is the cardinal recipient of the pathological insult. Organization of the central nervous system (CNS) motor system is complex. The systematized concept of Kuypers (12) is particularly useful for explaining the clinical and pathological features of ALS. Kuypers emphasized that in order to gain a functionally meaningful understanding of the motor system, the termination patterns of various descending pathways to the spinal motoneurons and the interneurons should be defined. In the monkey, and therefore probably in humans, three major termination patterns of descending motor pathways have been recognized, and their controls on motor functions as their final common pathways after directly or indirectly synapsing with lower motor neurons are summarized in Figure 1. In addition to the well-documented direct corticospinal (or pyramidal) tract from the upper motor neurons (Fig. 1A), there are two groups of brainstem fibers which terminate in the spinal gray intermediate zone and indirectly synapse with motoneurons via interneurons. They are (a) anteromedial (Fig. 1B) and lateral brainstem pathways (Fig. 1C); both receive premotor and precentral cortical fibers, respectively. The lateral pathway originates mainly in the contralateral red nucleus, descends in parallel to the direct corticospinal tract, and is therefore termed the indirect corticospinal tract. Its fibers terminate on interneurons in the contralateral posterolateral intermediate zone, whereas the direct corticospinal tract fibers monosynaptically terminate at the contralateral anteroposterolateral and bilateral anteromedial intermediate zones, as shown in Figure 1A and 1C. The anteromedial brainstem pathway originates in many brainstem nuclei, including the interstitial nucleus of Cajal, superior colliculus, vestibular complex, and bulbar medial reticular formation, and primarily terminates in the anteromedial intermediate zones of the spinal gray bilaterally (Fig. 1C). It is important to recognize that the nerve fibers of the anteromedial pathway distribute rather diffusely throughout the anterolateral funiculi of the spinal cord before they synapse indirectly with α motoneurons. This anatomical concept is crucial to understanding the diffuse

A) Descending Corticospinal Pathway (DCP)

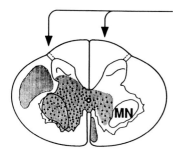

From: Motor & premotor cortex

Via: Direct Corticospinal tract

Contralaterally to:
-posterior lateral interneurons
-motoneurons (MN)

Bilaterally to:
-anteromedial interneurons

Control: Capacity for independent
use of distal extremities
and fingers

B) Anteromedial Brainstem Pathway (ABP)

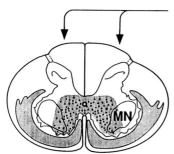

From: Interstitial N of Cajal:
Med. vest. N: Sup. collic.:
Bulbar med. RF

Via: Anteriolateral columns

Bilaterally to: Anteromedial
interneurons & MNs

Control: Axial and proximal extremity muscles: Head
and trunk: to maintain
erect posture

C) Lateral Brainstem Pathway (LBP)

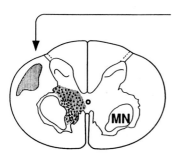

From: Red nucleus: Bulbar
lat. RF

Via: Indirect Corticospinal tract

Contralaterally to: posterolateral interneurons

Control: Flexion of distal ex-
termity muscles and distal
reflex movements

Figure 1 Three major motor pathways of primate.

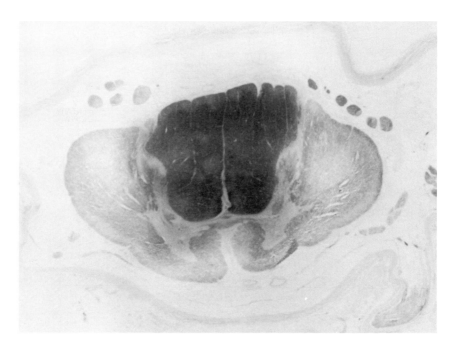

Figure 2 Low cervical spinal cord from a sporadic ALS case showing a remarkably well-preserved posterior column in contrast to diffuse myelin pallor in the anterolateral columns with accentuation in the corticospinal tracts.

degeneration of anterolateral funiculi commonly seen in the ALS spinal cord (Fig. 2).

Lower motoneurons in the anterior horns throughout the spinal cord as well as the brainstem (cranial nerves III–VII, IX–XII) innervate corresponding skeletal muscle. A motoneuron, more specifically an α motoneuron, innervates the bundle of extrafusal striated muscle fibers and forms the motor unit, whereas γ motoneurons innervate intrafusal muscle fibers. The major part of synaptic input to α and γ motoneurons is contributed by interneurons of the intermediate zone in the spinal cord. In addition, α motoneurons in primates also receive direct or monosynaptic terminations from descending systems, including the corticospinal fibers and some of the brainstem pathway fibers, as well as from group Ia muscle spindle afferents.

AXONAL TRANSPORT IN THE MOTOR SYSTEM

Pertinent to the discussion of pathology in ALS is the concept of axonal transport and primary impairment of axonal transport or "axostasis" (13,14). The mo-

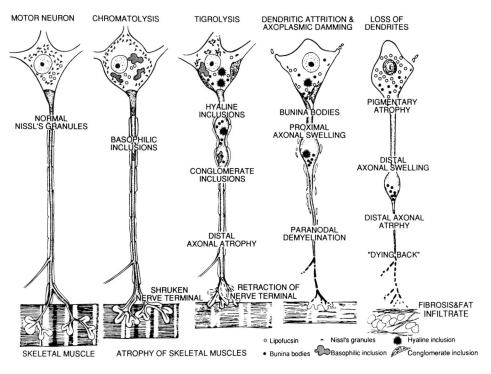

Figure 3 Hypothetical evolution of ALS as a disease of primary "axostasis."

toneurons, both Betz cells and anterior spinal neurons, are among the largest cells in the human body. The reason for the large cell body is obvious, for the motoneuron has to maintain the integrity of its dendritic branches, which often extend more than 1 cm, and its axon, which projects more than 100 cm from the cell body. Within the axon are different types of perpetual flow through which the cell body provides structural and functional proteins to the periphery and receives feedback signals. Two major types of orthograde transport include: (a) the fast (400 mm/day) (bidirectional also), which transports membrane-associated proteins and glycoproteins, and (b) the slow (a few mm/day), which transports a network of interconnected microfilaments, microtubules, and neurofilaments as component "a" (0.1–2 mm/day) and a large complex of soluble proteins as component "b" (2–4 mm/day) (15). In addition, there is retrograde axonal transport which carries both endogenous (amino acids, nerve growth factor) and exogenous (tetanus toxin, polio, herpes simplex, rabies viruses, horseradish peroxidase lectins, etc.) substances from the terminal axons to the cell body at a rate of over 75 mm/day. Pertinent to the possible etiology of ALS is the concept of "suicide transport" where a neurotoxic factor is transported by retrograde transport and selectively kill the neurons that transport the factor (16). Selective alterations in axonal transport induce predictable patterns of axonal pathology. Impairment of slow transport in axons may lead to neurofilament accumulation and axonal swelling proximal to the site of impairment (13,17,18). The resulting proximal axonopathy may induce distal axonal atrophy as well as secondary demyelination (19,20) consistent with central distal axonopathy (21) or "dying back" degeneration, as depicted in Figure 3. There is ample evidence that the basic properties of axonal transport in the CNS are different from those of large peripheral sensory or motor axons (22,23). Accordingly, a certain cytopathological difference should exist between the upper and lower motor neurons in ALS. Transneuronal degeneration from the upper to lower motor neurons may be expected from an impairment in axonal transport analogous to the denervation atrophy of skeletal muscles in ALS.

MACROSCOPIC PATHOLOGY OF ALS

In many cases, both the brain and spinal cord will appear normal except for the alterations related to the normal aging processes. In some cases, selective atro-

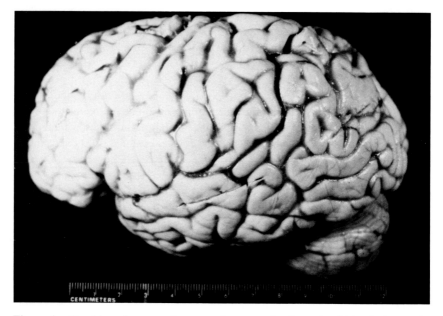

Figure 4 Atrophic and narrowed precentral motor strips (arrowheads) in the brain of a sporadic ALS case.

phy of the precentral gyri (Fig. 4), first described by Kohler and Pick in 1879 (24), may be conspicuous. Generalized atrophy of the spinal cord may be noted only in very chronic forms, but atrophic and grayish anterior spinal nerve roots in contrast to normal-appearing posterior spinal nerve roots are common features. Sclerotic discoloration and shrinkage of lateral corticospinal tracts may be detected on cut surfaces of chronic ALS spinal cords. Perhaps most striking is the atrophied, distal skeletal muscles, which are usually shrunken, pale, and fibrotic.

MICROSCOPIC PATHOLOGY OF ALS

The cardinal and characteristic histopathological features of ALS include:

1. Loss of large motoneurons of the motor cortex, brainstem, and spinal cord accompanied by focal astrogliosis.
2. "Senescent changes," including pigment atrophy, lipofuscinosis, and dendritic fragmentation and loss.
3. Various cytoplasmic inclusions associated with diverse perikaryal alterations, including chromatolysis, trigolysis, neuronophagia, and vacuolation.
4. Proximal and distal axonopathy with axonal spheroids.
5. Tract degeneration, including corticospinal tracts, descending brainstem pathways, and ascending tracts.
6. Secondary degeneration of motor nerve fibers, motor end-plates, and skeletal muscle fibers (see Chapter 7).

Motoneuron Loss

Motoneuron loss in the cortex, brainstem and spinal cord varies from case to case, and the literature on this is extremely inconsistent. One way to explain the inconsistency is to consider that the disease process in ALS may start at any of the motoneuron groups, be it in the motor cortex, bulbar motor nuclei, or spinal cord, and spread eventually to other motoneuron groups of different levels with diverse intensity. Premature death of motoneurons is in keeping with the concept of "abiotrophy" and "dying back" (25); however, motoneuron loss in ALS is more likely a selective loss of pathogenetic significance. Loss of Betz cells in the motor cortex was first described by Charcot and Marie (3). They demonstrated and also documented the degeneration of corticospinal tracts from the motor cortex down to the internal capsule, peduncles, pons, medulla oblongata, and spinal cord.

Scattered foci of patchy astrocytosis have been described in the second to third layers of the motor cortex in 8 of 11 ALS cases (26,27). We were unable to verify this particular finding; instead, marked astrocytosis confined to the motor subcortex, deep from the Betz cell layer, and intensifying along the gray-white junction (Fig. 5a,b) has been noted in relatively young ALS patients (aged 32–52

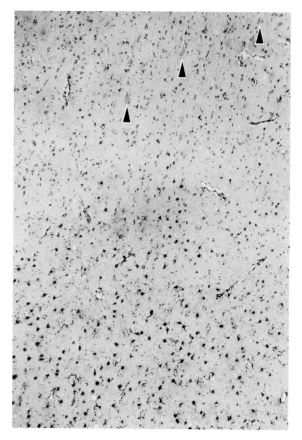

Figure 5a   Diffuse hypertrophic astrocytosis in the deep gray-white junction in the motor cortex with a few remaining Betz cells (arrowheads). × 50. GFAP immunostain.

years); foci of patchy astrocytosis are seen only in association with early or late senile degeneration. The reason for this topistic distribution of reactive astrocytosis is unclear, however; as will be discussed later, the astrocytosis may be related to distal axonal swelling and degeneration of Betz cells. Myelin sheaths are relatively well preserved in the white matter of ALS motor subcortex, supporting the concept of "dying back" axonopathy.

It has been debated if the motor cortex is singularly involved or if a more diffuse involvement of the entire frontal cortex occurs (6). We have seen cases of ALS where Betz cells of the motor cortex are well preserved as well as cases in which anterior spinal motoneurons are relatively well preserved. This variation may be due to tissue sampling since the motor system involvement in ALS

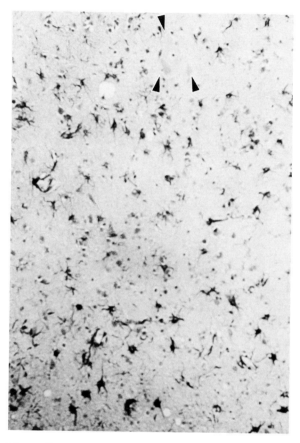

Figure 5b Higher magnification showing a leftover Betz cell (arrowheads) and hypertrophic astrocytes primarily at the deeper gray-white junction. ×200. GFAP immunostain.

has seldom been uniform and symmetrical. In the motor cortex, Davison (28) found involvement of the Betz cells with complete and continuous degeneration of the pyramidal tracts in only 12 of 42 ALS patients; Friedman and Freedman (29), in only one-third of 50 patients.

Of interest is the fact that among motoneuron groups at the same level, certain groups are more susceptible or more resistant to the disease process. In the brainstem, XII, nucleus ambiguus, and the V and VII motor nuclei are most susceptible, whereas III, IV, and VI nuclei are rarely involved (10). In the spinal cord, there is a tendency to involve motoneurons of the posterolateral group but

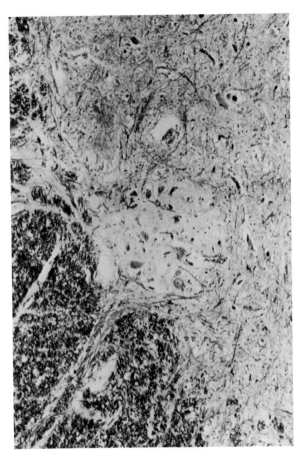

Figure 6a   Well-preserved small neurons in Onuf's nucleus while all the large α motoneurons disappeared in the sacral (S2) cord of an ALS patient. ×200. Klüver-Barrara
stain.

cases with predominant involvement of the anteromedial group have been
known. Here again, the different termination patterns of each descending motor
pathway must be taken in the consideration.

Selective preservation, which is often dramatic, of Onuf's nuclei in the sacral
(S2) cord (Fig. 6a) is well correlated with the clinical feature of well-preserved
vesicorectal function in ALS patients (30). Of great interest is the recent report
of well-preserved Onuf's nuclei in both acute and chronic cases of poliomyelitis
(31). While one may infer that viral-specific receptor protein may exist on certain
motoneuron groups, a recent immunohistochemical study has indicated that
Onuf's neurons are more akin to autonomic neurons than motoneurons (32).

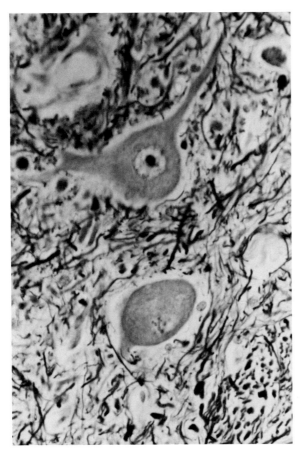

Figure 6b Rounded motoneuron with a marked loss of dendrites and aggregates of Bunina bodies in the cytoplasm. × 500. Bielschowsky stain.

Similarly, the well-preserved extraocular muscles in ALS patients are consistent with sparing of the corresponding bulbar nuclei, although rare cases of ALS with ophthalmoplegia as well as pathological findings in the oculomotor nuclei have been known (33–35). This selective sparing of motor nuclei is speculated by Weiner (36) to be due to the inherent absence of androgen receptors in neurons of those motor nuclei.

"Senescent Changes" in ALS

The most consistent and readily discernible microscopic finding is "accumu-lation" of lipofuscin granules in atrophied perikarya, the so-called "pigment

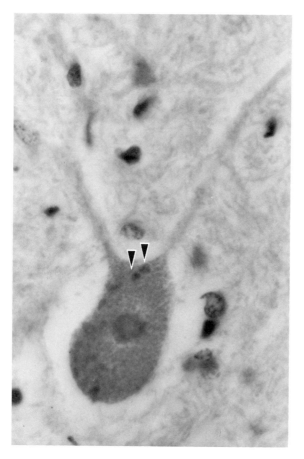

Figure 7a   Concurrence of hyaline inclusions in the center and two Bunina bodies (arrowheads) in the cytoplasm of a spinal motoneuron as visualized by immunostaining for ubiquitin. ×600. AEC immunostaining with hematoxylin counterstain.

atrophy." This change can be misinterpreted as a "senescent change" since these wear-and-tear pigments are characteristically present in neurons, particularly neurons of the aged. Lipofuscin granules also ostensibly increase in quantity in any atrophic mammalian cells, for example, myofibers in brown atrophy and adrenal cortex cells in brown degeneration. Hence, an apparent increase of lipofuscin granules at the expense of lost cytoplasmic components, including Nissl granules in neuronal perikarya, must not be construed as a phenomenon closely related to senescence. In motoneurons of ALS, it is the perikaryal atro-

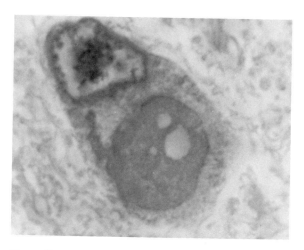

Figure 8e

larger (4–16 μ in average diameter) than Bunina bodies (Fig. 8b). They tend to occur in relatively well-preserved motoneurons of juvenile or young adult ALS patients. They were described in detail by Nelson and Prensky (52) as RNA-rich inclusions and are probably identical to those described in sporadic juvenile ALS cases by others (51,53–55). We described large basophilic inclusions in familial ALS cases of a father and son who died, both at the age of 33 (45), and an adult male of 31 years of age from Australia (56). Rarely, both eosinophilic and basophilic inclusions coexist in the cytoplasm of the same neurons. Of great interest is the description in the original article by Bunina (46) of the dimension of the inclusions measuring 5–20 μ in diameter, which suggest the possibility of overlying the next type of eosinophilic inclusions, hyaline inclusions. Indeed, the basophilic inclusions aggregating to become a single rounded inclusion with or without a central core resembling Lewy-body or hyaline inclusion may be encountered (Fig. 8c,d,e). Electron microscopy of basophilic inclusions (45,55) revealed aggregates of fuzzy microtubules, with outer diameter of 12–15 nm, closely associated with ribosomes and rough endoplasmic reticulum.

Hyaline inclusions, described first by Hirano et al. (57) and later by others (58–61) are thought to occur only in familial ALS. They consist of a hyaline-like, poorly stainable substance with an occasional central core which stains basophilic but is seldom concentrically laminated (Fig. 9a). They measure up to 3 or 5 μ in diameter, rarely resemble Lewy bodies, and are surrounded by a clear zone or halo. Twelve of eighty-two cases demonstrated this inclusion, including three PMA cases, seven sporadic ALS, and two familial ALS cases (45). In 10 of these, they were seen in association with Bunina bodies. Hyaline inclusions

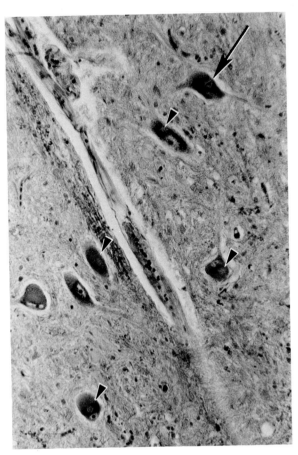

Figure 9a   Five out of seven anterior motoneurons showing an ill-defined hyaline inclusion in the cytoplasm (arrowheads); one of them with central refractile eosinophilic Bunina bodies (arrow) with the hyaline inclusion. ×200. H&E stain.

were commonly observed in sporadic ALS by others (62–65). It has been suggested that hyaline inclusions along with large proximal axonal spheroids may be more prominent and abundant in ALS patients with shorter clinical courses (66). Many histochemical characteristics of these inclusions overlap (67,68), and an inescapable impression is gained that three inclusions are interrelated and both basophicilic and hyaline inclusions may terminate as Bunina bodies, comparable to autophagic vacuoles. Immunohistochemically, the hyaline inclusions are strongly decorated by ubiquitin (69–75) in both sporadic and familial ALS (Fig. 9b). By comparing the histochemical, immunohistochemical, and ultrastructural

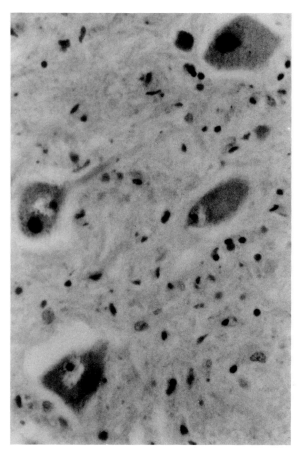

Figure 9b Three large motoneurons of the anterior horn of an ALS patient, each containing the hyaline inclusion, which is intensely decorated with antiubiquitin antibody. ×500. AEC immunostain with hematoxylin counterstain.

characteristics of these inclusions, one may propose the following scheme of evolution as: basophilic > hylaine > eosinophilic (Bunina), as summarized in Figure 3.

Prevalence of basophilic inclusions described in unusually young adults or juvenile patients is in keeping with this scheme that this inclusion represents the early stage in evolution of the intracytoplasmic inclusions.

Hyaline conglomerate inclusions, first described by Schochet et al. (76) in a sporadic ALS case and later by Hughes and Jerome (77) in a sporadic ALS case are relatively rare in ALS. This inclusion (Fig. 10a and 10b) was found in only

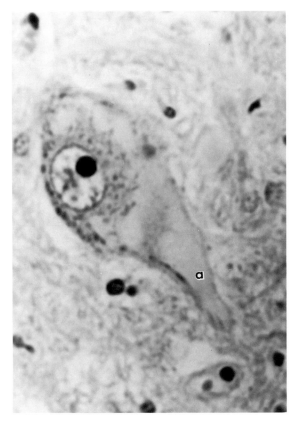

Figure 10a   Multiple conglomerate hyaline inclusions in the cytoplasm and proximal axon (a and b) with a larger axonal spheroid (A) in the vicinity of the motoneuron soma with multiple foci of axoplasmic damming. × 1100. H&E stain.

2 of 82 cases reviewed (45). The clinical features (one sporadic ALS and one familial PMA) did not differ much from those of the other sporadic ALS patients. Previous electron microscopy indicates that hyaline conglomerate inclusions consist mainly of neurofilaments and thus may be interpreted as not cytoplasmic inclusions in a strict sense, but a focal intracytoplasmic accumulation of regurgitated axoplasmic components. Such an intracytoplasmic accumulation has been described not only in motoneurons, but also in other neurons, including those in pontine reticular formation of a sporadic ALS case (78). Although it is possible that such a neurofilamentous aggregate is secondary to hyperproduction, it is more likely that it is secondary to the retrograde "axoplasmic damming"

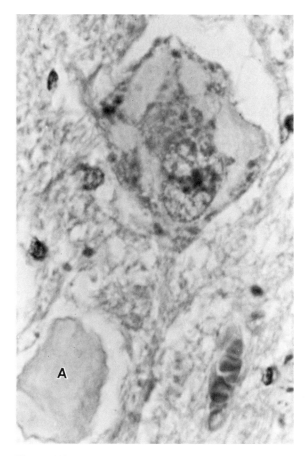

Figure 10b

due to an impairment in slow anterograde axonal transport. This would explain why phosphorylated neurofilament epitopes at distal axons tend to accumulate in the perikarya of ALS motoneurons (63,66–68,79,80). Apparently, this type of retrograde intracytoplasmic damming of phosphorylated neurofilaments with axonal spheroid formation (Fig. 10b) is not specific for ALS; it is found also in control anterior horn cells (68). Similar, if not identical, intracytoplasmic conglomerate inclusions have been induced in the upper motor neurons of IDPN-intoxicated monkeys where the inclusions are composed of whorled neurofilaments (Fig. 11) with mitochondria suggestive of an intracytoplasmic turbulence secondary to axoplasmic damming (81).

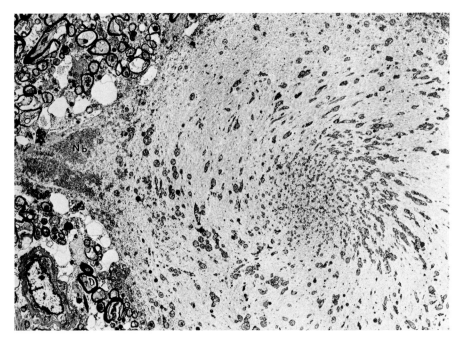

Figure 11 The major part of a motoneuron perikaryon from an IDPN-intoxicated monkey is replaced by a whorl of neurofilaments and mitochondria pushing Nissl's bodies (Nb) to the periphery. ×15,000.

Proximal and Distal Axonopathy in ALS

Large, proximal axonal swellings were first described by Carpenter (82) in 11 cases of subacute ALS (with clinical involvement of 10 months or less) and later by us in two ALS patients who died 4 and 11 months after onset (83). A direct connection between the proximal axonal swelling and the perikarya has been unequivocally demonstrated (Fig. 12a) (84,85). Similar axonal swellings could be induced by a single injection of the chemical IDPN (β-β'-iminodipropionitrile), a toxic dimer crystallized from *Lathyrus odoratus* (neurolathyrism). An intraaxonal or primary impairment of axonal transport has been suspected as the pathogenesis of the resulting axonopathy, and the concept of primary axostasis was proposed (13,14). Indeed, the selective impairment affects the slow component of the orthograde axonal transport (19,20,86) without affecting the fast component nor the retrograde transport (19,87) has been demonstrated. Since the concurrence of both proximal axonal spheroids and Bunina bodies may occa-

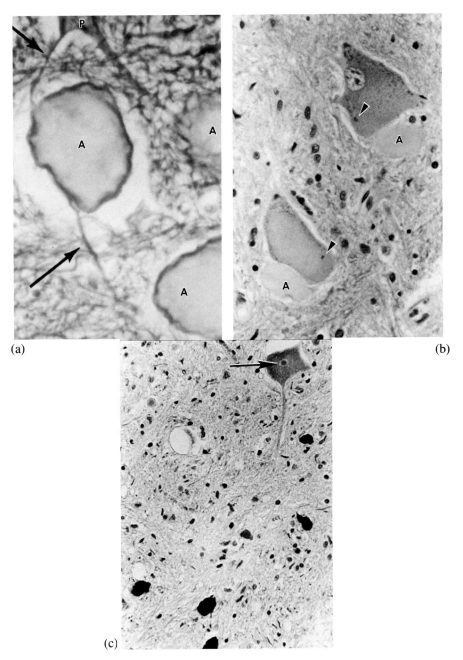

(a)

(b)

(c)

Figure 12 (a) Proximal axonal spheroids (A); one is connected to a perikaryon (P) through a proximal segment (arrow) and to a distal segment of axon (arrow). × 1200. Bodian stain. (b) Two slightly chromatolytic motoneurons each with a Bunina body (arrowhead) and a proximal axonal spheroid (A). × 800. H&E stain. (c) Immunostained anterior horns of a sporadic ALS case for phosphorylated neurofilament (200 kDa) showing several intensely stained axonal spheroid and negatively stained perikaryon with a negatively stained hyaline inclusion (arrow). × 250. AEC with hematoxylin counterstain.

sionally be present (Fig. 12b), it is tempting to pathogenetically correlate the role of intracytoplasmic inclusions in inducing the impairment of the axonal flow with a "dying back" degeneration of both upper and lower motor nerve fibers. Alternatively, a primary insult resulting in axostasis may predispose to the formation of intracytoplasmic inclusions with subsequent dying back. Immunohistochemistry of various neurofilament subunits (Fig. 12c) in axonal spheroids indicates neurofilament proteins of axonal or phosphorylated type and fails to suggest any posttranslational abnormalities (67,79,88–90).

Tract Degeneration

Corticospinal Tract Degeneration

Tract degeneration is most commonly found in the corticospinal tracts of the ALS spinal cord (Fig. 13). The extent of this degeneration, however, is not consistently correlated with the clinical manifestation of pyramidal signs. The involvement may be asymmetrical (91), yet clinically, the atrophy and pyramidal signs may be fairly symmetrical. Many authors have reported patients with pyramidal tract signs in the absence of corticospinal tract involvement at autopsy; the reverse has also been reported (10,29). A few authors considered that pyramidal degeneration starts in the internal capsule and the cortical lesions are attributable to the outcome of ascending degeneration. The credit for the first description of the entire pyramidal tract degeneration is given to Kojewnikoff (92), who described degeneration occupying the anterior third quarter of the posterior limb of the internal capsule in horizontal section (Fig. 14a). Later, this restricted area of pyramidal tract degeneration (Fig. 14b) was reconfirmed by Hirayama et al. (93), who corrected the traditional misconception for the topographic location of pyramidal tracts that largely originated from Dejerine's description (94). In general, the pyramidal tract involvement is uneven at various levels, as stressed by Bertrand and Van Bogaert (6). Of 37 ALS cases studied by Davison in 1941, 12 showed total pyramidal degeneration from the motor cortex to the spinal cord, two from the cerebral peduncle, seven from the pons, 12 from the medulla, and in four cases, the degeneration was limited to the spinal cord (28). Of 45 cases examined by Brownell et al., less than half demonstrated complete pyramidal degeneration from the cortex and in 10 the pyramidal degeneration was undetectable (7). Among 36 "classical" ALS cases, the same authors noted variable spinal tract degeneration: (a) no pyramidal degeneration in eight, (b) degeneration in pyramidal tracts alone in eight, (c) both pyramidal and anterolateral column involvement in 17, and (d) both pyramidal and anterolateral column involvement with some posterior column degeneration in three. This variation in involvement of the corticospinal tracts as well as the anteromedial brainstem pathway can be explained, in part, by the involvement of different motoneuron

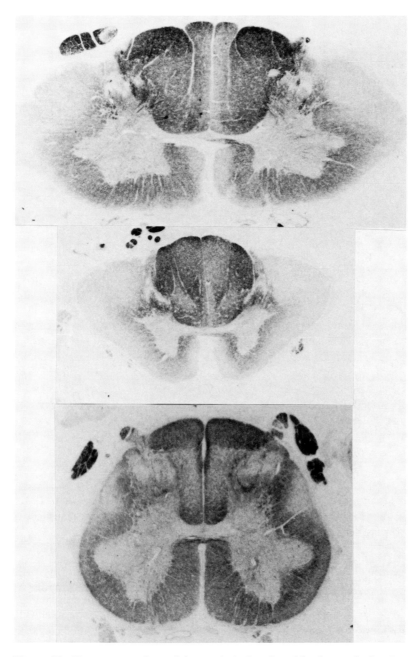

Figure 13 Transverse sections of the cervical, dorsal, and lumbar cords showing tract degeneration in the anterolateral, posterior spinocerebellar, corticospinal, and gracile tracts. Note involvement of Flechsig's middle root zone in the dorsal column of both dorsal and lumbar cords from a specific ALS case. Also note markedly atrophic spinal roots in contrast to well-myelinated posterior roots.

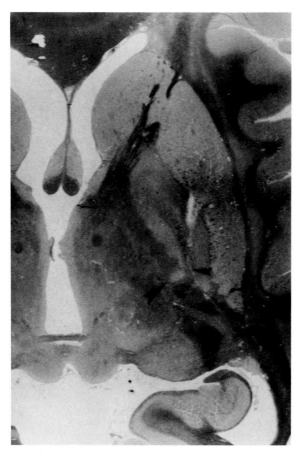

Figure 14a   Horizontal section of an ALS brain through the posterior commissure showing the spot of degeneration in the third quadrant of the internal capsule (arrowheads) corresponding to the direct corticospinal tract. × 2. LFB and Bodian stain.

groups (cortical, bulbar, and spinal) in the organizational scheme of Kuypers. Furthermore, it is of critical importance to recognize and distinguish clinicopathological substrates for indirect and direct corticospinal tract degeneration because these two tracts may be independently involved. Such a clinicopathological differentiation can be best discussed by comparing ALS with Strümpell's disease or Friedreich's ataxia.

However, the corticospinal tract degeneration emanating from the different levels of the CNS cannot be readily explained. In this regard, the findings of giant axonal spheroids collected segmentally along the corticospinal tracts in

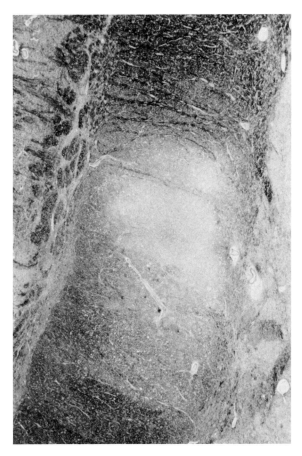

Figure 14b A higher magnification of the adjacent section stained for myelin showing focal myelin pallor and vacuolar changes. × 20. Klüver-Barrera stain.

internal capsules (Fig. 15a and 15b), cerebral peduncles, and medullary pyramids in two ALS cases from Guam and two sporadic cases with the clinical courses ranging from 7 months to 2 years may provide a plausible explanation (95,96). Those giant axonal spheroids, which are immunoreactive for neurofil aments and ubiquitin (Fig. 14c and 14d), provide additional evidence of an impairment in both distal and proximal axonal transport in ALS. Because the axonal transport profiles are different in the upper from the lower motoneurons, formation of these distal axonal spheroids in the upper corticospinal tracts is likely to be pathogenetically similar to, but different from, that for the spheroids formed at the proximal axons of spinal motoneurons. One may speculate that

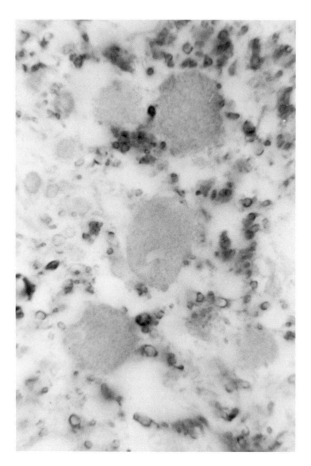

Figure 15a Large axonal spheroids in the third quadrant of the posterior limb of internal capsule from a sporadic ALS case. Compare the sizes of myelinated axons and spheroids. ×500. LFB–H&E stains.

precursors or components of these spheroids in the upper corticospinal tracts might have originally derived from either Betz cells or upper brainstem neuron somas, be carried distally, aggregated, and conglomerated until they could no longer be transported farther, and culminated in central distal axonopathy (21).

Selective involvement and loss of large myelinated motor fibers has been reported by several authors at anterior spinal roots (97,98) or peripheral motor axons (99) and at various levels of the corticospinal tract pathway (93). This selective involvement of large motoneuron axons implies that a certain physi-biochemical property unique to large motoneurons, which is potentially shared

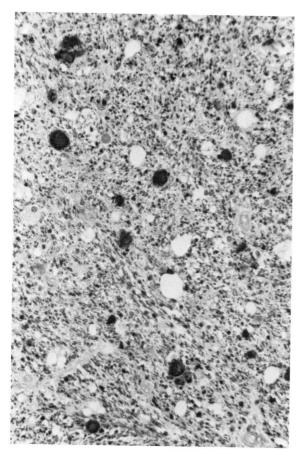

Figure 15b An adjacent section from (a), immunostained for phosphorylated neurofilament (200 kDa) showing many spheroids intensely decorated. × 150. AEC–hematoxylin stain.

by some large sensory neurons, renders them susceptible to such an axonopathy. This hypothesis may be applicable to certain large sensory neurons, such as those in Clarke's columns or large reticular neurons of the brainstem, and may further explain involvement of these systems in ALS, as described below.

Anterolateral Column Degeneration

The relatively common observation of symmetrical and diffuse myelin pallor in the anterolateral columns in the ALS spinal cord, especially of the cervical cord (Fig. 2), has puzzled neuropathologists for many years. This finding can now be explained on the basis of degenerating anteromedial brainstem pathway. The anteromedial pathway is poorly defined in humans and the pathological implication has been scarce. This generic pathway comprises many tracts, including reticulospinal, vestibulospinal, and interstitiospinal, all of which originate from brainstem reticular neurons.

Pale basophilic globose cytoplasmic inclusions (Fig. 8a and 8b) were found to distribute in motoneurons of the motor cortex, brainstem, and spinal cord of three young male adults (aged 31, 32, and 33 years, respectively) with ALS who died after relatively short courses (7, 15, and 12 months, respectively). The basophilic inclusions served as a convenient marker for the neurons, which were selectively involved before they might eventually disappear (56). Distribution of those inclusions in the brainstem reticular neurons was almost identical in all three ALS cases. Among the median, medial, and lateral groups of reticular formation in the brainstem, the median raphe or serotonergic reticular neurons were intact and showed no inclusions, while both the medial and lateral reticular neurons displayed prominent basophilic inclusions readily detectable in hematoxylin and eosin sections. Additionally, both the medial and lateral vestibular neurons and, to a lesser extent, the neurons in the interstitial nucleus of Cajal contained basophilic inclusions, as depicted in Figure 16. Two of the three ALS cases showed distinct myelin pallor in the anterolateral spinal funiculi corresponding to the anteromedial pathway. Thus, both the pathway and its neuronal origin appeared preferentially affected and provided a plausible explanation for the hitherto mystified myelin pallor of anterolateral spinal funiculi in ALS. Neuronal loss in the brainstem reticular formation has seldom been mentioned in ALS. The reason for the rare documentation of the neuronal degeneration in the brainstem reticular neurons may be due to difficulty in quantitation and localization of reticular neurons involved. The correlation of neuronal degeneration in reticular formation and its tract degeneration becomes feasible when such affected neurons display the specific change of intracytoplasmic basophilic inclusions (Fig. 8a–e). Loss of reticular neurons and gliosis in the pontine reticular formation as well as periaqueductal gray (interstitial nucleus of Cajal) has been noted in two sporadic ALS cases; the spinal cords showed severe diffuse degeneration of the anterolateral funiculi (100). Hyaline conglomerate neurofilamentous inclusions have been reported in bulbar reticular neurons from a case of sporadic ALS (78). Similarly, a marked loss of neurons and astrogliosis were described in the pontine reticular formation in a case of familial ALS by Tabuchi et al. (101).

Spinocerebellar and Clarke's Column Degeneration
Degeneration of the spinocerebellar tracts and Clarke's columns has been described and perhaps overemphasized in the past as a characteristic pathological

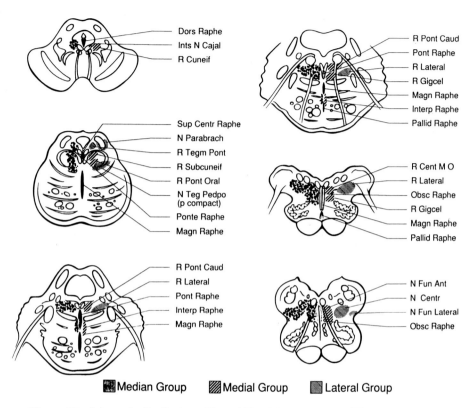

Dors Raphe
Ints N Cajal
R Cuneif

R Pont Caud
Pont Raphe
R Lateral
R Gigcel
Magn Raphe
Interp Raphe
Pallid Raphe

Sup Centr Raphe
N Parabrach
R Tegm Pont
R Subcuneif
R Pont Oral
N Teg Pedpo (p compact)
Ponte Raphe
Magn Raphe

R Cent M O
R Lateral
Obsc Raphe
R Gigcel
Magn Raphe
Pallid Raphe

R Pont Caud
R Lateral
Pont Raphe
Interp Raphe
Magn Raphe

N Fun Ant
N Centr
N Fun Lateral
Obsc Raphe

▓ Median Group ▨ Medial Group ▨ Lateral Group

Figure 16 Schematic distribution of basophilic globose inclusions ▓ in the lateral and median reticular neurons sparing the median (serotonergic) group; a composite of three ALS cases.

feature unique to familial ALS. Earlier reports on the pathological findings in familial ALS (57–60,102,103) contended that the spinocerebellar tract, posterior column, and motor system degeneration was a unique pathoanatomical entity at variance with sporadic ALS. However, many cases of sporadic ALS with spino-cerebellar degeneration (Fig. 13) have since been reported (7,77,91,104–107), some with Clarke's column involvement (100,108). In 12 sporadic ALS cases, Averback and Crocker (106) found loss of over one-third of the neurons in the Clarke's column. A recent study with a surface marker selective for neurons in the Clarke's column has demonstrated relative absence in the majority of spino-cerebellar neurons in five sporadic ALS cases studied (109). Degeneration of the posterior spinocerebellar tracts has been related to a primary disease of Clarke's column as best exemplified in Friedreich's ataxia. In ALS too, neurons in Clarke's columns are involved showing numerical reduction and are suspected to underlie the posterior spinocerebellar tract degeneration (25). Furthermore, many pathognomonic microscopic findings of lower motoneurons in ALS, e.g., proximal axonal swellings, axonal globules, Bunina bodies, and neuronal loss, have been recently reported in Clarke's columns in sporadic ALS (105,108). Accordingly, although clinically not manifest, it is fair to include spinocerebellar degeneration as a rare or late concomitant of the motoneuron system degeneration in sporadic ALS. In familial ALS, the phenotypic expression of the degeneration tends to be complete or "total" in the early stage (110).

Posterior Column Degeneration

Sensory complaints in ALS patients are not uncommon (111), but are usually not accompanied by corresponding histopathological findings in the sensory tracts. Posterior column degeneration, especially of the fasciculus gracilis, is common with aging. It has been estimated that approximately 5% of autopsied spinal cords from the population over the age of 65 will show posterior column degeneration. Posterior column degeneration in sporadic ALS has seldom been described in recent papers, probably because its specificity might be doubted, although many earlier reports described the presence of such a degeneration (102). The involvement of the middle root zone of Flechsig in the lumbar cord (Fig. 13) was considered characteristic for posterior column involvement in familial ALS; however, this finding simply means that the long and large nerve fibers for proprioception are not entirely spared in ALS. As expected, in many review articles on pathology of ALS, one finds occasional descriptions of the posterior column degeneration (7,8,10,45,112). The findings, however, were dismissed as coincidental rather than an unusual variant of ALS by some of those authors. A recent morphometric study suggests otherwise. Kawamura et al. (113) described a marked reduction in large cyton populations (54%) on studying lumbar (L5) spinal ganglion cytons in five sporadic cases of ALS. The findings were interpreted to correspond to both posterior column and spinocerebellar tract degenerations reported in both sporadic and familial ALS. The organization and function of the dorsal columns have recently been redefined. Accordingly, the dorsal columns have a major role in certain motor controls by transferring peripheral inputs to the motor cortex (114). Hence, one can no longer completely dissociate the dorsal columns from the motoneuron system.

Basal Ganglia Degeneration

Mild diffuse degeneration is said to be common in the basal ganglia, including the thalamus and substantia nigra (9), while Castaigne et al. reported 16 of 19 atypical ALS cases with basal ganglia involvement (8), though extrapyramidal signs were clinically absent. In rare instances, basal ganglia lesions with corresponding extrapyramidal signs have been described in sporadic ALS cases. Bertrand and Van Bogaert (6) described diffuse involvement of both the cerebral cortex and basal ganglia. Involvement of the thalamus has occasionally been mentioned (115,116) as well as of the substantia nigra (8,117,118). With the Marchi technique, which presumably is more sensitive in picking up degenerated fibers, Smith (119) noted degenerated fibers in the thalamus, the subthalamus, the globus pallidus, the substantia nigra, the prerubal field, the preaqueductal gray, the superior colliculus, and the brainstem reticular formation. Thus Marchi staining may be a useful tool for studying subtle involvement of the lateral and anteromedial brainstem pathways. In keeping with the concept of the "total" ALS (109), to be discussed below, it is of paramount importance to recognize the degeneration of neuronal groups from which the brainstem pathways emanate. Rare ALS cases with both thalamic and substantia nigra involvement have been postulated as a separate disease from ALS (115). The nosological and semiological position of ALS cases with involvement of basal ganglia and other systems has not been decided. Those motoneuron diseases in association with olivopontocerebellar, striatonigral or nigrospinodentate degenerations have, for the present, been conveniently lumped into the group of multiple system diseases (120).

Pathology of Atypical ALS and Other MND
The characteristic pathological features in each of the three major groups of atypical ALS (i.e., familial ALS, ALS in Guam, or in the Kii Peninsula of Japan, and Strumpell's familial spastic paraplegia) will be briefly discussed.

Familial ALS Inheritance patterns of familial ALS have been mainly of autosomal dominant transmission. Three different patterns of histopathological heterogeneity are known (121) and are not at variance from those in sporadic ALS. They are involvement of: (a) anterior horn cells with pyramidal tracts, (b) anterior horn cells without pyramidal tracts, and (c) such motor system changes plus spinocerebellar tracts, Clarke's columns, and posterior columns.

In addition to the characteristic features of sporadic ALS, Engel et al. (102) described a unique pathological feature in three members of an autosomal dominant familial ALS. It was characterized by demyelination in the midroot zones of the posterior spinal columns. The pattern of the degeneration is similar to that in tabes dorsalis except no disturbance of proprioception was detected in those patients. The spinocerebellar tracts were also involved. This clinically silent ascending degeneration is by no means the characteristic or essential pathological concomitant of familial ALS, since many familial ALS cases later reported did not show this ascending degeneration. It should be again emphasized that the posterior column degeneration may occur as a normal aging process and also as a common finding in patients of severe inanition. Furthermore, in compression neuropathy of posterior spinal roots, large-caliber proprioceptive fibers would be preferentially involved and produce midroot zone degeneration. In addition, posterior column involvement has been described in many sporadic ALS cases [one by Lawyer and Netsky (10), three by Brownell et al. (7), and three by Castaigne et al. (8)]. Among our 82 cases, there were three sporadic ALS cases which showed the midroot zone posterior column degeneration; this was considered a complication rather than a pathoanatomical concomitant of ALS (45). Combined posterior column and spinocerebellar tract degeneration has also been described in sporadic ALS cases [one by Hughes and Jerome (77), two by Brownell et al. (7), and one by Page et al. (104)]. These findings may be prominent in the absence of clean-cut pyramidal tract degeneration (122). At any rate, the ascending tract degeneration in ALS, if it exists, should not be severe and should be considered a minor histopathological concomitant; otherwise, it may be difficult to differentiate ALS from other heredofamilial motoneuron diseases such as spastic familial paraplegia, Charcot-Marie-Tooth disease, or Friedreich's ataxia.

Western Pacific ALS   Neurofibrillary tangles (NFT) in both brain and spinal cord, unassociated with senile plaques, were characteristic features in all 70 Guam ALS patients studied (39,123). They were compared with 90 sporadic ALS cases in New York City where NFT were either completely absent or their number was negligible. The neurons affected were not necessarily those of the motor system and included the hippocampal gyrus, amygdaloid nucleus, hypothalamus, substantia innominata, and locus ceruleus. Similar findings were reported in ALS of Kii Peninsula in Japan (46). NFT unassociated with senile plaques was also the characteristic feature in the Guam Parkinsonism dementia (PD) complex (39). A control study on 69 members of the Guamanian Chamorro without dementia, ALS, or Parkinsonism by Anderson et al. disclosed that NFT occurred at a very high rate and at an early age in this population and suggested that while a causal relationship between the NFT and Guamanian ALS or PD exists, it may not be direct (41). By comparing histopathological findings in 20 ALS cases from Western Australia and those among 22 Guamanian ALS cases, Tan et al. concluded that NFTs are not a feature of ALS (124).

Familial Spastic Paraplegia, Strümpell's Disease   What clinicopathological characteristics may differentiate direct from indirect corticospinal tract degeneration? This hypothetical question is asked in order to address the confusing issues and features previously encountered in ALS, e.g., primary lateral sclerosis without amyotrophy (125) or familial ALS without lateral sclerosis (122). The issue is best discussed and explained by presenting a case of the "pure" form of familial spastic paraplegia (FSP) or Strümpell's disease and by corroborating it with the clinicopathological features of FSP previously reported.

Case Report:

Clinical history: A 63-year-old white woman, who died after a 1-week history of "flu," was first hospitalized at the age of 45 years for evaluation of a slowly progressive decline in the strength and control of her lower legs since her teens. By age 32, she was confined to a wheelchair, but despite the lower extremity disability, use of her hands and arms were not impaired. She was able to continuously play the piano, write letters, knit endlessly, and kept her cheerful disposition. In her early 40s, however, she became increasingly taciturn, withdrawn, and irritable, probably because she developed increasing problems with fecal incontinence, became obsessed with "germs" and "contaminations," and developed compulsive hand washing. By this time, there was virtually complete paralysis of the legs, but she continued to use her hands and arms with remarkably good facility.

Except for moderate dorsal kyphoscoliosis and muscle atrophy of the lower extremities, the general examination was unremarkable. Neurological examination revealed normal cranial nerve functions and slurred speech. The patient was unable to stand and the lower extremities showed bilateral heel cord shortening and moderate equinovarus deformity. In contrast, strength and coordination of the upper extremities were intact. Babinski sign was bilaterally positive; deep tendon reflexes were hypoactive in the upper extremities, absent in the ankles, and bilaterally hyperactive in the knees. Sensory examination revealed loss of vibratory sensation below the iliac crests, but sensation was otherwise intact. Her second hospitalization 11 years later, at the age of 56, was for drainage of large abscesses in the buttocks. At the time, in addition to markedly hyperactive knee jerks, urinary incontinence and spotty hypesthesia were recorded. The third hospitalization, a year later, was for recurrent dysphagia, and for the first time, moderate spasticity and hyperreflexia in both upper extremities were noted. Her final hospitalization at age 63 was for a 1-week history of "flu" with lethargy and she died 2 hr after admission. Family history was remarkable in that at least three other members, including her brother, father, and paternal uncle, suffered from a similar disease with the onset in the teens in three (including the present patient) and at late middle age in the fourth. Each had a normal life span and died from unrelated illness.

Brain autopsy: The brain (1100 g) showed mild generalized cortical atrophy and ventricular dilatation. An old superficial cortical contusion (1 cm across) was noted over the left inferior temporal gyrus. The spinal cord appeared markedly small and showed mild grayish discoloration of the spinal roots, especially of the posterior. Microscopically, a striking pattern of degeneration in corticospinal-tracts and dorsal columns was seen (Fig. 17a). The corticospinal tract degeneration became noticeable below the medulla, reached maximum intensity at the

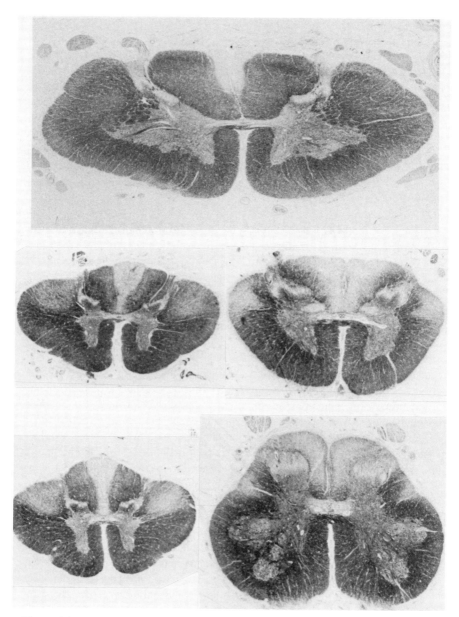

Figure 17a Sections of cervical, thoracic, and lumbar cord indicating degeneration of the indirect corticospinal and gracile tracts. Note the contour of the degenerated corticospinal tracts smaller and more dorsally localized than the direct corticospinal tract as seen in Figure 13. Klüver-Barrera stain.

phied. Thus, the brainstem neurons of the anteromedial pathways most probably terminate monosynaptically with lower motoneurons.

If the direct corticospinal tracts are primarily involved, distal muscle weakness and atrophy, especially of the finger muscles and distal flexor muscles, would be more evident. Pathologically, the lateral motoneuron group should be more severely affected transynaptically, since many receive monosynaptic terminations of direct corticospinal tract fibers. Thus, clinical features in the subtypes of ALS may be correlated with the degeneration patterns of both descending motor pathways and the termination patterns in given ALS cases, though admittedly they are never clear-cut and often overlap.

SUMMARY

While a certain personally biased view may inevitably be included in the foregoing discussion, emphasis has been placed on the following:

In light of the recently elucidated anatomical organization of primate motor systems by Kuypers, pathoanatomy of ALS must be reevaluated individually in ALS cases according to the clinical symptomatology referrable to the termination patterns in the intermediate zones and anterior horns, as well as the patterns of descending tract degeneration.

Clinicopathological correlation becomes feasible if one corroborates the given descending motor pathway degeneration with its clinical features as exemplified for the indirect corticospinal tract degeneration in Strümpell's disease or PLS.

Diffuse myelin pallor and degeneration of anterolateral funiculi in the spinal cord in ALS can be explained by involvement of the anteromedial brainstem pathway. Other tract degenerations are explained by the concept of "total" degeneration as visualized in ALS patients whose lives were sustained beyond the previously "terminal" point.

The basic pathomechanism involved in ALS may start in different neuronal groups (motor cortex, bulbar, and spinal) with corresponding descending motor pathways and induce proximal or central distal axonopathy in the subservient nerve fibers, characteristic of the "dying back" degeneration.

Such an axonopathy may be closely related to an impairment of axonal transport secondary to formation of various intracytoplasmic and intraaxonal inclusions described in motoneurons from ALS patients of all subtypes.

Three major types of neuronal inclusions (i.e., basophilic, hyaline, and Bunina) may represent different phases in the pathogenetic evolution of ALS process, whereas hyaline conglomerate inclusions may be formed secondary to retrograde axoplasmic damming.

The recent elucidation of "total" histopathological manifestations in long-term survivors maintained by life support strongly suggest that degeneration of both spinocerebellar tracts and dorsal columns is a slow pathoanatomical concomitant of sporadic ALS also. In familial ALS, the rate of ascending tract degeneration is merely faster than that in sporadic ALS.

More data from immunohistochemistry, electron and immunoelectron microscopy on the inclusion bodies in well-fixed specimens from ALS cases with relatively short clinical course and postmortem time are needed to elucidate the pathogenesis involved in ALS.

ACKNOWLEDGMENT

The author thanks Dr. Janet Miles for her review and comments on the manuscript and Mrs. Sharon Sminchak for her skilled secretarial assistance.

REFERENCES

1. Aran FA. Recherches sur une malade non encore décrite du systéme musculaire (atrophie musculare progressive). Arch Gén Méd 1850;24:5–35, 172–214.
2. Erb WA. Spastic syphilitic spinal paralysis. Lancet 1902;2:969–974.
3. Charcot JM, Joffroy A. Deux cas d'atrophie musculaire progressive avec lésions de la substance grise et des faisceaux antérolatéraux de la molle épiniére. Arch Physiol (Par) 1869;2:354–367, 629–649, 744–760.
4. Charcot JM, Marie P. Deux nouveaux cas de la sclérose latérale amyotrophie suivis d'autopsie. Arch Neurol 1885;10:1–35, 168–186.
5. Gowers WR. A manual of diseases of the nervous system. London: Churchill, 1888.
6. Bertrand I, Van Bogaert L. La sclérose latérale amyiotrophique (anatomie pathologique). Rev Neurol 1923;32:779–806.
7. Brownell B, Oppenheimer DR, Hughes JT. The central nervous system in motor neuron disease. J Neurol Neurosurg Psychiatry 1970;33:338–357.
8. Castaigne P, Lehermitte F, Cambier J, et al. Étude neuropathologique de 61 observation de sclérose latéral amyotrophique: Discussion nosologique. Rev Neurol 1972;127:401–414.
9. Colmant HJ: Die Myatrophische Lateralsclerose. Handbuch Spez Path Anat Histol (Henke-Lubarsch), Vol. 13. Berlin-Gottingen-Heidelberg: Springer-Verlag. OHG 1958:2624–2692.
10. Lawyer T Jr, Netsky MG. Amyotrophic lateral sclerosis: A clinicoanatomic study of 53 cases. Arch Neurol 1953;69:171–192.
11. Hirano A, Iwata M. Pathology of motor neurons with special reference to amyotrophic lateral sclerosis and related diseases. In Tsubaki T, Toyokura Y, eds. Amyotrophic lateral sclerosis. Tokyo: University of Tokyo Press, 1979:107–133.
12. Kuypers HGJM. The anatomical organization of the descending pathways and their contribution to motor control especially in the primates. In: Desmedt JE, ed.

New developments in electromyography and clinical neurophysiology, Vol. 3. Basel: S Karger, 1973:38–68.

13. Chou SM, Hartmann HA. Axonal lesions and walzing syndrome after IDPN administration in rats. With a concept . . . "axostasis". Acta Neuropathol 1964;3: 428–450.

14. Chou SM, Hartmann HA. Electron microscopy of focal neuroaxonal lesions produced by B-B′ iminodipropionitrile (IDPN) in rats. Acta Neuropathol 1965;4: 590–603.

15. Lasek RJ. Polymer sliding in axons. J Cell Sci 1986: (Suppl 5):161–179.

16. Wiley RG, Blessing WW, Reis DJ. Suicide transport: Destruction of neurons by retrograde transport of recin, abrin and modeccin. Science 1982;216:889–890.

17. Troncoso JC, Price DL, Griffin JW, Parhad IM. Neurofibrillary axonal pathology in aluminum intoxication. Ann Neurol 1982;12:278–283.

18. Gajdusek DC. Hypothesis: Interference with axonal transport of neurofilament as a common pathogenetic mechanism in certain diseases of central nervous system. N Engl J Med 1985;312:714–719.

19. Griffin JW, Hoffman PN, Clark AW, et al. Slow axonal transport of neurofilament proteins: Impairment by B-B′-iminodipropionitrile administration. Science 1978;202:633–635.

20. Griffin JW, Watson DF. Axonal transport in neurological disease. Ann Neurol 1988;23:3–13.

21. Thomas PK, Shaumburg HH, Spencer PS, et al. Central distal axonopathy syndrome: Newly recognized models of naturally occurring human degenerative diseases. Ann Neurol 1984;15:313–314.

22. Reh TA, Redshaw JD, Bisby MA. Axons of the pyramidal tract do not increase their transport of growth-associated proteins after axontomy. Mol Brain Res 1987;2:1–6.

23. Oblinger MM. Biochemical composition and dynamics of the axonal cytoskeleton in the corticospinal system of the adult hamster. Metabol Brain Dis 1988;3:49–64.

24. Kohler O, Pick L. Über die progressiven Spinaleramyotrophien. Ztschr Nervenh 1879;5:169.

25. Cavanagh JB. The "dying back" process. Arch Pathol Lab Med 1979;103:659–664.

26. Kamo H, Haebara H, Akiguchi I, Kameyama M, Kimura H. Peculiar patchy astrocytosis in the precentral cortex of amyotrophic lateral sclerosis. Clin Neurol 1983;23:974–981.

27. Kamo H, Haebara H, Akiguchi I, Kameyama M, Kimura H, McGeer P. A distinctive distribution of reactive astroglia in the precentral cortex in amyotrophic lateral sclerosis. Acta Neuropathol (Berl) 1987;74:33–38.

28. Davison C. Amyotrophic lateral sclerosis: Origin and extent of the upper motor neuron lesion. Arch Neurol Psychiatry 1941;46:1039–1056.

29. Friedman AP, Freedman D. Amyotrophic lateral sclerosis. J Neurol Ment Dis 1950;111:1–11.

30. Mannen T, Iwata M, Toyokura Y, et al. Preservation of a certain motoneuron

group of the sacral cord in amyotrophic lateral sclerosis: Its clinical significance. J Neurol Neurosurg Psychiatry 1977;40;464–469.

31. Kojima H, Furuta Y, Fujita M, Fujioka Y, Nagashima K. Onuf's motoneuron is resistant to poliovirus. J Neurol Sci 1989;93:85–92.

32. Katagiri T, Kuzikai T, Nihei K, Honda K, Sasaki H, Polak M. Immunocytochemical study of Onuf's nucleus in amyotrophic lateral sclerosis. Jpn J Med 1988;17: 23–28.

33. Takahata N, Yamanouchi T, Fukatsu R, et al. Brain stem gliosis in a case with clinical manifestations of amyotrophic lateral sclerosis. Folia Psychiatr Neurol Jpn 1976;30:41–48.

34. Harvey DG, Torack RM, Rosenbaum ME. Amyotrophic lateral sclerosis with ophthalmoplegia: A clinicopathologic study. Arch Neurol 1979;36:615–617.

35. Akiyama KH, Tsutsumi H, Onoda N, et al. An autopsy case of sporadic amyotrophic lateral sclerosis with sensory disturbances and ophthalmoplegia. Byori to Rinshou 1987;5:921–927 (Japanese).

36. Weiner LP. Possible role of androgen receptors in amyotrophic lateral sclerosis. Arch Neurol 1980;37:129–131.

37. Juergens SM, Kurland LT, Okazaki H, Mulder DW. ALS in Rochester, Minnesota 1925–1977. Neurology (NY) 1980;30:463–470.

38. Mulder DW: The clinical syndrome—What does it tell us of etiology? Int Congress ALS, Kyoto Meeting Abstract, 1987:33.

39. Hirano A. Progress in the pathology of motor neuron diseases. Progress in neuropathology, Vol. 2 (Zimmerman H, ed.). NY: Grune & Stratton, 1973:181–215.

40. Shiraki H, Yase Y: Amyotrophic lateral sclerosis in Japan. In: Handbook of clinical neurology, Vol 22, Chapter 16 (Vinken PJ, Bruyn GW, eds. 1975:353–419.

41. Anderson FH, Richardson EP Jr, Okazaki H, et al. Neurofibrillary degeneration on Guam: Frequency in Chamorros with no known neurological disease. Brain 1979;102:65–77.

42. Mandybur TI, Nagpaul AS, Pappas Z, Niklowitz WJ. Alzheimer neurofibrillary changes in subacute sclerosing encephalitis. Ann Neurol 1977;1:103–107.

43. Hammer RP Jr, Tomiyasu U, Scheibel AB. Degeneration the human Betz cell due to amyotrophic lateral sclerosis. Exp Neurol 1979;63:336–346.

44. Carpenter S, Karpati G, Durham H. Dendritic attrition preceeds motor neuron death in amyotrophic lateral sclerosis (ALS). Neurology 1988;38 (Suppl 1):252.

45. Chou SM. Pathognomy of intraneuronal inclusions in ALS: In: Tsubaki T, Toyokura Y, eds. Amyotrophic lateral sclerosis. Tokyo: University of Tokyo Press 1979:135–176.

46. Bunina TL. On intracellular inclusions in familial amyotrophic lateral sclerosis. AH Neuropat Psikhit Korsakov 1962;62:1293–1299.

47. Hirano A. Pathology of amyotrophic lateral sclerosis. In: Gajdusek DC, Gibbs CJ, eds. Slow, latent and template virus infection. Washington, DC: NINDB, 1965: 23–37.

48. Hart MN, Cancilla PA, Frommes S, Hirano A. Anterior horn cell degeneration and

Bunina-type inclusions associated with dementia. Acta Neuropathol (Berl) 1977;38:225–228.

49. Tomonaga M, Saito M, Yoshimura M, Shimada H, Tohgi H. Ultrastructure of the Bunina bodies in anterior horn cells of amyotrophic lateral sclerosis. Acta neuropathol (Berl) 1978;42:81–86.

50. Okamoto K, Hirai S, Marimatsu M, Ishida Y. The Bunina bodies in amyotrophic lateral sclerosis. Neurol Med (Tok) 1980;13:133–141.

51. Wohlfart G, Swank RL. Pathology of amyotrophic lateral sclerosis: Fiber analysis of the ventral roots and pyramidal tracts of the spinal cord. Arch Neurol Psychiatry 1941;46:783–799.

52. Nelson JS, Prensky AL. Sporadic juvenile amyotrophic lateral sclerosis. Arch Neurol 1972;27:300–306.

53. Berry RG, Chambers RA, Duchett S, Terrers R. Clinicopathological study of juvenile amyotrophic lateral sclerosis. Neurology 1969;19:312.

54. Tsujihata M, Hazama R, Ishii N, et al. Ultrastructural localization of acetylcholine receptor at the motor endplate: Myasthenia gravis and other neuromuscular diseases. Neurology (Minneap) 1980;30:1203–1211.

55. Oda M, Akagawa N, Tabuchi Y, Tanabe H. A sporadic juvenile case of the amyotrophic lateral sclerosis with neuronal intracytoplasmic inclusions. Acta Neuropathol (Berl) 1978;44:211–216.

56. Chou SM, Tan N, Kakulas BA. Involvement of anteromedial brainstem pathway in ALS: Its neuropathologic implication. Neurology 1988;36 (Suppl 1):252.

57. Hirano A, Kurland LT, Sayre GP. Familial amyotrophic lateral sclerosis. Arch Neurol 1967;16:232–243.

58. Metcalf CW, Hirano A. Clinicopathological studies of a family with amyotrophic lateral sclerosis. Arch Neurol 1971;24:518–523.

59. Takahashi K, Nakamura H, Okada E. Heredity amyotrophic lateral sclerosis. Arch Neurol (Chic) 1972;27:292–299.

60. Tanaka S, Yase Y, Yoshimasu H. Familial amyotrophic lateral sclerosis. Ultrastructural study of intraneuronal hyaline inclusion material. Adv Neurol Sci 1980;24:386–387.

61. Tanaka J, Nakamura H, Tabuchi Y, Takahashi K. Familial amyotrophic lateral sclerosis: Features of multisystem degeneration. Acta Neuropathol (Berl) 1984;64: 22–29.

62. Delisle MB, Carpenter S. Neurofibrillary axonal swellings amyotrophic lateral sclerosis. J Neurol Sci 1984;63:241–250.

63. Munoz DG, Greene C, Perl DP, Selkol DJ. Accumulation of phosphorylated neurofilaments in anterior horn motoneurons of amyotrophic lateral sclerosis patients. J Neuropathol Exp Neurol 1988;47:9–18.

64. Kuroda S, Kuyama K, Morioka E, Ohtsuki S, Nanba R. Sporadic amyotrophic lateral sclerosis with intracytoplasmic eosinophilic inclusions. A case closely akin to familial ALS. Neurol Cir (Tok) 1986;24:31–37.

65. Kato T, Katagiri T, Hirano A, Sasaki H, Arai S. Sporadic lower motor neuron disease with Lewy body-like inclusions: A new subgroup? Acta Neuropathol 1988;76:208–211.

66. Chou SM. Immunoreactivity of neurofilament epitopes in motor neurons of subacute ALS. J Neuropathol Exp Neurol 1987;46:375.

67. Chou SM. Immunocytochemical characterization of inclusions in motoneurons of subacute ALS. In: Tsubaki T, Yase Y, eds. Kyoto Japan, International conference of amyotrophic lateral sclerosis. 1987:232.

68. Leigh PN, Dodson A, Swash M, Brion JP, Anderton BH. Cytoskeletal abnormalities in motor neuron disease. Brain 1989;112:521–535.

69. Leigh PN, Anderson BH, Dodson A, Gallo JM, Swash M, Power DM. Ubiquitin deposits in anterior horn cells in motor neuron disease. Neurol Lett 1988;93: 197–203.

70. Lowe J, Lennox G, Jefferson D, Morrell K, Maguire D, Gray T, Landon M, Doherty FJ, Mayer RJ. A filamentous inclusion body within anterior horn neurons in motor neuron disease defined by immunocytochemical localization of ubiquitin. Neurosci Lett 1988;94:203–210.

71. Chou SM. Motoneuron inclusions in ALS are heavily ubiquitinated. J Neuropathol Exp Neurol 1988;47:334.

72. Murayama S, Ookawa Y, Nori H, et al. Immunocytochemical and ultrastructural study of Lewy body–like hyaline inclusions in familial ALS. Acta Neuropathol 1989;78:143–152.

73. Murayama S, Mori H, Ihara Y, Bouldin TW, Suzuki K, Tomonaga M. Immunocytochemical and ultrastructural studies of lower motor neurons in amyotrophic lateral sclerosis. Ann Neurol 1990;27:137–148.

74. Kato T, Katagiri T, Hirano A, Kawanami T, Sasaki H. Lewy body–like hyaline inclusions in sporadic motor neuron disease are ubiquitinated. Acta Neuropathol (Berl) 1989;77:391–396.

75. Sasaki S, Kamei H, Yamane K, Murayama S. Swellings of neuronal processes in motor neuron disease. Neurology 1988;38:1114–1118.

76. Schochet SS, Hardman JM, Ludwig PP, Earle KM. Intraneuronal conglomerates in sporadic motor neuron disease: Light and electron microscopy. Arch Neurol 1969;20:548–553.

77. Hughes JT, Jerrome D. Ultrastructure of anterior motor neurons in the Hirano-Kurland-Sayre type of combined neurological system degeneration. J Neurol Sci 1981;13:389–399.

78. Kondo A, Iwaki T, Tateishi J, Kirimotok K, Miromoto T, Oomura I. Accumulation of neurofilaments in a sporadic case of amyotrophic lateral sclerosis. Jpn J Psychiatr Neurol 1986;40:677–684.

79. Kurisaki H, Ihara Y, Nukina N, Toyokura Y. Immunocytochemical study of ALS spinal cords using an antiserum to 22 K-peptide of neurofilament and antibodies to tubulin. Clin Neurol 1983;23:1013.

80. Mannetto V, Sternberger NH, Perry G, Sternberger LA, Gambetti P. Phosphorylation of neurofilaments is altered in amyotrophic lateral sclerosis. J Neuropathol Exp Neurol 1988;47:642–653.

81. Chou SM. Selective involvement of both upper and lower motoneurons in (B-B′-iminodipropionitrile) intoxicated monkeys. J Neuropathol Exp Neurol 1983;42: 309.

82. Carpenter S. Proximal axonal enlargement in motor neuron diseases. Neurology (Minneap) 1968;18:841–851.
83. Chou SM, Martin JD, Gutrecht JA, et al. Axonal balloons in subacute motor neuron disease. J Neuropathol Exp Neurol 1970;29:141–142.
84. Sasaki S, Yamane K, Sakuma H, Maruyama S. Sporadic motor neuron disease with Lewy body-like hyaline inclusions. Acta Neuropathol 1989;78:555–560.
85. Sasaki S, Murayama S, Yamane K, Sakuma H, Takeishi M. Swelling of proximal axons in a case of motor neuron disease. Ann Neurol 1989;25:520–522.
86. Chou SM, Klein R. Autoradiographic studies of protein turnover in motor neurons of IDPN-treated rats. Acta Neuropathol 1972;22:183–189.
87. Kuzuhara S, Chou SM. Retrograde axonal transport of HRP in IDPN-induced axonopathy. J Neuropathol Exp Neurol 1981;40:300.
88. Gambetti P, Shecket G, Ghetti B, Hirano A, Dahl D. Neurofibrillary changes in human brain: An immunocytochemical study with a neurofilament antiserum. J Neuropathol Exp Neurol 1983;42:69.
89. Schmidt ML, Carden MJ, Lee V M-Y, Trojanowski JQ. Phosphate dependent and independent neurofilament epitopes in the axonal swelling of patients with motor neuron disease and controls. Lab Invest 1987;56:282–294.
90. Dickson DW, Yen SH, Suzuki KI, Davies P, Garcia JH, Hirarro A. Ballooned neurons in selective neurodegenerative disease contain phosphorylated neurofilament epitopes. Acta Neuropathol (Berl) 1986;71:216–223.
91. Swash M, Scholtz CL, Vowles G, Aingram D. Selective and asymmetric vulnerability of corticospinal and spinocerebellar tracts in motor neuron disease. J Neurol Neurosurg Psychiatry 1988;51:785–789.
92. Kojewnikoff A. Cas de sclérose amyotrophique La degenerescence de foisceaux pyramidaux se propgeant u transers tout éncéphale. Arch Neurol Sci 1883;6:357.
93. Hirayama K, Tsubaki T, Toyokura, Okinaka S. The representation of the pyramidal tract in the internal capsule and basis pendunculi. Neurology (Minneap) 1962;12:337–342.
94. Dejerine J. Anatomie des Centres Nerveux. Paris rueff 1901;II(1):128–137, 232–235.
95. Chou SM, Kuzuhara S, Gibbs CJ JR., Gajdusek DC. Giant axonal spheroids along corticospinal tracts in a case of Guamanian ALS. J Neuropathol Exp Neurol 1980;39:345.
96. Chou SM, Huang TE. Giant axonal spheroids in internal capsules of amyotrophic lateral sclerosis brains revisited. Ann Neurol 1988;24:168.
97. Tsukagoshi H, Yanagisawa N, Ogucki K, et al. Morphometric quantitation of the cervical limb motor cells in controls and in amyotrophic lateral sclerosis. J Neurol Sci 1979;41:287–297.
98. Sobue G, Sahashi K, Takahashi A, et al. Degenerating compartment and functioning compartment of motor neuron loss. Neurology (Cleve) 1983;33:654–657.
99. Dyck RJ, Stevens JC, Mulder DW, et al. Frequency of nerve fiber degeneration of peripheral motor and sensory neurons in amyotrophic lateral sclerosis: Morphometry of deep and superficial peroneal nerve. Neurology (Minneap) 1975;25:781–785.

100. Hayashi H, Nagashima K, Urano Y, Iwata M. Spinocerebellar degeneration with prominent involvement of the motor neuron system: Autopsy report of a sporadic case. Acta Neuropathol 1986;70:82–85.

101. Tabuchi TK, Takahashi K, Tananka J. Familial ALS with ophthalmoplegia. Clin Neurol 1983;23:278–287 (Japanese).

102. Engel KW, Kurland LT, Latzo I. An inherited disease similar to amyotrophic lateral sclerosis with a pattern of posterior column involvement. An intermediate form. Brain 1959;82:203–220.

103. Tanaka J, Nakamura H, Tabuchi Y, Takahashi K. Familial amyotrophic lateral sclerosis: Features of multisystem degeneration. Acta Neuropathol (Berl) 1984;64: 22–29.

104. Page RW, Moskowicz RW, Nash RE, Roesmann U. Lower motor neuron disease with spinocerebellar degeneration. Ann Neurol 1977;2:524–527.

105. Averback P, Crocker P. Abnormal proximal axons of Clarke's columns in sporadic motor neuron disease. Can J Neurol Sci 1981;8:173–175.

106. Averback P, Crocker P. Regular involvement of Clarke's nucleus in sporadic amyotrophic lateral sclerosis. Arch Neurol 1982;39:155–156.

107. Takasu T, Mizutani T, Sakamaki S, Tsuchiya N, Kamei S, Kohzu H. An autopsy case of sporadic amyotrophic lateral sclerosis with degeneration of the spinocerebellar tracts and the posterior column. Ann Rep Neurodig Dis Res Committee in Japan, 1985:94–100.

108. Okamoto K, Yamazaki T, Yamaguchi H, Shooji M, Hirai S. Pathology of Clarke's nucleus in sporadic amyotrophic lateral sclerosis. Clin Neurol 1988;28:536–542.

109. Williams C, Kozlowski MA, Hinton DR, Miller CA. Degeneration of spinocerebellar neurons in amyotrophic lateral sclerosis. Ann Neurol 1990;27:215–225.

110. Hayashi H, Kato S. Total manifestations of amyotrophic lateral sclerosis: ALS in the totally locked-in state. J Neurol Sci 1989;93:19–35.

111. Mulder DW. Motor neuron disease. In: Dyck RJ, et al., eds. Peripheral neuropathy, Chapter 38. Philadelphia: Saunders, 1975:709–770.

112. Malamud N. Amyotrophic lateral sclerosis. In: Minckley J, ed. Neuromuscular disease, pathology of nervous system, Vol 1. 1968:712–725.

113. Kawamura Y, Dyck PJ, Shimono M, et al. Morphometric comparison of the vulnerability of peripheral motor and sensory neurons in amyotrophic lateral sclerosis. J Neuropathol Exp Neurol 1981;40:667–675.

114. Davidoff RA. The dorsal columns. Neurology 1989;39:1377–1385.

115. Bogaert L van, Martin L, Martin J. Sclérose latérale amyotrophique avec dégénerescence spinocérébelleuse et délire épileptique. Acta Neurol Psychiatr Belg 1965;65:845–872.

116. Kosaka K, Mehrein P. Myotrophische Lateralsklerose kombiriert mit Degeneration in Thalmus und der Substania nigra. Acta Neuropathol (Berl) 1978;44:241–244.

117. Bonduell M. Amyotrophic lateral sclerosis. In: Vinken PJ, Bruyn GW, eds. Handbook of clinical neurology, Vol 22, Chapter 13. Amsterdam: North-Holland, 1975: 281–338.

118. Serratrice GT, Toga M, Pellisier JF. Chronic spinal muscular atrophy and pallidonigral degeneration: Report of a case. Neurology 1983;33:306–310.

119. Smith M. Nerve fiber degeneration in the brain in amyotrophic lateral sclerosis. J Neurol Neurosurg Psychiatry 1960;23:269–282.

120. Oppenheimer DR. Diseases of the basal ganglia, cerebellum, and motor neurons. In: Adams JH, Corsellis JAN, Duchen LW, eds. Greenfields neuropathology, 4th ed. 1984:699–747.

121. Horton WA, Eldridge R, Brody JA. Familial motor neuron disease: Evidence for at least three different types. Neurology 1976;26:460–465.

122. Power JM, Horoupian DS, Shaumburg HH, Wetherbee AL. Documentation of a neurological disease in a Vermont family 90 years later. J Can Sci Neurol 1974; 1(2):139–140.

123. Kurland LT, Brody JA. Amyotrophic lateral sclerosis Guam type. In: Vinken PJ, Bruyn GW, eds. Handbook of clinical neurology, Vol 22, Chapter 14, 1975: 339–351.

124. Tan N, Kakulas BA, Masters CL, et al. Observation on the clinical presentation and the neuropathological findings of ALS in Australia and Guam. In: ALS in Asia and Oceana: Proc 6th Asian and Oceanian Congress of Neurol ALS Workshop, 1984:31–40.

125. Younger DS, Chou SM, Hays AP, et al. Primary lateral sclerosis: A clinical diagnosis re-emerges. Arch Neurol 1988;45:1304–1307.

126. Behan WMH, Maia M. Strümpell's familial spastic paraplegia: Genesis and neuropathology. J Neurol Neurosurg Psychiatry 1974;37:8–20.

127. Harding AE. Classification of the hereditary ataxias and paraplegias. Lancet 1983;1:1151–1155.

128. Strümpell A. Beiträge zur Pathologie der Rückermarks. Arch Psychiatr Nervenkrank 1880;10:676–717.

129. Strümpell A. Über eine bestimmte Form der primaren kombinierten systemerkrankung des Rückenmarks. Arch Psychiatr Nervenkrank 1886;17:227–238.

130. Strümpell A. Die primäre Seitenstrangsklerose (spastische Spinalparalyse). Deutsch Zeit Nervenheilk 1904;27:291–339.

131. Schwartz GA, Liu C-N. Hereditary (familial) spastic paraplegia. Arch Neurol Psychiatry 1956;75:144–162.

132. Hirano A, Llena JF, Streifler M, Cohn DF. Anterior horn cell changes in a case of neurolathyrism. Acta Neuropathol (Berl) 1976;35:277–283.

133. Zülich KJ: Pyramidal and parapyramidal systems in man. In: Zülich KJ, Creutzfeldt O, Galbraith GC, eds. Cerebral localization. An Otfrid Foerster Symposium. Berlin-New York-Heidelberg: Springer-Verlag, 1975:32–47.

134. MacKay RP. Course and prognosis in amyotrophic lateral sclerosis. Arch Neurol (Chic) 1963;8:117–127.

7

Fine Structural Study of Sporadic and Familial Amyotrophic Lateral Sclerosis

Asao Hirano and Shuichi Kato

Montefiore Medical Center and Albert Einstein College of Medicine
Bronx, New York

INTRODUCTION

This chapter reviews the characteristic fine structural features of the anterior horns of cases of either sporadic or familial amyotrophic lateral sclerosis (ALS). Chromatolytic neurons, Bunina bodies, and spheroids observed in sporadic ALS will be described, as will be the Lewy body–like inclusions and cordlike swollen neuronal processes characteristic of familial ALS with posterior column and spinocerebellar tract involvement.

PATHOLOGY OF ANTERIOR HORNS

The significant pathology of the anterior horns in ALS has long been known to involve the loss of motoneurons and the atrophy of remaining neurons. However, detailed investigation of an ALS case with a short clinical course revealed certain identifiable early pathological alterations of the disease, including chromatolytic neurons, Bunina bodies, and spheroids (1). Thereafter, these changes were observed in many other cases of ALS (2).

The fine structural study of chromatolytic neurons demonstrates the dispersion and diminution of the characteristic well-developed stacks of rough endoplasmic reticulum (3,4). In some chromatolytic neurons there are abnormal accumulations of 10-nm neurofilaments as well as of dense bodies, lipofuscin granules, and mitochondria (5,6).

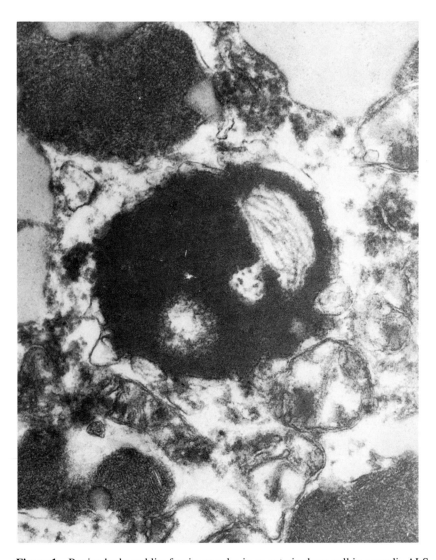

Figure 1   Bunina body and lipofuscin granules in an anterior horn cell in sporadic ALS.
× 33,000.

Bunina bodies are small eosinophilic granules found in anterior horn neurons
in ALS (7,8). They consist of irregularly shaped accumulations of dense, granular material with vesicular rims. They have no limiting membrane. Small islands of 10-nm neurofilaments or other cytoplasmic components are sometimes
found in the interior (Fig. 1). Their border is associated with cytoplasmic or-

ganelles, including vesicles, endoplasmic reticulum, mitochondria, etc. (3,4,9–11). The simultaneous presence of annulate lamellae was reported in the same neuron (12,13). Some workers have considered autophagic vacuoles as Bunina bodies (9,14).

Several eosinophilic granules showing a different fine structure are also seen in anterior horn neurons of non-ALS patients. They include certain lipid granules, altered mitochondria, accumulations of certain crystalloids, Hirano bodies, and distended rough endoplasmic reticulum (15) as well as other structures (16,17).

Spheroids are argentophilic bodies larger than 20 μ in diameter within the axons of lower motor neurons (18). They consist of the accumulation of interwoven bundles of 10-nm neurofilaments with characteristic side arms (1,3,4) (Fig. 2). Scattered mitochondria, vesicles, and fragments of smooth endoplasmic reticulum are commonly found among the bundles of neurofilaments.

The connection between the spheroid and the cell body is difficult to demonstrate in most ALS cases although it has been shown in a few cases of motor neuron disease (18,19). In one case of lower motor neuron disease, the spheroids were shown to be focal swellings of proximal axons, particularly in the distal portion of the initial segment and in the first internode of the myelinated axons (19,20). In addition, spheroids are found in the perikarya of some anterior horn cells as well as in the myelinated axons (3,21).

The pattern of filamentous accumulation in spheroids is not unique to ALS. Similar accumulations of 10-nm neurofilaments have been observed in a variety of different conditions unrelated to ALS in both experimental animals (22–28) and humans (29–32).

The familial cases of ALS show at least two major pathological forms (33). One of them is accompanied by posterior column and spinocerebellar tract involvement (33–35). Investigation of two cases of the "C" family and another case with this form of familial ALS showed two characteristic alterations of anterior horn neurons: intracytoplasmic Lewy body–like hyaline inclusions and cordlike swollen neuronal processes (33,36,37). These two alterations were also found in other cases of familial ALS with posterior column and spinocerebellar tract involvement (35,38,39).

The fine structural study of the "C" family reveals that in contrast to the spheroids composed of interwoven bundles of neurofilaments mentioned above, the cordlike swollen neuronal processes are filled with neurofilaments that run parallel to the long axis of the processes (40) (Fig. 3). Dense structures are sometimes observed within the large parallel bundles of neurofilaments. They are composed of ill-defined dense, granular and fibrillar materials (40) (Fig. 4).

Lewy body–like hyaline inclusions consist of focal accumulations of randomly oriented 10-nm neurofilaments intermingled with ill-defined coarse linear structures associated with dense granules (40). These granule-associated linear

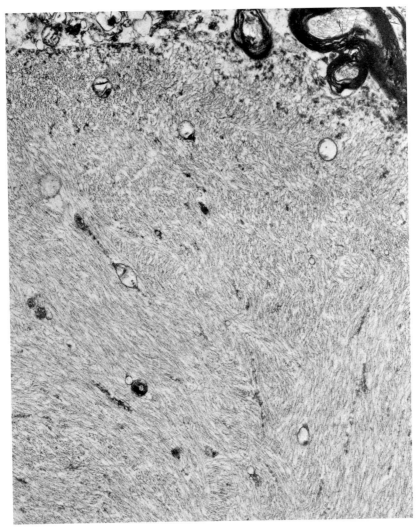

Figure 2   Portion of a spheroid in an anterior horn in sporadic ALS, showing prominent interwoven bundles of neurofilaments intermingled with scattered organelles. × 10,000.

structures may be identical to the dense structures within the cordlike swollen neuronal processes.

Many similar inclusions are seen in rare cases of sporadic lower motor neuron disease (14,41–44) and sporadic ALS (6,14). Accumulation of granule-associated linear structures identical to those shown in the inclusions and in the swollen

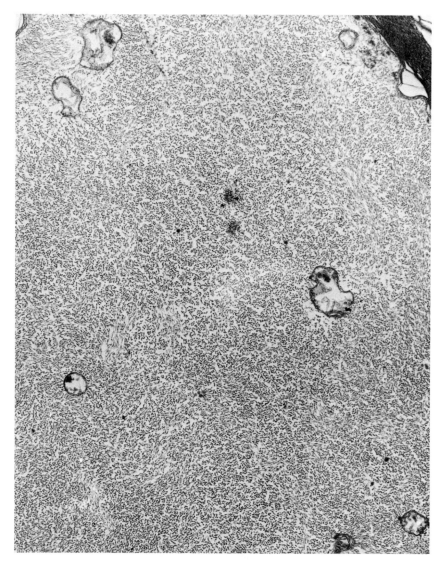

Figure 3 Cross-section of a cordlike swollen axon in the anterior horn containing parallel compactly arranged neurofilaments in familial ALS with posterior column and spinocerebellar tract involvement. Compare to Figure 2. ×20,000.

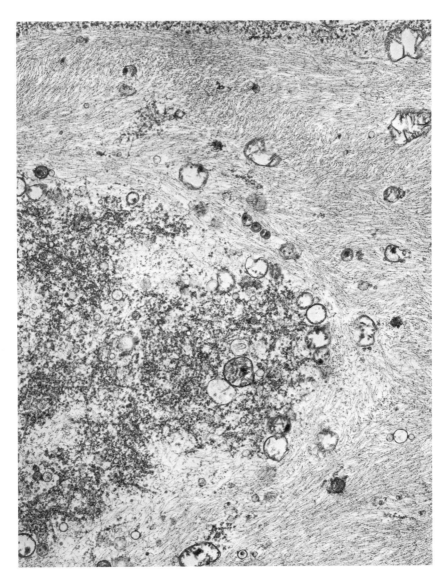

Figure 4   Area of dense structure, corresponding to a Lewy body–like inclusion surrounded by abundant neurofilaments and scattered mitochondria in familial ALS with posterior column and spinocerebellar tract involvement. × 15,000.

processes in familial ALS with posterior column and spinocerebellar tract involvement may also be observed in some of these cases. Furthermore, although it is rare, essentially identical granule-associated linear structures have been observed in a few cases of sporadic classical ALS (21). Therefore, the granule-associated linear structures are apparently not a specific alteration of familial ALS. Recently, positive immunoreactivity to antiubiquitin antibody has been reported in similar granule-associated fibrillary structures in several cases of familial ALS (39).

Another characteristic feature of ALS is the basophilic inclusions in juvenile cases (14,45). The fine structure of the inclusion consisted of ribosome-associated linear structures (45).

PATHOLOGY OF THE SKIN

Aside from the alterations in the anterior horns, the pathology of the skin has recently been described in several cases of ALS by Ono et al. (46). Electron microscopy revealed that the collagen fibers became thinner as the disease progressed, and that the collagen bundles were separated by much more amorphous materials (46). The amorphous material was shown to be composed of band "g" by two-dimensional gel electrophoresis (47). These fine structural findings were not observed either in controls (46) or in spinal muscular atrophy (48). The authors stated that these alterations of the skin might be unique and characteristic to ALS.

ACKNOWLEDGMENT

We are grateful to Dr. H. M. Dembitzer for reviewing the manuscript.

REFERENCES

1. Inoue K, Hirano A. Early pathological changes of amyotrophic lateral sclerosis. Autopsy findings of a case of 10 months' duration. Neurol Med (Tok) 1979;11: 448–455.
2. Nakano I, Donnenfeld H, Hirano A. A neuropathological study of amyotrophic lateral sclerosis. With special reference to central chromatolysis and spheroid in the spinal anterior horn and some pathological changes of the motor cortex. Neurol Med (Tok) 1983;18:136–144.
3. Hirano A, Inoue K. Early pathological changes of amyotrophic lateral sclerosis. Electron microscopic study of chromatolysis, spheroids and Bunina bodies. Neurol Med (Tok) 1980;13:148–160.
4. Hirano A. Aspect of the ultrastructure of amyotrophic lateral sclerosis. In: Rowland LP, ed. Advances in neurology, Vol. 36. Human motor neuron diseases. New York: Raven Press, 1982:75–88.

5. Hirano A, Donnenfeld H, Sasaki S, Nakano I, BArtfeld H. The fine structure of motor neuron disease. In: Rose FC, ed. Research progress in motor neuron disease. London: Pitman, 1984:328–348.

6. Kusaka H, Imai T, Hashimoto S, Yamamoto T, Maya K, Yamasaki M. Ultrastructural study of chromatolytic neurons in an adult-onset sporadic case of amyotrophic lateral sclerosis. Acta Neuropathol 1988;75:523–528.

7. Bunina TL. On intracellular inclusions in familial amyotrophic lateral sclerosis. Korsakov J Neuropathol Psychiatry 1962;62:1293.

8. Hirano A. Pathology of amyotrophic lateral sclerosis. In: Gajdusek DC, Gibbs CJ Jr, Alpers M, eds. Slow, latent, and temperate virus infections. NINDB monograph No. 2. Washington, DC: US Department of Health, Education, and Welfare, 1965: 23.

9. Hart MN, Cancilla PA, Frommes S, Hirano A. Anterior horn cell degeneration and Bunina-type inclusions associated with dementia. Acta Neuropathol 1977;38:225–228.

10. Asbury AK, Johnson PC. Pathology of the peripheral nerve. Philadelphia: Saunders, 1978:250.

11. Sasaki S, Hirano A, Donnenfeld H, Nakano I. An electron microscopic study of Bunina bodies. Neurol Med (Tok) 1983;19:317–324.

12. Tomonaga M, Saito M, Yoshimura M, Shimada H, Tohgi H. Ultrastructure of the Bunina bodies in anterior horn cells of amyotrophic lateral sclerosis. Acta Neuropathol 1978;42:81–86.

13. Okamoto K, Hirai S, Morimatsu M, Ishida Y. The Bunina bodies in amyotrophic lateral sclerosis. Neurol Med (Tok) 1980;13:133–1411.

14. Chou SM. Pathognomoy of intraneuronal inclusions in ALS. In: Tsubaki T, Toyokura Y, eds. Amyotrophic lateral sclerosis. Baltimore: University Park Press, 1979:135–176.

15. Hirano A. Neurons, astrocytes, and ependyma. In: Davis RL, Robertson DM (eds). Textbook of neuropathology. Baltimore: Williams & Wilkins, 1985:1–91.

16. Hirano A, Llena JF, Streifler M, Cohn DF. Anterior horn cell changes in a case of neurolathyrism. Acta Neuropathol 1976;35:277–283.

17. Sasaki S, Hirano A. Observation of Bunina-like bodies in anterior horn cells. Neurol Med (Tok) 1984;20:39–45.

18. Carpenter S. Proximal axonal enlargement in motor neuron disease. Neurology 1968;18:842–851.

19. Sasaki S, Maruyama S, Yamane K, Sakuma H, Takeishi M. Swellings of proximal axons in a case of motor neuron disease. Ann Neurol 1989;25:520–522.

20. Sasaki S, Kamei H, Yamane K, Maruyama S. Swelling of neuronqal processes in motor neuron disease. Neurology 1988;38:1114–1118.

21. Hirano A, Donnenfeld H, Sasaki S, Nakano I. Fine structural observations of neurofilamentous changes in amyotropohic lateral sclerosis. J Neuropathol Exp Neurol 1984;43:461–470.

22. Chou SM, Hartmann HA. Axonal lesions and waltzing syndrome after IDPN administration in rats with a concept "axostasis." Acta Neuropathol 1964;3:428–450.

23. Chou SM, Hartmann HA. Electron microscopy of focal neuroaxonal lesions pro-

duced by β-β'-iminodipropionitrile (IDPN) in rats. I. The advanced lesions. Acta Neuropathol 1965;4:590–603.

24. Griffin JW, Price DL. Proximal axonopathies induced by toxic chemicals. In: Spencer PS, Schaumburg HH, eds. Experimental and clinical neurotoxicology. Baltimore: Williams & Wilkins, 1980:161–178.

25. Cork LC, Griffin JW, Choy C, Padula CA, Price DL. Pathology of motor neurons in accelerated hereditary canine spinal muscular atrophy. Lab Invest 1982;46:89–99.

26. Higgins RJ, Rings DM, Fenner WR, Stevenson S. Spontaneous lower motor neuron disease with neurofibrillary accumulation in young pigs. Acta Neuropathol 1983;59:288–294.

27. Anthony DC, Giangaspero F, Graham DG. The spatio-temporal pattern of the axonopathy associated with the neurotoxicity of 3,4-dimethyl-2,5-hexanedione in the rat. J Neuropathol Exp Neurol 1983;42:548–560.

28. Troncoso JC, Price DL, Griffin JW, Parhad IM. Neurofibrillary axonal pathology in aluminum intoxication. Ann Neurol 1982;12:278–283.

29. Sasaki S, Okamoto K, Hirano A. An electron microscopic study of small argyrophilic bodies in the human spinal cord. Neurol Med (Tok) 1982;17:570–576.

30. Clark AW, Parhad IM, Griffin JW, Price DL. Neurofilamentous axonal swellings in the lumbosacral spinal cord of normal man. J Neuropathol Exp Neurol 1982;41:379 (Abstract).

31. Kusaka H, Hirano A. Fine structure of anterior horns in patients without amyotrophic lateral slerosis. J Neuropathol Exp Neurol 1985;44:430–438.

32. Shintaku M, Hirano A, Llena JF. Some unusual ultrastructural changes in the neuronal processes and somata of the spinal cord in chronic multiple sclerosis. J Clin Electron Microsc 1989;22:177–182.

33. Hirano A, Kurland LT, Sayre GP. Familial amyotrophic lateral sclerosis. A subgroup characterized by posterior and spinocerebellar tract involvement and hyaline inclusions in the anterior horn cells. Arch Neurol 1967;16:232–243.

34. Engel WK, Kurland LT, Klatzo I. An inherited disease similar to amyotrophic lateral sclerosis with a pattern of posterior column involvement. An intermediate form? Brain 1959;82:203–220.

35. Takahashi K, Nakamura H, Okada E. Hereditary amyotrophic lateral sclerosis. Histochemical and electron microscopic study of hyaline inclusions in motor neurons. Arch Neurol 1972;27:292–299.

36. Nakano I, Hirano A, Kurland LT, Mulder DW, Holley PW, Saccomonno G. Familial amyotrophic lateral sclerosis: Neuropathology of two brothers in American "C" family. Neurol Med (Tok) 1984;20:458–471.

37. Kato T, Hirano A, Kurland LT. Asymmetric involvement of the spinal cord involving both large and small anterior horn cells in a case of familial amyotrophic lateral sclerosis. Clin Neuropathol 1987;6:67–70.

38. Tanaka S, Yase Y, Yoshimasu H. Familial amyotrophic lateral sclerosis. Ultrastructural study of intraneuronal hyaline inclusion material. Adv Neurol Sci (Tok) 1980;24:386–387 (Abstract).

39. Murayama S, Ookawa Y, Mori H, Nakano I, Ihara Y, Kuzuhara S, Tomonaga M.

Immunocytochemical and ultrastructural study of Lewy body–like hyaline inclusions in familial amyotrophic lateral sclerosis. Acta Neuropathol 1989;78:143–152.

40. Hirano A, Nakano I, Kurland LT, Mulder DW, Holley PW, Saccomanno G. Fine structural study of neurofibrillary changes in a family with amyotrophic lateral sclerosis. J Neuropathol Exp Neurol 1984;43:471–480.

41. Kuroda S, Kuyama K, Morioka E, Ohtsuki S, Namba R. Sporadic amyotrophic lateral sclerosis with intracytoplasmic eosinophilic inclusions. A case closely akin to familial ALS. Med (Tok) 1986;24:31–37.

42. Mizusawa H, Hirano A. Lower motor neuron disease associated with a focal onion bulb formation in an anterior spinal root. Neurol Med (Tok) 1987;26:309–311.

43. Kato T, Katagiri T, Hirano A, Sasaki H, Arai S. Sporadic lower motor neuron disease with Lewy body–like inclusions: A new subgroup? Acta Neuropathol 1988;76:208–211.

44. Sasaki S, Yamane K, Sakuma H, Maruyama S. Sporadic motor neuron disease with Lewy body–like hyaline inclusions. Acta Neuropathol 1989;78:555–560.

45. Oda M, Akagawa N, Tabuchi Y, Tanabe H. A sporadic juvenile case of the amyotrophic lateral sclerosis with neuronal intracytoplasmic inclusions. Acta Neuropathol 1978;44:211–216.

46. Ono S, Toyokura Y, Mannen T, Ishibashi Y. Amyotrophic lateral sclerosis: Histologic, histochemical, and ultrastructural abnormalities of skin. Neurology 1986;36:948–956.

47. Ono S, Hashimoto K, Shimizu T, Mannen T, Toyokura Y. Amyotrophic lateral sclerosis: Electrophoretic study of amorphous material of skin. J Neurol Sci (in press).

48. Ono S, Mannen T, Toyokura Y. Differential diagnosis between amyotrphic lateral sclerosis and spinal muscular atrophy by skin involvement. J Neurol Sci 1989;91:301–310.

8

Pathology—Muscle and Nerve

Mark R. Glasberg*

Henry Ford Hospital
Detroit, Michigan

Clayton A. Wiley

University of California—San Diego
La Jolla, California

MUSCLE BIOPSY

Amyotrophic lateral sclerosis (ALS) is diagnosed on the basis of a typical history and physical examination. Electromyographic (EMG) examination is performed in order to confirm the clinical impression. Therefore, the need for a muscle biopsy in order to make a diagnosis of ALS occurs only infrequently.

However, muscle biopsy in the evaluation of ALS patients is useful in confirming involvement of the lower motor neuron. In choosing a muscle to biopsy, one should either evaluate for extent of disease, such as biopsying the quadriceps muscle, in a patient with prominent weakness, atrophy, and fasiculations in the upper extremities, or biopsying a moderately weak muscle, to rule out disorders that can mimic a motor neuron disease, such as inclusion body myositis or a mixed myopathic-neuropathic disorder. The latter two, predominantly myopathic disorders, may present at times like a spinal muscular atrophy, with diffuse, often asymmetrical, muscle weakness, without upper motor neuron signs.

In addition, muscle biopsy can exclude the possibility of vasculitis, which on rare occasions may clinically resemble ALS. Also, it is helpful in differentiating between cervical spondylosis and ALS. In patients with diffuse weakness and atrophy of the upper extremities, denervation atrophy in a quadriceps muscle biopsy, even at a time that the quadriceps is clinically and electrically uninvolved, helps substantiate a diagnosis of ALS rather than cervical spondylosis.

Present affiliation: Riverside Methodist Hospital, Columbus, Ohio.

One should, in general, not biopsy a muscle that has advanced atrophy and fasiculations or has marked denervation by EMG criteria, since that invariably just confirms neurogenic changes. In ALS, there are almost always pathological abnormalities of any muscle biopsied, whether or not clinical weakness is apparent (1).

DENERVATION AND ITS PATHOLOGICAL FEATURES

Many disease processes lead to denervation of skeletal muscle. The only feature they have in common is that they adversely affect the lower motor neuron somewhere between its cell body in the anterior horn of the spinal cord and the neuromuscular junction. The changes that occur in the muscle biopsy can be identified as neuropathic; however, the changes are nonspecific in the sense that the specific neuropathy cannot be identified. Lesions of the upper motor neuron do not cause changes of denervation, but may result in nonspecific disuse atrophy. Often, however, the rate of involvement or chronicity of a neurogenic disease can be predicted on the basis of a muscle biopsy. In ALS, although the changes of denervation atrophy are nonspecific, usually denervation is quite marked in comparison to reinnervation.

Denervating diseases can strike the neuron at various levels. The lower motor neuron has extensively branching axons and the motor unit may contain as many as 2000 fibers in the same muscle. If the neuron is destroyed at the level of the cell body, as in polio myelitis, all the muscle fibers innervated by the neuron become denervated. Much more commonly, however, is the occurrence of a given motor unit incompletely denervated in a random fashion, such as occurs in ALS. This is because the lesion occurs either in branches of the axon at varying distances from the cell body or because the cell body has a sublethal insult and cannot support its entire motor unit (2). When a given muscle fiber is no longer innervated by its motor neuron, it becomes atrophic and has an angular appearance.

Initially the process is extremely random, but if it is relentless as in ALS, adjacent fibers eventually become denervated as more and more fibers become atrophic and the angular atrophic fibers appear in small groups. The denervated fibers, in contrast to fiber-type atrophy, are dark with NADH-TR (3) or nonspecific esterase reactions (Fig. 1) (4), whether the fibers are type I or type II with the ATPase stain.

Since the patterns remain constant under pathological conditions, the ATPase reaction is more reliable for fiber typing (5). As standard neuropathic conditions generally affect both type I and type II fibers, atrophy confined to one fiber type suggests a process other than denervation. For an individual fiber, the end-stage of this process may be atrophy so extreme that the sarcoplasm is barely recognizable in cross-section. The fiber may consist of clusters of pyknotic nuclei,

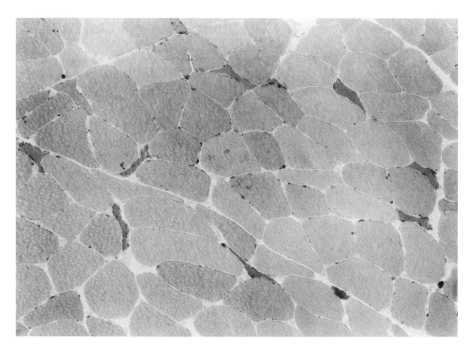

Fig. 1 Esterase-positive angular atrophic fibers. Nonspecific esterase. × 200.

attached by tiny portions of sarcoplasm that are almost completely absent of myofibrils. These pyknotic nuclear clumps are easily recognizable in hematoxylin and eosin stains. As denervation progresses, the angular atrophic fibers tend to become arranged in first small and then large groups (Fig. 2) and remaining fibers may become hypertrophed, often showing evidence of fiber splitting. In about 30–40% of cases of denervation, occasional fibers undergo a peculiar type of alteration in the central portion of the fiber, known as a target fiber (Fig. 3) (6). This consists of decreased staining in the central portion of the fiber, with an increased oxidative rim around the area of pallor. At this early stage the myofibrils may remain intact; therefore, the only way the fibers may be consistenly identified is with an oxidative enzyme reaction such as NADH-TR. As the central portion of the fiber continues to degenerate and the myofibrils become disorganized, the abnormality can be recognized with other stains, including modified Gomori trichrome and nonspecific esterase, and ATPase reactions. Target fibers occur virtually always in type I fibers. Fibers that are similar, but do not have the ring of increased oxidative activity, are called targetoid fibers (7) (Fig. 3). These also involve type I fibers but they are less specific for neuropathic

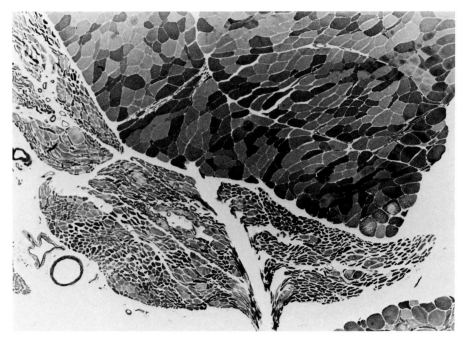

Figure 2 Large grouped atrophy. ATPase, pH 9.4. ×40.

diseases. The targetoid fiber is identical to a central core. However, in central core disease many more fibers are involved.

The third pattern seen in neuropathies is changes in fiber distribution. Under normal circumstances there is a checkerboard configuration to the fiber-type distribution. In the biceps or quadriceps muscle, about one-third of the fibers are type I, one-third type IIa, and one-third type IIB. In denervating conditions, there is a secondary process of a reinnervation through collateral sprouting of new nerve endings from regenerating nerve fibers (8). If the new nerve sprout is the same fiber type as the previous nerve, the muscle fiber will maintain its staining characteristic. However, if the new nerve is a different type, the muscle fiber will change its staining properties to that of the new type. When there is a chronic process of denervation with reinnervation, surviving motor units become fewer and larger, a phenomenon long recognized by the electromyographer. As the process continues, the muscle fibers in a given area tend to acquire the same fiber type because the motor units are enlarging and a given neuron is taking over all the fibers. This leads to a change in distribution pattern of the fiber, known as "fiber-type grouping" (Fig. 4) (9). These fibers show no other abnormality to indicate that a denervating condition is going on, and no signs of denervation will

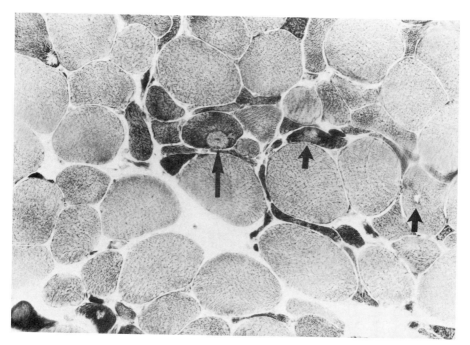

Figure 3 Target fiber (large arrow) and targetoid fiber (small arrows). NADH-TR. ×200.

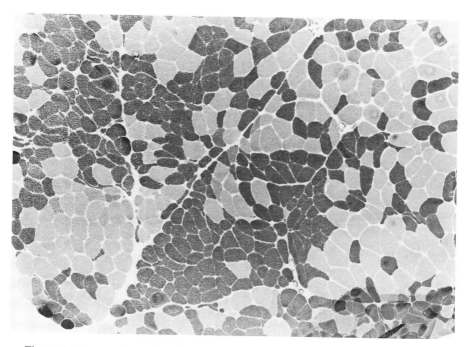

Figure 4 Groups of type I and type II fibers. ATPase, pH 9.4. ×200.

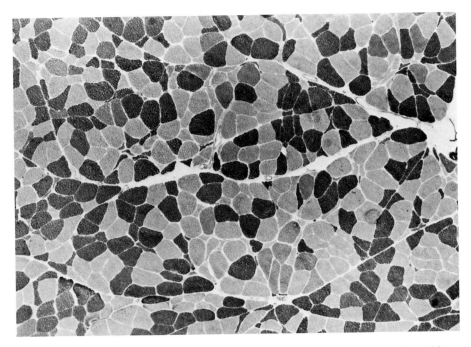

Figure 5 Small groups or clusters of type I and type II fibers. ATPase pH 9.4. × 100.

be detected with routine stains, if reinnervation is keeping place with denervation. With histochemical stains such as ATPase, however, this distribution abnormality is striking and is pathognomonic for a neuropathic process. When the disease is rapidly progressive, as in ALS, the pace of denervation is faster than reinnervation and eventually those initially reinnervated become denervated, resulting in groups of angular atrophic fibers. Generally, when fiber-type grouping occurs in ALS, there are small or incomplete groups of fiber types (Fig. 5).

Occasionally in ALS, there are "myopathic" changes in addition to the characteristic findings of denervation. These consist of degenerating, regenerating, and necrotic fibers, and eventually focal increase in endomesial connective tissue (3) (Fig. 6). These patients often have moderate elevations in creatinine phosphokinase determinations, reflecting the injury and breakdown of muscle fibers. These changes are mild in comparison with neuropathic features, and the mechanism of these changes is unclear. However, when it does occur in ALS, especially in association with many hypertrophied fibers and large-fiber-type grouping, it tends to indicate a better prognosis. However, if degenerating fibers occur in association with many esterase-positive angular atrophic fibers, groups

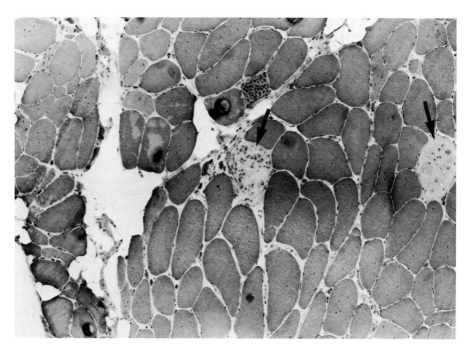

Figure 6 Necrotic fibers with reactive macrophages (arrows). Modified Gomori trichrome. × 100.

of atrophic fibers, and very little fiber-type grouping, prognosis may be even poorer than usual, owing to very rapid denervation.

ILLUSTRATIVE CASES

Case 1

A 60-year-old man presented with a 6-month history of diffuse atrophy, weakness, and fasiculations of the upper extremities. Reflexes were brisk, but no definite pathological reflexes were noted. Sensory examination was normal. EMG showed denervation and reinnervation in proximal, intermediate, and distal muscles in both upper extremities and was negative in the lower extremities. Computed tomography scan of the cervical spine showed spondylotic changes without spinal cord encroachment. However, quadriceps muscle biopsy revealed many esterase-positive angular atrophic fibers indicative of recent or ongoing denervation (Fig. 1). Therefore, presence of denervation atrophy in a quadriceps muscle biopsy helps substantiate a diagnosis of ALS rather than cervical spondylosis, in this patient.

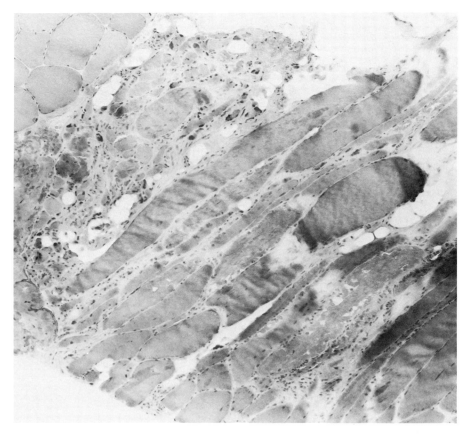

Figure 7   Degenerating-regenerating muscle fibers, variation in fiber size, and increased endomesial connective tissue. Modified Gomori trichrome. × 100.

Case 2

A 76-year-old man presented with a history of progressive weakness, affecting primarily lower extremities, over 2 years. There were no sensory or bulbar symptoms. On physical examination there was diffuse motor weakness and atrophy, predominantly in the lower extremities with hypoactive reflexes. EMG showed evidence of widespread denervation in all four limbs, consistent with a disorder of anterior horn cells. There was no evidence of a generalized peripheral myopathy; however, there was a left ulnar sensory neuropathy. Clinical impression was of progressive muscular atrophy form of ALS. However, muscle biopsy revealed a mixed myopathic-neuropathic disorder (Figs. 7,8). Over the next 4

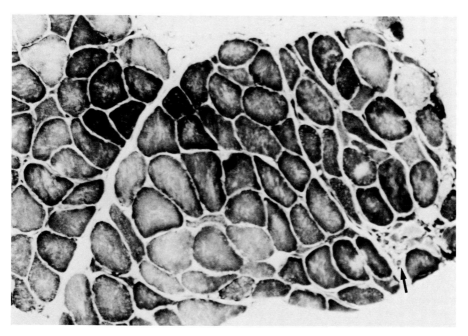

Figure 8 Moth-eaten fibers and small-group atrophy (arrow). NADH-TR. × 100.

years, there was very slowly progressive muscle weakness in the lower extremities, without upper extremity or bulbar involvement.

Case 3

A 55-year-old woman presented with bilateral lower extremity weakness of 4 years' duration. More recently, there had been weakness of upper extremities with development of dysarthria. On physical examination, there was spastic dysarthric speech, with an atrophic, fasiculating tongue, weakness of pterygoid and lower facial muscles, milk weakness in the upper extremities, and marked weakness in the lower extremities. Fasiculations were noted in the shoulder girdle muscles bilaterally. Reflexes were brisk in the upper extremities and absent in the lower extremities. Jaw jerk was hyperactive. EMG showed diffuse denervation in three limbs, consistent with ALS. Laboratory studies included a rheumatoid factor of 10,240 and an immune complex screen of 528 µg/ml. The patient was felt not to have rheumatoid arthritis. A muscle biopsy showed perivasculitis with prominent inflammation and marked atrophy of both fiber types (Fig. 9). The patient was started on high-dose corticosteroids and had a course of five plasmaphoreses, without clinical improvement.

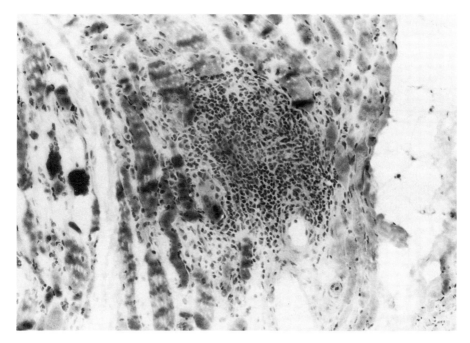

Figure 9   Perivascular inflammation and fiber atrophy. Modified Gomori trichrome.
×200.

PERIPHERAL NERVE BIOPSY

Pathological evidence of non–motor system involvement in ALS is well established (10). There are decreased numbers of large myelinated fibers and more
frequently degenerating fibers in sensory nerves, as well as increased frequency
of segmental demyelination and subsequent remyelination (11). Studies of sural
and common peroneal nerve biopsies by Bradley et al. in ALS patients confirmed
considerable reduction in total myelinated nerve fibers (12). Indications for a
sural nerve biopsy in ALS include a monoclonal gammopathy, a concomitant
sensory or sensorimotor polyneuropathy, abnormal serological studies suggestive of vasculitis, and a significantly high anti-Gm1 ganglioside antibody titer.
Sural nerve biopsies in 22 ALS patients at Henry Ford Hospital (1985–1990)
have demonstrated a mild degree of nerve fiber dropout and axonal degeneration
and regeneration in 17 cases (Fig. 10). In chronic cases, there is also demyelination secondary to long-standing axonal degeneration (Fig. 11). There are occasional small epineurial perivascular inflammatory cell infiltrates. However,
inflammation is most likely secondary to nerve fiber degeneration, rather than

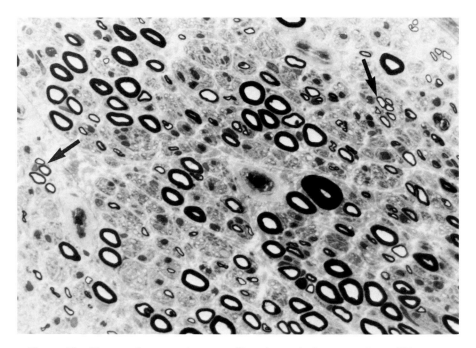

Figure 10   Clusters of regenerating nerve fibers (arrows). Paragon stain. ×900.

indicating a primary inflammatory polyneuropathy. Axonal neuropathy, although frequently present in sural nerve biopsies of ALS, is generally of a minor degree.

APPLICATION OF MOLECULAR BIOLOGY TO THE STUDY OF NEUROMUSCULAR DISEASE

Recent advances in studies of noninherited myopathies have employed techniques that are likely to be applicable to degenerative neuromuscular disorders like ALS. The molecular biology revolution has also led to important new insights into genetic myopathies (e.g., Duchenne's dystrophy) (13). Delineation of the structural gene for dystrophin has advanced our understanding of the pathogenesis of Duchenne's muscular dystrophy to a degree unimaginable a decade ago. Similar studies of mitochondrial myopathies will show similar advances within the next few years. Studies of noninherited myopathies are now also benefiting from the techniques of molecular biology.

Traditionally, identification of infectious etiologies of myopathies was restricted to seroepidemiological analysis, electron microscopy, or tissue culture

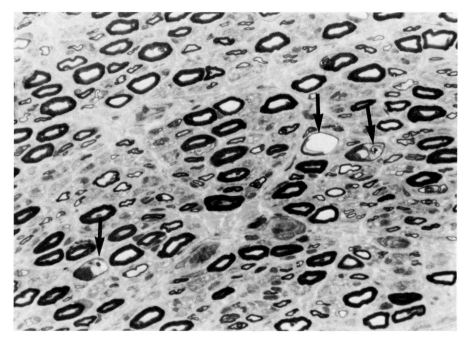

Figure 11 Demyelinating nerve fibers with axonal degeneration (arrows). Paragon stain. ×900.

recovery of infectious agents. A variety of different viruses (paramyxoviruses, orthomyxoviruses, picornaviruses, and retroviruses) have been readily linked on the basis of seroepidemiological data to inflammatory myopathies. In a much smaller fraction of human cases, virus has been recovered from muscle biopsy or autopsy specimens. In one or two cases electron microscopy has identified subcellular particles compatible with viral-infected myocytes (14).

While the paucity of data directly identifying viral infection is certainly due in part to sampling problems, the above techniques are suited for specificity and not sensitivity. Now there are a variety of new techniques for sensitively identifying infectious agents within tissue specimens. The first technique to be developed was a direct extension of immunocytochemistry used for identifying normal cellular antigens. Immunocytochemistry employs either antisera or monoclonal antibodies to specifically tag antigens in situ. The specificity offered by the antibody permits screening of large tissue sections. Using this technique, several animal and human viruses have been localized to myocytes both in vivo and in vitro. A disadvantage of immunocytochemistry in detecting viral infections is that many antibody probes are directed against surface proteins, which in viral infections can be notoriously variable. Additionally, preservation of antigen is another critical limiting factor to the utility of immunocytochemistry. However, since routine muscle studies employ frozen material, sensitivity is seldom compromised by fixation.

A newer technique, in situ hybridization, has recently been employed in the analysis of muscle disease. In situ hybridization requires the cloning of a nucleic acid sequence specific to the offending agent. Sequences complimentary to viral message or genomic nucleic acids are then tagged with a radioactive label and allowed to anneal to tissue sections suspected of harboring the infectious agent. The probe is then visualized using autoradiography with development of photographic grains above regions of radioactive decay. While technically more difficult to perform, this method offers several advantages over immunocytochemistry. First, one is not restricted to surface molecules, but can examine messages for intracellular proteins that are not under immunological pressure for mutation. Second, the radioactive probe can be made very hot and should in theory offer greater sensitivity. This second advantage is perhaps off set by not being able to take advantage of the biological amplification of many proteins translated off of one messenger RNA molecule.

More recently the development of the polymerase chain reaction (PCR) has offered the theoretical limits of sensitivity for identifying foreign agents (i.e., one genomic copy of nucleic acid) (15). While it is beyond the scope of this chapter to specifically detail the methodology of PCR, the sensitivity of the procedure derives from the investigator-controlled amplification of specific nucleic acid sequences. By choosing primer oligonucleotides complementary and flanking a specific nucleic acid sequence, an investigator can, within minutes, amplify a rare infectious agent to detectable levels. The specificity of the technique derives from constructing a specific probe for a nucleic acid sequence that resides *between* the flanking sequences used in the amplification procedure.

We have recently published how these techniques can be used in the study of human muscle and spinal cord disease (16). Patients infected by human T-cell leukemia virus-I (HTLV-I) develop a variety of neuromuscular diseases (17). The majority of chronically infected individuals do not develop disease; however, subjects of patients develop a spectrum of neuromuscular abnormalities (18). The reason for interindividual differences is possibly determined by immunological control of viral infection (e.g., variations in major histocompatibility genes). One subset of patients develop a chronic relapsing polymyositis. We have employed PCR to show direct HTLV-I infection within involved muscle tissues. Additionally, we have employed immunocytochemistry and in situ hybridization to identify myocytes themselves to be infected (17). This suggests that HTLV-I causes polymyositis by chronically infecting myocytes, which are then subjected to immunological surveillance and destruction.

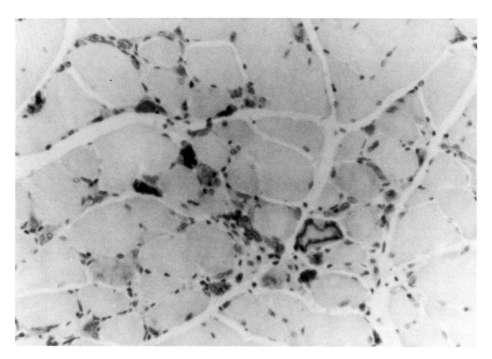

Figure 12 Immunocytochemical staining of skeletal muscle of a transgenic mouse carrying the HTLV-I *tax* transgene. Fascicles of normal appearing myofibers are interrupted by atrophic oxidative myofibers intensely stained for the *tax* transgene product. As all cells of the transgenic mouse contain the *tax* gene, selective expression within oxidative myofibers must be due to specific cellular transcription factors unique to oxidative myofibers. This finding is consistent with the hypothesis that viral infection of muscle can depend on cellular transcription factors as much as cell surface receptors. Counterstained with hematoxylin. × 400.

The utility of molecular biology is not limited to simple identification of offending agents within neuromuscular tissue. It is now possible to design experiments to ask specific questions regarding the pathogenesis of the neuromuscular disease. Having identified HTLV-I infection of myocytes, an immediate question is why is muscle specifically infected? The easiest assumption would be that muscle expresses a specific viral receptor. But in the case of HTLV-I, the viral receptor is uniquitously expressed on the surface of most human cells. Therefore, the reason TLV-I preferentially infects human muscle must reside at some stage beyond binding to the myocyte surface.

To address these questions in collaboration with Dr. Michael Nerenberg, we examined mice in which a specific and critical regulatory gene of HTLV-I (*tax*) was inserted into mouse lines transgenically (19). By inserting this gene into the mouse genome, we avoid questions of cellular surface receptors for the virus and can study transcriptional control of viral gene expression. These studies have shown that in mice that all cells contained the viral *tax* gene, skeletal muscle preferentially expressed and accumulated the gene product (Fig. 12). This implies that the reason muscle is infected in vivo is not because of selective expression of a surface receptor, but rather because the myocytes' transcription machinery selectively promotes expression of the viral sequences. These observations suggest an entirely different way of looking at the pathogenesis of viral infection and hint at what the future has in store for studies of neuromuscular disease.

REFERENCES

1. Engel WK, Brooke MH: Muscle biopsy in ALS and other motor neuron disease. In: Norris Jr. FH, Kurland LT, eds. Motor neuron diseases: Research on amyotrophic lateral sclerosis and related disorders, Vol 2. New York: Grune & Stratton, 1969: 154–159.
2. Arbrustmacher VW: Skeletal muscle in denervation. Pathol Ann, 1982.
3. Engel WK, Brooke MH, Nelson PG. Histochemical studies of denervated or tenotomized cat muscle. Ann NY Acad Sci 1966;138:160.
4. Ringel SP, Bender AN, Engel WK. Extrajunctional acetylcholine receptors. Alterations in human and experimental neuromuscular disease. Arch Neurol 1976;33: 751.
5. Brooke MH, Kaiser KK. Muscle fiber types: How many and what kind? Arch Neurol 1970;23:369.
6. Resnick JS, Engel WK. Target fibers—Structural and cytochemical characteristics and their relationship to neurogenic muscle disease and fiber types. In: Milhorat AT, ed. Exploratory concepts in muscular dystrophy and related disorders. Amsterdam: Excerpta Medica International Conference Series No. 147, 1967:255.
7. Schmitt HP, Volk B. The relationship between target, targetoid and targetoid/core fibers in severe neurogenic atrophy. J Neurol 1975;210:167.
8. Karpati MD, Engel WK. "Type grouping" in skeletal muscle after experimental reinneration. Neurology (Minneap) 1968;18:447.
9. Brooke MH, Engel WK. The histologic diagnosis of neuromuscular diseases: A review of 79 biopsies. Arch Physiol Med Rehabil 1966;47:99.
10. Kawarmura Y, Dyck PJ, Shimono M, et al. Morphometric comparison of the vulnerability of peripheral motor and sensory neurons in amyotrophic lateral sclerosis. J Neuropathol Exp Neurol 1981;40:667–675.
11. Dyck PJ, Stevens JC, Mulder DW. Frequently of nerve fiber degeneration of periphal motro and sensory neurons in amyotrophic lateral sclerosis. Neurology (Minneap) 1975;25:781–785.
12. Bradley WG, Good P, Rassool GC, Adelman LS. Morphometric and biochemical studies of peripheral nerves in amyotrophic lateral sclerosis. Ann Neurol 1983;14: 267–277.

13. Myology. New York: McGraw-Hill, 1986.
14. Gamboa ET, Eastwood AB, Hays AP, Maxwell J, Penn AS. Isolation of influenza virus from muscle in myoglobinuric polymyositis. Neurology 1979;29:1323–1335.
15. PCR protocols: A guide to methods and applications. San Diego: Academic Press, 1990.
16. Bhigjee AI, Wiley CA, Wachsman W, et al. HTLV-I associated myelopathy: Clinical pathological correlation with localization of provirus to spinal cord. Neurology 1991 (in press).
17. Wiley CA, Nerenberg M, Cros D, Soto-Aguilar M. HTLV-1 polymyositis in a patient also infected with the human immunodeficiency virus. N Engl J Med 1989;320:992–995.
18. Bhigjee AI, Kelbe C, Haribhai HC, et al. Myelopathy associated with human T cell lymphotropic virus type I (HTLV-I) in Natal, South Africa. A clinial and investigative study in 24 patients. Brain 1990;113:1307–1320.
19. Nerenberg MI, Wiley CA. Degeneration of oxidative muscle fibers in HTLV-1 tax transgenic mice. Am J Pathol 1989;135:1025–1033.

9

Neurophysiological Studies in Amyotrophic Lateral Sclerosis

Erik V. Stålberg

University Hospital
Uppsala, Sweden

Donald B. Sanders

Duke University
Durham, North Carolina

INTRODUCTION

The classical electromyographic (EMG) signs of amyotrophic lateral sclerosis (ALS) are denervation and reinnervation in the absence of evidence of other pathological processes that may cause similar EMG changes. The combination of denervation and reinnervation in three anatomically unrelated sites with normal sensory nerve conduction is strongly suggestive of motor neuron disease (MND). Because of the random loss of motor axons, maximal motor conduction velocity values may be slightly reduced.

In this chapter, we will discuss the role of conventional EMG and nerve conduction studies in the diagnosis of MND. Some results obtained from other neurophysiological techniques used to explore the physiology of the motor unit in MND will also be presented. The neurophysiological abnormalities do not describe the basic defect in ALS but they do add to our understanding of the disease.

Motor neuron diseases are characterized by involvement of the lower and upper motor neuron in varying degrees, typically without evidence of involvement of other pathways. Concomitant with lower motor neuron degeneration, there is axonal loss and denervation of corresponding muscles. The degeneration is usually diffuse throughout the spinal cord, but evidence of focal predominance and subsequent spread has been reported (1).

The clinical examination is routinely supplemented by a neurophysiological evaluation to confirm the presence of widespread lower motor neuron involvement and to exclude other possible diagnoses, according to the following principles:

Denervation should be present in three anatomically separate areas (usually three limbs).
Denervation should be distributed without relationship to spinal segments or peripheral nerves.
Sensory nerve conduction velocities should be normal.

For many years (2) the most commonly used electrophysiological techniques for these purposes have been EMG and nerve conduction studies. The combination of findings from these techniques usually demonstrates the presence of abnormalities characteristic of MND and differentiates it from conditions with which it can be confused clinically.

ELECTROMYOGRAPHY IN MOTOR NEURON DISEASE COMPARED TO FINDINGS IN HEALTHY SUBJECTS

The conventional EMG investigation with concentric or monopolar needle electrodes is commonly performed in three steps: with the muscle at rest, to detect various kinds of spontaneous activity; during slight voluntary contraction, to study details of the motor unit action potential; and during strong contraction, to study firing rates and the number of motor units that can be activated.

During Rest

Normal

The normal muscle at rest is electrically silent, except for occasional fasciculations, which are seen particularly immediately after physical exercise.

In the end-plate zone of normal muscle, two types of spontaneous activity may occur that must be distinguished from fibrillation potentials. One, called end-plate noise, is related to the spontaneous release of acetylcholine. The other type of end-plate activity, called end-plate spikes, shows waveforms that are characteristic of single muscle fiber action potentials but have no initial positive-going phase, indicating that they originate at the end-plate zone. End-plate spikes probably represent muscle action potentials triggered by mechanical stimulation of the terminal nerve branch by the EMG needle.

Denervation

When a muscle fiber is denervated, e.g., due to degeneration of the anterior horn cell or the axon or due to neuromuscular blockade, e.g., with botulinum toxin, extrajunctional receptors develop, and the sensitivity to acetylcholine increases (3). The muscle fiber becomes hyperexcitable and spontaneous activity such as *positive waves* and *fibrillation potentials* occur (Fig. 1). Because of this hyperexcitability, spontaneous activity in one muscle fiber may sometimes trigger activity in an adjacent fiber and locked fibrillation potentials occur. In more chronic situations, groups of denervated muscle fibers may activate each other giving rise to so called *complex repetitive discharges* (4).

Fibrillation potentials persist for a long time in a denervated muscle fiber, probably until the fiber is reinnervated or undergoes fibrosis.

Motor Neuron Disease

All the above findings of denervation are seen in MND. In addition, *fasciculations* are typically seen (5), but are not pathognomonic or even always pathological, since they may be seen in healthy subjects, particularly after exercise. All visible fasciculations can be recorded by EMG, but fasciculation potentials may also be recorded by EMG in muscles in which clinical fasciculations cannot be seen. In MND, fasciculations may originate distally in the nerve terminal (6,7) or more proximally, indicating abnormal membrane properties in the nerve trunk (8). Single-fiber EMG studies demonstrate that fasciculations in MND represent motor unit potentials (MUPs) with markedly increased jitter and fiber density, findings that are also seen in voluntarily activated MUPs in this disease (9).

During Slight Voluntary Activity

During slight voluntary activation, all muscle fibers in an activated motor unit discharge synchronously. The action potentials from individual muscle fibers in a motor unit summate and generate so-called motor unit potentials (MUPs). The MUP is produced by the temporal and spatial summation of action potentials from muscle fibers that lie within an area of about 2.5 mm from the electrode (10). This area does not always cover the entire motor unit territory, which extends 2–10 mm. The configuration of the MUP depends on the number of muscle fibers that lie within the studied area of the motor unit, on the distribution of muscle fiber diameters, on the action potential conduction in the terminal nerve tree, and on the distribution of motor end-plates.

Normal

The normal MUP is bi- or triphasic, has an amplitude between 50 and 500 μV, and a duration of 5–15 msec, depending on muscle, age, and type of recording electrode. The MUP shape is nearly constant in consecutive discharges.

Reinnervation

In muscles undergoing active reinnervation, the MUP parameters follow a characteristic sequence of changes. Within days after denervation, the reinnervation

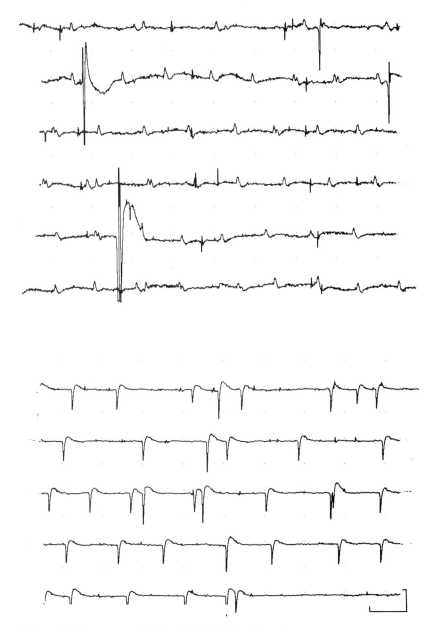

Figure 1   Spontaneous EMG activity in ALS. Fibrillations and fasciculation (top), positive waves (bottom). Calibration 5 msec/div, 200 μV/div.

starts. New intramuscular nerve sprouts from surviving axons reach the dener-vated muscle fibers in large numbers and form contacts with the muscle fibers within weeks. The surviving motor unit incorporates the new fibers by means of so-called collateral sprouting. There is no evidence that a degenerated ventral horn cell can regenerate. The reinnervated muscle fibers will assume the same histochemical characteristics as those of the reinnervating motor unit. Since a denervated fiber is typically reinnervated from the nearest nerve terminals, the fibers in the reinnervated motor unit tend to cluster, producing so-called fiber-type grouping in muscle biopsies. The phase of ongoing reinnervation is char-acterized by increasing duration and increasing amplitude of the MUPs, reflect-ing the increasing number of muscle fibers in the motor units under study (Fig. 2). The MUPs are polyphasic or complex owing to increased time dispersion among action potentials generating the MUP. Late components may be seen since the newly formed poorly myelinated nerves and the reinnervated muscle fibers, which are probably atrophic, conduct their impulses more slowly than do the original parts of the motor unit. There is an abnormal variability in the shape of the MUPs at consecutive discharges, due to uncertain impulse transmission in newly formed nerve sprouts and motor end-plates. This is most pronounced during ongoing reinnervation, particularly during the first 3 months after a nerve lesion.

In later stages, more than 3–6 months after an acute denervating lesion, the pattern changes. The main component of the MUP shows increased amplitude, area, and duration. Often there continues to be an increased proportion of poly-phasic or complex MUPs. The neuromuscular transmission improves and the MUPs are now relatively stable in shape at consecutive discharges.

Motor Neuron Disease

In MND, where denervation and reinnervation processes are taking place in parallel, the MUPs have increased amplitude and duration and are complex or polyphasic. Motor units recently involved in reinnervation will produce unstable MUPs. Therefore, an EMG picture dominated by a high proportion of unstable MUPs indicates a rapidly progressive process.

During Strong Voluntary Contraction

Normal

In order to study the firing pattern and density of electrical activity of the muscle that reflect the total number of activated motor units, the EMG is analyzed during strong voluntary contraction. The firing rates of individual motor units increase and new motor units are recruited as the force increases. This produces a so-called interference pattern. With increasing force of contraction, the EMG

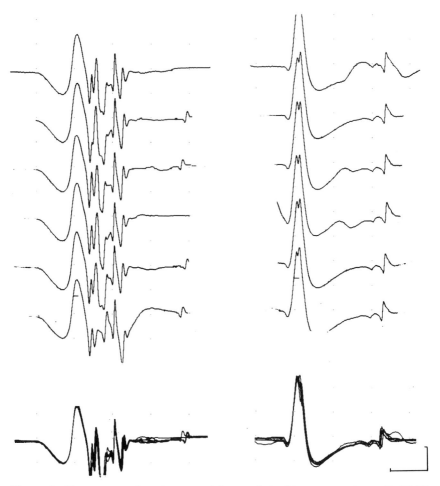

Figure 2 Two motor unit action potentials recorded with a concentric needle EMG electrode from the biceps muscle of a patient with ALS. Six oscilloscope sweeps for each recording are displayed rastered (above) and superimposed (below). One of them (left) is polyphasic and demonstrates variations in the waveforms between consecutive discharges with blocking in a late component. The other (right) is more stable in shape. Calibration 5 msec/div, 200 μV/div.

interference pattern becomes increasingly dense. In normal muscle this EMG signal will fill up the screen at maximum contraction, leaving no baseline visible on the oscilloscope trace, producing a so-called full or dense interference pattern. The maximal amplitude of the signal peaks, i.e., the amplitude of the signal envelope, increases due to the fact that later-recruited motor units usually have

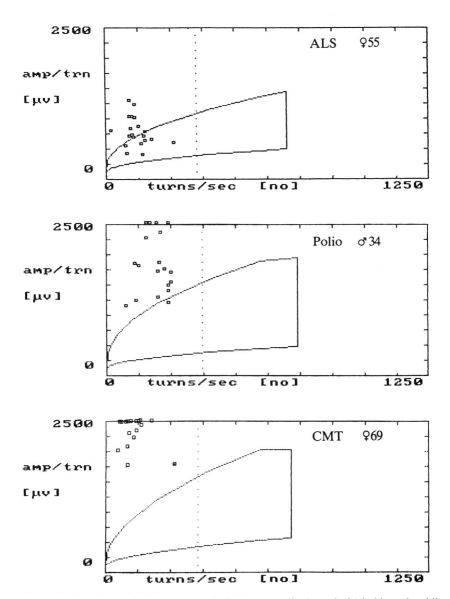

Figure 3 Interference EMG pattern analysis (turns/amplitude analysis) in biceps brachii muscle from three different patients with neurogenic conditions. Note the low number of turns and high amplitudes in relation to the age-matched normal distribution (indicated area). CMT, Charcot-Marie-Tooth disease.

greater MUP amplitude and also because of the increasing statistical probability of occurrence of larger motor units as the sample size increases.

Motor Neuron Disease

In MND, the recruitment of additional motor units during increasing force occurs later in relation to force development than in normal muscle and the interference pattern is reduced compared to normal, owing to the loss of active motor units. The signal envelope amplitude is increased because the MUPs are larger. The interference pattern may be analyzed quantitatively with different methods. So-called turns/amplitude analysis (11–13) shows high-amplitude peaks and a reduced number of turns/sec or reduced fullness of the pattern at full effort in MND. Interference pattern analysis may be used both for diagnosis and to quantitate the severity of involvement (Fig. 3).

NERVE CONDUCTION STUDIES IN MOTOR NEURON DISEASE

In MND, the motor and sensory nerve conduction velocities are normal in preserved axons. Denys (14) reported that measurements of *maximal* motor nerve conduction velocity (MCV) showed a slowing by an average 11% in ALS patients compared with controls. This has been assumed to be due to the loss of the large, fast-conducting axons since these have the strongest influence on the motor velocity values obtained in routine nerve conduction velocity studies. The fact that slowing was not seen until severe atrophy had developed was considered to speak against the possibility that there is preferential early involvement of large axons. It is more likely that there is random loss of axons. At the stage when large, rapidly conducting axons were also lost, the MCV became reduced.

The distal latencies of motor nerve conduction are prolonged, also in correlation with the degree of atrophy (14). Prolongation of distal latencies was found more often in the median than in the ulnar or peroneal nerves. When the distal latency of a nerve was prolonged, the amplitude of the muscle response was low and the MCV reduced. Slow conduction in new sprouts or conduction block in distal nerve branches (15) may contribute to the prolonged distal latencies, but is not considered of major importance. A more likely explanation is that the distal slowing is due to "dying back" of the distal portions of the motor nerves. However, it is unclear why such changes are less marked in long nerves such as the peroneal than in the median or ulnar nerves.

The sensory nerve conduction velocities and amplitudes are normal in MND. This is an important finding which helps to differentiate ALS from axonal neuropathies.

For the correct interpretation of nerve conduction studies in patients with suspected ALS, some factors must be given special attention. Note that cooling may reduce nerve conduction velocity in the cold segment and thus simulate a neuropathy. Patients with muscle atrophy may have cold limbs because of heat loss and reduced heat production with inactivity. Therefore, all nerve conduction studies must be performed under temperature control. Special attention must be paid to the M-wave amplitude. It should be remembered that a slow MCV in the presence of a low M-wave amplitude can also be seen in peripheral neuropathies. Sensory nerve studies are essential in the investigation of patients with suspected MND. Since pure motor nerve neuropathies do occur and can produce the same nerve conduction findings as MND, the ultimate diagnosis will depend on the clinical presentation as well as the EMG findings.

DIFFERENT FORMS OF MOTOR NEURON DISEASES

The EMG pattern in various forms of MND varies in relation to the rate of progression and type of involvement (upper or lower motor neuron) and predominant distribution. EMG findings point to principal changes in the motor unit rather than giving a diagnostic label (16).

In *ALS*, both upper and lower motor neurons are involved. Weakness and atrophy frequently begin locally, producing a clinical pattern suggesting a peripheral nerve or root lesion. EMG studies at this point usually demonstrate widespread neurogenic abnormalities. As the disease progresses, weakness and atrophy spread and EMG ultimately demonstrates neurogenic abnormalities in all muscles except ocular and sphincter muscles, which are also clinically spared.

The EMG examination usually begins with investigation of a weak, atrophic muscle. This will usually confirm that denervation is present. However, if the muscle is severely affected and fibrotic, it may be difficult to interpret the results. In such cases, investigating a moderately affected muscle may give more specific information.

If an EMG pattern compatible with denervation and reinnervation is present in one muscle, muscles innervated by different nerves and different spinal segments should be examined to determine the distribution of the abnormality. Distal and proximal muscles should be studied. To support the diagnosis of MND, three separate anatomical locations should show signs of denervation, e.g., muscles in three limbs or in two limbs and the bulbar area. It may often be valuable to study a muscle innervated by a cranial nerve, e.g,. the tongue, sternocleidomastoid, digastric, or masseter muscles. To study the tongue, the electrode may be introduced into its lateral margin with the tongue protruded from the mouth. The tongue is then slowly retracted into the mouth while the EMG electrode is allowed to follow. In this way relaxation may be achieved (although this is not always true) and fibrillation potentials and positive waves can be studied. Another approach is to introduce the electrode into the base of the tongue from below the chin in the midline. With this approach it is easier to relax the tongue. Fibrillation potentials, positive waves, and fasciculations may be detected. Slight and strong contraction can also be obtained.

In *progressive muscular atrophy*, denervation and reinnervation are widespread, bulbar muscles are not involved, and there are no electrophysiological signs of upper motor neuron involvement, such as irregular firing pattern, increased F-wave occurrence, or H reflexes outside the S1 segment.

In *progressive bulbar palsy*, the oropharyngeal muscles are involved early and EMG studies show more denervation in these muscles than in limb muscles.

Juvenile progressive bulbar palsy (Fazio-Londe syndrome) produces rapidly progressive weakness of the tongue, face, and pharyngeal muscles in a clinical pattern similar to bulbar myasthenia gravis (17). Neuromuscular transmission may be abnormal in these muscles because of rapid denervation and immature reinnervation, and strength may improve after administration of cholinesterase inhibitors. EMG examination demonstrates fibrillations and large, complex, unstable MUPs in involved muscles.

In the hereditary form of *spinal muscular atrophy* (Kugelberg-Welander syndrome) the EMG changes often indicate slow progression, seen as high-amplitude, long-duration, relatively stable MUPs. No signs of upper motor neuron involvement are present.

The condition that exists in patients who have had *poliomyelitis* can contribute greatly to our understanding of MND. The pathophysiology of this disease, loss of anterior cells without significant changes elsewhere in the nervous system, is similar to the sporadic type of MND. However, it does differ from these conditions in an important way; namely, it results from an acute monophasic attack on the motor neuron pool. Patients who have had poliomyelitis in the remote past sometime complain of new progressive weakness, fatiguability, and other symptoms. These symptoms could be due to the effects of wear and tear, aging, cardiovascular disease, and so on, superimposed on the residua of poliomyelitis. These factors may also affect patients with MND. In patients with various types of neurogenic diseases, it may be difficult to distinguish between changes due to the primary disease and those superimposed from other factors. Studies of patients who have had poliomyelitis may provide important information about the nature of these secondary effects.

Patients with postpolio sequelae show an EMG pattern of chronic neurogenic changes which are often asymmetrical and usually widespread. In some patients who have had polio in the remote past, spontaneous activity suggesting ongoing denervation may be seen, even in the absence of clinical evidence of progression (18). The motor unit potentials are usually relatively stable. Single-fiber EMG (SFEMG) shows signs of pronounced reinnervation, sometimes in muscles that are clinically strong and symptomatically uninvolved by the initial disease process. Macro EMG reveals that the motor unit size may be increased by more than 5 times, similar to findings in patients with MND (19).

DIFFERENTIAL DIAGNOSIS OF NEUROPHYSIOLOGICAL FINDINGS SEEN IN MND

The neurophysiological findings in ALS merely reflect changes in the motor unit produced by denervation and reinnervation. In individual muscles these findings are similar in various generalized neurogenic conditions, such as MND and axonal neuropathy; segmental lesions, such as spinal stenosis; or more localized lesions, such as radiculopathies, nerve entrapment, or peripheral nerve trauma. Depending on the point during the time course when the examination is performed, the EMG findings in MND may even simulate polymyositis or myasthenia gravis. Therefore, before the diagnosis of MND can be made, other conditions that may give similar neurophysiological findings must be excluded. It should be noted that the following refers mainly to the interpretation of the neurophysiological findings. Clinically, there may be other differential diagnostic considerations.

Peripheral Nerve Disease

In order to exclude *polyneuropathy*, motor and sensory nerve conduction studies should be performed in arm and leg nerves. The EMG changes of denervation and reinnervation are typically most pronounced distally in neuropathies and the facial and pharyngeal muscles are spared. In MND there is equal involvement of proximal and distal muscles and frequent involvement of bulbar muscles.

In *demyelinating neuropathy*, motor and sensory conduction velocities are significantly reduced, the F-wave latencies are prolonged, and the duration of the sensory responses may be increased. This type of neuropathy causes varying degrees of axonal degeneration, and therefore only slight signs of denervation and reinnervation may be seen on EMG.

In *axonal neuropathies*, the nerve conduction velocities are normal or slightly reduced and the M-response amplitude is reduced as in MND, reflecting loss of innervated muscle fibers. The amplitude of sensory nerve action potentials is correspondingly reduced, reflecting the loss of sensory axons.

Recently, much attention has been paid to an acquired, multifocal demyelinating neuropathy that at least initially affects only motor nerve fibers and presents with clinical features resembling MND (20–22). These patients do not have upper motor neuron signs and the disease usually follows an indolent course. There is some evidence that this represents a variant of inflammatory neuropathy which may improve after immunosuppressive therapy. Neurophysiological studies demonstrate multifocal conduction blocks (not seen in MND), predominating proximally, involving motor nerve fibers solely or predominantly, with evidence of widespread denervation and reinnervation. The frequency with which conduction abnormalities are found is determined by the number of motor nerves tested, indicating the value of testing many motor nerves in these patients.

In *radiculopathies* and *local nerve entrapment*, neurogenic changes are found in the distribution of roots, peripheral nerves, or their branches. In the latter case, the sensory nerve action potential amplitude is reduced since sensory nerve fibers are involved distal to the dorsal root ganglion.

In *spinal stenosis* the neurogenic changes are more widespread than in most other radiculopathies. In *cervical myelopathy*, atrophy of hand muscles and upper motor neuron signs in the lower limbs may simulate MND. In both these conditions the denervation changes are usually restricted to a few segmental levels and are not found in facial muscles. Sensory root involvement may be indicated by abnormal findings in somatosensory evoked potentials.

Other Conditions

In exceptional cases of MND with very rapid progression, the MUPs may not be significantly increased in amplitude or duration but show instability and polyphasicity. This may sometimes lead to the EMG differential diagnosis of *polymyositis*, which also shows fibrillation potentials and small MUPs in its acute phase.

Myasthenia gravis is only rarely suspected in the early stage of MND, though fatiguability and the absence of sensory symptoms may raise the question in some patients. If upper motor neuron signs are missing, the resemblance to myasthenia gravis sometimes leads to neurophysiological testing of neuromuscular function. In both conditions disturbed synaptic transmission is seen, but in MND there are usually clear signs of ongoing reinnervation, which will differentiate the condition from myasthenia gravis.

OTHER NEUROPHYSIOLOGICAL TECHNIQUES TO INVESTIGATE MOTOR NEURON DISEASE

Additional information about the motor unit in MND can be obtained by some other electrophysiological techniques. The place of electrophysiology in ALS research was recently reviewed (23).

Single-Fiber EMG

The technique is described in detail elsewhere (24). Two parameters measured by SFEMG are useful in studying the process of reinnervation.

Fiber Density

Fiber density (FD) represents the average number of muscle fibers within a small area (300 μm radius) of the motor unit (Fig. 4). When reinnervation occurs due

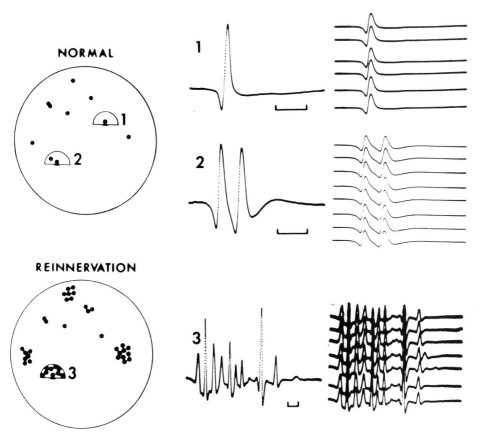

Figure 4 The principle of fiber density measurement in SFEMG. The muscle fibers in one motor unit are indicated as small solid circles, and the uptake area of the recording electrode is represented as a half-circle. In the normal muscle (1 and 2), only action potentials from one or two fibers are recorded. In reinnervation (3) many fibers are recorded owing to increased fiber density in the unit. Time calibration 1 msec. [From Stålberg and Trontelj (24), with permission.]

to collateral sprouting, which is the only type of reinnervation that takes place in MND, the surviving motor units innervate adjacent denervated muscle fibers. This causes fiber grouping and therefore the FD increases. The FD is increased before the conventional MUP parameters show definite signs of motor unit enlargement.

FD has been found to be increased in 65–85% of the investigated muscles from patients with MND (25) (Figure 5, Table 1). Even clinically normal mus-

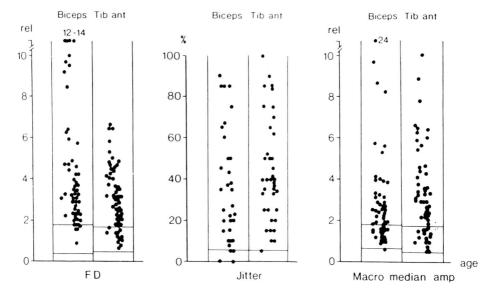

Figure 5 Fiber density, jitter (% of pairs with increased jitter), and macro median amplitude in biceps and tibialis anterior muscle from patients with MND. ±2 SD from control values is indicated for each muscle. Each dot represents one patient.

cles often show increased FD. For example, in patients with predominantly bulbar symptoms FD is usually increased in limb muscles. This indicates that involvement is more widespread than is clinically apparent. The distribution of elevated FD values indicates that there is different involvement among different spinal segmental levels as well as asymmetrical involvement of the motor neuron pool at one spinal cord level (1). In MND the fiber density is not increased to the same extent as in more slowly progressive motor neuron disorders such as spinal muscular atrophy. This could be due to different degrees of denervation or to reduced reinnervation capacity, but is most likely simply due to there being insufficient time for a reinnervating motor neuron to form a dense motor unit before it undergoes denervation itself (26).

Jitter

The jitter parameter measured by SFEMG characterizes the impulse transmission in the peripheral part of the motor unit. During the early phase of reinnervation, e.g., after partial nerve section, impulse transmission in terminal nerves and newly formed motor end-plates is very uncertain, producing abnormally increased jitter and intermittent transmission blocking. In the later stages of reinnervation, the impulse transmission becomes more normal as the newly formed

Table 1 Comparison of EMG Findings in 82 Patients
with MND

	Studies abnormal (%)
Tibialis anterior muscle:	
SF-EMG	100
↑ Jitter	91
↑ Fiber density	67
EMG[a]	96
Biceps brachii muscle:	
SFEMG	92
↑ Fiber density	85
↑ Jitter	78
EMG[a]	84

[a]Abnormal spontaneous activity, motor unit potentials, or recruitment.

nerve terminals and neuromuscular junctions mature. In MND, where denervation and reinnervation are taking place continuously, there is insufficient time for
these structures to mature. Increased jitter and blockings are typical findings,
seen in some muscles in 90% of all ALS patients (25,27) (Fig. 5, Table 1).
Increased jitter and impulse blocking are particularly pronounced in patients with
MND with rapidly progressing symptoms.

The increase in jitter seems to be related mainly to the degree of reinnervation,
and usually both FD and jitter are increased in MND. Exceptionally we have
seen abnormal jitter in muscles with normal FD (27). It has been suggested that
there is early and etiologically important involvement of the motor end-plate in
ALS (28,29), but so far this has been difficult to confirm electrophysiologically.

REPETITIVE NERVE STIMULATION

A decrementing response to repetitive nerve stimulation may be seen in MND,
particularly in atrophic muscles (30,31), corresponding to the findings of increased jitter (Fig. 6). Denys and Norris (30) found a decrementing response to
slow repetitive stimulation (2 Hz) in 67% of 55 patients with ALS. The decrement was of the order of 3–12%, with the higher values being found in atrophic
muscles. The largest decrement was 27.7% in one patient. The decrement was
similar to that in myasthenia gravis, in that it occurred at low stimulation frequencies, showed postactivation facilitation and exhaustion, and was less
marked after local cooling and after administration of edrophonium (Tensilon).
The reason for the decrement was not studied in detail, but it was speculated that

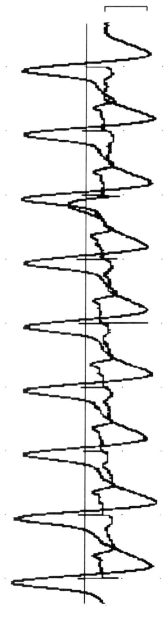

Figure 6 Repetitive nerve stimulation test in a patient with ALS. Recordings were made from the abductor pollicis brevis muscle, which was severely weak and atrophic, while stimulating the median nerve at the wrist at a frequency of 3/sec. The area of the 4th response is 85% of the first. Calibration 1 mV/div.

it could be related to the immaturity of structures during reinnervation or morphological changes at the neuromuscular junction, such as enlargement of the end-plates, retraction of presynaptic terminals, or other factors causing less effective neuromuscular transmission. The decrement was more pronounced in muscles showing frequent fasciculations. Both these phenomena may be related to the activity of the denervation/reinnervation process.

One may ask whether any of the weakness and fatiguability in patients with ALS could be due to defective neuromuscular transmission. The neuromuscular transmission may be improved by cholinesterase inhibitors, but only occasionally does this improve function significantly (32). The disturbed neuromuscular transmission mainly, although not necessarily exclusively, reflects a reparative phenomenon of reinnervation, which counteracts the weakness, rather than a primary defect that would cause weakness. As mentioned above, increased jitter is only exceptionally seen in muscles in the absence of signs of reinnervation. Most of the weakness is therefore probably due to loss of muscle mass owing to denervation rather than to abnormal neuromuscular transmission. Recently it has been shown that twitch tension in motor units in MND is less than the corresponding electrical activity (Macro MUP amplitude) would suggest (33).

CORTICAL STIMULATION

In some patients upper motor signs may dominate the early stages. EMG methods here may show little change. Cortical stimulation may be used to study the central motor pathways. Electrical stimulation was initially used for this purpose (34) though later magnetic stimulation was used, being virtually free of discomfort (35,36). In a recent summary of 40 ALS patients Eisen et al. (37) showed that magnetic stimulation was abnormal in nearly all patients, because of either low amplitude or prolonged latencies in at least one of three arm muscles. In patients with predominantly upper motor neuron signs, no responses could be elicited. In patients with mixed upper and lower motor neuron signs, the latencies were prolonged and the amplitude was often less than 15% of normal values. This was considered to indicate significant loss of cortical motor neurons.

In the appropriate clinical setting, small-amplitude, modestly prolonged motor responses to magnetic stimulation make the diagnosis of MND likely even when EMG findings are sparse. Patients with other myelopathies must be studied further before the above-mentioned findings can be considered unique for MND.

TECHNIQUES TO INVESTIGATE THE NUMBER AND SIZE OF MOTOR UNITS

The balance between the denervation and reinnervation processes in MND determines the neurophysiological and clinical dynamics of the disease. One way to express this electrophysiologically would be by measuring the size of reinnervated motor units. Such measurements would mainly reflect the reinnervation capacity of the motor units but would be affected by the degree of denervation and the time for maturation, which are factors that must be considered in the interpretation. What methods can be used to obtain this information? In conventional EMG, the amplitude and duration of MUPs are not particularly reliable indicators of motor unit size because they do not reflect the electrical activity from the entire motor unit but only from muscle fibers within a restricted area of its territory. SFEMG gives information about the local density of muscle fibers but not about total motor unit size. To estimate the motor unit size other methods must be applied. Two such methods are so-called motor unit counting and Macro EMG.

Motor Unit Counting

Motor unit potentials may be recorded either during slowly increasing stimulus strength, as in so-called motor unit counting techniques (38,39), or by means of spike-triggered surface recordings (40). These techniques have been used not only to determine the size of individual motor units, but to estimate the number of motor units in a muscle (41,42). They have also been used to follow ALS patients over time (39,43). In assessing the validity of these techniques one should ask if only single axons are being stimulated and if there is a bias toward measuring certain types of motor units owing to the relationship between axon diameter and the excitability threshold and the difficulties in detecting contributions from small motor units. Regardless of methodological details, comparisons between repeated investigations in the same patient may give sufficiently accurate results to be of great clinical usefulness.

Two factors make surface recordings less versatile. First, many proximal muscles are difficult to investigate with the stimulation technique since the nerves to these muscles are inaccessible. The spike-triggered technique eliminates this problem. Second, the surface electrode cannot reliably record from motor units located deep in large muscles, which therefore cannot be studied accurately. This is a problem common to both techniques.

Macro EMG

Another way to obtain a nonselective recording from all fibers in a motor unit is by means of so-called macro EMG (44) (Fig. 5). Recordings are made from the cannula of a modified single-fiber electrode. The amplitude and area of the macro motor unit potential (MUP) reflect the number and size of muscle fibers in the entire motor unit. The fiber density is also measured with this technique and is of great value in interpreting the results.

In ALS the macro MUP is usually much larger than in peripheral neuropathies. The largest individual macro MUPs in ALS patients we have seen was 57 times normal in biceps brachii and 25 times normal in anterior tibial muscles. This is similar to the size of macro MUPs seen following poliomyelitis and in spinal muscular atrophy (SMA) and corresponds to the studies of McComas et al. (39), who found surface-recorded MUP amplitudes to be increased 40 times in ALS.

It has been questioned whether reduced reinnervation capacity contributes to the progressive nature of motor neuron disease. These findings indicate that the surviving motor neurons in ALS have a good capacity for reinnervation, although the brief survival time of the reinnervated motor units may prevent full functional maturity.

Muscles in which the average macro MUP amplitude has increased two- to fourfold, corresponding to a loss of 50–70% of the neurons, are of interest in ALS studies. These muscles may still have relatively well-preserved strength. Using a motor unit counting technique, Hansen and Ballantyne (38) found a normal-amplitude M response even in muscles in which up to 50% of the motor units had been lost, in which case the remaining motor units had doubled their size. McComas et al. (39) showed that the twitch tension of the total muscle became abnormally low only after 90% of the motor units had been lost. This indicates that there is a high degree of functional compensation for the loss of neurons.

NEUROPHYSIOLOGICAL MONITORING OF DISEASE PROGRESSION

It is often desirable to follow the dynamics of disease over time (45). Some methods for quantitation, such as measurements of *strength during maximal voluntary contraction*, depend on patient cooperation and may therefore give inaccurate results. These measurements reflect both upper and lower motor neuron involvement.

A few quantitative neurophysiological techniques have been used to monitor MND. All of them have shortcomings, and therefore it may be necessary to use combinations of different methods to obtain accurate information.

SFEMG and Motor Unit Parameters

EMG can be used not only for the diagnosis of MND, but also to obtain information about the dynamics of the disease. This information may be obtained from one investigation or by serial examinations performed as the disease progresses. In each investigation, indications of the amount of denervation, the degree of reinnervation, and the speed of progression of the disease may be obtained.

When the disease progresses rapidly, fibrillations are abundant. Since there is insufficient time for all nerve sprouts and newly formed motor end-plates to mature, the FD is only moderately increased, jitter is increased, and the degree of blocking is high. The MUPs are very unstable, reflecting the increased jitter and blocking that are better seen with SFEMG. The MUPs are polyphasic but their amplitude and duration are only moderately increased (30).

When the disease progresses more slowly, the FD may be higher, and the jitter and blocking are less abnormal. In muscles with slower progression, the MUPs are generally more stable and of higher amplitude.

M-Wave Amplitude

The combined effects of denervation, muscle fiber atrophy, and compensatory reinnervation determine the M-wave amplitude in individual muscles. It does not reflect upper motor neuron involvement. The M-wave amplitude seems to be one of the best electrophysiologic indicators of clinical status in ALS. Measurement of the M-wave is noninvasive and easy to perform in both distal and proximal muscles. For maximal reliability, the electrode positions and temperature of the tested muscle must be standardized.

Interference Pattern

The fullness of the interference pattern, analyzed quantitatively, has also been used to measure and follow the severity of denervation in motor neuron disease (13). When increasing loss of motor neurons, the interference pattern becomes progressively less full. This parameter reflects both upper motor neuron and lower motor neuron function (Fig. 7).

Motor Unit Counting

The technique of motor unit counting has also been used to study the progressive loss of motor units in patients with ALS. It is still unclear whether the method gives the correct number of axons or a relative estimate. In either case, the data obtained may be used to follow changes within one patient. Despite the limitations of the method, it has a major advantage over other techniques in that it measures the loss of motor units and not the combinations of denervation and reinnervation, as do the others.

Macro EMG

Macro EMG has been used in longitudinal studies in ALS, in postpolio syndromes, and in other neuropathic conditions. The size of the motor unit, as

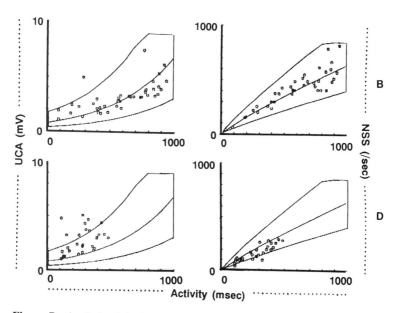

Figure 7 Analysis of the interference pattern in the right biceps muscle (A,B) and left biceps muscle (C,D) of a patient with ALS (13). The strength and interference pattern analysis were normal in the right biceps; there was moderate weakness in the left biceps, the activity (a measure of the "fullness" of the EMG signal) was reduced and the amplitude of the largest spikes in the signal was increased. UCA, upper centile amplitude (a measure of amplitude of the largest spikes in the signal); NSS, number of small segments (a measure of the high-frequency components in the signal).

indicated by the macro MUP amplitude, changes over time. This is due to ongoing reinnervation as a response to earlier denervation. It is therefore an indirect measure of severity of denervation. It has also been used as a recording method for the motor unit counting technique (46).

Longitudinal Macro EMG Studies in ALS

Initially the fiber density increases in parallel with the size of the motor units as reflected by the macro EMG amplitudes (Fig. 8). The FD usually remains high thereafter. For methodological reasons, it is difficult to quantitate further increases when the values have become very high. Measurement of FD is therefore not useful in following very pronounced changes in the motor unit. However, macro EMG provides useful information about motor unit size even in severely affected muscles. Sometimes an initial increase in macro MUP amplitude is followed by a reduction in both macro MUP amplitude and strength of muscle

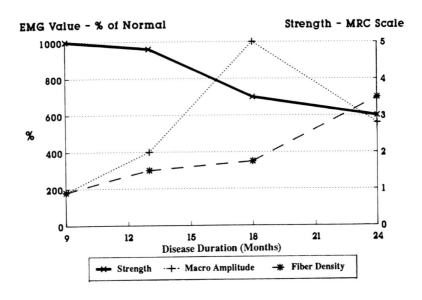

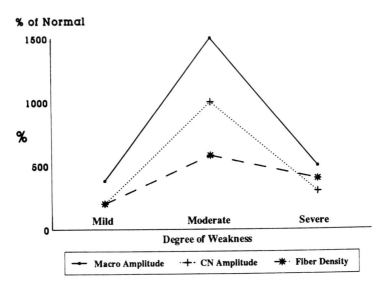

Figure 8   Changes in strength and EMG findings in the biceps muscle of a patient with ALS as the disease progressed over 15 months. (Bottom) EMG findings in the biceps muscle of 30 patients with ALS compared to the weakness in the tested muscle.

contraction. Whether this is due to loss of the largest motor units, a concept supported by some morphometric studies of the spinal cord (47) but not by others (48), or to deterioration of the large reinnervated motor units is not settled.

One reason for loss of large motor units may be that all muscle fibers in large, dense motor units cannot become reinnervated after denervation of that unit. This explanation is based on the view that fibers in one motor unit can only be reinnervated by overlapping motor units, i.e., from nerve terminals represented in the same fascicles as the denervated motor unit. This is suggested from the findings of scanning EMG (49), a technique used to map the electrophysiological cross-section of the motor unit. The findings indicate that the territory of a reinnervating motor unit does not increase very much from normal. Correspondingly, findings from rat muscles (50) show that a given motor unit is unable to expand outside the fascicles where it was originally represented. Physical hindrance for collateral sprouting or insufficient triggering signals from fibers outside the fascicular borders are both possible explanations for these spatial restrictions in reinnervation. Thus, a dense motor unit that completely occupies the fascicles where it was originally represented may not be reinnervated at all after it subsequently becomes denervated. This will cause grouped atrophy in the muscle biopsy. These most dense motor units, probably with the highest macro MUP amplitudes, will disappear as the disease progresses and the average macro MUP size will decrease.

Another possible explanation for a fall in MUP size is that the surviving motor unit reaches a state of relative metabolic insufficiency in which the motor neuron can no longer support all its distal fibers, and peripheral deterioration takes place. This may occur if there are reinnervation attempts beyond the capacity of the normal motor neuron or the neuron becomes sick.

CHANGES OUTSIDE THE MOTOR UNIT IN MOTOR NEURON DISEASE

Although the principal changes in MND occur in the motor unit, there are reports indicating functional changes in other parts of the nervous system.

Studies of *central sensory pathways* by means of somatosensory evoked potentials have shown abnormalities in about half the ALS patients studied, whereas brainstem auditory and visual-evoked potentials show fewer abnormalities (51–54).

The autonomic nervous system does not show any major changes in MND, although our findings of slight abnormal RR-interval variation in many patients may indicate subtle involvement (55) (Fig. 9).

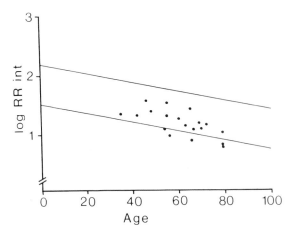

Figure 9 Autonomic function tested with heart rate variation during deep breathing in patients with ALS. Reference values plotted as two lines (±2 SD). A few of the patients fall outside the normal values. Log RR int = logarithmic value of RR intervals. [Modified from Nogues and Stålberg (55).]

CONCLUSION

In this chapter we have shown how neurophysiological techniques can be useful in the diagnosis, in quantifying the degree of involvement, and in assessing the dynamics of MND. They will hopefully continue to add significant information to further understanding of the condition.

REFERENCES

1. Swash M, Schwartz MS. Staging motor neurone disease: Single fibre EMG studies of asymmetry, progression and compensatory reinnervation. In: Rose FC, ed. Research progress in motor neurone disease. London: Pitman, 1984:123–140.

2. Lambert EH. Electromyography in amyotrophic lateral sclerosis. In: Norris FH, Kurland LT, eds. Motor neuron diseases. New York: Grune & Statton, 1969: 135–153.

3. Thesleff S, Ward MR. Studies on the mechanism of fibrillation potentials in denervated muscle. J Physiol (Lond) 1975;244:313–323.

4. Trontelj J, Stålberg E. Bizarre repetitive discharges recorded with single fibre EMG. J Neurol Neurosurg Psychiatry 1983;46:310–316.

5. Denny-Brown D, Pennypacker JB. Fibrillation and fasciculation in voluntary muscle. Brain 1938;61:311.

6. Forster FM, Alpers BJ. Site of origin of fasciculations, in voluntary muscle. Arch Neurol Psychiatry 1944;51:264–267.

7. Conradi S, Grimby L, Lundemo G. Pathophysiology of fasciculations in ALS as studied by electromyography of single motor units. Muscle Nerve 1982;5:202–208.

8. Brown RJ, Johns RJ. Abnormal motor nerve excitability. Johns Hopkins Med J 1970;127:55–63.

9. Janko M, Trontelj JV, Gersak K. Fasciculations in motor neuron disease: Discharge rate reflects extent and recency of collateral sprouting. J Neurol Neurosurg Psychiatry 1989;52:1375–1381.

10. Nandedkar SD, Barkhaus Pe, Sanders DB, Stålberg E. Analysis of the amplitude and area of the concentric needle EMG motor unit action potentials. Electroenceph Clin Neurophysiol 1988;69:561–567.

11. Willison RG. Analysis of the electrical activity in healthy and dystrophic muscle in man. J Neurol Neurosurg Psychiatry 1964;27:386–394.

12. Stålberg EV, Chu J, Bril V, Nandedkar S, Stålberg S, Ericsson M. Automatic analysis of EMG interference pattern. EEG Clin Neurophysiol 1983;56:672–681.

13. Nandedkar S, Sanders DB, Stålberg EV. Automatic analysis of the electromyographic interference pattern. Part II. Findings in control subjects and in some neuromuscular diseases. Muscle Nerve 1986;9:491–500.

14. Denys EH. Anterior horn cell diseases viewed by the clinical electromyographer. AAEE 28th ann meeting. Portland, OR, 1981:25–31.

15. Stålberg E, Thiele B. Transmission block in terminal nerve twigs: A single fibre electromyographic finding in man. J Neurol Neurosurg Psychiatry 1972;35:52–59.

16. Stålberg E, Fawcett PRW. Electrophysiological methods for study of the motor unit in spinal muscular atrophy (SMA). In: Gamstorp IH, Sarnat B, eds. Progressive spinal muscular atrophy. New York: Raven Press, 1984:111–134.

17. Albers JW, Zimnowodski S, Lowrey CM, Miller B. Juvenile progressive bulbar palys. Acta Neurol 1983;40:351–353.

18. Halstead LS, Wiechers DO. Late effects of poliomyelitis. Miami, FL: Symposia Foundation, 1985.

19. Einarsson G, Grimby G, Stålberg E. Post polio syndrome. Muscle Nerve 1989;13: 165–171.

20. Parry GJ, Clarke S. Multifocal aquired demyelinating neuropathy masquerading as motor neuron disease. Muscle Nerve 1988;11:103–107.

21. Pestronk A, Cornblath DR, Ilyas AA, Baba H, Quarles RH, Griffin JW, Alderson K, Adams RN. A treatable multifocal motor neuropathy with antibodies to GM1 ganglioside. Ann Neurol 1988;24:73–78.

22. van den Bergh P, Logigian EL, Kelly J. Motor neuropathy with multifocal conduction blocks. Muscle Nerve 1989;11:26–31.

23. Bradley WG. Recent views on amyotrophic lateral sclerosis with emphasis on electrophysiological studies. Muscle Nerve 1987;10:490–502.

24. Stålberg E, Trontelj J. Single fibre electromyography. Old Woking, Surrey, UK: Mirvalle Press, 1979.

25. Stålberg E, Sanders DB. The motor unit in ALS studied with different neurophysiological techniques. In: Rose FC, ed. Research progress in motor neurone disease. London: Pitman, 1984:105–122.

26. Stålberg E. Capability of motor unit sprouting in neuromuscular disorders. AAEE didactic program, 34th annual meeting, San Antonio, 1987:33–39.

27. Massey JM, Sanders DB, Nandedkar SD. Sensitivity of various EMG techniques in motor neurone disease. Electroenceph Clin Neurophysiol 1985;61:S74–S75.

28. Appel SH. A unifying hypothesis for the cause of amyotrophic lateral sclerosis, Parkinsonism and Alzheimer's disease. Ann Neurol 1981;10:499–505.

29. Festoff BW. Neuromuscular junction macromolecules in the pathogenesis of amyotrophic lateral sclerosis. Med Hypotheses 1980;6:121–131.

30. Denys EH, Norris FH. Amyotrophic lateral sclerosis: Impairment of neuromuscular transmission. Arch Neurol 1979;36:202–205.

31. Bernstein LP, Antel JP. Motor neuron disease: Decrementing responses to repetitive nerve stimulation. Neurology 1981;31:202–204.

32. Aquilonius S-M, Askmark H, Eckernas S-A, Gillberg P-G, Hilton-Brown P, Rydin E, Stålberg E. Cholinesterase inhibitors lack therapeutic effect in amyotrophic lateral sclerosis. A controlled study of physostigmine neostigmine. Acta Neurol Scand 1986;73:628–632.

33. Konstanzer A, Dengler R, Heese S, Elek J, Wolf W. Weakness of motor units (MUs) in late amyotrophic lateral sclerosis (ALS). Electroenceph Clin Neurophysiol 1990;75:S744.

34. Merton PA, Morton HB. Stimulation of the cerebral cortex in the intact human subject. Nature 1980;285:227.

35. Barker AT, Freeston IL, Jalinous R, Jarratt JA. Magnetic stimulation of the human brain and peripheral nervous system: An introduction and results of an initial clinical evaluation. Neurosurgery 1987;20:100–109.

36. Mills KR, Murray NMJ, Hess CW. Magnetic and electrical transcranial brain stimulation: physiological mechanisms and clinical applications. Neurosurgery 1987;20: 164–168.

37. Eisen A, Shytbel W, Murphy K, Hoirch M. Cortical magnetic stimulation in amyotrophic lateral sclerosis. Muscle Nerve 1990;13:146–151.

38. Hansen S, Ballantyne JP. A quantitative electrophysiological study of motor neurone disease. J Neurol Neurosurg Psychiatry 1978;41:773–783.

39. McComas AJ, Sica REP, Campbell MJ, Upton ARM. Functional compensation in partially denervated muscles. J Neurol Neurosurg Psychiatry 1971;34:453–460.

40. Stålberg E. Electrogenesis in human dystrophic muscle. In: Rowland LP ed. Pathogenesis of human muscular dystrophies. Amsterdam-Oxford: Excerpta Medica, 1976;570–587.

41. Brown WF, Strong MJ, Snow R. Methods for estimating numbers of motor units in biceps-brachialis muscles and losses of motor units with aging. Muscle Nerve 1988;11:423–432.

42. Strong MJ, Brown WF, Hudson AJ, Snow R. Motor unit estimates in biceps-brachialis in amyotrophic lateral sclerosis. Muscle Nerve 1988;11:415–422.

43. Liedholm LJ, Stålberg E. PC based method for estimating the number of axons in human motor nerves implemented for routine use. Electroenceph Clin Neurophysiol 1990;76:2.

44. Stålberg E, Fawcett PRW. Macro EMG changes in healthy subjects of different ages. J Neurol Neurosurg Psychiatry 1982;45:870–878.

45. Rose CF. Problems in neurological clinical trials. London: Demos, 1989.
46. De Koning P. Functional and electrophysiological evaluation of damaged peripheral nerve: Neurotrophic actions of org. 2766. Thesis, Utrecht, 1987.
47. Kawamura Y, Dyck PJ, Shimono M, Okazaki H, Tateishi J, Doi H. Morphometric comparison of the vulnerability of peripheral motor and sensory neurons in amyotrophic lateral sclerosis. J Neuropathol Exp Neurol 1981;40:667–675.
48. Tsukagoshi H, Yin Q, Yamada M, Wada Y, Furukawa T, Yanagisawa N. Morphometric study on the spinal cord of amyotrophic latersclerosis: Quantification of the number and size of anterior horn cells of the cervical cord. In: Tsubaki T, Yase Y eds. Amyotrophic lateral sclerosis. Recent advances in research and treatment. Amsterdam: Excerpta Medica, 1988;119–124.
49. Stålberg E. Single fiber EMG, macro EMG, and scanning EMG. New ways of looking at the motor unit. CRC Crit Rev Clin Neurobiol 1986;2:125–67.
50. Kugelberg E, Edstrom L, Abruzzese M. Mapping of motor units in experimentally reinnervated rat muscle. J Neurol Neurosurg Psychiatry 1970;33:319–329.
51. Cosi V, Poloni M, Mazzini L, Callieco R. Somatosensory evoked potentials in amyotrophic lateral sclerosis. J Neurol Neurosurg Psychiatry 1984;47:857–861.
52. Bosch EP, Yamada T, Kimura J. Somatosensory evoked potentials in motor neuron disease. Muscle Nerve 1985;8(7):556–562.
53. Matheson JK, Harrington HJ, Hallett M. Abnormalities of multimodality evoked potentials in amyotrophic lateral sclerosis. Arch Neurol 1986;43:338–340.
54. Radtke RA, Erwin A, Erwin CW. Abnormal sensory evoked potentials in amyotrophic lateral sclerosis. Neurology 1986;36(6):796–801.
55. Nogues M, Stålberg E. Automatic analysis of heart rate variation. Part II. Findings in patients attending an EMG laboratory. Muscle Nerve 1989;12:1001–1008.

10
Neuroimaging Studies in Amyotrophic Lateral Sclerosis

John M. Hoffman and Orest B. Boyko

Duke University Medical Center
Durham, North Carolina

W. Kent Davis

Rex Hospital
Raleigh, North Carolina

INTRODUCTION

Amyotrophic lateral sclerosis (ALS) is a form of motor neuron disease (MND) representing a heterogeneous group of progressive degenerative diseases affecting the voluntary motor system. Pathologically, the cerebral cortex, pyramidal structures, brainstem, anterior horn cells, and spinal cord can be involved (1). ALS affects, to varying degrees, the upper motor neuron, lower motor neuron, and bulbar motor neuron (2).

The differential diagnosis of syndromes causing a similar clinical picture includes toxin exposure (3), remote effects of neoplasia (4), hypoglycemia (5), and cervical spondylosis and spinal cord tumor. The majority of neuroradiological studies are obtained in ALS patients to exclude an anatomical etiology for the patient's signs and symptoms.

With the advent of computed tomography (CT), magnetic resonance imaging (MRI), and positron emission tomography (PET), imaging studies in ALS patients have been performed in an attempt to better understand and define neuroanatomical and metabolic pathophysiology in this disease.

The purpose of this chapter is to initially describe the usefulness of standard radiological studies (plain radiographs, myelography, CT, and MRI) in evaluating the patient with signs and symptoms of ALS. Neuroimaging studies specifically examining the anatomical, biochemical, and metabolic consequences (PET) of ALS will also be reviewed.

SKELETAL RADIOGRAPHY

For many years skeletal radiography was used to investigate patients with clinical signs and symptoms suggestive of ALS. Numerous patients with an ALS-like syndrome secondary to multiple-level radiculopathy as well as myelopathy were described in the medical literature. These particular individuals typically have significant degenerative disc disease involving both the cervical and lumbosacral spine. These patients typically complain of pain, however, which is atypical in ALS. The clinical history and neurological examination often show abnormalities in all extremities. For many years the initial examination of choice was that of plain films of the cervical and lumbosacral spine. Often, significant degenerative disease was documented and the patient was further evaluated with myelography, particularly when myelopathy was present. The typical skeletal radiographic abnormalities noted included foraminal narrowing secondary to spurring, spondylosis, and spondylolisthesis. An example of these particular abnormalities is shown in Figure 1. When widespread extensive disease of this type is observed in both the cervical and lumbosacral region, it can be extremely difficult to differentiate ALS from multiple-level radiculopathy and myelopathy.

Despite the advances in available imaging technology, plain radiographs of the cervical and lumbosacral spine can provide important information and remain the first step in neuroimaging of spinal disorders.

MYELOGRAPHY

The development of myelography in the 1930s made it possible to better examine the external anatomy of the spinal cord and nerve roots (Fig. 2). This became important in defining surgically correctable lesions. Initial studies were performed with oil-soluble iophendylate (Pantopaque). This myelographic agent has been associated with complications, including arachnoiditis (6). In the 1970s water-soluble contrast agents such as metrizamide (Amipaque) became available. This agent is water soluble and, unlike Pantopaque, does not require complete removal at the completion of the study. This agent has also been associated with side effects such as nausea, vomiting, headache, decrease in seizure threshold, or overt seizures; however, these are easily managed (7–9). With the advent of CT in the 1970s it became possible to do postmyelographic CT procedures (Fig. 2e) with the water-soluble contrast agent. Again, the critical issue in examining the patient with presumed ALS with neuroradiological procedures was to exclude the possibility of tumor, disc herniation (Fig. 3), degenerative disease (Figs. 4 and 5), syringohydromyelia, or other abnormalities that would cause a syndrome mimicking the signs and symptoms of ALS. It is possible to detect spinal cord or nerve root atrophy in ALS patients; however,this is extremely difficult because of the normal variation of these anatomical structures.

COMPUTED TOMOGRAPHY

The development of CT in the 1970s also allowed for detailed cross-sectional anatomical evaluation of the brainstem and spinal cord (10). The ability of CT to fully evaluate and rule out other causes for ALS-like signs and symptoms is well documented. Numerous publications have described the applications as well as limitations of CT techniques when examining the spine (11–13). Various techniques, including thin cuts (1.5–3 mm) with computerized reformatting of images in the coronal and sagittal projections, can often be helpful. One of the major improvements in CT studies of the spine and craniocervical junction region occurred after the introduction of metrizamide. This agent provided excellent CT-myelogram studies. Numerous reports then appeared in the medical literature describing the utility of the technique (14). Several reports of the use of CT in syringomyelia (Fig. 6) and syringohydromyelia appeared (15–17). The evaluation of paraspinal and intraspinal tumors was facilitated (18,19) (Fig. 7). The ability to localize and evaluate spinal stenosis (Figs. 1, 5, and 8), spondylosis, and herniated nucleus pulposus (Fig. 9) was also much improved (20,21).

With the advent of MRI, the number of spinal CT and CT-myelogram procedures performed has fallen precipitously. However, in situations where MRI is not available, CT still provides excellent-quality images and can be important in limiting the differential diagnosis in individuals with ALS-like signs and symptoms.

MRI

The first report of MRI abnormalities in patients with ALS was reported by Goodin et al. in 1988 (22) (Fig. 10). The investigators studied a total of five individuals with proven ALS. The individuals had axial brain MRI scans. Partial T1-weighted and T2-weighted images were obtained in contiguous 5-mm axial slices. In two patients, increased signal intensity was noted on the T2-weighted images extending from the motor cortex through the corona radiata into the posterior limb of the internal capsule and into the cerebral peduncles and brainstem. Another individual had white-matter signal abnormalities localized in the posterior limb of the internal capsule. The remaining two individuals had completely normal MRI scans. The investigators noted that the pattern of signal abnormality on MRI was similar to the histological findings of ALS patients where degeneration of the pyramidal system could be traced along the cortical spinal tracts into the posterior limb of the internal capsule and eventually into the motor cortex. In one of the largest pathological series of ALS patients, Lawyer and Netsky showed demyelination of the pyramidal tract in the brainstem up to the level of the internal capsule (23). Goodin et al. postulated that lesions found on MRI corresponded to the specific neuropathological changes known to occur in the white matter of ALS patients. The distribution of the abnormalities was confined to the cortical spinal tract in the same distribution as seen on postmortem examples.

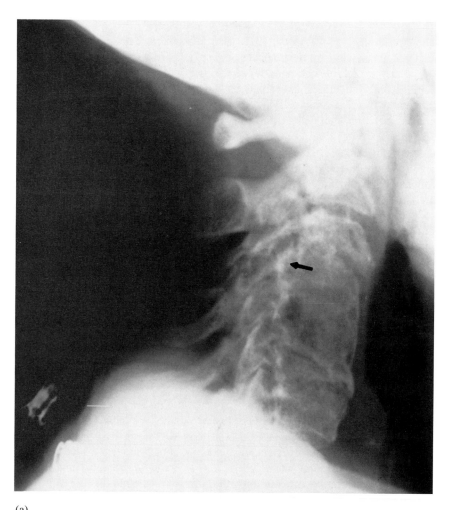

(a)

Figure 1 Sixty-five-year-old woman with rheumatoid arthritis who noted progressive weakness of the lower extremities. Examination revealed significant lower extremity weakness with minimal upper extremity weakness. No obvious sensory abnormalities were appreciated. (a) Lateral cervical plain film shows marked osteopenia and degenerative changes of the vertebral bodies with loss of the disc space at C3–4 and possible bony fragment in the spinal canal at C4 (arrow). (b) Axial noncontrast cervical spine CT at the C3–4 level demonstrates degenerative change of the vertebral body with evidence of bone fragment within the epidural space and compression of the thecal sac and cervical cord (arrows). (c) Midline sagittal multiplanar GRASS (MPGR) image (TR = 40 msec; TE = 20 msec, with 15° flip angle) demonstrates myelographic effect (hyperintense CSF). There is loss of normal disc space signal at C3–4 with posterior subluxation of C4 and better visualization of bony fragment impinging and compressing the cervical cord. There is posterior ligamentous hypertrophy (arrow).

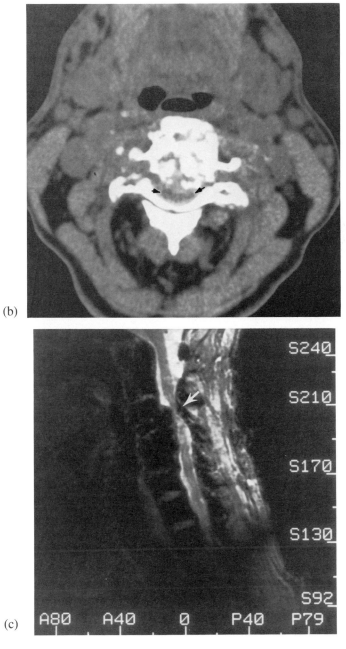

(b)

(c)

Figure 1b and c.

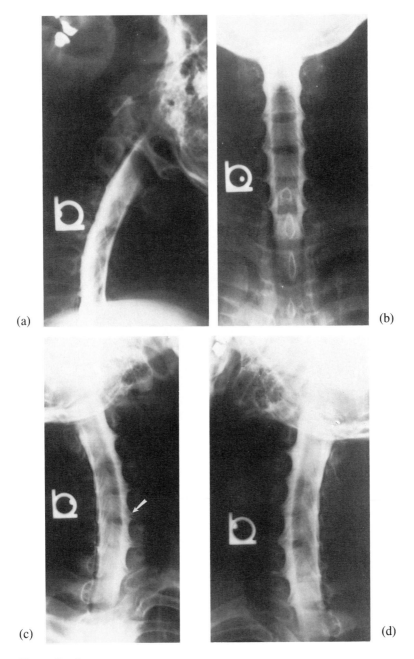

(a)

(b)

(c)

(d)

Figure 2a–d.

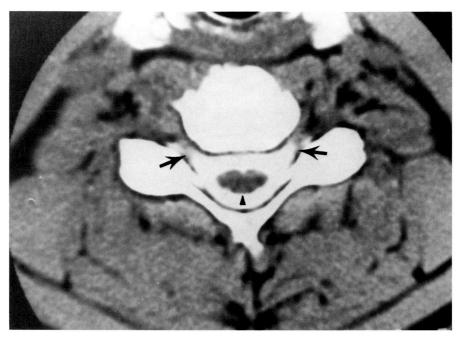

(e)

Figure 2 Normal cervical myelogram. (a) Lateral view of the cervical cord demonstrates no evidence for cord atrophy or enlargement and there is no evidence for anterior extradural defects. (b) Anteroposterior view of the cervical cord demonstrates normal cervical cord silhouette with normal bilateral filling of the nerve root sleeves and no evidence for nerve root sleeve filling defects. (c) Oblique cervical spine film demonstrates normal filling of the nerve root sleeves (arrow). The nerve roots themselves appear as normal filling defects in the sleeves. (d) Oblique lateral view of the cervical cord demonstrates normal filling of the nerve root sleeves. (e) Axial CT scan after intrathecal contrast administration demonstrates normal cervical cord silhouette (arrowhead) and normal filling of the nerve root sleeves (arrows) without evidence for anterior extradural defect or compression of the thecal sac.

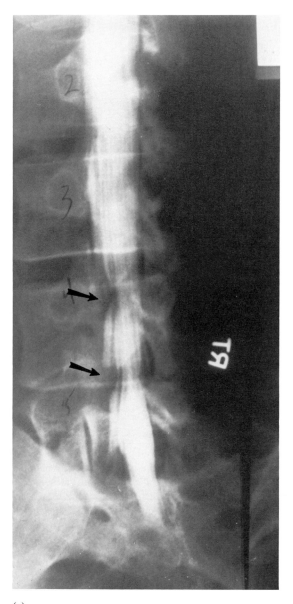

(a)

Figure 3   Patient with lower extremity weakness but no associated sensory complaints. (a) Oblique lumbar myelogram plain film shows extradural defect and poor filling of the nerve roots at L3–4 and L4–5 (arrows). (b) Sagittal T2 intermediate weighted MR image (TR = 2000 msec, T = 35 msec) shows herniated discs at L3–4 and L4–5 (arrows).

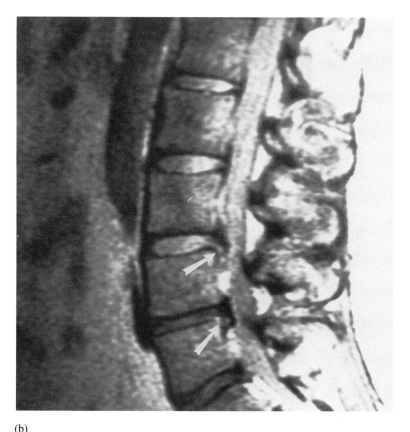

(b)
Figure 3b.

The importance of the information obtained from the MRI studies of the brain confirm more extensive central nervous system changes than previously suspected in ALS.

The role of MRI in evaluation of the spine in patients with ALS-like signs and symptoms is undisputed. The detail, contrast resolution, and quality of images are superb. It is possible to describe atrophy or very focal pathology (24). A recent report describes bilateral degeneration of the corticospinal tracts in spinal cord specimens from ALS patients. High signal intensity was noted on both T1- and T2-weighted images (25). MRI has essentially replaced CT and myelographic studies in centers where it is available. Again, the spinal MRI study is obtained to rule out tumor (Figs. 7 and 11), spondylosis (Figs. 1 and 4), syrin-

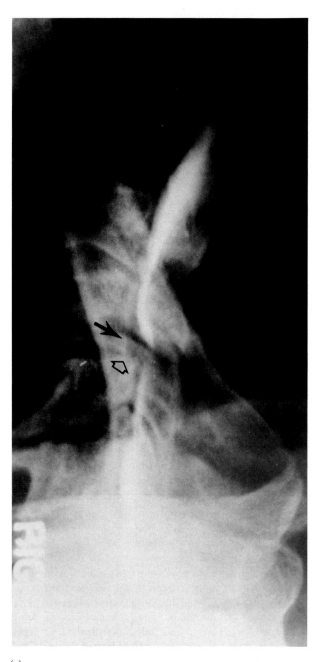

(a)
Figure 4a

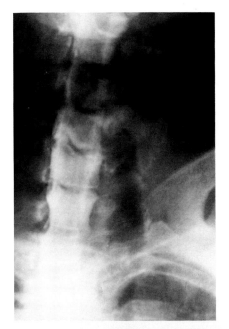

(b)

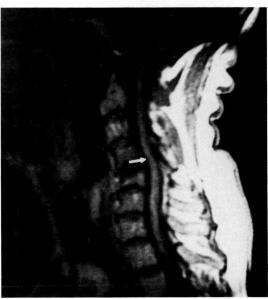

(c)

Figure 4 Seventy-seven-year-old man with insidious onset of left leg and arm weakness. There was progressive difficulty with bilateral finger dexterity. (a) Lateral cervical spine plain film after intrathecal contrast administration shows anterior extradural defect (arrow) centered at the C4–5 disc space. There is very mild retrolisthesis of C5 (open arrow). (b) Oblique cervical myelogram plain film shows lack of filling of the right C4–5 nerve root, and confirmation was made by CT of a bone spur impinging on the nerve root causing the lack of filling of the nerve root sleeve. (c) Compression of the cord is better demonstrated on midsagittal T1-weighted MR image (TR = 500 msec: TE = 20 msec) (arrow). Both bone spur and bulging disc were involved in the cord compression.

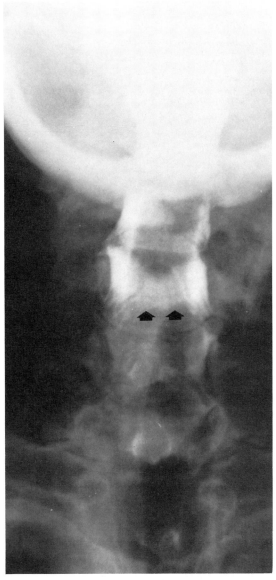

(a)

Figure 5 Sixty-eight-year-old man with progressive weakness and atrophy of the right hand. The patient had a long history of neck pain. (a) Anterior cervical myelogram after C1–2 puncture shows poor opacification of the subarachnoid space inferior to C5–6 due to partial block of subarachnoid contrast flow (arrows). Postmyelogram CT (b) demonstrates marked facet hypertrophy bilaterally and marked bony hypertrophy anterior to the thecal sac. Patients with spondylytic change are placed in a hyperextended position for myelography, which can accentuate spondylytic compression of the thecal sac. The patient's cervical spine is in a neutral position during CT scanning.

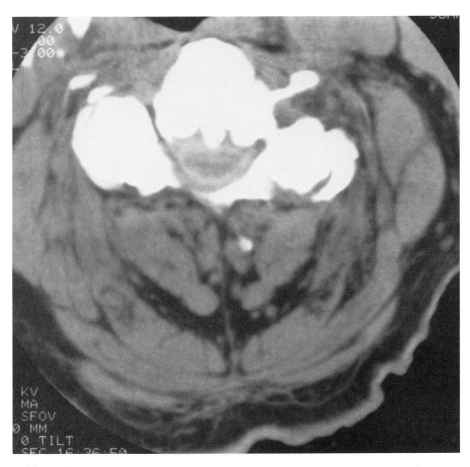

Figure 5b.

gomyelia (Fig. 6), or another anatomical lesion (Fig. 3) that causes ALS-like signs and symptoms. Typically, however, the spinal cord appears entirely normal despite profound motor weakness in the ALS patient (Figs. 12 and 13). An interesting recent MRI observation is the loss of normal shape, size, internal structure, and position of the tongue in ALS patients (26).

PET STUDIES IN ALS

Several studies have examined the effects of ALS on cerebral blood flow and glucose metabolism using PET (27–30). It has been hypothesized that neuropathological changes observed in ALS should correlate with the local cerebral

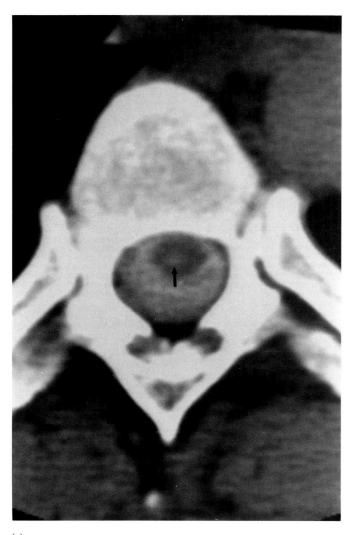

(a)
Figure 6 Thirty-five-year-old man with progressive spastic paraparesis without any sensory complaints. Examination confirmed diffuse lower extremity weakness, hyperreflexia, and no sensory level. (a) Postmyelogram CT after 6-hr delay demonstrates thoracic cord atrophy with central cord hyperattenuation (arrow) representing contrast diffusion into a central cord syrinx. (b) Midsagittal cervical MR image (TR = 500 msec: TE = 20 msec) demonstrates normal cervical cord, but at the C7–T1 disc space level (top arrow) is a central signal hypointense to the cord but isointense with surrounding CSF, which extends inferiorly to the T2 disc space level (bottom arrow). (c) Sagittal T1-weighted thoracic MRI (TR = 500 msec: TE = 20 msec) shows further extension of central cord syrinx into the midthoracic level (arrows) with thoracic cord atrophy. Central cord syrinx often presents with cord expansion on MRI.

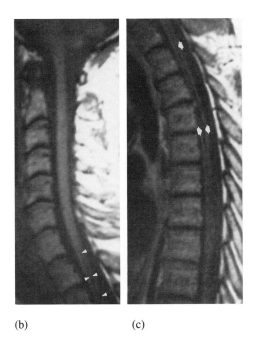

(b)   (c)

metabolic rate for glucose (LCMRGLc) using ^{18}F-2-fluoro-2-deoxy-D-glucose (FDG) and PET. LCMRGLc is felt to reflect neuronal synaptic metabolic activity in normal adults (31–34) (Fig. 14). Since ALS involves selected loss of motor neurons (35), large pyramidal cells in the motor cortex, and cortical spinal tract degeneration, there should be a resultant decrease in LCMRGLc, which should correlate with regional neuronal cell loss (Figs. 15 and 16). The FDG-PET studies to date have had conflicting results. Initial studies performed by Dalakas showed widespread reductions in LCMRGLc even in brain regions not considered to be associated with motor function (26,27). An investigation by Hoffman et al. (29) did not show such widespread LCMRGLc reductions in motor or nonmotor regions. In fact, only a few cortical regions showed a significant ($p <$ 0.05 reduction in LCMRGLc) (Table 1). An unusual finding noted in the investigation by Hoffman et al. was the observation that increasing weakness correlated with a decline in LCMRGLc of the precentral gyrus. This particular finding was felt to be consistent with observations by Munsat et al. of symmetrical and linear loss of motor neurons in ALS (35). In the middle frontal gyrus, however, increasing weakness was associated with increasing LCMRGLc. It was postulated that the finding may represent increasing metabolic activity of motor association cortex in response to primary loss of pyramidal cells. A similar pattern was observed when the deep tendon reflex changes were correlated with LCM

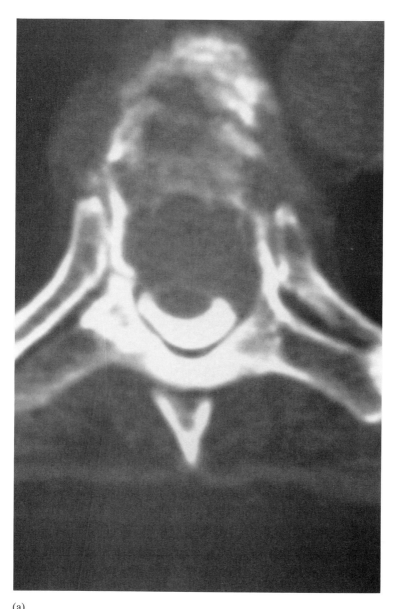

(a)

Figure 7 Forty-seven-year-old woman with progressive lower extremity weakness. Axial CT scan (a) shows lytic change with paraspinal soft tissue mass and epidural extension of tumor with compression of the thecal sac and cord secondary to tumor. (b) Sagittal MRI multiplanar GRASS (MPGR) (TR = 400 msec: TE = 20 msec: flip angle = 15°) shows plasmacytoma extending from the vertebral body into the epidural space (arrows) with compression and draping of the thoracic cord over the epidural mass. There is marked cord compression. Incidental note is made of a second focus of abnormal marrow signal in a lower vertebral body (inferior arrow) presumed to represent another focus of tumor.

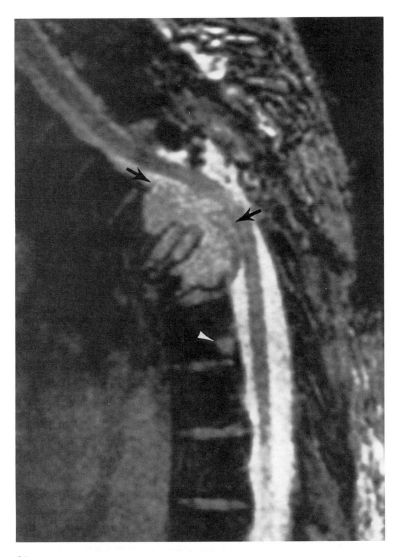

(b)
Figure 7b.

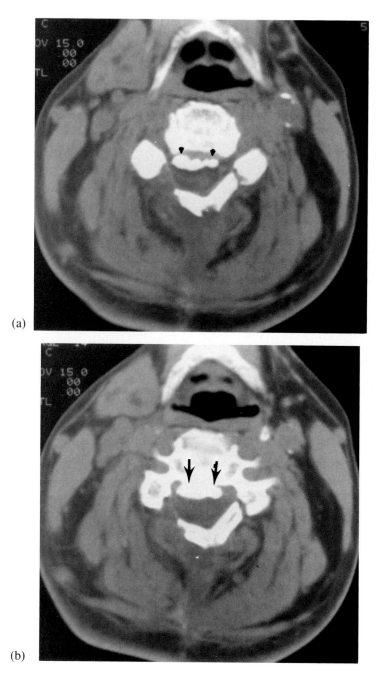

(a)

(b)

Figure 8a and b.

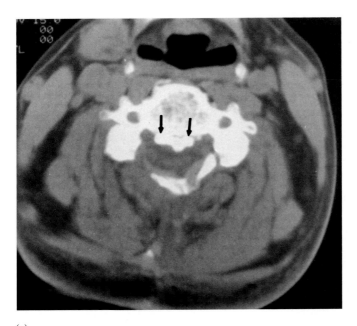

(c)

Figure 8 Fifty-eight-year-old woman who noted onset of left arm numbness, right leg weakness, and gait instability after a motor vehicle accident. Examination was significant for normal sensory examination, diffuse upper extremity weakness, proximal lower extremity weakness, lower extremity increased deep tendon reflexes, and right extensor plantar response. Axial CT scans at the C3–4 disc space level without administration of contrast demonstrates significant bony proliferation and deposition along the posterior longitudinal ligament (arrows) with compression of the thecal sac.

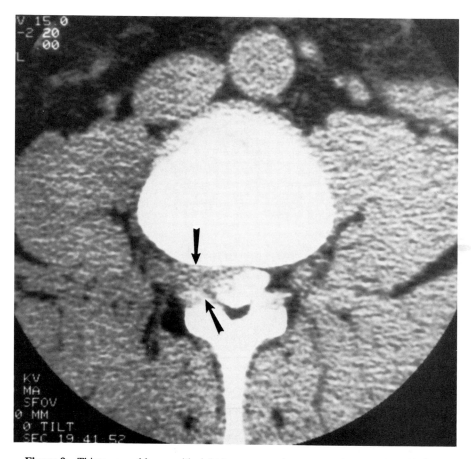

Figure 9 Thirty-year-old man with right lower extremity motor and sensory complaints. Axial CT scan after myelography demonstrates thecal sac to be compressed on the right side secondary to soft tissue density representing herniated disc material (arrows) with nerve root compression.

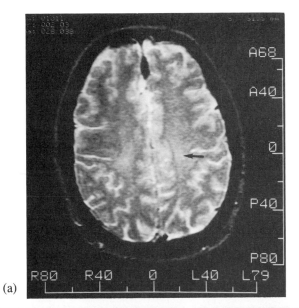

(a)

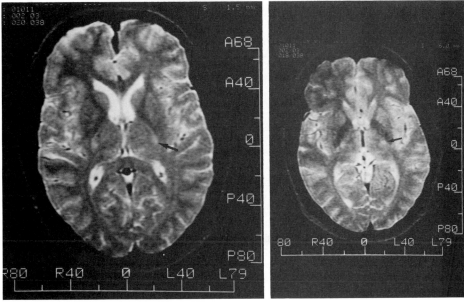

(b)   (c)

Figure 10a–c. Legend on p. 258.

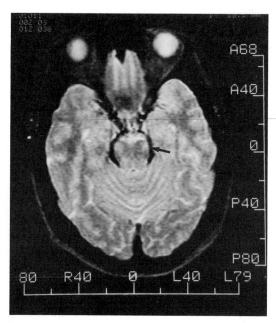

(d)

Figure 10   T2-weighted magnetic resonance images from a 41-year-old man with ALS (echo time = 80 msec; repetition time = 1,900 msec; 1.5-Tesla field strength). Four axial views are shown: (a) at the level of the centrum semiovale; (b) level of the lateral ventricles; (c) level of the thalamus, (d) level of the pons. Focal and symmetrical areas of increased signal intensity (arrows on the left hemisphere only) can be followed from the cortex through the posterior limbs of the internal capsule and into the pons. [From Goodin et al. (22), used with permission of author and publisher.]

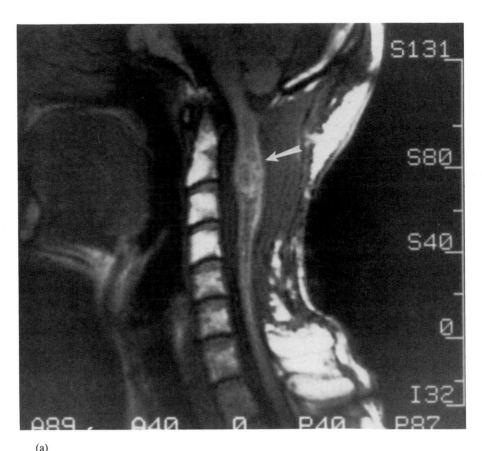

(a)

Figure 11 Forty-five-year-old man who initially noted neck stiffness. His initial neu-rologic examination, however, revealed quadraparesis and increased deep tendon re-flexes. Sagittal (a) and axial (b) T1-weighted MR images after intravenous administration of Gd-DTPA contrast agent demonstrates cord expansion at C2–3 with a central mass and peripheral enhancement representing a primary cervical cord neoplasm. A tumor cavity is noted as well as central cord hypointense signal superior and inferior to the enhancing mass (arrow). Incidental note is made of hyperintense T1 signal in the cervical 2, 3, and 4 vertebral bodies representing radiation changes.

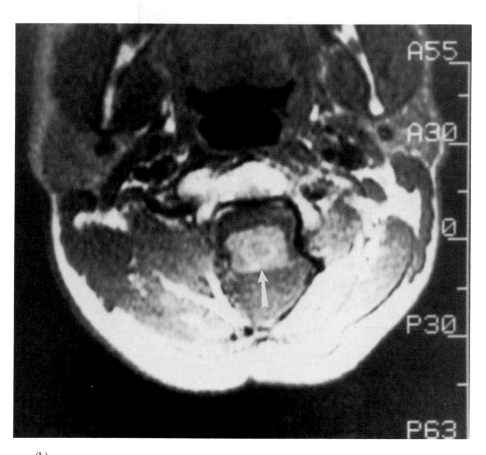

(b)
Figure 11b

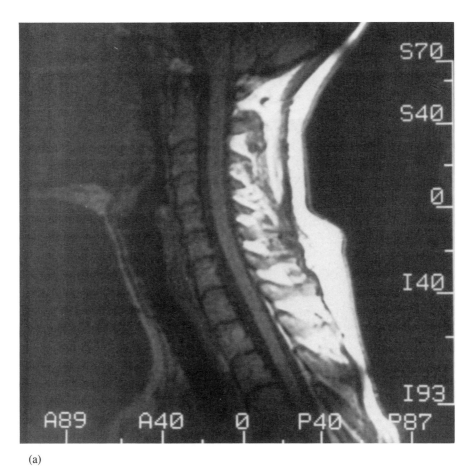

(a)

Figure 12   Fifty-year-old woman with progressive left hand and foot weakness. Neurological examination reveals normal sensation, diffuse weakness of the distal left upper and lower extremities, bilateral extensor plantar responses, and EMG evidence of diffuse denervation. By clinical and EMG evidence patient was diagnosed as having ALS. Midsagittal T1-weighted image (a) (TR = 500 msec: TE = 20 msec), and (b) axial multiplanar GRASS (MPGR) (TR = 500 msec: TE = 20 msec: 15° flip angle) shows no definite evidence for cord atrophy in this ALS patient.

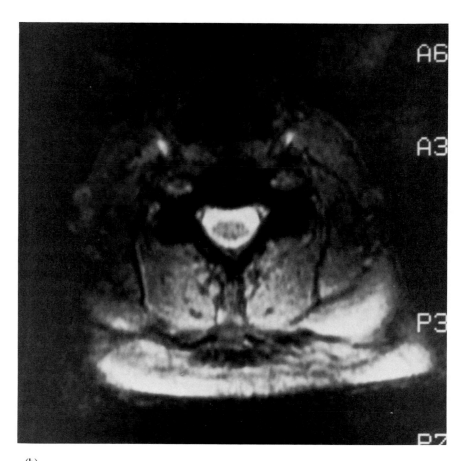

(b)
Figure 12b

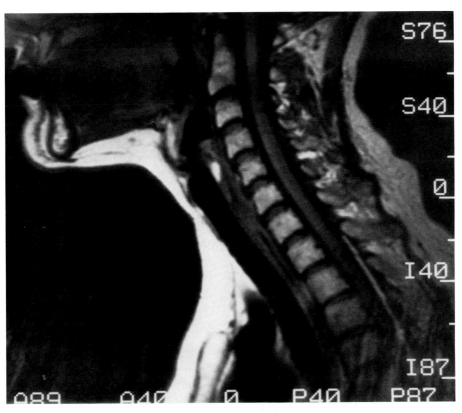

Figure 13   Patient with unequivocal ALS with prominent upper extremity weakness and muscle atrophy. Midsagittal T1-weighted MR image (TR = 500 msec: TE = 20 msec) shows normal contour of the cervical cord without evidence for cord atrophy. Despite the patient's prominent upper extremity involvement, no obvious cord pathology was appreciated on MRI.

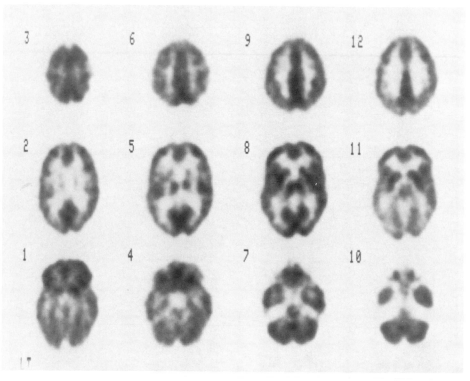

Figure 14 FDG-PET images of local cerebral metabolic rate of glucose (LCMRGLc) obtained on the Neuro-Ecat tomograph. Twelve emission images adequately sample the entire brain. This particular individual is approximately the same age as the ALS patients described in Figures 15 and 16. This is a normal study.

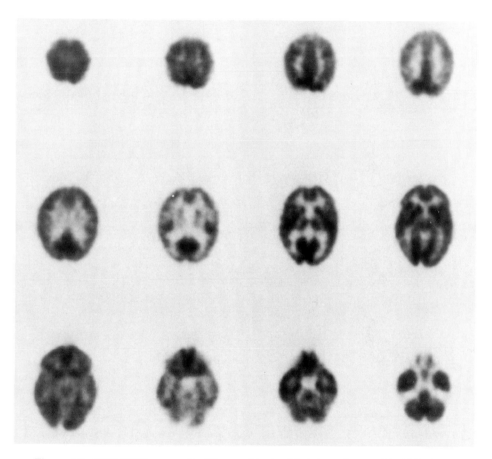

Figure 15 FDG-PET images of a 65-year-old wheelchair-bound man with ALS. Note the symmetrical FDG uptake without focal or global reduction.

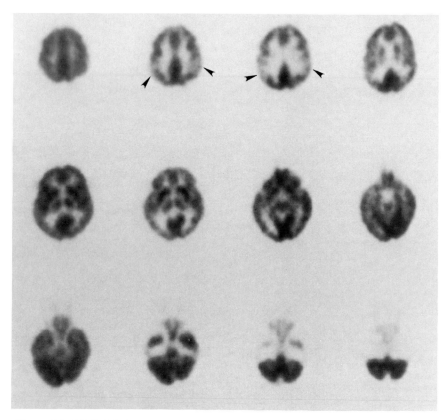

Figure 16 FDG-PET images of a 62-year-old man with severe ALS. Patient is wheel-chair-bound and clinically has prominent bulbar involvement. There is minimal reduction in parietal FDG uptake (arrows); however, the LCMRGLc value is within two standard deviations of the mean of an age-matched control population for this brain region.

Table 1 Cerebral Metabolic Rate of Glucose (Weighted Normalized)

Brain region	Left brain		Right brain	
	MND	Control	MND	Control
Precentral gyrus	1.02 ± 0.05	1.03 ± 0.03	0.96 ± 0.05*	1.01 ± 0.04
Lateral superior frontal gyrus	0.98 ± 0.10	1.01 ± 0.08	0.95 ± 0.11	0.99 ± 0.09
Medial superior frontal gyrus	1.15 ± 0.13	1.06 ± 0.14	1.11 ± 0.14	1.08 ± 0.14
Middle frontal gyrus	1.12 ± 0.08	1.07 ± 0.07	1.10 ± 0.08	1.07 ± 0.05
Inferior frontal gyrus	1.11 ± 0.08	1.06 ± 0.03	1.03 ± 0.07	1.00 ± 0.05
Superior parietal lobule	0.97 ± 0.10	0.94 ± 0.11	0.95 ± 0.09	0.95 ± 0.09
Inferior parietal lobule	1.04 ± 0.05	1.04 ± 0.07	1.02 ± 0.06	1.02 ± 0.05
Middle temporal gyrus	1.02 ± 0.07*	0.92 ± 0.05	1.00 ± 0.11	0.92 ± 0.05
Head caudate	1.20 ± 0.05*	1.29 ± 0.05	1.25 ± 0.06*	1.33 ± 0.04
Body caudate	1.22 ± 0.08	1.20 ± 0.14	1.20 ± 0.10	1.21 ± 0.10
Thalamus	1.23 ± 0.09	1.28 ± 0.06	1.26 ± 0.09	1.30 ± 0.06
Vermis-cerebellum			0.85 ± 0.13	0.97 ± 0.04
Dentate-cerebellum	0.81 ± 0.09*	0.93 ± 0.04	0.81 ± 0.11*	0.94 ± 0.04
Superior lobule cerebellum	0.72 ± 0.09	0.80 ± 0.03	0.70 ± 0.09*	0.81 ± 0.05
Midbrain			0.95 ± 0.08	0.93 ± 0.07
Pons			0.71 ± 0.09	0.78 ± 0.04
Frontal white matter	0.77 ± 0.03*	0.70 ± 0.65	0.80 ± 0.04*	0.72 ± 0.03

Weighted nomalized mean LCMRGlc values for right and left brain in MND and control subjects. Significant difference ($p < 0.05$) between MND and control values is denoted by * (not corrected for multiple comparisons).

RGLc. It is possible that when larger patient groups are studied with newer higher-resolution tomographs, focal precentral gyrus metabolic abnormalities may be noted correlating with neuronal cell loss.

REFERENCES

1. Hughs JT. Pathology of amyotrophic lateral sclerosis. In: Rowland LP, ed. Human motor neuron disease. New York: Raven Press, 1982:61–74.

2. Bonduelle M. Amyotrophic lateral sclerosis. In: Vinken PJ, Bruyn GW, eds. Handbook of clinical neurology, Vol 22. Amsterdam: North Holland, 1975:281–338.

3. Adams CR, Ziegler DK, Lin JT. Mercury intoxication simulating amyotrophic lateral sclerosis. JAMA 1983;250:642–643.

4. Schold SC, Cho E-S, Somasundaram M, Posner JB. Subacute motor neuronopathy: A remote effect of lymphoma. Ann Neurol 1979;5:271–287.

5. Danta G. Hypoglycemic peripheral neuropathy. Arch Neurol 1969;21:121–132.

6. Kieffer SA, Binet EF, Esquerra JV, Hartman RP, Gross CE. Contrast agents for myelography: Clinical and radiological evaluation of Amipaque and Pantopaque. Radiology 1978;129:695–705.

7. Baker RA, Hillman BJ, McLennan JE, Strand RD, Kaufman SM. Sequelae of metrizamide myelography in 200 examinations. Am J Radiol 1978;130:499–502.

8. Hauge O, Falkenberg H. Neuropsychologic reactions and other side effects after metrizamide myelography. Am J Neuroradiol 1982;3:229–232.

9. Skalps IO. Adhesive arachnoiditis following lumbar radiculopathy with water-soluble contrast agents. Radiology 1976;121:647–651.

10. Meschan MA. The vertebral column and spinal cord. In Meschan MA, ed. An atlas of anatomy basic to radiology. Philadelphia: Saunders, 1975.

11. Roub LW, Drayer BP. Spinal computed tomography: Limitations and applications. Am J Radiol 1979;133:267–273.

12. Keating JW, Nadell JMD, Luciano E. Fourth generation computed tomographic scanning of the spinal cord. In Post MJD, ed. Computed tomography of the spine. Baltimore: Williams & Wilkins, 1984.

13. Lee BCP, Kazam E, Newman AD. Computed tomography of the spinal cord. Radiology 1978;128:95–102.

14. Dublin AB, McGahan JP, Reid MH. The value of computed tomographic metrizamide myelography in the neuroradiological evaluation of the spine. Radiology 1983;146:79–86.

15. Batnitzky S, Price HI, Gaughan MJ, Hall PV, Rosenthal SJ. The radiology of syringohydromyelia. Radiographics 1983;3(4):585–610.

16. Bonafe A, Manelfe C, Espagno B, Guiraud B, Rascol A. Evaluation of syringomyelia with metrizamide computed tomographic myelography. J Comput Assist Tomogr 1980;4(6):797–802.

17. Resjo IM, Harwood-Nash DC, Fitz CR, Chuang S. Computed tomographic metrizamide myelography in syringohydromyelia. Radiology 1979;131:405–407.

18. Nakagawa H, Huang YP, Malis LI, Wolf BS. Computed tomography of intraspinal and paraspinal neoplasms. J Comput Tomogr 1977;1(4):377–390.

19. Tadmor R, Cacazorin ED, Kieffer SA. Advantages of supplementary CT in myelography of intraspinal masses. Am J Neuroradiol 1983;4:618–621.

20. Williams AL, Haughton VM, Daniels DL, Grogan JP. Differential CT diagnosis of extruded nucleus pulposus. Radiology 1983;148:141–148.

21. Grogran JP, Hemminghytt S, Williams AL, Carrera GF, Haughton VM. Spondylolysis studied with computed tomography. Radiology 1982;145:737–742.

22. Goodin D, Rowley H, Olney RK. Magnetic resonance imaging in amyotrophic lateral sclerosis. Ann Neurol 1988;23:418–420.

23. Lawyer T, Netsky M. Amytrophic lateral sclerosis. A clinicoanatomic study of fifty-three cases. Arch Neurol Psychiatry 1953;69:171–192.
24. Norman ND, Mills CM, Brant-Zawadski M, Yeates A, Crooks LE, Kaufman L. Magnetic resonance imaging of the spinal cord and canal: Potentials and limitations. Am J Neuroradiol 1984;5:9–14.
25. Carvlin MJ, Fielding R, Ragan SS, Muraki A, Manz HJ, Schellinger D, Hackney DB. MR imaging of amyotrophic lateral sclerosis: Results of a high resolution study of spinal cord specimens. Radiology 1989;173(Suppl):84.
26. Cha CH, Patten BM. Amyotrophic lateral sclerosis: Abnormalities of the tongue on magnetic resonance imaging. Ann Neurol 1989;25:468–472.
27. Dalakas M, Hatazawa J, Brooks R, Di Chiro G. Lowered cerebral glucose utilization in amyotrophic lateral sclerosis. Ann Neurol 1987;22:580–586.
28. Hatazawa J, Brooks RA, Dalakas MC, Mans L, DiChiro G. Cortical motor sensory hypometabolism in amyotrophic lateral sclerosis: A PET study. J Comput Assist Tomogr 1988;12(4):630–636.
29. Hoffman JM, Mazziotta JL, Hawk TC, Sumida R, Phelps ME. Normal cerebral glucose utilization in amyotrophic lateral sclerosis. J Nucl Med 1988;29(5):821.
30. Langen KJ, Ludolph AC, Kuwert T, Bottger IG, Kemper B, Feinendegen LE. Glucose metabolism in amyotrophic lateral sclerosis: Relation to clinical and neuropsychological status. J Cereb Blood Flow Metab 1989;9(Suppl 1):524.
31. Greenberg JH, Reivich M, Alavi A. Mapping of functional neuronal activity in man with ^{18}F-fluorodeoxyglucose. Neurology 1979;29:545.
32. Phelps ME, Huang SC, Hoffman EJ, Selin SC, Sokoloff L, Kuhl DE. Tomographic measurements of local cerebral metabolic rate in humans with (f-18) 2-fluoro-2-deoxyglucose: Validation of method. Ann Neurol 1979;6:371–388.
33. Huang SC, Phelps ME, Hoffman EJ, Sideris K, Selin CJ, Kuhl DE. Non-invasive determination of local cerebral metabolic rate of glucose in man. Am J Physiol 1980;238:E69–E82.
34. Mazziotta JC, Phelps ME, Miller J, Kuhl DE. Tomographic mapping of human cerebral metabolism: Normal unstimulated state. Neurology 1981;31:503–516.
35. Munsat TL, Andres PL, Finison L, Conlon T, Thibodeau L. The natural history of motor neuron loss in amyotrophic lateral sclerosis. Neurology 1988;38:409–413.

11

Caring for Patients with Amyotrophic Lateral Sclerosis

David Goldblatt

University of Rochester School of Medicine and Dentistry
Rochester, New York

> My days are like a shadow that declineth; and
> I am withered like grass.
>> Psalms 101:11
> A Day! Help! Help! Another Day!
>> Emily Dickinson
> What fortitude the Soul contains. . . .
>> Emily Dickinson

INTRODUCTION

Elisabeth Kübler-Ross delineated five stages through which a person may pass in succession while coping with terminal illness (1). A century earlier, Emily Dickinson had described five successive requests that arise in the heart of any person whose life is thwarted by chronic illness—or by Life itself.

> The Heart asks Pleasure–first–
> And then–Excuse from Pain–
> And then–those little Anodynes
> That deaden suffering–
>
> And then–to go to sleep–
> And then–if it should be
> The will of its Inquisitor
> The liberty to die– (2)

I have chosen those words of the poet, who so well understood pain and suffering (3,4) as the outline for this chapter, but the work of the practitioner who pioneered our modern understanding of death and dying should be recalled, and

271

her five stages (denial and isolation, anger, bargaining, depression, and acceptance) should be compared with Dickinson's five apothegms.

PLEASURE

The wish for a pleasant life—natural in a healthy person—does not vanish at the onset of amyotrophic lateral sclerosis (ALS), which begins so quietly and so painlessly that it it usually mistaken at first for more innocent problems, nor does that wish disappear when the diagnosis is considered and, eventually, established. A doctor called me recently to say that he has ALS, the disease from which his father had died rather rapidly. The doctor–patient was asking about investigative studies, but what was really uppermost in his thoughts was the good life he has been leading: he described horseback riding, his practice of medicine, his home. There was joy in the telling.

Another doctor whom I saw in consultation had wheedled out of his neurosurgeon the possibility that his leg cramps and twitches might mean ALS and had been devastated by that opinion, which was tentative and, happily, also incorrect. He spoke at greatest length about skiing, something it was easy to describe to a stranger, easier than saying, ''I love my family, I love the sunlight, I love life.''

How may a physician respond to a patient's heartfelt question, ''How can I continue to enjoy living if I am dying?'' The answer is, ''You're not dying of ALS; you are living with it.'' The patient must be told, ''Take life a day at a time.'' But these are trite sayings. How can the doctor persuade the patient to believe in them? When the patient's thoughts are governed by denial, when the plea for continuation of a normal, pleasant life is on the patient's lips, he cannot.

My colleague, Robert Griggs, remarking on how difficult it is for the doctor who first makes the diagnosis of ALS to continue to maintain rapport with the patient, suggested to me that, most often, referring the patient to another physician for continuing care is the most practical solution. Another of my mentors, Robert Joynt, counts ''Don't shoot the messenger'' among his store of wise sayings. Unable to be angry at a disease, patients do get angry at the person who first informs them about the presence of an illness that is untreatable, progressive, and ultimately fatal. To move toward developing a successful way of managing progressive illness, the patient does not need to give up pleasure, but it must come from different, often deeper sources. Yet another physician, whom I saw the day before writing these words, first discovered his problem recently when he began to have trouble tossing up the ball for his tennis serve (all these doctors worked hard in their practice, I might add; this man was continuing to do so). He said, ''I've forgotten about the tennis; I just want to be able to go on taking care of my patients.'' Although untrue at a deeper level, such a declaration does provide a template for action. The family should attempt to hold the patient to his intentions in a supportive way.

The challenge to family and friends, after the diagnosis has been established, is to maintain a pleasurable relationship with someone who has been told he has a fatal disease, without false jocularity or brushing aside of concerns that caregivers have not yet developed the skills to address. The celebrated case of Dr. Rabin (5) makes the point that he was distressed by his isolation from fellow–physicians who had a hard time acknowledging that this could happen to "one of us."

Careful reading of the article he wrote, soon after diagnosis, reveals that he was unwilling to indicate to others his need for help and his readiness to accept it. I remember one of my own patients who told me about a good Samaritan who helped him up when he had fallen in the road. There was a simple difference between that encounter and the one recounted by Rabin, in which a colleague saw him stumble and fall, but pretended not to notice and went on: My patient asked for help. Dr. Rabin did not. Moreover, as judged by what he wrote, Dr. Rabin mistakenly substituted a consultant in a far-off clinic for someone who would be "his doctor." He blamed the consultant for not telling him everything he needed to know to prepare for what was to come, whereas the best advice for patients is "Don't borrow trouble": don't live so much in the future that you dwell on what will, or may, happen and neglect the pleasures of today. In this way the early "denial and isolation" of Kübler-Ross and the "pleasure-asking" of Dickinson are related ideas pertaining especially to the early stage of adjustment to illness.

EXCUSE FROM PAIN

Kübler-Ross tells of a dying physician who recalled wondering why it was not an old man he knew, who was "of no earthly use," instead of the doctor himself, who had to die (1, p. 44). In the wish to relieve their own pain, patients may inflict it on those closest to them, not just in fantasy but by becoming "difficult patients." Because this happens early in the course of illness, when families, also, are unpracticed in carrying for a chronically ill person, and at a time when the patient's dependence on others is more psychological than physical, it may generate resentment and rejection.

Given the chance (and this means separate interviews with patient and caregiver, despite the almost universal desire of the spouse, especially the wife, to accompany the patient into the examining room), the patient and those emotionally close to him will admit to behaviors of which they are ashamed and for which they may need forgiveness, if they can be forgiven. From my own life experience in caring for my mother, during her dementing illness, I know how hard it may be for the caregiver to come to terms with his own failings in that area. (I am not alone in this; I have heard it from others who do fine as professional caregivers, but who lapse badly when called on to play that role in their own family.)

It is unforgivable that any professional—aide, nurse, doctor, therapist—should ever do anything the least bit cruel or hurtful to a patient under his or her care. More leniency is required toward a family member who slips from saintliness under the constant strain and the sleep deprivation that often accompany home care of an ailing relative. Just acknowledging to the family, who often say to the doctor, "I don't know how you do it [take care of patients with ALS]," that *theirs*, not yours, is the demanding job may be very helpful in recharging their emotional batteries—and avoiding assault and battery!

A way that families seek "excuse from pain" for the patient is by saying to the doctor, "Don't tell him." (Perhaps I have more often heard that directive or request in relation to a female patient.) When I was in training, that was an accepted way of dealing with patients, to "spare them," but it is a course doomed to failure; the truth is bound to leak out, and all that is accomplished if a doctor says, "I don't know what you have" or uses one of the many euphemistic terms and explanations for "motor neuron disease" is that the patient loses confidence. Whatever he has is obviously getting worse; not understanding that it is *inevitable* that he will get worse only frustrates him more.

How and when to tell the patient what is wrong is, nonetheless, vitally important. There is a differential diagnosis for ALS, considered elsewhere in this volume. In clinical medicine, there are always some diagnoses on the list that are really absurd in a given case, and it is wrong to string along the patient who has clear-cut ALS by adding yet another negative laboratory finding to those that have already legitimately been obtained. A mildly elevated lead level, for example, provides no useful approach to treatment and only confuses the patient. Therefore, do a thorough investigation, get second opinions if there is any doubt (but not when an inexorable progression of fully developed signs and symptoms makes that fruitless), and then tell the patient that the problem is not the diagnosis but what comes next: doing the best we can, together, to keep the patient functional as long as possible.

ANODYNES

To alleviate the suffering associated with ALS, it is necessary first to define what suffering is and is not. "Suffering," Eric Cassel has pointed out, "can include physical pain but is by no means limited to it" (6). Pain, indeed, does not come to mind immediately when most people, including physicians, think of ALS, although pain has to be listed among the important physical effects of the disease (7,8). Within suffering, then, the caregiver can attend to the "boundaries of pain" (as Emily Dickinson called them), the definable attributes of pain, related to immobility, altered posture, and, probably, variably important, intrinsic changes caused by the disease within the nervous system itself.

"Suffering," says Cassel, "is ultimately a personal matter," and his first task is to define the "person" (6). (Those of us who assume that we can skip that definition will do well to read his thoughtful analysis of what does constitute a person, in which he emphasizes that mind and body cannot be separated. This is especially important when we realize that ALS, even more than a high spinal cord transection or, I suspect, an infarct in the basis pontis, can bring a human being close to being a disembodied mind.)

Second, Cassel speaks of the "threat" of suffering—the future-oriented, "impending" aspect. It is in this area that egregious failures occur in the proper management of ALS patients, and it will receive attention below.

Cassel's third, and last, major point is that "suffering can occur in relation to any aspect of the person" (6, p. 640). I have previously discussed the simplest case, in which a man with ALS who valued his manual skills above all other aspects of his existence took his own life when he lost his dexterity (9).

In what we can only hope is an overstatement, Cassel contends, "The relief of suffering, it would appear, is considered one of the primary ends of medicine by patients and lay persons, but not by the medical profession" (6).

That indictment can go both ways: why should lay persons *have* to look to physicians to bring about the relief of suffering, when it is in the power of every person to impose or improve suffering—or just to ignore it. Auden's great poem, "Musée des Beaux Arts," begins, "About suffering they were never wrong,/ The Old Masters" and makes the point not only that the world is indifferent to suffering, but that indifference creates suffering out of mere misfortune.

There is an extraordinary group of articles in the journal *Literature and Medicine* (10–14) which you *must* read if you want to enlarge your thinking about your role in caring for ALS (if you are a patient, trying to help yourself; a family member; a doctor or other professional caregiver). Since I am writing this article from the only viewpoint I really understand, I was astonished and enlightened to learn that what was, for me, the "smoothly-written" account and summary of how a physician did her best to help an elderly man and his wife cope with his ALS became the cause of a critic's anger—even of an accusation that, by giving "inferior medical care" the doctor had contributed to the deaths of both patient and spouse (12).

I was, and am, angry about what a professor of English had to say about how a doctor ought to take care of her patient (and, obviously, to the extent that the shoe fits, about how I should take care of mine). No doubt about it: when he talks about the doctor as "martyr–hero," the shoe pinches. I am sure (and I already knew this) that the mythologizing of the physician by his patient is a payoff and a bribe that the doctor too readily accepts. I also know, however, that to imbue one's physician with power is to fashion an amulet to ward off death. The

Table 1 Symptomatic Management of ALS (a Personal-Opinion List)

Problem	Strategies, equipment		Comment
	Useful	Rarely useful or unnecessary	
Upper-limb weakness	Universal strap (hand); functional hand splint; enlarged handles for pen, key, utensils, doorknobs; Velcro closures on shoes and clothing; zipper pulls; pliers; plate guard; rocker knife; drinking straw; long-handled sponge (to wrap toilet paper around); electric toothbrush; Water Pik; jogging outfit (loosely fitting); range-of-motion exercises (shoulder especially)	Ballbearing feeder; Mestinon treatment; exercise program (active)	Shoulder subluxation and frozen shoulder benefit from referral to a physical therapist; hand problems should be addressed by an occupational therapist
Lower-limb weakness	Ankle-foot orthosis (AFO) (posterior plastic splint, readymade); walker with wheels; lightweight folding wheelchair with footrests; electric scooter and wheelchair; Jobst cushion; eggcrate cushion; bedside commode; raised toilet seat; cane with large rubber tip	Long leg braces; single-shank or double-shank braces attached to shoe; elastic stockings, diuretics (for edema); quad cane; crutches	Plastic AFOs are useful even for transfers of nonambulatory patients (who are not using Hoyer lifter); expense of fitted splints (which will need to be revised as atrophy progresses) is not justified; AFOs are not useful when severe spasticity exists
Neck and trunk weakness	Soft cervical collar; electric hospital bed; alternating-pressure mattress with pump; reclining chair; chair with high seat and back	Plastic orthopedic collar; Philadelphia collar; Somi brace (forehead to shoulders); lumbosacral corset or body jacket; lift-seat chair; waterbed; high-backed or reclining wheelchair	More elaborate devices for head support are uncomfortable; chin support interferes with eating; corsets are difficult to put on; lift chairs are usually useful for only a short time; patients cannot turn or be turned easily on a waterbed

Dysphagia	Avoidance of crumbly foods (nuts, popcorn, potato chips); coarsely chopped food (food processor); pudding-consistency foods; percutaneous endoscopic gastrostomy with large-caliber Silastic tube; percutaneous gastrostomy under fluoroscopy; cool liquids	Puréed, dispersible foods; hot foods or liquids; thickeners for liquid; milk and milk products; cricopharyngeal myotomy, with or without feeding pharyngostomy; esophagostomy; surgical gastrostomy under local or general anesthesia; nasogastric tube (N-G)	Milk often causes troublesome phlegm; alternatives to gastrostomy have drawbacks: N-G tubes are small and easily clogged; pharyngostomy stoma may spew saliva, etc., when patient coughs; Foley catheter in stomach (rubber) quickly disintegrates
Dysarthria and dysphonia	Writing tablet; Magic Slate; letter board; picture book for communication; typewriter (with rubber-tipped pencil to push keys); electronic communicators (with LED display and voice synthesizer)	Electrolarynx; palatal lift prosthesis; ETRAN system (transparent plastic letter board)	Dysphonia is rarely as much of a problem as dysarthria; patients must be forced to give up ineffective verbal communication in favor of written, etc. (they naturally cling to speech when it has lost communicative usefulness); caregivers must not guess, fill in, or complete a phrase for a patient
Drooling	Portable suction apparatus; amitriptyline, 10–75 mg/day; methscopolamine (Pamine), 2.5 mg up to t.i.d.; terrycloth bib and washcloth (held in mouth while working)	Facial tissue (it makes a mess); ligation of salivary ducts; radiation of salivary glands; tympanic neurectomy	Dry mouth at night is as much of a problem as daytime drooling; a glass of water or an atomizer spray at the bedside may help, as does "artificial saliva." Patients differ: some have no problem with milk or ice cream
Mucus (phlegm) Bad breath	Avoidance of milk products; sparing use of anticholinergics Meticulous dental hygiene (easy to say, hard to achieve); breath fresheners, if feasible		Breath is a subject that needs frank discussion (the patient likely will be unaware of what a "turnoff" a foul mouth odor is)

Table 1 Continued.

Problem	Strategies, equipment		Comment
	Useful	Rarely useful or unnecessary	
Sexual dysfunction	Rechanneling of interests and energies when the patient has become seriously disabled	Antispasticity drugs (baclofen, diazepam)	We have attempted to explore attitudes of patients directly and by questionnaire without much success (i.e., without much discussion forthcoming)
Pain (back, joints)	Proper transfer techniques; passive range-of-motion exercises; analgesics, narcotics	Body braces; tricyclic antidepressants	A minority of patients have widespread pain; frozen shoulder and back pain are common
Constipation	Increase in daily water intake (try for 8 glasses/day); fruits and other high-fiber materials; eliminate diuretics, including caffeine-containing beverages; suppositories, disimpaction, enemas	Stool softeners; bulk-forming medicines unaccompanied by high water intake	Weakness of glottic closure and abdominal muscles makes this one of the most distressing problems

physician must not defeat that strategy, since there is always something to be done for the patient, even if it is not what he would like to be able to do, and that is the message the patient needs to hear (Table 1).

An example of what the doctor can do came recently when I received an inquiry from a patient who lives in another city. He was writing to those of us who have been identified with ALS (including the authors of other chapters in this book) to ask what we thought of the question "Does a positive attitude influence the progress of the disease or help to bring about plateauing of symptoms?" More important than the answers themselves, which, of course, cannot be more than impressionistic, is the fact that the doctors queried took time to give full replies. I often say that the only thing I have to give to my patients is my time. Evidently, others feel the same way.

An immediate question from the person who has been diagnosed as having ALS—even if he "knows" that there is no effective treatment for the disease— is "What can I do? Isn't there something I can take or do that will at least slow it down?" Diet, exercise, and drugs are the means usually considered. Patients often develop their own ideas about foods they should eat, or avoid, and they take vitamins. Since various practitioners such as chiropractors can "prescribe" vitamins, they may become expensive placebos or worse. (Although large doses of pyridoxine are harmful to peripheral nerves, I have not seen a case of sensory neuropathy in an ALS patient that was caused by "megavitamin" treatment, but that is a poor argument in favor of such treatment.) Various amino acids are presently under investigation for the treatment of ALS. Whether or not they ultimately prove useful, the anecdotal evidence that other investigators and I have shared suggests that, as used by patients in uncontrolled, personal trials, amino acids are not beneficial and may even have temporary adverse effects.

Exercise is another controversial topic (15). Attempts have been made to analyze the effect of exercise on the progression of the disease, since a hypothetical case can be made for performing it (to maintain strength and mobility and to promote collateral sprouting of motor axons) and for avoiding it (to conserve strength for vital functions and to prevent exhaustion of motor neurons.)

It is clear that exercise cannot retard the progression in a rapidly advancing case. As one of my patients said, "My disease hit me going 50 miles an hour, and it never let up." This man's son, an Olympic athlete and coach, set up a sensible program of vigorous exercise that he and his father performed regularly, but it was not long before it had to be abandoned in the face of the patient's advancing debility.

Drugs prescribed by physicians fall into two categories: those used for symptomatic improvement, usually slight at best (such as baclofen, pyridostigmin, and amitriptyline) (8), and those intended to halt progression, which can be further subdivided into those that are known to be ineffective (such as steroids) and those that have not yet proved to be so (such as deprenyl) (16). In recent years, controlled clinical trials have been conducted, as discussed elsewhere in this volume by the editor. My personal experience has been limited to a single double-blind, placebo-controlled trial of cyclosporine, not yet completely analyzed or published at the time of this writing. This trial was prompted by the favorable findings reported by Appel et al. after a pilot study (17) and was carried out under the direction of Appel, in four centers including the University of Rochester. The only observations from that study that I wish to report here as being relevant to the care of patients pertain to those men who, by random assignment, received placebo: the protocol called for 1 year of either placebo or cyclosporine, to be followed by an open trial of cyclosporine for those who wished to take it. Of those who received placebo (but did not yet know that fact when they answered our questionnaire), five of the eight who had an opinion believed that they had actually received placebo during the first phase of the clinical trial. Nevertheless, they had positive comments about having participated in the study: support, altruistic contribution, a sense of "doing something," "a sense of hope for the time being," "a positive mental attitude," "a thread of hope"—those were some of their comments.

SLEEP

In her line "And then to go to sleep," Emily Dickinson shows her profound understanding of the progression toward death in someone fatally ill: it translates directly into the depression that Kübler-Ross characterizes first as "reactive" and then "preparatory." Cheering up, she says, may serve for the former, but preparatory grief is "usually a silent one . . . a time when too much interference from visitors who try to cheer him up hinders [the patient's] emotional preparation rather than enhances it" (1, p. 77).

An important difference between ALS and terminal cancer is the more protracted time course of ALS; it is only for a short time that the patient should have to enter fully into this stage of quiet withdrawal. At many times, prior to this, he will certainly have contemplated his death and moved toward acceptance of it, but he will perceive that, without an accurate prediction as to how long he will live, he must not give up too early. A trap that doctors fall into is trying to give a precise estimate of survival to a patient or a family member (who will likely let the patient know it in one way or another). The patient outlives the predicted length of survival and asks (at least subconsciously), "What do I do now?"

It is reprehensible for the doctor to "show off" by recounting all the possible problems of ALS, and it is also wrong to be talked into being too precise in making a prediction. Forecasting a short survival time for someone who has every likelihood of living for several more years is a great disservice, but it is done all the time.

THE LIBERTY TO DIE

Life-sustaining and life-prolonging treatments requiring consideration in ALS are enteral feeding by means of a tube and respiration assisted or supported by the use of a ventilator. Our concern here is with both methods and, especially, the physician's obligation to guide the patient in making a "right" choice.

Within the patient-autonomy model of medical care increasingly espoused in our affluent society, the cost in dollars of heroic treatment has dropped in rank among the factors influencing a decision to treat (18). (The cost of tube feeding is small, but the cost of supportive ventilation is high and becomes extremely high when the patient must remain for months or even years in an intensive care unit, a setting more suitable for short-term care of the critically ill, but potentially salvageable patient.)

A skillful, experienced gastroenterologist can easily perform a percutaneous, endoscopically guided gastrostomy. An alternative method of percutaneous gastrostomy involves filling the stomach with air by means of a nasogastric tube, permitting the radiologist to identify the positions of the stomach, the liver, and the bowel. After percutaneous introduction of the gastrostomy tube, the nasogastric tube is withdrawn.

In either case, a large-caliber Silastic feeding tube should be installed, which will not disintegrate in the gastric juice or become sticky and distorted at its proximal end and is easily unclogged if it does become obstructed. It can be connected to various delivery systems from an Asepto syringe to a plastic feeding bag with either simple gravity flow or delivery regulated by a kangaroo pump. Some tubes must be removed by repeat endoscopy, and the recommending physician needs to decide whether the possible need to repeat the procedure in a year or so is of practical significance. The daily cost of prepared tube feedings is competitive with the cost of nutritious meals, and their convenience is obviously greater than that of preparing food to be swallowed by the severely dysphagic patient.

These things being true it is unconscionable not to offer the patient tube feeding, although I know that not all physicians do so. The alternatives to gastrostomy as just described have been surgical gastrostomy under general or local anesthesia, esophagostomy, feeding pharyngostomy (with or without cricopharyngeal myotomy), or simple nasogastric tube feeding, usually with a small-caliber tube. None of these is as satisfactory in my opinion (19). They need to be mentioned mainly because they may have soured the physician on enteral alimentation, whereas newer experience gives a more favorable impression.

Why, then, would a patient refuse a feeding tube? Recently, one of my own patients did so. His case is worth considering.

Robert was 58, divorced, with two grown daughters. He loved the wilderness, and when his hands forced him to give up his work as a carpenter, he set off for the West, in his recreational vehicle, to see again the snow-covered peaks and mirror lakes he had so often photographed. On his return from past trips, he would share his lonely travels with others, presenting slide shows of uncommon quality at meetings of senior citizen groups and at fraternal lodges.

This time he returned only when his weakness compelled it. His younger daughter took him in and he struggled with all the problems that ALS can create: impaired limb function, breathing, speaking, and swallowing. Somewhat unusually, he became completely aphagic at a time when his speech was still understandable. He decided he had had enough, he refused tube feeding despite all arguments, but he was afraid to die at home, where he was often alone while his daughter was at work. He was also frightened of a nursing home. No place in a hospice program was available for him.

I admitted him to the hospital. He felt no hunger but he was dry and thirsty. The resident told him he might develop a painful neuropathy or other complications of avitaminosis, and he accepted intravenous fluid with supplemental vitamins but no calories. Of course, he also refused any type of ventilatory assistance.

He lived for a month in the hospital, cachectic, and finally dying of respiratory failure. In his last days, he was given morphine to allay anxiety. He had talked to everyone, including his mother, who was still searching for a cure for her son and was clipping items from the newspapers concerning unrelated ''breakthroughs'' in medical care. He himself wanted to do nothing but sleep. At last he became briefly delirious from hypoxia and drug, and he died quietly. At the funeral service, the patient's family showed his beautiful slides of the wildflowers and the mountains.

Robert had fulfilled all the criteria for rational refusal of treatment, as summarized recently by Peterson under five headings: urgency, effect of illness, certainty of the consequences, conflicts between desires, and the opportunity for deliberation (20).

A decision about tube feeding in this case did not have to be made quickly, although patients with ALS can die suddenly if they have undergone a considerable decline in body weight. A tendency to aspirate food that complicates chronic dysphagia does, however, pose the hazard of pneumonia or possibly a fatal choking spell, although that must be very rare. (Surgical procedures can be performed to close off the trachea from the pharynx, when the patient cannot talk and a permanent tracheostomy is acceptable. My experience is limited to one patient, who was miserable, apparently because there was a tiny leak past the site of closure. I do not plan to encourage another patient to undergo such radical surgery.)

Urgency and, indeed, a crisis mentality too often accompany the decision to ''go on the respirator'' (21). Talking to a patient about respiratory failure is the most trying task a doctor has to perform, not from a technical viewpoint—the function of breathing hardly needs to be explained—but because the patient knows that he is being asked to choose, ultimately, between living and dying. In many parts of the world, the patient has no choice between life and death. Either ventilatory aids are unavailable or the physician, who decides for the patient, thinks it is wrong in some way to offer breath support to a person with ALS. In the United States, however, it should be possible for any patient who wants it to have a ventilator—and equally possible to refuse it or to have it stopped. That is "patient autonomy," the model of care that U.S. physicians now tend to support, in theory, over the paternalism of 19th-century medicine (18). But if the doctor is *practicing* 19th-century medicine—offering only symptomatic treatments and psychological support in the face of progressive and ultimately fatal illness—should he not be wise enough to know how miserable his patient will be on a respirator and spare him that final suffering?

I think not. I cannot accurately predict how well or poorly a given patient will do with a respirator, and even if I foresee misery, I have no right to decide not to offer every patient the same opportunity. I am assuming that no additional problem, such as dementia, is present that supersedes even ALS in importance. If it is decided that the patient has the right to know his choices, the art is to present the concept in a reasonable way, at the right times.

I say "times" advisedly: I certainly don't think it is right to badger a patient into accepting life support. I have seen what happens when the family keep after the patient until he finally gives in to something he does not want. By the same token, it is not fair to the patient to get that "little talk" about life support over with too soon. Ask healthy people if they would want to live hooked up to a respirator if they had to, and very few will say yes. Ask the patient in the early stages of ALS and you will get the same answer. Yet, when the time comes, some accept artificial prolongation of life. The process of making a decision must be respected, and the patient must be allowed to change his mind. In a crisis of respiratory distress it should then be possible to adhere to the predetermined plan, whether that is starting the ventilator or providing comfort only, with the use of oxygen and sedation.

While I believe in autonomy, I also realize that patients deserve guidance based on experience. A recent newspaper article makes the point. The headline read, "Weather was bad, so pilot asks passengers: New York or Chicago?" Reportedly, a show of hands supported the decision to go ahead during bad weather, but the plane was actually forced to land short of its New York City destination. Two passengers from Chicago were incredulous at what happened but reported that the majority of passengers were from New York or headed there on business and carried the vote to go ahead despite the bad storms. I am afraid that I often see too much of that pilot in myself.

Before tracheostomy, ideally, the patient has had time to progress through trials of noninvasive techniques: the intermittent positive pressure breathing apparatus, two or three breaths hourly while awake; the cuirass (chest-shell) negative-pressure ventilator; a "raincoat" or "Poncho-wrap," negative-pressure machine; and nasal-access, positive-pressure ventilation.

Reasoning and planning are commendable (21), but the physician has to expect that, when dyspnea develops, a predetermined course may be overthrown. With the support and understanding of the family, it may be possible even then to make the patient comfortable, but everyone must understand that, when an ambulance is called, the emergency medical technician cannot be handed a "living will" and told just to make the patient comfortable. Resuscitative measures *will* be taken. (It is useful for the patient and family to know, also, that oxygen, even at a low flow rate, may prove lethal unless mechanical ventilation is used. More than once, the ambulance crew have administered the coup de grace to a patient with restrictive lung disease.)

In the emergency room, the same rules normally apply. What can be done is done for (or to) the patient, unless there are explicit instructions to the contrary. If the physician who is thoroughly familiar with the patient's wishes is there, or able to direct those who are, it may still be possible to avoid intubation. Again, knowing the answers to the "what ifs"—what if you had a collapsed lung or pneumonia, and we had some hope of getting you off the machine?—is necessary, and the patient's wishes should be documented.

How well will this work? Consider this recent case: An elderly woman with ALS, who remained ambulatory with a cane, had good use of her hands, and showed only slight bulbar involvement, was becoming increasingly dyspneic, with interrupted sleep and walking limited by shortness of breath. We had a long discussion, she, her husband, and I, in which she expressed an adamant opposition to any form of ventilatory support. This was a woman who had been through a lot, including successful treatment for breast cancer, and I thought that she was making a decision as rationally as anyone I have known.

That evening, she was in the emergency room, and the resident reported to me that she was having an anxiety attack characterized by increased shortness of breath. His analysis proved true, as judged by the fact that, months later, although she is now even more short of breath, she has never had to come to the hospital because of it. Instead, she successfully underwent percutaneous gastrostomy, a measure she did accept, but continues not to want a ventilator.

Heironymus (22), in a practical treatise on mechanical ventilation, wrote, "With respect to present day intensive care, including the use of artificial ventilation, therapy should be continued until all possible evidence indicates that a salvageable patient with a functioning central nervous system cannot be obtained. The persistent attempt, be it done with cognizance or in ignorance, to reverse the irreversible is no less wrong than prematurely judging the patient to be unsalvageable. One of the most difficult decisions is knowing when to stop." Because of the lengthy period of time during which the patient with a poorly functioning and weakening nervous system may stay on the ventilator with ALS, as compared with the setting of the intensive care unit, these questions may not receive the attention they need. Things may be left to drift along, and, eventually, the patient may become unable to communicate wishes, even by eye signals. We have discussed this issue fully elsewhere (23,24).

DEATH

"This disease is beyond my practice," says the doctor confounded by the sleepwalking Lady Macbeth. "I think, but dare not speak." Later, Macbeth, receiving news of his wife's death, remarks, "She should have died hereafter." He means nothing more than "She would have died at some time or other" (25). The doctor hesitates to express himself. The husband has no feelings to express, is at that moment incapable of experiencing emotion, and sees life itself as "signifying nothing." He is like the Stranger in Camus's novel, who reports, "Mother died today," as if he were commenting on the weather.

It is wrong for the doctor ever to step aside from his role as a counselor even when illness so overwhelms his patient that he, and those who normally care most deeply about him, are robbed of feeling: that is certainly a state of living death for all of them. If the doctor washes his hands of such a desperate situation, his hands (like those of Lady Macbeth) will never be clean (Table 2).

We must try to restore emotion, we must encourage the patient to live: it is the duty of caregivers, including the nurse and the physician, to be ardent advocates for life. We are sustainers and teachers: those are the origins of our names. But we must ultimately respect his "liberty to die."

I do not want to overstate my position. I do not claim that, whenever a human being becomes incapable of sustaining his or her own life independently, we should permit him to die (9). What I do believe is that when loss of enough strength to breathe is what brings down the curtain on the drama of life—when a person has become extensively paralyzed and that person's mind is made up in favor of death—the decision belongs to the patient and will, at the close of life, restore to him the power that disease has so cruelly stolen.

Emily Dickinson speaks of the "will" of an "Inquisitor," but, even among persons who believe in a deity, there are those who believe also that God has left decisions concerning daily life in the hands of men (26).

Society has accepted the idea that the patient may decide to discontinue treatment that artifically prolongs life. The courage to act on that decision is the courage of the patient. For all others involved, other emotions are appropriate—love, admiration, sadness, and faith among them—but not fear, repugnance, or, worst of all, the absence of *any* emotion (24). We are not Macbeth, we are not the Stranger. *We care for our patients*, in all the ways that those words may be understood.

Table 2   Care of the ALS Patient—A Physician's Checklist

Have you and the patient both fully accepted the diagnosis as correct?

Has the patient been given opportunity to understand what is happening to his body? (Not all patients want details.)

Does the patient know what ALS will *not* do?

Did you give the patient literature that includes information about local and national organizations concerned with ALS care and research? (See below)

Did you make referral to the regional clinic sponsored by the Muscular Dystrophy Association or other groups that provide benefits to patients, such as loan and purchase of equipment and supplies?

Has the patient consulted a lawyer who is knowledgeable about Medicaid and Medicare? This is especially important if supported ventilation is an option the patient may choose.

Has the patient made a will and planned his estate?

Is the patient's primary physician comfortable with following him as the disease progresses? If not, to what extent is the neurologist willing to assume primary responsibility?

Does the family understand the prognosis, including the variable length of survival?

To what extent can home care be provided?

Have you addressed the fears of the family, including contagion, genetic transmission, and harms they may inadvertently cause?

Have you ensured that the patient will not feel abandoned? Have you arranged periodic contact (not p.r.n.)?

When the patient has died, have you expressed condolences to the family and attended services? Have you opened the door for continued contact with the family? Have you made them feel that something positive has come from his life and from his illness?

Agencies Providing Services to ALS Patients (National)

ALS Association
21021 Ventura Blvd., Suite 321
Woodland Hills CA 91364

Muscular Dystrophy Association
810 Seventh Ave.
New York, NY 10019

A patient who wishes to participate in research may write to the National Headquarters of MDA providing details of his or her illness. The patient's name will be sent to all investigators doing ALS clinical research under MDA sponsorship, and the investigator will get in contact with a patient who might be suitable to participate.

AFTERWORD

The patient who dies loses the world; the family loses the patient but also the caregivers—those outside the family and also those who resume other roles *within* the family structure. Often, when a parent dies, the adult children behave childishly, creating rifts that may be slow to reunite.

The doctor can now help by at least letting the family know that he or she will continue to be available to them. Occasionally it is to examine a son who develops fasciculations. Or it may be to acknowledge a gift of money or of equipment no longer needed by the patient but useful to someone else.

Whenever possible (and it is possible if you make the effort), go to the funeral home or to the church service. It is very rewarding to be welcomed by the family at such a time. It is not out of place to be there as a reminder of the long struggle: that memory is uppermost in everyone's mind. You may learn something you never knew about your patient, and you will give all who were involved with his life a chance to say goodbye to you. You are acknowledging what they did for the one who has died; they are doing the same for you. You will feel rededicated, and that is what other patients need from you.

REFERENCES

1. Kübler-Ross E. On death and dying. New York: Macmillan, 1969.
2. Poem 536, reprinted by permission of the publishers and the Trustees of Amherst College from The Poems of Emily Dickinson, Thomas H. Johnson, ed., Cambridge, MA: The Belknap Press of Harvard University Press, Copyright 1951, © 1955, 1979, 1983 by the President and Fellows of Harvard College.
3. Cody J. After great pain—The inner life of Emily Dickinson. Cambridge, MA: Harvard University Press, Belknap Press, 1971.
4. Goldblatt D. Kinsmen met a night—Otfrid and Emily. Semin Neurol 1983;3:409–411.
5. Rabin D. Compounding the ordeal of ALS—Isolation from my fellow physicians. N Engl J Med 1982;307:506–509.
6. Cassel EJ. The nature of suffering and the goals of medicine. N Engl J Med 1982;306:639–645.
7. Newrick PG, Langton-Hewer R. Motor neurone disease: Can we do better? A study of 42 patients. Br Med J 1984;289:539–542.
8. Newrick P. Motor neurone disease. In: Tallis R, ed. The clinical neurology of old age. Chichester: Wiley, 1989:151–160.
9. Goldblatt D. All at once, and nothing first. Semin Neurol 1984;4:111–112.
10. Banks JT. A controversy about clinical form. Lit Med 1986;5:24–26.
11. Barnard D. A case of amyotrophic lateral sclerosis. Lit Med 1986;5:27–42.
12. Rabkin E. A case of self defense. Lit Med 1986;5:43–53.
13. Smith DH. The limits of narrative. Lit Med 1986;5:54–57.
14. Hunter KM. Making a case. Lit Med 1988;7:66–79.

15. Sanjak M, Reddan W, Brooks BR. Role of muscular exercise in amyotrophic lateral sclerosis. Neurol Clin 1987;5:251–268.
16. Goldblatt D. Treatment of amyotrophic lateral sclerosis. In: Griggs RC, Moxley RT, III. Adv Neurol 1977;17:265–283.
17. Appel SH, Stewart SS, Appel V, et al. A double-blind study of the effectiveness of cyclosporine in amyotrophic lateral sclerosis. Arch Neurol 1988;45:381–386.
18. Clements CD, Sider RC. Medical ethics' assault upon medical values. JAMA 1983;250:2011–2015.
19. Hillel AD, Miller R. Bulbar amyotrophic lateral sclerosis: patterns of progression and clinical management. Head Neck 1989;11:51–59.
20. Peterson LM. Refusing medical treatment. Perspect Biol Med 1988;31:454–460.
21. Hudson AJ, Jr. Outpatient management of amyotrophic lateral sclerosis. Semin Neurol 1987;7:344–351.
22. Heironymus TW. Mechanical artificial ventilation, 2nd ed. Springfield, IL: Charles C Thomas, 1971:10.
23. Goldblatt D. Decisions about life support in amyotrophic lateral sclerosis. Semin Neurol 1984;4:104–110.
24. Goldblatt D, Greenlaw J. Starting and stopping the ventilator for patients with amyotrophic lateral sclerosis. Neurol Clin 1989;7:789–806.
25. Garrison GB, ed. Shakespeare—Major plays and the sonnets. New York: Harcourt, Brace, 1948:860.
26. Kushner HS. When bad things happen to good people. New York: Avon, 1983.

12

Communication Technology for Disabled Persons

Erich E. Sutter

Smith-Kettlewell Eye Research Institute
San Francisco, California

COMMUNICATION AS PART OF REHABILITATION

While there is, at this time, no known cure for amyotrophic lateral sclerosis (ALS), much can be achieved in helping the patient with effective rehabilitation. The most important factor in successful use of rehabilitation technology is the mental attitude of the patient and those close to him. It is extremely difficult to cope with the severe progressive disabilities caused by this disease. Patients show a variety of reactions and attitudes. At one extreme, some patients are totally unable to deal with the disease and the resulting disabilities, rejecting all help and assistive devices. At the other extreme, some patients fiercely and courageously fight to continue an active life using all the means that can be mobilized. Coping with the situation may be most difficult for patients who have been very independent and self-reliant.

One of the most severe consequence of progressive neurological diseases is the impairment and eventual loss of the ability to communicate. The patient is slowly robbed of all active participation in social interactions, loses control over his environment, and is forced into a state of complete passivity. In each patient, the disabilities are manifested somewhat differently and progression may take a different course. The requirements for successful rehabilitation vary enormously, not only between persons, but also in the same person over time. To meet these varying needs, a large variety of devices have been developed and are now commercially available.

Much in human activity depends on a person's ability to communicate. This is even more true for persons with severe disability. Choosing the right device and properly fitting it to the user is extremely important. Anticipating future changes in the capacities of the patient should be part of a long-range rehabilitation program. Ideally, this can be formulated through the use of a series of devices that are mutually compatible, so that a minimum of retraining is necessary in the transition from one to the other.

The task of matching each disabled person with the proper communication system is a challenge. It requires experience, interdisciplinary expertise, a keen ability to observe, and sensitivity to the disabled person's need and preferences.

DEVICES FOR THE COMMUNICATIVELY DISABLED

The Physical Interface

Our brains connect with the outside world and communicate with man and machine in many ways. We speak, write, and type to express our thoughts, and we also communicate with facial expressions and gestures. In addition, moving about we control our environment by manipulating light switches, operating appliances, and so forth. With progressive neurological disease this range of abilities becomes more and more limited. In the early stages, one function may be taken over by another. This substitution is initially easy, but later it may require special training or the use of sophisticated electronic devices.

When control over the extremities fails but speech remains intact, it is possible to perform many functions of the body by means of robotics (mechanical devices controlled by speech input). Speech recognition through microprocessor technology has made tremendous progress during the last decade. These systems are trained not only to recognize a person's voice, but also to recognize specific words. While the vocabulary that can be recognized is still very limited, speech recognition devices that control the environment have been shown to be very useful.

As ALS progresses, the production of speech may become extremely difficult or impossible. This can happen rather suddenly when the patient is placed on a respirator or insidiously as the pharyngeal muscles and tongue are affected. Often the person can still move his lips, and an experienced lip reader can serve as an interpreter. This mode of communication can be very efficient but requires a skilled interpreter, a resource not always available. When lip reading is not an option, speech has to be substituted by other available motor responses. If some control over a hand remains, the person may be able to write or type on a standard keyboard. However, the available motor responses are often too limited or too weak to operate devices designed for the general population. The disabled person may be able to perform only a few movements to operate specially designed switches or other controls. Under these conditions, the communication rate drops drastically. For example, a person operating a keyboard with 64 keys transmits six bits of information with every stroke ($2^6 = 64$); when this person operates a single switch, he transmits only one bit. A key stroke is thus equivalent to six consecutive switch operations. When a person's movements are severely limited, it becomes crucial to choose the most efficient of the available motor responses for communication so that the most information can be communicated in a short period of time. Strategies must be developed to enhance the communication rate. First, we find the most efficient motor response, to interface the brain with the outside world; i.e., we select a suitable communication channel. Then, strategies are developed for efficient use of this channel.

In this electronic age the most important communication link for the disabled person is no longer direct speech with other persons, but rather a computer. Today computers can supplant many motor functions of the human body. They can produce speech, directly operate appliances, and control the environment through robotics. Interfacing the disabled person with a computer may be the most important, but also the most difficult, step in rehabilitation.

When there is still enough motor control left to efficiently touch or point to one item out of many, a device that permits direct selection may be the best choice. The larger the selection of choices a patient can handle, the larger the amount of information that can be transmitted by each of his movements. The principles of ergonomic design that apply here are basically the same as those used in the construction of a normal typewriter or computer keyboard. For the latter, the number of keys and their layout has been determined by the anatomy and physiology of the human hand. In the case of the typewriter, the keys are assigned letters of the alphabet. The computer keyboard may have several levels of key functions, depending on the application.

The typewriter illustrates the consequences of less than optimal ergonomic design. Almost all typewriters use the QWERTY key assignment, even though research has shown that significantly better performance can be reached with the DVORAK keyboard. The cost of replacing existing equipment and changing old habits has prevented the change to a more efficient keyboard. For the disabled, the choice of the proper ergonomic design is even more important, since the equipment is so essential in the person's daily life, and changing to a different design can be extremely frustrating.

Keyboards can be designed for access by finger, hand, or foot. Head-pointing devices are often efficiently used by ALS patients for use in combination with mechanical keyboards. To facilitate the use of a keyboard with a head pointer or mouth stick, special key guards, i.e., masks with holes that can be placed on top of the keyboard, are employed. Key guards help guide the pointer to the individual keys.

Head pointers do not have to be mechanical. A light-sensitive detector with a very narrow field of view can be mounted to the head. It detects and identifies the light source at which it is aimed and is often used with lighted targets such as light-emitting diodes (LEDs). This principle can also be used to point to a spot on a computer screen. The detector identifies the location on the screen by the time it is scanned by the electrode beam.

Another approach to head pointing involves ultrasonic sensors mounted on a head rest to sense the head position. This method has been successfully applied to control the speed and direction of wheelchairs.

When all other modes of pointing fail, a person's gaze can also be used for direct selection of targets. However, many technical problems are associated with this concept. When the patient can still operate a single switch efficiently and with good reaction time, devices designed to make the most out of such simple movements may be preferable.

Keyboard Encoding

Computer keyboards are basically designed for selection of one key at a time (an exception is key modification, e.g., by simultaneous depression of the control key). If this restriction is dropped, the same number of functions can be accessed by means of a much smaller keyboard. With this approach the fingers strike chords as on a piano, hence the name chordic keyboards. With all possible combinations of simultaneous depressions of five keys (one for each finger of a hand), one can generate the functions of an ordinary set of 32 keys ($2^5 = 32$). If both hands are used simultaneously, 1024 functions can be generated with 10 keys. Keyboards of this type are commonly used by court stenographers and for braille embossing. Mainly two types of such keyboards are used by professional stenographers: the British Palantype and the American Stenograph (1). With these devices a skilled stenographer can type 120–200 words/minute. The same principle can be exploited in rehabilitation when a person cannot move the arms to access the keys of an ordinary keyboard. The hands may now rest in a fixed position with each finger over a key. Clearly, mastering such keyboards is more difficult, since it requires memorizing the encoding of the key functions.

Temporal Encoding

In many cases the range of movement of the extremities and the head may no longer be sufficient for any of the techniques discussed above. Often only one or two small movements may remain under control of the patient. This is usually sufficient to allow operation of a switch. In such cases temporal encoding of the key functions is necessary. Many different encoding schemes are presently being used. Such binary encoding is complicated by the fact that switch closure/nonclosure is used not only to signal, e.g., yes/no, but also to indicate whether information is being transmitted. This problem has been solved in various ways.

In Morse code two types of switch closures are being distinguished: short and long, while no closure means no transmission. Morse code is not used much in rehabilitation, for two main reasons. Mastering Morse requires a lot of practice learning a new code. In addition, Morse is mainly designed for transmission of written language and requires spelling of words. Because of the high degree of redundancy in written language, Morse is inherently inefficient.

In other approaches the problem is solved by means of two switches. The patient views a matrix of keys. He can use one switch to move a pointer to the right key and a second switch to affirm his choice. There are many variations to this approach that cannot be discussed here. In principle, they all represent different schemes of temporal encoding of information.

When the patient is only able to operate a single switch, auto-scan systems are most useful. Here the device does the temporal encoding by moving the pointer sequentially from one key to the next and the user only needs to depress the switch when the pointer is on the selected item. In most such systems the keys are arranged in rows and columns. The scan proceeds vertically until the user selects the row and then horizontally until he selects the desired element. The scan rate can be adjusted according to the user's reaction time and skill. This type of system is presently the most widely used method of communication for the severely disabled. Some users have achieved remarkable communication rates using this type of equipment.

These designs are far from optimal if one considers information theory concepts alone. Simple scanning and selection of the time interval when the proper item is accessed is a highly inefficient method of binary temporal encoding. For example, in scanning a set of 16 elements, only one out of the 16 time intervals can be selected during a scan; i.e., only a small subset of the possible binary codes of length 16 is being used. If all possible binary codes were allowed, the length of the code could be reduced to four time intervals ($2^4 = 16$). The reasons why more efficient encoding schemes are not being used are related to ergonomic design. It is important to take into account not only information flow, but also the structure of the information to be transmitted and the capabilities and preferences of the person transmitting it. In this regard, scanning of a simple matrix of labeled keys is usually preferable over more efficient schemes.

To exploit the best residual movement for the switch operation often requires specially designed switches. Various models of switches operated by the foot, knee, eyebrow, and puff of breath are now commercially available. Sometimes creative adaptations are necessary to utilize small, relatively weak movements.

Communication by Gaze
Often a disabled person's gaze is the most efficient and reliable means remaining to transmit information. This is particularly true for patients with advanced ALS. There are various ways this ability can be used to communicate. A simple and

useful method is to look to the side to indicate no and straight ahead for yes. This yes/no response combined with a sensible query can efficiently satisfy a patient's most urgent needs. In one approach to gaze communication, commonly used sentences are arranged in several columns and posted on the wall in front of the patient. With a few questions, the patient's choice is first narrowed down to a specific column and next to a sentence in the column. While such simple approaches serve their purpose, they do not permit patients to fully express their thoughts and feelings. Clearly, spelling out words and sentences by means of the query technique and yes/no answers is too cumbersome to be practical. Only one bit of information is transmitted with each question and answer. However, much more efficient uses of a person's gaze are possible. Instead of responding to a two-alternative choice, the patient can, in principle, select one out of a large number of items using his gaze. The difficulty is to establish exactly which item he is looking at. In a simple and inexpensive approach called "eye transfer," or ETRAN, this task is performed by a human observer. It usually employs a transparent board with engraved letters. The board is placed between the patient and the observer. Looking at the patient's eyes through the board, the observer can quite reliably determine the gaze direction and identify the selected item (Fig. 1). The most severe limitation of this approach is not only that it requires another person, but also that for efficient operation the observer has to develop a skill. ETRAN boards thus do not contribute to the user's independence. In addition, the number of symbols that can be reliably communicated in this manner is too limited.

There have been various attempts to overcome the problems of limited vocabulary and need for an observer inherent in such simple gaze communication systems. The human observer is replaced by optoelectronic devices and microprocessors. Most approaches use some form of eye tracking to establish the line of gaze and determine the visual target. This seems to be an easy and obvious solution. However, its implementation poses numerous technical problems that are difficult to solve. Since the eye is a small globe mostly hidden under the lid, it is hard to measure its angle of rotation. There are two ways to accomplish this: by means of head-mounted detectors or stationary video cameras focused on the user's eye. If head-mounted detectors are used, the head position also has to be measured to calculate the line of gaze to a fixated target, unless the selectable targets are mounted on the head (2). Accurate eye tracking using stationary cameras usually requires stabilization of the head by means of a bite bar or, at least, a chin rest. Without severe restriction of head movements, the spatial resolution, i.e., the number of distinguishable targets, is relatively low. This head restriction is unacceptable for long-term, daily use. The technology that would permit both accurate eye tracking and freedom of head movement is presently too expensive for the rehabilitation market.

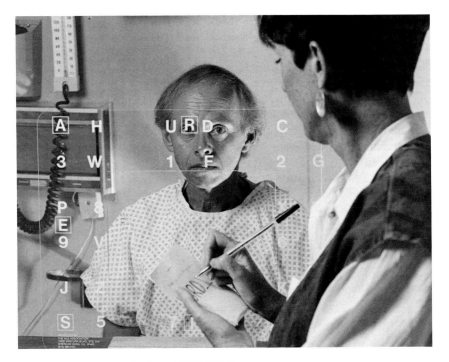

Figure 1 An eye transfer board (ETRAN) in use.

Several of the eye-tracking techniques mentioned above have been explored over the past 10 or 15 years. Some have led to marketable products (e.g., Eye Typer* and Cedric†). Both these systems tolerate only very small head movements.

Communication Strategies

So far we have focused on the problem of establishing a communication channel for the disabled person, i.e., designing a physical interface with the person's brain. Equally important is the design of the interface with the person's mind. Solving this part of the problem requires the development of special techniques for efficient use of the new communication channel once it is established. Both, the architecture and structural organization of the communication aid and the

---

*"Eye Typer" is a trademark of Sentient Systems Technology, Inc.
†The Cedric communicator is manufactured by Santech Pty Ltd., Australia

capabilities and structural properties of the mind that operates it have to be taken into account. It is important to know what the primary use of the aid will be and what degree of complexity the patient can handle. Higher communication rates are usually tied to increased complexity that, in turn, requires longer training periods to achieve proficiency.

Communication with others is based on language that structurally is not ideally suited to the communication needs of the disabled. Written and spoken language contains a great deal of redundancy that enhances the reliability of communication. This redundancy is already evident from the fact that with an average word length of five letters per written word there are over 10 million possible letter combinations, while the number of words used by the average person is, at best, in the tens of thousands. This redundancy can be sacrificed for greater speed when information flow is slow. For instance, communication rates can be greatly increased by means of a symbolic representation of language using a relatively small number of symbols. Another approach to reduce the number of choices employs semantic information whereby a symbol can have a context-dependent meaning (3). An example of such a system is Minspeak (4). While these approaches are useful in accelerating casual conversation, they are not suitable for serious writing.

Communication rates with row/column scanning devices can be enhanced through proper key assignment. Since the scan always starts from top left, the most frequently used letters or symbols should be placed in the neighborhood of this corner. The best assignment for spelling systems has been carefully studied, and the findings have been incorporated in commercially available scanning devices.

Optimal key assignment in various types of systems depends on the user and sometimes on the particular use, such as the context of a conversation. In some systems the assignment of some keys can be changed by the user. In another approach the system uses statistical analysis of word usage to modify key assignment. Rarely used keys are reassigned to words that were frequently spelled. In addition, predictive systems have been developed that attempt to finish words that are being spelled on the basis of a few letters (5) or sentences based on the first few words and syntactic information. One or several predictions are displayed for affirmation by the user. These systems have the disadvantage that the user has to interupt his actions to read the predictions. This requires an additional expense in time and effort that partially offsets the gains achieved through prediction.

Users differ greatly in their abilities, background, and intended use of their communication system. In many cases efforts have been made to make the systems programmable so they can be customized if necessary. It is clear, however, that the linguistic problems involved in optimizing the performance for a specific user are extremely difficult (6).

A LOOK INTO THE FUTURE

Communication System Using Bioelectrical Signals from the Brain

When confronted with persons with extreme disability, one is motivated to think about new ways of interfacing these individuals with the outside world. A new interface system could take advantage of the brain's own internal communication system. Sensory input from the environment, muscle responses of the human body, thinking, and other mental processes are all accompanied by bioelectrical signals from the central nervous system that can be detected on the scalp. These signals are components of the electroencephalogram (EEG). They represent a direct link of the brain with the outside world that does not depend on the ability of the body to respond. These signals, thus, have great and as yet untapped potential as an alternate communication channel. However, before they can be put to use in rehabilitation, we have to learn enough about the underlying mechanisms to reliably interpret these signals. This knowledge has proven very elusive.

Consider the possibility of direct detection of human thought from scalp signals. This problem bears some similarities to speech recognition, which was discussed in the previous section. It has taken many years of research and development to achieve reliable speech recognition of a small vocabulary of known words in a known language. Even today's most advanced speech recognition techniques fail in the presence of significant noise contamination. In the case of brain signals, we presently do not know the "language" of human thought, and contamination by noise from other brain functions and from muscle activity outside the skull is very high. It does not appear likely that persons will soon directly communicate their thoughts by means of brain waves. However, more modest applications of brain signals in rehabilitation have been investigated. Repeated attempts have been made to utilize the P300 component, a positive wave associated with novel or anticipated events (oddball events) (7). The user is presented with a sequence of choices. The selection is detected by the associated P300 response. The feasibility of this approach has been demonstrated, but it is presently too slow to be practical (8).

Another approach to communication by means of brain signals is outlined in the following section. It has been explored in our laboratory and led to useful communication rates (9). The example may provide some insight into the possibilities as well as the present limitations in the use of brain signals for communication.

The Brain Response Interface (BRI)

The Concept

Our best understanding of brain signals is confined to a few relatively simple components of the electroencephalogram (EEG) called sensory evoked potentials. Some uses of these brain signals are possible now, allowing us to develop a simple, but practical application for gaze communication. Our approach does not use eye tracking, but uses the responses from the human brain to identify the selected target. It determines the target by analyzing small electrical signals called visual evoked potentials (VEPs) that originate from the visual cortex of the brain. Since the visual system itself does most of the work, it is possible to take advantage of its great sensitivity and adaptability. We have termed our gaze communication method brain response interface (BRI). The most important advantages of this approach are that it leaves the user with complete freedom of head movement and works over a wide range of environmental conditions. It requires little or no calibration or adjustment during operation and does not interfere with the use of eyeglasses.

The largest VEPs are recorded from the back of the head where the primary visual areas of the cerebral cortex are located. The observed signals change in response to changes in the visual stimulus. The signals evoked by such changes reflect certain properties of the stimulus, but it is not possible at this time to identify the object viewed by a person from these signals alone. However, it is possible to determine which one of a number of similar stimuli a person is directly looking at, simply on the basis of the size of the response generated. The signal evoked by a small stimulus increases enormously the closer to the center of the visual field it is located. This emphasis of the center of our vision starts already in the eye, in the light-sensitive layer of the retina, and becomes progressively more pronounced in successive stages of visual processing. The density of retinal cones, the light-sensitive elements responsible for daylight vision, is much higher at the very center. With a contact lens electrode it is possible to detect small electrical signals from the retina (ERG signals) which are proportional to the cone density. With new recording techniques we are now able to image these local responses across the visual field. Figure 2 shows such a three-dimensional representation of the local responses for the central 23°. The response peak corresponds to the center of the visual field.

When the signal reaches the visual cortex of the brain, a further enhancement of the center has taken place. The cortical surface area allocated to processing of the center of the visual field is extremely large. Signals from the visual cortex derived with an electrode pair pasted to the scalp on the back of the head reflect this magnification. Figure 3 shows the response density obtained with the imaging technique for the central 23° of the visual field. This visual evoked response from the brain is exquisitely tuned to the center of the visual field. The signal is very small and contaminated with noise, but given enough signal averaging time, it is possible in most individuals to distinguish visually fixated targets with an accuracy better than 1° (or less than 1 in. on a computer screen 2 ft away).

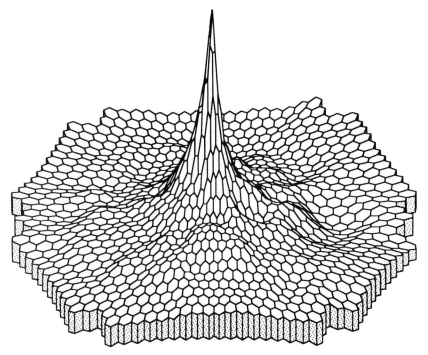

Figure 2 Local responsiveness of the human retina measured under daylight conditions. The peak response density corresponds to the center of the visual field (center of gaze). The plot extends to 23° eccentricity.

What complicates the problem somewhat is the fact that there are several representations of the visual field on the cortex of the brain. Because the cortex is convoluted, their respective signals can cancel each other. The curvature of these representations varies considerably from person to person such that electrode placement for best central response has to be determined for each individual.

A Prototype System

Based on the above scientific background, a prototype communication system was designed and constructed that allows its user to randomly access a considerable number of targets by means of his gaze. It consists of an 8 × 8 matrix of rectangular fields displayed on a computer monitor. Each field represents a key that can be operated by one's gaze. It is labeled with the corresponding function.

To generate evoked responses the fields are independently stimulated. Several different modes of stimulation are available: flicker, alternation between two

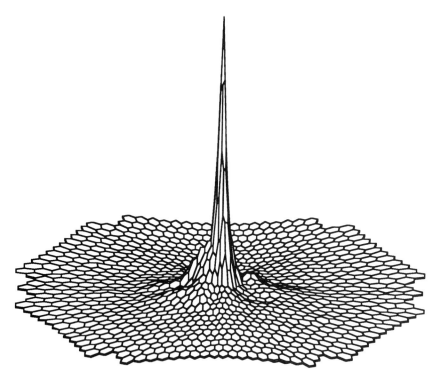

Figure 3 Response of the visual cortex of the human brain to small flickering stimuli within the central 23° of the visual field. The responses were derived from an electrode pair pasted to the scalp over the visual cortex. Note that the cortical response density falls off much faster with eccentricity than the retinal response (Fig. 2).

colors, and color reversal of a fine pattern of checks of two different colors. The mode is selected depending on the magnitude of the responses of the user and his personal preference. Alternation between equally bright red and green is most frequently used since it generates a large signal and appears to be least disturbing to most users.

Through analysis of a single signal derived from the scalp, the BRI system has to determine which one of the stimulus fields generates the largest response. This is not easy because of the great noise contamination of the signal mainly due to muscle activity. It requires application of special signal analysis techniques which involve simultaneous stimulation of all the targets. To extract the signal from the noise, the system makes use of the special response characteristics of each person, which is determined ahead of time.

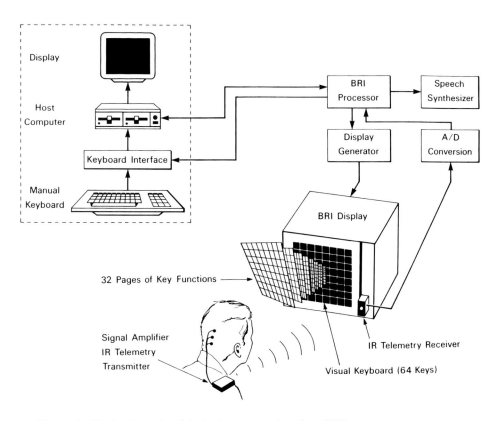

Figure 4 Block schematic of the brain response interface (BRI).

The BRI is implemented with a modern high-speed microprocessor. A block schematic of the prototype system is shown in Figure 4. The 64 gaze-addressable keys are displayed on a color monitor. Each key has 32 levels of key functions. Through a serial port, the BRI processor is connected with a synthesizer for generation of high-quality speech. Special function keys permit the user to switch between different speech modes (no speech, speech after each word, or speech after each sentence). Through a special keyboard interface the user has access to a personal computer and uses commercial software for word processing and other tasks. The BRI processor can also directly interface with a universal remote control for access to video and audio equipment. A special overlay of key functions provides the user with complete control over household appliances.

The 32 levels of key functions can be used to implement various techniques that accelerate communication. The following simple scheme was implemented for evaluation of the prototype: the first screen the user sees contains the alphabet and the most frequently used words. If the desired word is not on the screen, the user selects the beginning letter. The BRI instantaneously switches to an overlay with words starting with this letter. This simple scheme gives the user access to approximately 700 of the most frequently used words with one or two key selections. Words not in this dictionary can be spelled out, since each screen also contains the alphabet. All 2048 key choices presently available on this prototype are programmable and modifiable by the user. Key choices can be letters, words, entire sentences, or controls for special devices.

The prototype system has been tested with almost 100 normal subjects and approximately 20 severely disabled persons. With most normal subjects, adequate response times of less than 3 sec could be achieved after an initial tuning of the system to the person's brain signals. This procedure lasts 10 min to 1 hr. In the evaluation with disabled persons, we encountered two major obstacles toward use in everyday life. First, the two most important etiologies, cerebral palsy and ALS, often cause EMG artifacts originating mainly from the neck musculature. In the case of cerebral palsy, they are due to involuntary athetoid movements, while with ALS, they originate from fasciculation, spontaneous oscillations of muscle fibers. Second, the placement and maintenance of the scalp electrodes by a relatively inexperienced nursing staff can lead to inadequate performance.

Both these problems can be solved with electrodes implanted in the space between the dura (thick membrane surrounding the brain) and the skull. No direct contact with the brain is required. With such intracranial electrodes, the brain signals are 5–10 times larger, while the bone shields the electrodes from muscle artifacts.

An ALS patient volunteered to test this system (10). Under local anesthesia, a small strip of biocompatible material with four platinum electrodes was slipped into the epidural space through a small hole in the skull. The best placement and orientation of the strip had been established through scalp recordings prior to the implantation. The electrode leads were tunneled under the scalp to a small exit hole in the neck region where they could be connected to a tiny telemetry transmitter. The signal quality remained stable for the entire evaluation until the death of the patient 11 months after the implant. Cause of death was unrelated to this project.

The volunteer subject was given a complete BRI communication system for use and evaluation in his home. It permitted him to communicate with high-quality synthetic speech (Dectalk, Digital Equipment Corp.), operate word-processing software on the host computer, and control his television set and VCR. Toward the end of the evaluation, the subject reached communication rates of

10–12 words/minute. He could operate the gaze-addressable keyboard with a mean access time of approximately 1.2 sec.

After the initial healing process, the implanted electrodes did not cause any discomfort, and the subject claimed not to be aware of the implant. However, the transcutaneous electrode leads do present a small risk of infection that could result in meningitis, necessitating removal of the electrodes. This risk can be eliminated through implantation of the amplifier-telemetry transmitter unit. At the time of our first implantation, the battery life of the available transmitter did not warrant implantation. With recent advances in telemetry technology, a unit with a battery life of 7–10 years has become available that could be used in future implants.

In the first evaluation with implanted electrodes, the BRI prototype has shown great promise. The subject still had some residual movement in his left knee that enabled him to operate conventional row/column scanning devices. However, with the BRI system, he could achieve significantly higher communication rates using his gaze alone. Many severely disabled persons have no motor control left for communication besides eye movements and are unable to use any of the presently available eye-tracking devices. For them, the BRI concept may represent the only hope to achieve an acceptable level of communication.

The BRI system represents the first practical application of signals from the central nervous system in rehabilitation. Certainly, many other and far more sophisticated applications of brain signals are possible. Through this project new techniques of signal derivation and transmission were tested that could be used to interface with other areas of the cerebral cortex. It is hoped that the success of the BRI concept will encourage research into new applications of neurosciences that will bring today's fast-advancing electronic technology to those who need it the most.

ACKNOWLEDGMENTS

The author thanks Ms. Lani Hardage, Ms. Charlette Schmidt, and Dr. Richard Smith for their assistance and helpful suggestions. The research presented in the last section was funded in part by NIH Grant EY06861, NIDRR Grant 133KH6003, and the Smith-Kettlewell Eye Research Institute.

REFERENCES

1. Arnott JL. A comparison of Palantype and Stenograph keyboards in high-speed speech output systems. Proceedings of the 10th Annual Conference on Rehabilitation Engineering (RESNA), 1987:106–108.

2. Demasco P, Horstmann H. A line of gaze communication system. Proceedings of the 10th Annual Conference on Rehabilitation Engineering (RESNA), 987:112–114.

3. Demasco P, McCoy K, Gong Y, Pennington C, Rowe C. Towards more intelligent interfaces: The use of natural language processing. Proceedings of the 12th Annual Conference on Rehabilitation Engineering (RESNA), 1989:141–142.
4. Baker B. Minspeak. Byte Sept 1982:186.
5. Foulds R, Soede M, van Balkom H, Boves L. Lexical prediction techniques applied to reduce motor requirements for augmentative communication. Proceedings of the 10th Annual Conference on Rehabilitation Engineering (RESNA), 1987:115–117.
6. Coleman CL, Cook AM, Meyers LS. Assessing non-oral clients for assistive communication devices. J Speech Hear Disord 1980;45:515–526.
7. Walter WG, Cooper R, Aldridge VJ, McCallum WC, Winter AL. Contingent negative variation: an electric sign of sensorimotor association and expectancy in the human brain. Nature 1964;203:380–384.
8. Farwell LA, Donchin E. Talking off the top of your head: Toward a mental prosthesis utilizing event-related brain potentials. Electroenceph Clin Neurophysiol 1988;70:510–523.
9. Sutter EE, Tran D. Communication through visually induced electrical brain responses. Proceedings of the 2nd International Conference: Computers for Handicapped Persons. Schriftenreihe der Oestereichischen Computer Gesellshaft 1990; 55:279–288.
10. Sutter EE, Pevehouse BC, Barbaro N. Intra-cranial electrodes for communication and environmental control. Proceedings of the Fourth Annual Conference: Technology and Persons with Disabilities. California State University, Northridge, 1988.

13

Legal Issues

Joseph M. Healey, Jr.

University of Connecticut School of Medicine
Farmington, Connecticut

INTRODUCTION

The various chapters in this book represent a tribute to the progress that has been made in understanding and treating amyotrophic lateral sclerosis (ALS) and in considering how the well-being, interests, and wishes of patients with ALS can be identified and respected. There has been an important shift in the biomedical and biosocial dimensions of caring for the patient with ALS. This shift from ignorance and fear to knowledge and compassion must also occur in addressing related legal issues. In many ways, the legal shift is already occurring. There are now options, where formerly there were none. There are alternative models of the health professional–patient relationship that offer greater self-determination to patients. There is the increased opportunity to control decisions at the end of life, permitting the patient's values and wishes to be respected. But much more remains to be accomplished. This chapter will examine the common legal problem areas that confront patients with ALS, their families, and their health professionals and will recommend strategies to anticipate and to deal with these areas of concern constructively. The goal of this chapter is to describe in general terms the problem areas, the principles involved, and strategies available to deal with them. Application to specific cases will require using these concepts in contexts that vary greatly from individual case to individual case in different states whose laws may vary. Discussion of relevant local and state law with one's own legal advisor is always a wise first step in developing one's own plan of action.

PROBLEM AREAS AND GUIDING PRINCIPLES

Many of the legal problem areas encountered in caring for a patient with ALS are similar to those encountered in any contemporary doctor-patient relationship. These include:

1. Assuring that the patient has access to an appropriate level and quality of health care, in therapeutic and experimental settings
2. Clarifying the nature of the doctor-patient relationship
3. Protecting the patient's right to self-determination as reflected in consent to treatment and refusal of treatment, generally, and in end-of-life decisions, specifically
4. Clarifying the role of family members in the patient's health care

Access to Appropriate Level and Quality of Care

The initial problem area for most patients is obtaining access to an appropriate level and quality of health care. First, this problem area is a reflection of the extent to which the American legal system views the health professional–patient relationship as a contractual relationship and does not recognize a legally enforceable right to health care. In those countries which have a national health system, a patient may possess a legal right to appropriate care. As a practical matter, there is no such legal right in the United States. Second, this problem area is further a reflection of the inadequacies of the mechanisms for financing health care that tend to fragment, rather than to integrate, the components of the health care delivery system. Whatever its sources, this problem area raises a number of legal issues for patients with ALS:

1. How to find the right health professional, capable of providing the appropriate level and quality of health services
2. How to obtain health care services consistent with appropriate professional standards
3. How to assure that guidelines for the protection of human subjects are followed when experimental therapies are considered

The American legal system views the relationship between health professional and patient as a contractual relationship—freely entered into by both parties and governed by the law of contracts. Under principles of contract law, both health professional and patient choose to establish a relationship and various rights and duties arise after the relationship has been established. It is the responsibility of the patient to seek the services of appropriate health professionals and to enter into relationships with them. Since there is no general duty to accept a person as a patient, health professionals are generally legally free to enter or not enter such a relationship. However, once a relationship has been initiated, a series of specific and implied legal duties arises from the contract. For example, health professionals are expected to possess the skills and expertise that they claim to possess and may be held legally accountable for their misrepresentations or for their failure to fulfill their contractual obligations. Patients have legal recourse to vindicate such rights (1).

Health professionals are expected to provide services consistent with appropriate professional standards. Patients may enforce their claims to such a level of care by using the malpractice system under which a patient may recover damages. To establish that malpractice has occurred, a patient must prove each of the following elements: (a) that the health professional owed a duty (including what the nature of the duty itself was); (b) that the conduct of the health professional breached the duty; and (c) that the breach of duty directly and proximately caused harm to the patient. It is important to recognize that the malpractice system does not provide a remedy for all injuries, but only for those that are the direct and proximate result of a breach of the health professional's duty to the patient (2).

The use of experimental treatments or procedures is subject to additional safeguards to assure protection of the patient–subject. Most human experimentation in the United States is subject to guidelines developed and enforced by the federal Department of Health and Human Services or the Food and Drug Administration. These regulations describe in detail the review process that precedes the enrollment of subjects in an experimental protocol and the requirements with respect to informed consent and confidentiality (3).

In summary, the responsibility for obtaining the services of appropriate health professionals rests with ALS patients and their supporters. However, once a relationship is begun, there are legal rights and duties which arise out of that existing relationship. ALS patients and their health professionals should know and understand these legal rights and duties.

The Nature of the Doctor-Patient Relationship

The second area of legal concern involves clarification of the model of the health professional–patient relationship upon which a specific relationship is based. At issue is the balance of rights and duties between the parties in the relationship. Part of the negotiation preceding the initiation of a relationship should include discussion of the alternative models and the implications of each for the relationship. In reviewing the challenge of establishing the balance of rights and duties between the parties, the President's Commission has provided a concise summary of the alternatives:

Two models of the patient-professional relationship have dominated the debate surrounding this challenge. For the sake of simplicity, while recognizing the cariacatures involved, these may be referred to as "medical paternalism" and "patient sovereignty." Medical paternalism is based on a traditional view of health professionals—typically physicians—as the dominant, authoritarian figure in the relationship, with both the right and the responsibility to make decisions in the medical best interests of the patient. In reaction to this view, some have sought to take over the physician's dominant position. Proponents of maximal patient sovereignty assign patients full responsibility for and control over all decisions about their own care. According to this view, practitioners should act as servants of their patients, transmitting medical information and using their technical skills as the patient directs, without seeking to influence the patient's decisions, much less actually make them.

Both positions attempt to vest exclusive moral agency, ethical wisdom, and decisionmaking authority on one side of the relationship, while assigning the other side a dependent role. In the view of the Commission, neither extreme adequately reflects the current nature and needs of health care. The debate has increasingly become an arid exercise, which the Commission believes should be replaced by a view that reflects the tremendous diversity of health care situations and relationships today. In this Report, the Commission attempts to shift the terms of the discussion toward how to foster a relationship between patients and professionals characterized by mutual participation and respect and by shared decisionmaking. The Commission believes such a shift in focus will do better justice to the realities of health care and to the ethical values underlying the informed consent doctrine (4).

For some patients, the model of medical paternalism is the most comfortable model. To the extent possible, patient wishes should be accommodated. However, especially in the period since the end of World War II, this model has been increasingly challenged by the compromise model endorsed by the President's Commission, which emphasizes shared decision making. Many patients are unaware that there is an alternative to the traditional model. At the very least, patients should know that an alternative model exists. The options should be clear, so informed negotiation can take place.

The model of the doctor-patient relationship influences such important questions as: (a) the respective roles of the doctor and patient in making decisions; (b) the patient's right of access to complete, accurate information; and (c) other patient rights, such as the right to have one's privacy and confidentiality respected.

The model of the relationship selected will influence the manner in which decisions are made for or by the patient. Medical paternalism is often used to justify limiting the role of the patient in decision making on the grounds that the health professional is in a better position to know what is in the patient's best interests. In such a relationship, the health professional's focus may also shift from the patient to other family members. Information may be withheld from a patient to spare the patient worry. The health professional becomes the active party while the patient is viewed as the passive recipient. In contrast, a model emphasizing shared decision making remains focused on the patient as decision maker and assures disclosure of current, accurate information to the patient, to permit the patient to take as active a role as is possible or desired. It is the patient who helps to determine what is best, not only the family or health professionals alone. Similarly, the patient is entitled to have personal information treated as confidential and to have rights of privacy respected. Access of others to such information should occur only with the knowledge and approval of the patient.

In summary, there is more than one model of the health professional-patient relationship. Patients with ALS should seek out relationships with health professionals that reflect the model of the relationship with which the patient is most comfortable. Patients have a legal right to participate actively in decisions affecting their health care and are free to terminate relationships with health professionals unwilling to respect their rights.

Protection of the Patient's Right to Self-Determination

It is a fundamental principle of American law that adult persons of sound mind have the right to determine what happens to their bodies. This principle is applied in the health care context through the concepts of consent and refusal of treatment. This problem area centers around how best to assure that patients receive health care of an appropriate quality, to the extent and in a manner consistent with the patient's wishes. The goal is to avoid the twin undesirable extremes of undertreatment and overtreatment of the patient. This problem area raises three issues for patients with ALS:

1. The nature of the right to consent
2. The nature of the right to refuse treatment, including life-sustaining treatment
3. Strategies that the currently competent patient may use in anticipation of future inability to communicate personal wishes

Health professionals have a legal obligation to obtain the informed, competent, and voluntary consent of a patient before treatment can be provided. Although the boundaries of the consent process are a matter of state law and there is a great deal of variety among the states, some general guidelines should be kept in mind. The requirement of informed consent imposes a legal duty on the health professional to provide sufficient information to permit the patient to make a choice. The consenting party must be competent, that is, an adult person of sound mind or a minor who is eligible under state law to make health care decisions. The consent must be voluntary, that is, not the result of fraud or deception by the health professional. As these dimensions of consent suggest, consent is a process rather than an event. It involves the assent of the party and not merely the obtaining of a signature. Its goal is to encourage active participation in health care decisions, not only to satisfy a technical legal obligation.

If the right to consent is to mean more than just the right to agree with one's health professional, it must also include the right to refuse treatment (5). It is now uniformly acknowledged that patients have a right to refuse treatment. Particular attention has been focused on whether the right to refuse treatment may be outweighed in certain circumstances by another, "compelling" interest. A second issue is whether there are limits with respect to which treatments may be refused. These issues are of particular interest in the context of ALS. A series of cases involving patients with ALS who sought to refuse respiratory support of artificial nutrition and hydration through a feeding tube has emerged during the past 15 years. In addition, the U.S. Supreme Court in 1990 decided a case involving the refusal of artificial nutrition and hydration by the surrogate of a patient in a persistent vegetative state. Although there remain variations from state to state, the outlines of public policy in this area finally seem to be emerging.

It is generally acknowledged that the right to refuse treatment is not an absolute right, but under certain circumstances may be outweighed by "compelling state interests." There is disagreement about the interests and when they apply, but most states would include among the interests that must be considered: (a) the state's interest in the preservation of life; (b) the state's interest in protecting third parties; (c) the state's interest in preventing suicide; and (d) the state's interest in maintaining the ethical integrity of the medical profession. Although some disagreement remains, most states acknowledge that an adult person of sound mind has the right to refuse treatment, including life-sustaining treatment, unless there is a compelling state interest in the case to outweigh the refusal. Virtually all the states have viewed respirators and artificial nutrition and hydration as forms of treatment that may be refused. In each of the four leading cases involving patients with ALS, the patient's right to refuse treatment or to have treatment refused in the patient's name was respected (6). None of the state's interest was found to be "compelling."

A degenerative disease such as ALS raises the possibility that decisions involving consent or refusal of treatment might have to be made when the patient is not capable of communicating his/her wishes. It is especially important that such patients use one or more of the available mechanisms to assure that the patient's wishes are known and followed. First and foremost, it is important for the patient to discuss with the attending health professionals the type and variety of decisions that are likely to occur. In most states, a patient can document express wishes about future decisions in a "living will," which provides instructions to the physician, family, and friends about how decisions should be made, if the patient cannot communicate directly. Second, many states permit a currently competent patient to empower a surrogate decisionmaker through the creation of a power of attorney or advanced designation of a guardian or conservator. Such a person would be given instructions about how the patient wishes desicions to be made. Use of one of these strategies provides the best assurance that the wishes of the patient will be known and followed (7).

The full implications of the U.S. Supreme Court's decision involving the removal of artificial nutrition and hydration from a patient in a persistent vegetative state are unclear (8). The majority of the Court emphasized the need for "clear and convincing evidence" of the patient's wishes. At the very least, this case underscores the need for patients to think over the decisions that might be faced in the future and to give as clear and explicit guidance as possible about how those decisions should be made.

The health professional's duty to respect a patient's right to refuse treatment or to have treatment withheld or withdrawn should be distinguished from two related, but very different, concepts: physician-assisted suicide and active, involuntary euthanasia. Both concepts received recent widespread publicity. Physician-assisted suicide received national attention in the late spring of 1990 when a retired Michigan pathologist connected a woman, allegedly suffering from Alzheimer's disease, to his "suicide machine" and allowed her to bring about her own death. This case raised questions about the extent to which doctors or other health professionals should be permitted to assist patients to commit suicide. Active, involuntary euthanasia was the subject of a controversial article in the *Journal of the American Medical Association* entitled, "It's Over, Debbie," which appeared in early 1988 (9). This case raised questions about the extent to which doctors or other health professionals should be permitted to take actions that directly and intentionally take the lives of their patients.

Traditionally, the common law regarded suicide as a felony and punished those who attempted it, those who actually committed it, and those who assisted in its commission. Although suicide has been decriminalized by virtually all states, a suicide attempt may still be the basis for a psychiatric or public health intervention, and many states continue to treat assisting suicide as a crime (10). Physicians who assist their patients in attempting suicide may find themselves accused of violating relevant sections of their state's criminal law. However, it should be emphasized that at least since the case of Karen Anne Quinlan in 1975, courts have routinely refused to consider the refusal of medical treatment as the equivalent of suicide (11). Therefore, respecting a patient's right to refuse treatment should not be construed as "assisting a suicide."

Active, involuntary euthanasia involves the intentional taking of a patient's life by a health professional and is subject to the criminal law's prohibition against homicide (12). Though there have been recent attempts to establish exceptions that would permit physicians under certain circumstances to engage in acts of this sort, there has been no change in the legal treatment of such conduct. Physicians who engage in such conduct remain potentially legally liable for their actions.

In summary, patients have a legal right of self-determination, which includes the right to accept or refuse treatment (including life-sustaining treatment) as long as the refusal is not outweighed by a compelling state interest. Patients should clearly articulate their wishes in a legally acceptable manner and should designate a surrogate decision maker in anticipation of being unable to communicate their wishes at some time in the future.

The Role of Family Members

The fourth legal problem area involves the extent to which family members or the next of kin are entitled to make decisions for a patient unable to make decisions for himself or herself. The law assumes that a person who has reached the age of adulthood (generally 18 years) is legally competent to make decisions alone, without the approval or involvement of others. Traditionally, it has been the responsibility of those who question the competence of another to demonstrate that the person is not capable of making decisions and to petition the appropriate court for appointment of a formal surrogate decision maker, such as a guardian or conservator. Until 1990, there had been a clear trend in the law away from the strict application of this requirement and toward allowing family members or the next of kin to serve as informal surrogates presenting either the patient's previously expressed wishes or a recommendation of what the informal surrogate judged to be in the patient's best interest. The relaxation of the requirement for the appointment of a formal surrogate was the result of several factors, especially the realization that family members are usually in the best position to know and to implement the wishes or best interests of the patient. Requiring the appointment of a formal surrogate imposes a financial and emotional burden, deemed unjustified by the remote possibility of an abuse of the patient's rights. The decision of the U.S. Supreme Court in the *Cruzan* case raises questions about how much authority can be vested in either formal or informal surrogates and is likely to stimulate reconsideration of requirements in this area on a state-by-state basis.

STRATEGIES FOR IMPLEMENTATION

Patients with ALS, members of their families, their friends, and their health professionals should take steps to implement preventive strategies that permit the identification, anticipation, and successful confrontation of these legal issues. A valuable initial step would be to assemble a working group of advisors with whom the various legal issues could be addressed. It is important, for example, to have access to legal counsel, capable of providing current, accurate information about the specific legal boundaries in the state in which the patient is located. Other participants might include a person designated to serve as surrogate if necessary, involved health professionals, family, and friends. Among the important steps to be taken in conjunction with these advisors are: (a) discussing the likely areas of concern and clarifying the patient's wishes; (b) documenting and implementing those wishes; (c) providing specific guidance for a surrogate to deal with foreseeable decisions that might have to be made when the patient is incapable; (d) providing general guidance for a surrogate to deal with decisions that are not foreseeable but might have to be made when the patient is incapable.

Discussion and Clarification

Guiding the preventive strategies should be a commitment to use the law in an anticipatory manner. It is important for the patient with ALS to review the specific areas of legal concern with appropriate counsel and to discuss them with those who will be involved in providing care and support to the patient. Among these people should be the person chosen to be the surrogate decision maker, involved health professionals, family members, and friends. Early discussion will help to bring these issues into the open at a time when there can be constructive consideration of the issues and when the wishes of the patient can be made clear. Among the specific areas of legal concern that should be discussed are the nature of the patient's wishes concerning (a) the extent of involvement in medical decision making; (b) the model of the doctor-patient relationship to be implemented; (c) access to information about the progress of the disease; (d) pursuit of experimental therapy; (e) level of respiratory support; and (f) the conditions under which treatment and support should be withheld or withdrawn. Patients should be aware of the options that exist and the extent to which existing options are exercisable and should discuss their wishes as clearly and concretely as possible.

Documentation and Implementation

Once patients have identified their wishes, appropriate documentation and implementation should follow. Patients should use whatever mechanisms are available within their state. These may include written instructions, such as a living will, the identification of a formal surrogate by using a power of attorney, or advanced designation of guardian or conservator; or identification of an informal surrogate (such as a family member) if permitted by state law. The patient's wishes should also be documented in the patient's record, so there will be no doubt, should decisions need to be made at a time when the patient's regular health professional is unavailable. Once known, the wishes of the patient should be implemented.

Specific Guidance

The patient should provide specific guidance for surrogates to deal with foreseeable decisions that might have to be made when the patient is incapable. Among the most common decisions are those involving the withholding or withdrawing of treatment, medication, respiratory support, or artificial nutrition and hydration. As an expression of self-determination, the patient should discuss the likely unfolding of the disease process, the potential decisions that are likely to arise, and how the patient would want such decisions to be made.

General Guidance

It is impossible to anticipate all the possible situations in which a surrogate might be called on to make decisions. Nonetheless, patients can provide general guidance for a surrogate to deal with decisions that are not foreseeable but might have to be made by a surrogate when the patient is incapable. This guidance should express the general principles that the patient wishes to influence such decisions. While not as useful as specific guidance, such guidance provides a base from which these decisions can reasonably be made.

CONCLUSION

The greatest achievement of 20th-century medicine has been the rise of medical power with medicine's improved capacity to confront many of the major causes of death and disability for those who lived and died in the early part of this century. While much has been accomplished, much more remains to be done. An important legacy of this era has been the recognition that increased medical power makes possible increased opportunity for choice where chance and fate once determined process and outcome. While much more remains to be uncovered about ALS and its prevention and treatment, there are now more choices about how patients with ALS can and should be cared for. The law provides support for those patients who wish to take more active roles in examining these options and in participating in making these choices. Health professionals, family members, and friends should encourage this positive use of the law as a force for enhancing the dignity and the self-determination of the patient with ALS.

REFERENCES

1. For an introduction to legal issues involved in patient access to health professionals, see Hall M, Ellman I. Health care law and ethics in a nutshell. St. Paul, MN: West, 1990:71–101.
2. For an introduction to medical malpractice, see Annas G. The rights of patients. Carbondale and Edwardsville: Southern Illinois University Press, 1989:239–257.
3. See, generally, Levine R. Ethics and regulation of clinical research, 2nd ed. New Haven and London: Yale University Press, 1988.
4. President's Commission for the Study of Ethical Problems in Medicine and Biomedical and Behavioral Research. Making health care decisions. Washington, DC: US Government Printing Office, 1982:36.
5. See, generally, President's Commission for the Study of Ethical Problems in Medicine and Biomedical and Behavioral Research. Deciding to forego life-sustaining treatment. Washington, DC: US Government Printing Office, 1983, and Weir R. Abating treatment with critically ill patients. New York and Oxford: Oxford University Press, 1989.
6. See *Satz v. Perlmutter*, 362 So. 2d 160 (Fla. App.) 1978; *Leach v. Akron General Medical Center et al.*, 68 Ohio Misc. 1 (Court of Common Pleas of Ohio) 1980; *In the Matter of Beverly Requena*, 213 N.J. Super 475 (Superior Court of New Jersey) 1986; *In the Matter of Kathleen Farrell*, 108 N.J. 335 (Supreme Court of New Jersey) 1987.
7. Current information about specific state statutes affecting decisions at the end of life may be obtained from Concern for Dying and the Society for the Right to Die, both of which are located at 250 W. 57th St., New York, NY 10107.
8. *Cruzan v. Director, Missouri Dept. of Health et al.* (No. 88-1503) decided June 25, 1990.
9. It's over, Debbie. *JAMA* 1988; 259:272.
10. President's Commission, note 5 above, p. 37.
11. *Ibid.*, note 78, p. 38.
12. *Ibid.*, p. 72. See also Singer PA, Siegler M. Euthanasia—A critique. Sounding Board, N Engl J Med 1990; 322:1881–1883.

RESEARCH STRATEGY

14

The Experimental Treatment of Amyotrophic Lateral Sclerosis

Richard Alan Smith

Center for Neurologic Study
San Diego, California

INTRODUCTION

With the advent of biotechnology the opportunity to treat amyotrophic lateral sclerosis (ALS) experimentally has been markedly enhanced. A variety of potent biologicals, including interferon, growth hormone, insulin-related growth factor, and nerve growth factor, have been synthesized using recombinant DNA methodology. Some of these enjoy advantages over previously available products, but increasingly, as in the instance of epidermal growth factor, they represent novel pharmaceuticals that have previously not been available for clinical use. As the understanding of cellular processes unfolds, even more dramatic therapeutic opportunities are envisioned. Cellular functions will be regulated at the level of translation using antisense RNA technology or defective genes will be repaired using viral vectors or a similar strategy. At some point, one of these efforts is certain to lead to a cure for ALS. If the results are dramatic in a small number of cases, it might seem unnecessary and possibly unethical to proceed with a double-blind, placebo-controlled trial. However, it is more likely that a new treatment will only slow the course of ALS or benefit only a certain class of patients, perhaps being beneficial early in the disease. Assuming this to be the case, researchers will need to conduct rigorous treatment trials to convincingly demonstrate that a treatment is beneficial.

On the surface, experimental treatment seems to be a rather straightforward proposition. By conventional wisdom, ALS is a progressive disease, running its fatal course over a finite period (1). If the disease seemed to stabilize or more persons than expected survived after treatment, a conclusion about the effect of treatment should be possible. On this basis, a steady stream of therapeutic claims have been made for a wide variety of compounds ranging from vitamins and dietary supplements to hormones and antivirals (2–5). Because none of these claims has been substantiated, a number of concerned investigators have suggested that standardization of trial design could advance research progress. This discussion touches on some of the complexities involved in the experimental treatment of ALS.

DEFINITION OF ALS

Recently, a committee was convened under the auspices of the World Health Organization (see Appendix) to promulgate the clinical criteria for the diagnosis of ALS (6). This exercise has proved necessary as the syndromic nature of ALS has been appreciated (7). These criteria, summarized below, permit the inclusion of like patients in treatment programs. For obvious reasons, a homogeneous group of patients is needed to test a treatment hypothesis. It is inconceivable, to be specific, that a therapy for classical ALS will benefit patients with motor neuron disease related to hexosaminidase deficiency or paraproteinemia.

Several levels of certainty have been incorporated into the definition of ALS. Assuming the criteria for this diagnosis is met, most, hopefully all, of the patients included in a trial would be expected to be correctly diagnosed. The strictest definition is included under the term "definite ALS." This includes certain anatomical and temporal characteristics. Over time, patients with definite ALS will exhibit both upper and lower motor neuron signs in muscle groups innervated from the brainstem, cervical, and lumbosacral spinal cord. Electrophysiological and laboratory tests should support the diagnosis, and the patient should be free of sensory and other findings that might ultimately be explained by another diagnosis. Obviously, the pool of patients available for enrollment in a trial will be limited if a strict definition of ALS is a requirement for inclusion. This may constrict the supply of patients to the point where a multicenter trial becomes necessary.

PROTOCOL

An important step toward formulating a treatment plan is the preparation of a protocol. While there are no absolute requirements dictating the content of this document, a protocol is a critical part of any research study. To the degree that it is a clear statement of the purpose of the study and the methods by which the study will be conducted and evaluated, it serves the interests of all the interested parties, including the investigators, the patients, and the overseers. As a general rule, the protocol should include the following:

1. Names of study chairperson, collaborating investigators, and institutional affiliations
2. Abstract
3. Scientific background
4. Objectives of the study
5. Experimental plan, including the matter of patient selection, type of patients to be excluded, drugs to be excluded, drug treatment plan, and clinical and laboratory parameters to be measured at the time of entrance to the study and during the course of the study.
6. Criteria for evaluating the effect of treatment
7. Conditions for stopping or modifying the study or removing patients from the study.
8. Course of action in the event of side effects
9. Statistical considerations
10. Patient consent
11. Investigator's responsibility, including the filing of case report forms, laboratory reports, and monitoring of drug usage
12. Confidentiality statement
13. Bibliography

INFORMED CONSENT

Patients with ALS are highly motivated to participate in experimental treatment trials. This is desirous for many reasons, but can have the effect of interfering with the process of informed consent. One could consider the example of experimental treatment as exaggerating the roles of both the patient and the physician. In the extreme, the patient may be seen as a helpless petitioner and the physician as an all-knowing, powerful provider of miracles (8). Although exaggerated, this sociological view of the prospective roles of patient and physician does lend itself to the view that the patient is at a great disadvantage when it comes to weighing the risks and benefits of a putative treatment. There are innumerable historical examples when patients have clearly suffered as a result of participation in experimental treatment (9). These egregious occurrences serve as a reminder that informed consent should be an integral part of the treatment process.

Fortunately, patients with ALS maintain their intellect, guaranteeing that lack of comprehension cannot interfere with the consent process. Nevertheless, it is clear that considerable effort needs to be made to assure that patients are aware of the nature of the experiment, the potential risks, including the occurrence of physical discomfort in some cases, and the expected benefits. Unfortunately, a signed consent form does not ensure that the patient has understood these matters. When even extraordinary measures have been made to inform patients and the process has been documented, there still remains a group of patients who are confused about the treatment, assuming that the doctor is providing standard care, rather than something experimental (10). While is it is not reassuring that such confusion exists, it reinforces the need to give consent a high priority. Although there may be some who argue that this is necessary to meet a minimal legal standard, this is a secondary consideration.

Ideally, physicians and others involved in a trial would be willing to spend time educating patients about the experiment and the demands that will be placed on them. This can be accomplished in a number of ways. In our experience a meeting with all the participants has been useful for communication with patients and their families. This provides patients with the support of a group, which may have the effect of empowering them in a relationship in which they may feel disadvantaged when alone. On another occasion, on a one-to-one basis, details of the experiment can then be reviewed and patients asked for their consent. This approach has the advantage of separating the consent process from the treatment process. All too often, patients sign consent forms while the physician and staff are waiting to begin their work. Whether or not the patient elects to participate, it must be clearly understood that participation in the experiment is not necessary to assure access to future care.

COMPLIANCE

Irrespective of the best intentions, it is common for all participants—patients, physicians, and staff—to fail to comply with the protocol requirements. Not surprisingly, compliance reports are often overstated when independently validated. Not only do patients overreport the amount of medication they take, they often fail to appreciate that their use of medication is erratic (11). It is important to recognize this problem when designing treatment trials to minimize this occurrence and make allowances for unavoidable breaches of responsibility. A number of commentators have discussed the many factors that may contribute to the problem of compliance (12). There are obvious social factors, such as education, cultural grouping, and social status, which may interfere with communication, but other factors more integral to the patient-physician relationship may be important. There is reason to believe that patients who feel thay are in partnership with their physician are more likely to take responsibility to follow the treatment regimen than those who remain passive participants (13).

To try to select patients who are most likely to comply in a treatment trial, a run-in period can be considered. In a recent nationwide trial of the effect of aspirin in reducing the risk of heart attack, volunteers were given medication for 18 weeks. Those who took less than two-thirds of their pills were subsequently dropped from the trial. The remaining participants achieved high compliance rates (14).

To keep the issue of compliance in mind, it is important to discuss this aspect of the trial at each follow-up visit. Failure to include this in the list of things to be evaluated unwittingly signals to the patient that this is not a priority of the study.

Several strategies are available to monitor compliance, although none are foolproof (15). Patients can be asked to fill out a daily log, and medication can be counted at each visit, sometimes indirectly by the return of empty bottles or packages, which can then be "exchanged" for new supplies. If feasible, the levels of medication can be monitored in the blood or spinal fluid. This is not without pitfalls because measurement can be hampered by the short half-life of the active ingredient, and if the interval between samplings is too great, it is not certain that the blood sample is representative for the entire period of treatment. Another problem arises when nonprescribed medication cross-reacts with the test drug, resulting in false positives. When this occurs in the placebo group, it can suggest "drop-ins" to the trial (16).

In some instances the test drug may work indirectly, as in the case of synthetic growth hormone (Protropin), which was recently tested in a multicenter treatment trial of ALS. Growth hormone is thought to exert all its biological effects through the induction of insulin-related growth factor (IGF-1). To monitor drug usage IGF-1 was measured in the serum at monthly intervals in both the treated and the placebo groups of the Protropin trial. Almost all patients receiving growth hormone experienced an increase in IGF-1, whereas there was little change in patients receiving placebo. However, a few placebo patients showed high IGF-1 baseline values (Fig. 1). At some point this might have provided misleading information.

Adding to the problem of compliance, ALS treatment trials are complicated by a high dropout rate. This could be interpreted as an indictment of the treatment trial paradigm. Most likely, ALS patients become quickly discouraged when a proposed treatment fails to slow the course of their disease. Olarte, among the first to comment on the problems associated with ALS trials, reported that 24 of 55 patients in a 1-year crossover trial dropped out (17). Another seven patients had reactions that necessitated their removal and six patients died. Only 19 of the original 55 patients completed the protocol. In the Protropin trial similar losses were noted. At the completion of a 12-month trial only 29 of the initial 77 patients remained. Approximately one-fourth of the total died and the remainder (38%) withdrew (8).

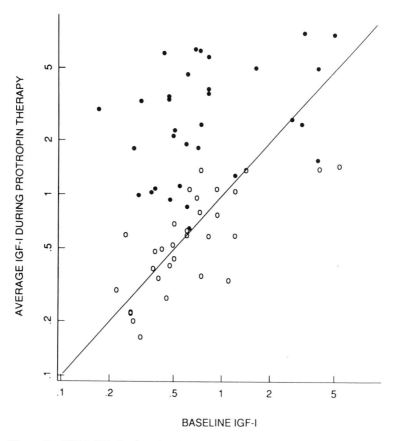

Figure 1 IGF-1 (U/ml) plotted at baseline and in response to treatment. The diagonal indicates "no change" in IGF-1. ○, Placebo treated; ●, Protropin treated.

PHARMACOLOGY

It is surprising to recall that drug therapy was almost entirely empirical until recently (18). Symptoms such as fever or pain were the barometer by which the effect of treatment was gauged. With the advent of antimicrobial therapy, blood levels of therapeutic agents were determined and found to be key determinants of therapeutic success. Unfortunately, the level of a drug in bodily fluids does not necessarily reflect concentrations at the site of action.

To the degree possible, it is important to have some idea of the processes that influence the absorption, distribution, metabolism, and elimination of drugs employed in treatment trials. These basic pharmacokinetic principles should be considered as they relate to the medication under study (19). The bioavailability of a drug relates to the extent to which the active ingredient is absorbed and becomes available at the site of action. Drugs given intravenously are considered to exhibit a 100% bioavailability because they immediately enter the general circulation. Drugs delivered orally, subcutaneously, or intramuscularly must be absorbed before they reach the general circulation. To determine the extent to which this occurs, the absolute bioavailability can be determined, although in a clinical setting this may not be practical.

Insight into the dosing requirements can be obtained by calculation of the elimination half-life, which is the time for plasma concentrations of the drug to decrease one-half during the elimination phase. As a general principle, steady-state concentrations can be achieved by dosing over a time span approximating five half-lives.

The clearance of a drug provides information about its elimination by the liver, kidney, and/or lung. Under the simplest paradigm, clearance is directly proportional to drug concentration in the blood. As an illustration of the importance of hepatic clearance, the example of dextromethorphan (DM) is noteworthy. This medication has been considered a putative therapy for the treatment of ALS and other neurological disease because of its action as an NMDA antagonist. The major pathways of DM metabolism are shown in Figure 2. The conversion of DM to dextrorphan is the principal route for DM elimination. Dextrorphan formation is accounted for, in large part, by the action of a single enzyme in the liver (cytochrome P4502D6) (20). However, in a small portion (6–8%) of the Caucasian population who are unable to express this specific cytochrome P450 enzyme the elimination of DM is impaired (21). To determine the pattern of cytochrome P4502D6 expression in an ALS population, patients and control subjects were compared after administration of a test dose of 60 mg of DM (Table 1). Eight hours later, a morning urine specimen was collected and frozen and an aliquot later used to measure the ratio of DM to dextrorphan. The vast majority of patients metabolized DM to dextrorphan efficiently (Table 1). Confirming the futility of conducting a treatment trial with DM in this group, undetectable to low (less than 20 ng/nl) serum levels of DM were found in patients treated with up to 120 mg/day of the drug. The few patients with a "slow" phenotype did achieve high serum levels (up to 325 ng/ml) of DM. The basis for the variability in serum levels was not apparently appreciated in a recent treatment trial in which patients with Huntington's disease were administered up to 1 g of DM a day (22).

It has been reported, however, that quinidine is a potent inhibitor of the cytochrome P4502D6 enzyme (23). Thus, the blockage of DM metabolism by quinidine was viewed as a reasonable approach to enhance its systemic delivery. When the phenotyping studies were repeated after the daily administration of 150

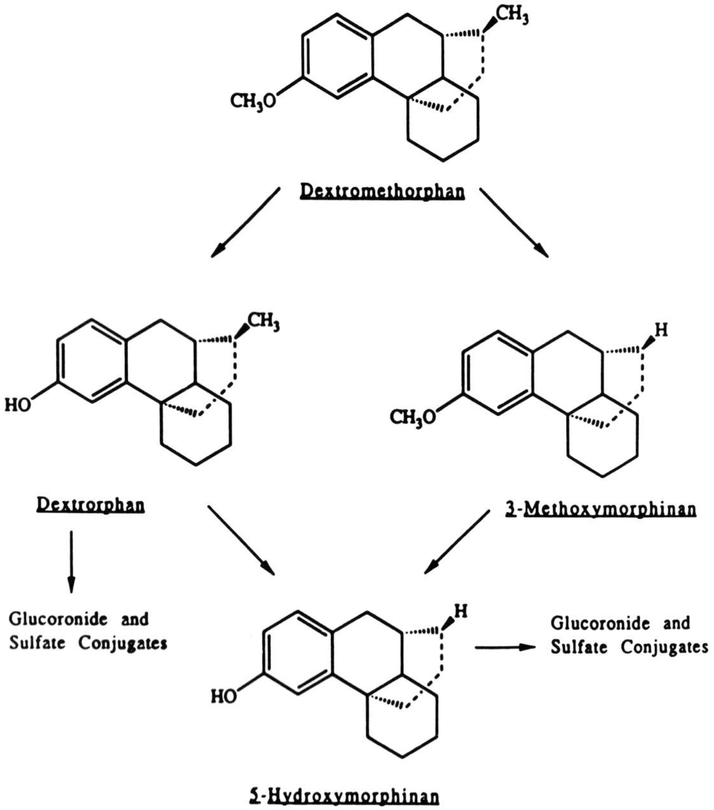

Figure 2 Degradation pathway for dextromethorphan.

mg quinidine, all ALS patients who were efficient metabolizers of DM became phenotypically poor metabolizers (Table 2) (24).

To establish that potentially therapeutic levels could be achieved with a treatment regimen consisting of both dextromethorphan and quinidine, a dose tolerance study was conducted (Table 3). Keeping the dose of quinidine constant, DM was increased weekly from 15 mg/day to a final dose of up to 120 mg/day. DM concentrations were monitored by the collection of blood samples in the morning. Using this regimen, serum levels of approximately 100–300 ng/ml were obtained for dextromethorphan (Table 3). Therapy was generally well tolerated in almost all patients, but a few noted fatigue, headaches, dizziness, insomnia, and diarrhea. However, the medication had to be temporarily discontinued in one instance when a patient developed a resting hand and head tremor.

Table 1 Cytochrome P-450 Phenotypes

Metabolic ratio

ALS		CONTROLS	
0.01	0.00	0.00	0.00
0.01	0.00	0.00	0.01
1.20	0.00	0.00	0.01
0.05	0.00	0.00	0.04
0.00	0.01	0.00	0.00
0.00	0.00	0.00	0.00
0.00	0.00	0.00	1.37
0.00	0.00	0.01	0.02
0.00	0.01	0.00	0.02
0.00	0.00	0.00	0.05
0.00	0.00	7.83	0.00
0.00	0.00	0.02	0.00
0.03	0.01	0.01	0.00
0.00	0.00	0.00	0.00
0.00	0.00	0.01	0.03
0.01	0.00	0.20	6.70
0.00	0.00	0.01	0.00
0.00	1.34	0.15	
6.49	0.04	7.12	
Total patients: 38		36	
% slow metabolizers: 8		11	
(MR > 0.30)			

Drug distribution is an important consideration, particularly in the case of neurological diseases in which the blood-brain barrier can limit the access of drug to the central nervous system. The example of interferon is a case in point. Based on its putative antiviral and immunomodulatory properties, interferons have been considered a possible treatment for ALS (25). There are three major classes of interferon (alpha, beta, and gamma) each of which exhibits its own pharmacokinetic peculiarities. Prior to undertaking an experimental treatment trial of ALS with alpha interferon, it was deemed useful to perform some preliminary pharmacokinetic studies with the idea that the results might influence the protocol design (26). Two doses (18×10^6 and 50×10^6 U) were chosen for intravenous administration after which simultaneous serum and spinal fluid was sampled serially. This could be readily accomplished in the case of spinal fluid because all the patients had an indwelling Ommaya reservoir. Maximal serum concentrations (C_{max}) were achieved at the end of each 10-min infusion

Table 2 Effect of Cytochrome Oxidase P450 Inhibition on Dextromethorphan Metabolism

	Metabolic ratio[a]	
Subject	DM	DM/quinidine
BC	0.02	1.58
LG	1.20	—
DG	0.00	1.42
AH	0.00	5.40
MH	0.00	24.99
WI	3.8	5.20
AJ	0.02	3.46
BK	0.01	0.25
EM	0.00	6.19
PM	0.00	0.42
CP	0.00	0.64
AR	0.00	0.85
MR	0.00	0.63

[a]A metabolic ratio > 0.30 indicates extensive metabolism.

Table 3 Serum Dextromethorphan Levels After Inhibition of Cytochrome P450[a]

	mg DM/day					
	15	30	45	60	90	120
BC	22.87	46.11	84.96	118.19	126.24	285.51
DG	25.80	48.88	76.18	—	97.97	223.99
AH	30.03	65.49	92.16	138.87	203.79	—
MH	20.11	30.19	49.04	78.78	105.58	164.15
WI	58.08	87.84	122.26	162.76	210.84	255.87
BK	52.01	66.46	95.48	124.73	118.80	—
AR	26.26	48.12	86.99	132.66	—	—
WW	33.76	103.00	57.43	105.30	192.67	230.02
DC	—	56.00	—	50.35	64.38	75.01

[a]Quinidine dose—150 mg/day.

(Table 4). Within 4 hr there was approximately a 3000% decrease in the concentration. This rapid distribution was followed by an apparent terminal elimination phase. Despite high peak serum levels of interferon, there were no measurable levels of interferon in the spinal fluid of subjects receiving 18×10^6 U (Table 5). Three of the four subjects who received a larger dose (50×10^6 U)

Table 4 Titers in Serum and CSF After Intravenous Infusion of rIFN

| | rIFN dose | | | |
| | 18×10^6 U | | 50×10^6 U | |
Time	Serum (pg/ml)	Ventricular CSF (pg/ml)	Serum (pg/ml)	Ventricular CSF (pg/ml)
0	<23[a]	<15	<16	<15
5 min	5440 ± 775	—	21,000 ± 940	—
10 min	9340 ± 945	—	38,000 ± 2150	—
15 min	5260 ± 1050	—	35,100 ± 3290	—
30 min	2570 ± 1050	<15	18,900 ± 2240	<15
60 min	1150 ± 400	<15	9,990 ± 870	50
2 hr	430 ± 190	<15	3,210 ± 250	45
4 hr	170 ± 60	<15	595 ± 155	35
8 hr	55 ± 35	<15	165 ± 60	20
12 hr	35 ± 20	<15	95 ± 60	15
24 hr	[b]	<15	30 ± 20	20
48 hr	[b]	<15	[b]	<15

[a]One subject had elevated baseline serum rIFN titers.
[b]An average was not computed when rIFN levels were undetectable in one or more subjects.
Data are $\bar{X} \pm SE$.

Table 5 Pharmacokinetic Parameters Following Systemic Administration of rIFN

Subject	C_{max}[a] (pg/ml)	$AUC_{0-8 hr}$ (pg·ml/hr)	$t_{1/2}$ (hr)	Total body clearance (ml/min)	Serum C_{max}/CSF C_{max} ratio
18×10^6 dose					
M.P.	9,230	2,770	1.2	650	
E.F.	10,400	6,750	3.1	267	
T.A.	6,720	2,910	1.2	619	
J.B.	11,000	10,300	7.3	175	
$\bar{X}$	9,340	5,680	1.9[b]	[c]	
±SE	945	1,800	—	—	
50×10^6 dose					
M.P.	38,000	32,800	3.0	152	
E.F.	43,400	35,100	6.4	142	610:1
T.A.	32,900	26,900	1.7	186	1100:1
J.B.	38,600	37,600	11.2	133	550:1
$\bar{X}$	38,200	33,100	3.4[b]	153	
±SE	2,150	2,300	—	12	

[a]Concentration at end of 10-min infusion.
[b]Harmonic mean $t_{1/2}$.
[c]Mean not determined (see text).

Table 6   Reaction to Chronic Intraventricular Administration of 5 × 10⁵ U
Leukocyte Interferon (PIF) to Subhuman Primates

Week	Temp. (°C)	Weight (kg)	Cell (#/mm³)[a]	Protein (mg%)[a]
1	37.60	8.36	33	12
	37.55	8.16	40	22
	38.27	8.00	40	31
2	38.46	7.99	23	37
	38.00	8.06	24	36
	38.60	8.04	44	45
3	38.40	8.20	244	54
	38.50	8.10	316	57
	38.75	8.04	171	59
4	38.55	8.17	247	66
	38.75	8.20	302	75
	37.25	8.07	252	54
5	38.60	7.99	292	72
	38.70	8.20	533	62
	38.50	7.94	387	55
6	38.20	8.04	407	45
	39.00	8.00	70	57
	38.20	8.15	477	52

[a]Cerebrospinal fluid.

had cerebrospinal fluid (CSF) concentrations ranging from 17 to 70 pg/ml. Based on these data, it was concluded that there was little distribution of interferon within the central nervous system in the case of systemically administered interferon. This seemed to preclude treating patients by this route of administration.

To determine whether intraventricular administration would be well tolerated, a decision was made to administer interferon by Ommaya reservoir to rhesus monkeys. Because recombinant interferon was not yet available for clinical studies, natural partially purified alpha interferon (PIF) was employed. Animals were treated with 5 × 10⁵ U of PIF three times a week for 6 weeks. Over this time, the CSF was monitored for cells and protein and the animals' weight and behavior were also assessed (Table 6) (27). Although there was a cellular response and some effect on the protein over the period of treatment, animals tolerated the therapy remarkably well. Their weight was stable and, on observation, their behavior did not appear to be adversely effected by the treatment.

After it was demonstrated that interferon could be safely administered intraventricularly to monkeys, the decision was made to do a parallel experiment in humans. Following intraventricular administration of 2.5 × 10⁵ to 1 × 10⁶ U of PIF, a stereotypic response consisting of fever, malaise, and loss of appetite

Table 7 CSF Interferon Titers After Intraventricular Administration of Leukocyte Interferon (PIF)

Time	2.5×10^5 U		5×10^5 U		1×10^6 U	
(hr)	V	L	V	L	V	L
0	<20	—	<20	—	<20	—
2	3500	—	3900[a]	—	3500	—
4	1925[a]	—	1400[a]	—	2000	—
8	<20	—	75[a]	—	350	350
12	—	—	<20	350	35	—
24	<20	—	<20	—	—	200
48	—	—	<20	—	—	—

[a]Average of two or more experiments.
V = ventricular CSF; L = lumbar CSF.

occurred approximately 2–4 hr after drug administration. With repeated injections, this response diminished in severity. After empirical observation, it was determined that patients could tolerate treatment indefinitely if the drug was administered every 72 hr (28). In contrast to systemic administration, high intraventricular levels of interferon were achieved (Table 7). The $t_{1/2}$ of intraventricularly administered drug was approximately 6 hr, a value that was similar for systemically administered interferon. Within 12 hr interferon had been cleared from the ventricular CSF, after which it appeared in the lumbar CSF, from which it could be detected for as long as 24 hr.

On theoretical grounds, it was assumed that interferon within the CSF would be distributed throughout the extravascular space of the brain. This seemed reasonable based on studies with horseradish peroxidase, which has been shown to widely stain the brain after injection into the CSF of animals (29). To document this, it was decided to attempt to map interferon in the brain by conducting further studies in rhesus monkeys (30). Since interferon acts like a hormone to induce an intracellular cascade of events, it was decided to look for a species of mRNA that codes for a protein (C56) specifically induced by interferon (31). One monkey was administered PIF intravenously and the other intracisternally. Approximately 6 hr later, both animals and a control were sacrificed, and the brain was removed, sectioned, and snap-frozen in dry ice. Following the extraction of RNA from these tissues and dot blotting on a nitrocellulose filter, specimens were hybridized with a radioactive probe for C56 protein (Fig. 2). After both intravenous and intracisternal administration, there was an induction of C56 protein in brain tissues, although the signal was greater in the sample taken from the intracisternally treated animal. These results were somewhat unexpected considering the pharmacokinetic data, leading one to reflect on the significance of the results for treatment trials with interferons. Under ideal circumstances, further work would have been done before settling on a treatment design, but in this circumstance it was ultimately decided to proceed with intraventricular treatment because interferon was not available in the amounts needed for systemic treatment. In short, pragmatic considerations often intrude on the design of treatment trials.

ASSESSMENT

To the degree that measurement is essential to any science, ALS treatment trials must incorporate an assessment paradigm. A meaningful and reliable end-point is essential for a worthwhile study. Explicit definition of the end-point is important for determining the size and duration of the trial and for ensuring that the proper measurements are taken and that follow-up evaluations are performed without bias. Historically, manual muscle testing or use of a clinimetric scale has been utilized to assess treatment outcome, but more recently, emphasis has been placed on the use of a quantitative neuromuscular examination. Several prospective studies have been performed to determine the correlation between these various modes of assessment. Kuther et al. found a good correlation between the results of manual versus transducer strength tests, although the methods differ in several respects (32). Transducer measurements can demonstrate a linear decline of strength whereas this is not the case with manual muscle testing. The use of manual tests and the Norris scale, which were well correlated, offer the advantage that no special equipment is required and that patients with advanced disease can still be monitored at home.

In setting up a trial it is necessary to validate the reproducibility of the test system. This becomes a bigger problem if one or more observers are going to be involved, which is often the case for multicenter trials. One can eliminate interobserver variability through the use of one examiner, usually a physical therapist, even in instances when centers are widely separated. In a recent trial, employing a physical therapist, test/retest correlations were determined for four aspects of the Tuft Quantitative Neuromuscular Exam (TQNE) (Fig. 4) (33). Raw data generated from the force measurements was converted to a mega score using a mathematical conversion (see Chapter 3). Comparing examinations that were separated by a 1–2-day interval, correlations of 0.97–0.98 were noted for all mega scores.

Brooks et al. pointed out regional differences in the progression of ALS, as judged by serial measurement of the TQNE (34). In the upper extremities, the shoulder and elbow flexors showed relatively linear decline over a 12-month period of observation. A similar change was noted for the knee flexors. In some muscle groups (for example, the shoulder and hip extensors), there was a steep decline of strength over the first 6 months of observation, but less of a change

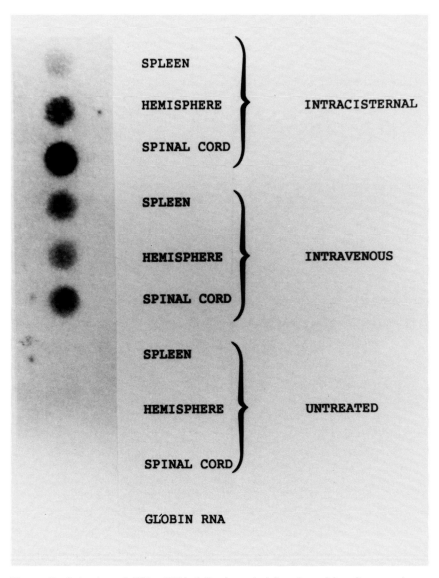

Figure 3 Induction of C56 mRNA following administration of interferon to rhesus monkeys.

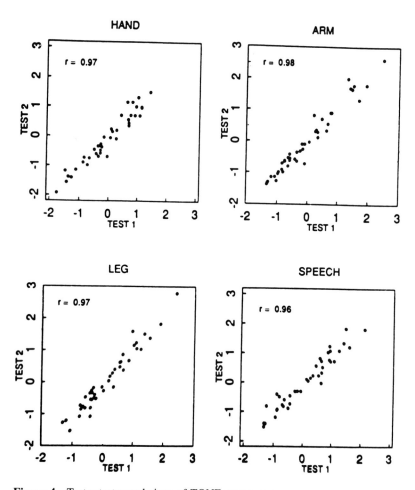

Figure 4   Test-retest correlations of TQNE megascores.

over the later period of observation. Appreciation of these differences may be important since the sample size needed for conducting treatment trials can be reduced if tests that seem to faithfully reflect the course of the disease are utilized.

To illustrate the use of the TQNE to monitor the effect of treatment, the following serial data, generated in the Protropin trial are illustrated. The use of the TQNE allowed for interval data on functional motor units to be quantitatively compared between the two treatment arms. For all megascores (hand, arm, leg, and speech), there was a downward trend between the placebo and growth

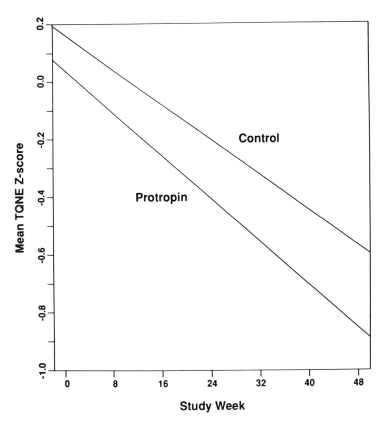

Figure 5 Effect of placebo and growth hormone on the course of ALS as determined by serial quantitative examinations (TQNE).

hormone–treated groups (Fig. 5). The decrease from visit to visit averaged 0.122 for the placebo patients and 0.149 for the Protropin group. This difference was not statistically significant. Because of the fact that losses occurred as the trial proceeded, some caution is warranted in displaying the data in this fashion. The implication is that patients who died or dropped out would have demonstrated similar decreases in their TQNE scores had they remained in the study.

Examining the data from this trial for interesting clinical correlations, it was noted that patients who demonstrated rapid loss of arm strength were more likely to drop out of the study or die (Fig. 6A) early. For those who survived (Fig. 6B), arm strength was relatively well maintained over the period of observation (censoring time). Considering the anatomical overlap of cervical segments innervat-

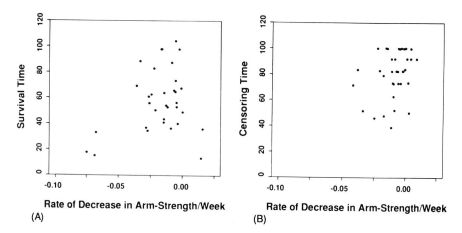

Figure 6 Survival time versus arm strength as determined by quantitative examination (TQNE). (A) Deceased; (B) survivors.

ing the arms and diaphragm, this correlation might be anticipated. However, this association is not absolute. There are rare patients with complete paralysis of the arms in whom the diaphragm is spared until late in the disease process. These patients may represent a variant of ALS or "benign focal amyotrophy" which has been described in Japan, and more recently elsewhere (35).

STATISTICS

The interpretation of clinical trials involves some type of comparison of results between the "intervention" group and a "control" group. Selection bias in the assignment of individuals to the study group or the control group or systematic biases between the groups must be recognized to ensure proper study design. Differences in diagnostic and staging procedures, supportive care, secondary treatments, or methods of evaluation and follow-up can all account for bias. Although stratification may obviate the chance of gross imbalances in prognostic factors related to response, this is generally not a consideration in ALS trials because of the size of the cohorts available for study. If genetic analysis identifies subgroups of the disease—which may be on the horizon—this sort of treatment may be indicated.

Three types of data are collected for each patient in a clinical trial:

1. Prognostic factors: Details of the patient's history at time of entry into the trial.
2. Treatment: the patient's assigned treatment and actual treatment received.

3. Response: Measures of the patient's response to treatment, including side effects.

There are three types of response data from clinical trials: qualitative response, quantitative response, and time to event. With qualitative responses, each patient is classified into one of several response categories according to some predefined evaluation criterion. For example, one might simply have dichotomous responses, "yes" or "no," "success" or "failure." More detailed classifications may give rise to more than two categories of response, and these categories might be ordered progressively. However, the use of a qualitative response classification engenders some loss of detail, or information, in evaluating each patient. When a reliable quantitative measure of response does exist, it is usually preferable to use its actual numerical value for each patient in the statistical analysis of results. If the main evaluation of therapy is in terms of the time to some major event (e.g., death or disease progression), then the statistical techniques of survival analysis are appropriate.

A randomized, double-blinded, placebo-controlled trial will minimize the possibility of bias. In its strictest form, all participants—patients, physician/evaluators, and data analysts—are unaware of the assignment of patients to the treatment or placebo arm of the trial. Although a crossover design in which the patients serve as their own control seems, on the surface, appealing, this design is not suitable for evaluating ALS. Because two disease intervals are being compared, these would have to be the same. For most variables the change over time is not absolutely linear, undermining the premise of comparability of the treatment and placebo period. More damning is the problem created by the possibility of a therapeutic effect that extends beyond the time that the drug is stopped. This would have the effect of contaminating the placebo arm of the trial. Although there may be statistical means for minimizing these problems, it is best to forego this approach.

The protocol for a clinical trial should specify the number of patients and the duration of follow-up planned. Statistical methods are generally used for sample size determination, based on the specific study objectives and the end-points used. These methods presume that at the conclusion of the trial, a statistical significance test will be performed comparing the treatment groups with regard to the major end-points. Statistical significance testing begins with the formulation of a study hypothesis stating that the different treatment groups in the clinical trial will differ in terms of outcome end-points. In performing statistical significance tests, it is assumed initially that the study hypothesis is false, and a null hypothesis is formulated stating that no such difference exists. Statistical methods are then used to calculate the p value, or probability of obtaining the observed results from the clinical trial if the null hypothesis were true (that is, if no true difference exists between the treatment groups). One typically rejects or

Table 8 Inherent Errors of Statistical Significance Testing

	Type I error	Type II error
Definition	Rejection of null hypothesis when no true difference exists	Failure to reject null hypothesis when a true difference indeed exists
Cause	Chance	Chance or a too small sample size
Likelihood of occurrence	Setting of significance level (e.g., 0.05 or 0.01) will indicate how large a type I error will be tolerated	Statistical techniques can estimate the magnitude of type II error, from the size of the groups, magnitude of the difference, and significance level of the statistical test

fails to reject the null hypothesis on the basis of the weight of evidence as summarized in the *p* value.

Two types of statistical errors may occur from the decision to reject or fail to reject the null hypothesis with a statistical significance test. If a null hypothesis is falsely rejected, that is, a difference between the treatment groups is declared when in fact no difference exists, this is known as a type I error. By tradition, one sets the probability of observing a Type I error at 0.05 or less. This is the significance (or alpha level) of the statistical test one is willing to tolerate in the experimental paradigm. The reverse of a type I error is a type II error, the failure to reject a null hypothesis when it indeed is false. The power of a statistical test is 1—the type II error, that is, the probability of correctly rejecting the null hypothesis when it indeed is false. The two error types are depicted schematically in Table 8.

Formulas typically exist to estimate the sample sizes needed on each arm of a clinical trial, once the investigator has specified the end-point (e.g., a single qualitative or quantitative outcome), the significance level of the statistical test to be used, the magnitude of the difference between the true effects of the treatments, and the desired power or probability of showing a statistically sig nificant difference between the treatment groups. Ideally, a clinical trial should have power of at least 0.8 of finding scientifically or clinically meaningful differences. Power increases with sample size. Calculations needed to make these determinations are included in basic texts of statistics (36).

One should bear in mind that the statistical analysis of results, no matter how cleverly done, can never rescue a poorly designed study. Clinical trials are heavily dependent upon good planning and proper execution as well as appro priate statistical analysis. Particular attention should be paid to obtaining adequate personnel and equipment and ensuring that the data are complete and correct.

Problems of patients being ineligible, not receiving their assigned treatment, or withdrawing from treatment are common in ALS studies. Clear-cut rules are needed to handle these events during the analysis of data accruing from clinical trials. A general recommendation is that as few patients as possible should be excluded from the analysis of each treatment group's results.

CONCLUSION

Considering that the cause of ALS is unknown and that no treatment has been shown to modify or arrest the course of the disease, the experimental treatment of ALS may ultimately make a unique contribution to our understanding of this presently incurable disease. Historically, most of the trials reported in the literature have been anecdotal (33). Recognition of this fact has led researchers to try to advance their research methodology. Although this will undergo further refinement and new strategies for evaluating the course of the disease will undoubtedly be forthcoming, enough work has been done to allow a putative therapy to be tested rather quickly. This should be particularly important to patients who have often had to wait years while investigators sort out the validity of a therapeutic claim. In our opinion, the research community has an obligation to patients to document the efficacy of treatment within a reasonable time. From our experience this can be done, at the outside, within 18 months. To accomplish this, multicenter treatment trials are likely to be necessary. Further, if a strict definition of ALS and a recent diagnosis are requirements for entry, it is likely that multicenter trials will be needed to rapidly assess drug treatment. In any one city it is difficult to identify a large number of patients who meet these requirements—even at major referral centers.

One of the most difficult issues to broach with patients is the subject of including them in a placebo-controlled trial. From the patients' perspective, they may only have one chance at stopping the disease process. To many of them, scientific niceties are irrelevant. Although this attitude is articulated by most patients, it has been our experience that patients are willing to participate in controlled trials if the need for doing so is explained to them. One way of reassuring the patients that they will not miss out if they are in the placebo group is to break the code midway in the trial to take an early look at the results. If convincing evidence for an effect is demonstrated, say within 6 months, it is reasonable to promise patients that the trial will be stopped and that all patients will be treated. If the interim results are negative, patients are willing to continue with the study because it is easy to account for the lack of a notable effect within 6 months. If one is looking for a dramatic difference in treatment effect, it may be possible to do trials with a small number of patients over a shorter period of time. This risks the chance of missing a partial therapeutic benefit. As a compromise, one can consider conducting trials with historical controls. This requires that a treatment center follow a representative group of untreated patients with a standardized assessment mode. Assuming that a later group of patients meets the same criteria and is followed in the same manner, the treated group can be compared with the historical controls. This approach is not without problems, but it does go a long way in meeting the objections of patients while allowing the investigator to gain experience with a treatment regimen. Unfortunately, the use of historical controls will never be a substitute for concurrent controls. Unavoidable factors, such as the fact that the referral base, the facilities, and the observors change with time, negate the comparability of the treatment and control groups.

Although it is hazardous to make research predictions, it is likely that the cause of ALS will be known before the end of the century. If this incriminates an altered growth factor or some similar problem, it may be possible to treat patients with an exogenously administered substance, as in the case of endocrine disorders for which hormonal replacement is now standard. Although it will have taken a long time to arrive at this point, considering that ALS was described in the middle of the last century, a therapy for ALS could be available in months if a simple protein proved to be the problem. Although basic research might lead to this, one of the many molecules being produced by the biotechnology industry could find application in the treatment of ALS. It will take insight to recognize this and careful clinical studies to document a benefit.

While it is ideas and the will to bring them to fruition that ultimately will lead to a cure for ALS, a lot more could be done to support these activities at both the local and the national level. At least one national funding agency refuses, as a matter of philosophy, to provide any support for treatment trials. Some of the costs that should be borne by third-party carriers are specifically excluded because of the experimental nature of ALS treatment. It is a rather curious circumstance that insurance carriers take full responsibility for the treatment of diseases attributable to self-indulgence, but refuse to provide even modest support for experimental treatment of a disease such as ALS.

Finally, the cause of ALS would be well served if the quality of a study rather than its result was emphasized by medical journals, which ultimately decide what is meritorious.

Although a breakthrough in the treatment of ALS is still ahead, it is clear that both patients and physicians benefit through participation in treatment trials. For patients, participation offers numerous satisfactions. While all hope to achieve some health benefit, their involvement usually transcends personal gain. Making a general contribution to research is often a reward in itself. For the physician, academic achievement may initially be an inducement to involve oneself in a treatment trial, but ultimately this gives way to a deeper purpose.

Inexplicably, the problem of ALS seems to draw many persons to greater involvement. Although one has to be cautious about metaphysical explanations for human behavior, it takes only a small leap of faith to conclude that a breakthrough in understanding or treating ALS may well have its origin in the relationship between patient and physician that is fostered through clinical research.

ACKNOWLEDGMENT

This chapter is dedicated to patients David Baker, William Doro, Warren Irwin, Colleen Kelley-Matthews, and John Stockton. The critical commentary of Jim Coziol and Peter Wedlund helped to clarify the sections dealing with statistics and pharmacology, respectively. Finally, this effort was generously supported by the Joseph Drown and Thagard Foundation.

APPENDIX
CRITERIA FOR DIAGNOSIS OF AMYOTROPHIC LATERAL SCLEROSIS (6)

Operational criteria to make the diagnosis of amyotrophic lateral sclerosis (ALS)* are required to ensure uniform inclusion of patients with ALS and uniform exclusion of other diseases. The criteria are sensitive to the fact that features of ALS may initially affect different regions of the central nervous system (cortical, brainstem, cervical, thoracic, and/or lumbosacral spinal cord motor neurons), yet manifest in their course in multiple segments within a region and in multiple regions of the central nervous system.

1. The diagnosis of ALS requires the *presence* of
   a. Lower motor neuron signs
   b. Upper motor neuron signs
   c. Progression, and . . .
2. The *absence* of
   a. Sensory signs
   b. Sphincter abnormalities
   c. Parkinson's disease

---

*"Amyotrophic lateral sclerosis" is used interchangeably worldwide as a specific type of progressive neurodegenerative disorder of the motor system and as a general group of these conditions with upper, lower, or mixed upper and lower motor neuron degeneration. The terms "motor neuron disease, motoneuron disease, etc." are used in the United Kingdom and elsewhere to denote the use of "amyotrophic lateral sclerosis" described above.

    d. Alzheimer's disease

    e. Other causes of ALS-like syndromes

    f. Anterior visual system abnormalities

3. The diagnosis is *supported* by

    a. Fasciculations in one or more regions or abnormalities in . . .

    b. Isokinetic/isometric strength tests

    c. Pulmonary function tests

    d. Speech tests

    e. Swallowing studies

    f. Muscle biopsy

    g. Normal nerve biopsy

4. The division into Definite, Probable, Possible, and Suspected cases defined below is based on the grouping of clinical signs from 1a and b in one or more regions (brainstem, cervical, thoracic, lumbosacral) of the central nervous system, together with 1c and 2. Clinical signs

Definite   Upper motor neuron (UMN) and lower motor neuron (LMN) signs in three regions (brainstem, cervical, lumbosacral), e.g., Charcot ALS.

Probable   UMN and LMN signs in two different regions and UMN signs rostral to LMN signs, e.g., UMN bulbar, LMN spinal; UMN and LMN bulbar, LMN spinal; etc.

Possible   UMN and LMN in one region or UMN in two or three regions, e.g., monomelic ALS; progressive bulbar palsy.

Suspected   LMN in two or three regions or other motor syndromes.

5. The diagnosis of Proven, Definite, Probable, Possible, and Suspected ALS is subject to the results of electrophysiological, laboratory, and pathological tests and may be confirmed, excluded, or upgraded and downgraded as defined below:

Electrophysiological, laboratory, or pathological tests

Proven   Confirmed by post mortem examination alone requiring the *presence* of:

LMN and UMN neuronal loss and neuronal atrophy, loss of Nissl substance and corticospinal tract degeneration

and the *absence* of:

other major CNS abnormalities,

extensive central chromatolysis,

active neuronaphagia,

Alzheimer's neurofibrillary changes,

abnormal storage material,

significant spongiform change and

extensive inflammation

Definite   Electrophysiological and laboratory tests are supportive or exclusionary; raise to Proven if confirmed by post mortem examination.

Probable   Electrophysiological and laboratory tests supportive or exclusionary; raised to Proven if confirmed by post mortem examination; raised to Definite by clinical or electrophysiological spread.

If appropriate correction of laboratory abnormality does not stabilize or improve condition and progression occurs, then laboratory exclusion is rescinded.

Possible   If appropriate correction of laboratory abnormality does not stabilize or improve condition and progression occurs, then laboratory exclusion is rescinded.

Suspected   Electrophysiological and laboratory tests are supportive or exclusionary; raised to Proven if confirmed by post mortem examination; raised to Possible, Probable, or Definite by clinical or electrophysiological spread. If appropriate correction of laboratory abnormality does not stabilize or improve condition and progression occurs, then laboratory exclusion is rescinded.

6. "ALS-like syndromes" present with the ALS phenotype as defined by 1–5 and must be excluded by appropriate laboratory tests:
   a. Spondylitic myelopathy
   b. Vascular
   c. Lymphoma
   d. Nontumor endocrine abnormalities
   e. Acute infection
   f. Postinfectious
   g. Monoclonal gammopathy
   h. Dysimmune
   i. Exogenous toxins
   j. Physical injury
   k. Genetic/acquired enzyme defects
7. "ALS variants" comprise clinical syndromes where the predominant presentation is that seen in sporadic ALS, but which includes one or more additional features such as:
   a. Geographic (Western Pacific, Guam, Kii, etc)
   b. Dementia
   c. Extrapyramidal signs
   d. Cerebellar degeneration
   e. Autonomic nervous system involvement
   f. Objective sensory abnormalities

REFERENCES

1. Mitsumoto H, Maurice RH, Chad DA. Amyotrophic lateral sclerosis, recent advances in pathogenesis and therapeutic trials. Arch Neurol 1988;45:189–202.
2. Quick DT, Greer M. Pancreatic dysfunction in patients with amyotrophic lateral sclerosis. Neurology 1967;17:112–116.
3. Festoff BW, Crigger NJ. Therapeutic trials in amyotrophic lateral sclerosis: A review. In: Mulder DW, ed. The diagnosis and treatment of amyotrophic lateral sclerosis. Boston: Houghton Mifflin, 1980:337–366.
4. Engel WK, Siddique T, Nicoloff JT. Effect on weakness and spasticity in amyotrophic lateral sclerosis of thyrotropin-releasing hormone. Lancet 1983;2:73–75.
5. Tyler HR. Double-blind study of modified neurotoxin in motor neuron disease. Neurology 1979;29:77–81.
6. Brooks BR, et al. Criteria for diagnosis of amyotrophic lateral sclerosis. World Neurol 1990;5(1):12.
7. Patten BM. The syndromic nature of amyotrophic lateral sclerosis. In: Cosi V, Kato A, Parlette W, Pinelli P, Poloni M, eds. Amyotrophic lateral sclerosis. New York: Plenum Press, 1987:99–107.
8. Smith RA, Jacoby S, Festoff B, et al. Influence of compliance and other human factors on treatment trials. In: Rose CF, ed. Amyotrophic lateral sclerosis. New York: Demos Publications, 1990:45–53.
9. Barber B. The ethics of experimentation with human subjects. Sci Am 1976:234(2): 25–31.
10. Epstein LC, Lasagna L. Obtaining informed consent. Arch Intern Med 1969;123: 682–688.
11. Kass, et al. Compliance with topical pilocarpine treatment. Am J Ophthalmol 1986;101:515–523.
12. DiMatteo MR, Robin N. Achieving patient compliance: The psychology of the medical practitioner's role. New York: Pergamon Press, 1982:8–28.
13. Kirscht P, Rosenstock, M. Patient's problems in following recommendations of health experts. In: Stone GC, Cohen F, Adler NE, eds. Health psychology: A handbook. San Francisco: Jossey Bass, 1980:189–215.
14. The Steering Committee of The Physicians' Health Study Research Group. Preliminary report: Findings from the aspirin component of the ongoing physicians' health study. N Engl J Med 1988;Jan 28:262–264.
15. Friedman LM, Furberg CD, DeMets DL. Fundamentals of clinical trials. Littleton: PSG, 1985:173–189.
16. Baron JA. Compliance issues/biological markers. In: Sestilli, MA, ed. Chemoprevention clinical trials: Problems and solutions. Bethesda, MD: National Cancer Institute, 1985.
17. Olarte MR. Therapeutic trials in amyotrophic lateral sclerosis. In: Rowland LP, ed. Human motor neuron diseases. New York: Raven Press, 1982:555–557.
18. Gladtke E. History of pharmacokinetics. In: Pecile A, Rescigno A, eds. Pharmacokinetics, mathematical and statistical approaches to metabolism and distribution of chemical drugs. New York: Plenum Press, 1986:1–8.
19. Wills RJ, Smith RA. Pharmacokinetics of interferons. In: Smith RA, ed. Interferon treatment of neurologic disorders. New York: Marcel Dekker, 1988:103–133.

20. Woodworth JR, Dennis RK, Moore MS, Rotenberg KS. The polymorphic metabolism of dextromethorphan. J Clin Pharmacol 1987;27:139–143.
21. Vetticaden SJ, et al. Phenotypic differences in dextromethorphan metabolism. Pharm Res 1989;6(1):13–19.
22. Walker FO, Hunt VP. An open label trial of dextromethorphan in Huntington's disease. Clin Neuropharmacol 1989;12:322–330.
23. Brinn R, Brosen K, Gram LF, Haghfelt T, Otton V. Sparteine oxidation is practically abolished in quinidine-treated patients. Br J Clin Pharmacol 1986;22:194–197.
24. Smith RA, Valderhaug KL, Wedlund P. The excitotoxin hypothesis: Therapeutic considerations in amyotrophic lateral sclerosis. In: Rose FC, Norris FH, eds. ALS, new advances in toxicology and epidemiology. Smith-Gordon, 1990:287–293.
25. Salazar AM, Gibbs CJ, Gajdusek DC, Smith RA. Clinical use of interferons: Central nervous system disorders. The handbook of experimental pharmacology. 1984:71.
26. Smith RA, Norris FH, Palmer D, Bernhardt L, Wills RJ. Distribution of alpha interferon in serum and cerebrospinal fluid after systemic administration. Clin Pharmacol Ther 1985;37(1):85–88.
27. Unpublished data obtained in collaboration with David G. Poplack (National Cancer Institute).
28. Smith RA, Norris NH. Treatment of amyotrophic lateral sclerosis with interferon. In: Smith RA, ed. Interferon treatment of neurological disorders. New York: Marcel Dekker, 1988:265–275.
29. Brightman MW, Prescott L, Reese TS. Intracellular junctions of special ependyma. In: Knigg KM, Scott DD, Kobayashi H, Ishii S, eds. Brain endocrine interaction. Basel: Karger, 1975.
30. Smith RA, Landel CP. Mapping the action of interferon on primate brain. In: Stewart WE, Schellekens H, eds. The biology of the interferon system. Amsterdam: Elsevier, 1986.
31. Chebath J, Merlin G, Benech P, Revel M. Nucl. Acids Res 1983;11:1213–1226.
32. Kuther G, Struppler A, Lipinski HG. Therapeutic trials in ALS—The design of a protocol. In: Cosi V, Kato A, Parlette W, Pinelli P, Poloni P, eds. Amyotrophic lateral sclerosis, therapeutic, psychological and research aspects. New York: Plenum Press, 1987:265–276.
33. Festoff BW, Melmed S, Smith RA. Therapeutic trial of recombinant human growth hormone in amyotrophic lateral sclerosis. In: Myelopathies, neuropathies et myopathies—Acquisitions recentes: Advances in neuromuscular diseases. Paris: Expansion Scientifique Française, 1988.
34. Brooks BR, Sufit RL, DePaul R, Tan YD, Sanjak M, Robbins J. Design of clinical therapeutic trials in amyotrophic lateral sclerosis. In: Rowlands LP, ed. Advances in neurology, amyotrophic lateral sclerosis and other motor neuron diseases. New York: Raven Press, 1991:521–546.
35. Oryema J, Ashby P, Spiegel S. Monomelic atrophy. Can J Neurol Sci 1990;17(2):124–130.
36. Snedecor GW, Cochran WG. Statistical methods. 7th ed. Ames: Iowa University Press, 1980.

15

Ethical Aspects of Experimental Treatment

Andrew Feenberg

San Diego State University
San Diego, California

INTRODUCTION

Patients with chronic, incurable diseases have a particularly tense relationship to modern medicine, which has increasingly deemphasized caring in favor of the very curing function that is deficient in their case. To make matters worse, they sometimes experience rejection from doctors who, because they are unable to offer a cure, discourage them from seeking medical care, including even symptomatic help and advice. For these patients, experimental treatment often symbolizes both hope and societal commitment to caring for their ills. It offers access to treatment of some sort on terms that are acceptable to many patients. Clinical trials are one way in which a highly technologized medical system can care for those it cannot yet cure. But is the medical institution prepared to assume this new responsibility? And if so, how? These are the questions to which this chapter is addressed.

THE REVOLT AGAINST ETHICAL REGULATION

The welfare of human subjects is usually discussed in terms of the need to protect patients from doctors more concerned with science than humanity. Codes of ethics and philosophical reflection generally focus on such matters as the patient's right to refuse to lend his or her body for use by others, the right to information about risks, the right to withdraw at any time, the right to treatment for complications arising out of experimental participation, and so on. In 1966 the Food and Drug Administration (FDA) issued strict regulations on human research, and since then the ethical climate surrounding such research has in fact changed for the better (Curran, 1969). These regulations were designed to achieve both ethical goals and consumer protection, the first, by protecting the rights of human subjects, and the second, by preventing the sale of drugs lacking scientific proof of safety and effectiveness.

The negative emphasis on rights is understandable, given the origins of our current conception of legitimate clinical research in revulsion against the abuse of patients and prisoners. Yet many chronically ill and dying patients resist protection and seek to enter experimental treatment programs even at the risk of being defrauded or injured by "quacks." These facts are well known in neurology where the diagnosis of incurable diseases such as amyotrophic lateral sclerosis (ALS) or multiple sclerosis (MS) is often the starting point for a lengthy and frustrating pursuit of experimental treatment or, in its absence, unconventional alternatives.

The widespread demand for participation is usually interpreted as a sign of irrationality. Paternalistic attitudes toward patients, rationalized by concern for their rights, has led to systematic dismissal of their desire to participate. After all, it is frequently said or implied, only desperation can explain why a sick person would want to join a scientific experiment he or she cannot understand and which has little likelihood of offering a cure (Ingelfinger, 1972, p. 466; Mackillop and Johnston, 1986, pp. 182–183). Hans Jonas writes that "everything connected with his condition and situation makes the sick person inherently less of a sovereign person than the healthy one. Spontaneity of self-offering has almost to be ruled out; consent is marred by lower resistance or captive circumstance . . ." (Jonas, 1969, p. 239).

Yet in recent years, it is precisely these "desperate" patients who have provoked a crisis of experimental medicine that promises to change it as radically as did the post–World War II reaction in favor of ethical procedures. The patients who are bringing this about are AIDS victims. They entered the medical arena at the height of a major political organizing drive in the homosexual community which left them better equipped to resist paternalism than any previous group of patients. Energies mobilized around social and political rights during the preceding decade were turned on the medical system, and networks of patient education and support arose on a scale never before seen in connection with any other disease. The result has been rapidly expanding access to experimental drugs and a drastic weakening of the shield of protections enforced by the FDA and other medical institutions with such pride until quite recently.

The collapse of barriers to the use of unproven drugs occurred gradually under intense political pressure from 1987 to 1989. The initial measures proposed by the FDA included accelerated administrative reviews of AIDS drugs (the "1AA review process''), the public announcement by the FDA of the legality of importing unapproved drugs for personal use, and an expanded program of "compassionate investigational new drug exemptions,'' or "treatment INDs,'' to make it possible to sell as-yet-untested drugs to dying victims of AIDS. These measures were all dismissed as electoral ploys by AIDS organizations, a criticism that was perhaps exaggerated for political effect.

Although the new regulations were not in fact very effective in opening access to new drugs, they did tend to shift the burden of proof from drug manufacturers to the FDA, a change noted with concern by Senator Edward Kennedy (Marwick, 1987, p. 3020). Kennedy was not wrong about the implications of the FDA's new policy. In June 1989, the Agency caved in completely and, in conjunction with the National Institute of Allergy and Infectious Diseases, instituted a new "parallel-track'' drug-testing system. Under this system, physicians were authorized to prescribe unproven drugs that had passed toxicity tests just as they would a licensed drug, simultaneously with the regular controlled studies. '' 'It's a great step forward,'' said Dr. Mathilde Krim, a founder of the American Foundation for AIDS Research. "It represents a new consensus on how to handle drug development for AIDS and life threatening diseases in general' '' (Kolata, 1989, p. B5).

The FDA resolved the political crisis over AIDS drug testing by issuing new rules, but Dr. Krim is certainly wrong to suggest that there is a consensus in favor of these rules. Rather, there is grave concern among researchers about the harm they may do both to patients and to the process of scientific evaluation of new drugs (Marwick, 1987, p. 3020; Reidenberg, 1987, pp. 599–560). Perhaps even more worrisome than drug company profiteering on unproven remedies at patients' expense is the possibility that scientific research will be crippled by the new system. How can patients be recruited to studies with placebo controls when they can obtain the same experimental drug with 100% certainty directly through their physician (Goyan, 1988, pp. 3052–3053)? How can drugs be compared when patients can obtain and use all of them at the same time? And how can the results of the rather informal parallel track by rigorously assessed?

These questions appear to be unanswerable today, but the new rules are probably less responsible for these obstacles to research than they appear to be. In fact compliance among patients in controlled trials was already breaking down before the new rules were issued (Barinaga, 1988, p. 485). In the long run, that trend would have had all the dire consequences brought on in the short run by the National Institutes of Health reforms. The problem is thus not really regulatory, but is due to a shift in the public perception of the balance between the scientific and the curative functions of clinical research.

That shift will force the research community to rethink the concept of informed consent by bringing it face-to-face with the extent to which the old system actually relied on the absence of alternative access to care and treatment to recruit patients to controlled trials. Medical science must respond to this unpleasant discovery by establishing a new framework for patient education and treatment within which recruiting for controlled trials can compete with the parallel track. That objective can be achieved, as I will show in the remainder of this chapter, only where medicine accepts fully its responsibilities toward patients with incurable diseases.

It would be a mistake to blame our current problems entirely on the AIDS crisis; rather, victims of AIDS are simply saying loud and clear, with political clout, what many patients and a few doctors had been saying for years. The message is simple: the desire to participate in programs of experimental treatment has been unfairly ignored to the detriment of large numbers of mentally competent patients with incurable diseases. These patients argue that exclusion from research diminishes their dignity, harms their physical and mental health more than would the experimental risks they might undergo, and thrusts them into the arms of unorthodox healers. Medicine, has been forced by the AIDS crisis to recognize this desire for experimental participation as a legitimate interest of patients which can no longer be paternalistically dismissed. Science will have to find new ways to adjust to the problems posed by this moral advance.

PARTICIPANT INTERESTS

We take it for granted that all interests are represented to some degree in the public debates that determine social policy and law in a democratic society. Yet in the case under discussion here, the expressed desire of a significant number of citizens was systematically dismissed, not so much because they were judged to be wrong as because they were not even granted the right to participate in the discussion in the first place. This sort of injustice may occur wherever wishes are subject to "interpretation" by professional agents, such as physicians or social workers, who are credited with the right to define the legitimately constituted "interests" of their clients. In this case, the agents delegitimated their clients' own self-expression by emphasizing such incapacitating factors as ignorance and irrational hopes. To recover a voice, the clients had to intervene through a political movement.

In the new climate of protest, it is sometimes suggested that we ought to reject professionalism altogether and affirm the absolute right of medical "consumers" to select whatever treatment they want (Illich, 1976, pp. 252–253). If this were the only alternative to the present system, the case for reform would indeed be weak given the very real knowledge differential between physicians and patients.

But there is another possibility that will be explored here: to preserve professionalism but in the context of enhanced knowledge sharing and patient initiative (Ladd, 1980, p. 1128). In this framework it is possible to give a legitimate form, as medicine understands it, to the expressed desire of so many patients for opportunities to participate in research. That reformulation also indicates the most responsible way for medical institutions to deal with demands they can no longer channel in the accustomed manner.

I will argue that the existing regulatory framework ignores important beneficial effects of experimental participation on the welfare of patients. These overlooked effects belong to the general class of incentives to participate in research, a subject treated in the literature with great caution because of the difficulty of distinguishing between positive benefits and subtle forms of coercion (Freedman, 1975). The slippery slope leading from compensation to compulsion is most difficult to negotiate in such cases as monetary rewards or shortened prison terms. Rarely, ethicists have rejected any appeal to extrinsic rewards, but most commentators insist, with due qualification, on "the right of the volunteer to volunteer" and to receive compensation for doing so (Edsall, 1969, p. 476).

In fact, I do not believe these cases to be directly relevant to our discussion, but they must be mentioned because it is sometimes claimed that the hope of cure is a "reward" sought by the sick on the same order as payment by a volunteer. This identification is confusing. To treat cure as a mere extrinsic reward overlooks the tragic dimension of the patient's dilemma in accepting the risks of experimental participation, reduces a moral sacrifice to a mere market relationship, and makes a fool of the patient who dies despite joining a research program.

I will call the specifically health-related incentives for patients to participate in clinical research "intrinsic" or "participant" interests. These interests arise naturally in the experimental context and include not only the hope of cure, but also access to physicians, test results, advice, and education about one's condition or disease. The importance of these concerns to volunteers is widely recognized although insufficiently studied. Cassileth found that over half his respondents gave the desire for the best medical care as their main reason for willingness to participate in research (Cassileth et al., 1982, pp. 968–970). In justifying the parallel track, Dr. Anthony Fauci of NIAID reportedly said that "many people join clinical trials for altruistic reasons and also to obtain the medical care that goes with participation—even knowing they may not receive the experimental drug" (Kolata, 1989, p. B5). In the next section, I will offer a fuller account of these surprising explanations for patients' desire to participate in research.

A more robust recognition of participant interests would not tell against moral restraint in recruiting poorly informed or incompetent individuals as subjects, nor would it detract from the principal purpose of experimentation, which must be the acquisition of new knowledge. However, within these limits, recognition of participant interests would affect the volume of opportunities to participate and the design of experiments.

Until recently, the supply of places was regulated entirely by scientific considerations without regard for the number of patients wishing to participate. Many physicians and philosophers considered the scarcity of places a blessing in disguise, since it prevented masses of presumably self-deluding patients from entering the experimental setting with unrealistic hopes. Whether justified or not, this attitude has proven untenable in the face of current protests. Instead of regulating the number of places in terms of statistical minimums required to determine effectiveness, places are now multiplied to serve participant interests.

This point has been made effectively in the political arena, but there remains a subtler implication of participant interests that is not yet sufficiently appreciated. Under the assumptions introduced here, experimental medicine has an *obligation* not simply to avoid harm so far as possible, but to serve patients while simultaneously serving science through appropriate experimental design. Certain designs further participant interests, while others frustrate them unnecessarily, independent of the scientific validity of the alternatives. It is a matter of ethics to chose designs and procedures that best serve participant interests within the limits of scientifically sound experimentation. Thus one commentator writes that the new FDA regulations create a situation in which "we need to consider alternative study designs that allow the patient maximum hope for cure and the opportunity for some control over his or her destiny" (Goyan, 1988, p. 3053).

But the argument must be carried even further once participation in research is recognized as a legitimate form of treatment. It is necessary to rethink the whole structure of care for those classes of patients whose involvement in research can be expected to increase dramatically in the coming years. The fact is that medical institutions rarely accept the heavy responsibility for patient education that could alone give meaning to informed consent. This flaw, which we have so long tolerated in our medical system, risks becoming a source of egregious abuse as access to clinical research broadens to include millions of sick individuals.

EXPERIMENTAL TREATMENT AS A FORM OF CARE

The key to legitimating participant interests within the professional framework is the determination that clinical research confers a properly medical benefit on subjects. But in the research situation, it is difficult, if not impossible, to guarantee that the likelihood of cure will outweigh risks. Even in the case of dying patients, where risk is of less concern, cure is such an improbable result of research that it is dishonest to hold up the tantalizing promise of success (Glaser and Strauss, 1965, pp. 1098–1100).

The conflict between patients' desires and their interests as interpreted by most physicians can only be resolved by discovering benefits of participation that are independent of success or failure in achieving cure. That approach in turn implies that medicine has benefits other than cure, a fact attested to by a voluminous literature which shows that patients place at least as great store on the ''caring'' functions of medicine as on actual healing (Powles, 1973, pp. 16–24). *If participation in research were seen as an effective dimension of ''caring,'' rather than as a defective mode of ''curing,'' it could be more easily justified.*

Fletcher and his collaborators found, for example, that what patients most valued in their doctor was compassion and availability rather than technical achievements (Fletcher et al., 1983). Studies of homeopathic and chiropractic medicine indicate that many patients today, especially those with chronic illnesses, seek alternative therapy because they miss these caring benefits in the conventional setting (Avina and Schneiderman, 1978; Kane et al., 1974). Dissatisfaction with scientific medicine may be explained by studies which show that the chronically ill are signified negatively in medical culture (Kuttner, 1978). Negative attitudes are sometimes signaled to the patients themselves, as in the case of one MS patient whose doctor reportedly said: ''You have multiple sclerosis; don't worry; get a book from the library and read about it; if you have any questions, call me'' (Hartings et al., 1976, p. 68).

The importance these studies attribute to ''caring'' might be taken to mean that patients reject the application of medical technology, but that would be a mistaken conclusion. Compassion is often expressed through the administration of medicine, even when it is known to be of little value. Powles writes:

> The almost exclusive concentration, within modern medical culture, on the technical mastery of disease is more apparent than real. For in addition to countering the challenges to human well-being on the biological level, this technology is serving also to meet the emotional and existential challenges that disease involves (Powles, 1973, p. 20).

Participation in clinical trials obviously possesses somewhat the same ''caring'' significance for physicians and patients as the commonplace prescription of symbolically charged, but marginally effective drugs.

These observations converge with our growing understanding of the so-called ''placebo effect,'' the most *predictable* benefit of experimental participation. If the placebo effect were recognized as a normal dimension of medical care, then experimental participation would fall into place as a form of treatment most particularly suited to patients with incurable diseases. Unfortunately, the very term connotes deception, which, even if it be to patients' benefit, reduces their dignity. We seem to have reverted to the dilemma of false hopes versus medical responsibilities.

But something very much like the placebo effect occurs constantly in medical practice without the deceptive administration of sugar pills or other fraudulent substitutes for ''real'' medicine. These results are due to what anthropologists call the "symbolic efficacy" of medicine, which is independent of its technical effectiveness and, in fact, explains much of its value in premodern societies (Levi-Strauss, 1968, p. 198).

In view of the widespread role of placebos, Shapiro and Morris accordingly propose the following definition: "any therapy or component of therapy that is deliberately used for its nonspecific, psychological, or psychophysiological effect, or that is used for its presumed specific effect, but is without specific activity for the condition being treated" (Shapiro and Morris, 1978, p. 371). This definition suits many aspects of doctor-patient interaction that have a generalized therapeutic effect through mechanisms that are still unclear (Brody, 1980, pp. 8–24). In fact, such phenomena are so commonplace there is a risk doctors will confuse nonspecific effects of care for specific effects of drugs and procedures (Shapiro and Morris, 1978, p. 397).

Howard Brody argues that since deception is not actually required to achieve the placebo effect, patients should not be deceived to obtain its benefits (Brody, 1980, p. 110). Thus even if the placebo effect is the principal source of benefits to patients in clinical research, that would not justify lying to them about the likelihood of success or enlisting them in incompetent or purely symbolic experiments "for their own good." The demand inscribed in all codes of experimental medicine that patients be honestly informed and research be scientifically sound stands as before, although the significance of the research may be quite different for scientists and patients.

A better understanding of the placebo effect can aid in the design of more therapeutically effective participation in research. Adler and Hammett analyze the placebo effect in terms of the therapeutic power of "meaning" supplied by a shared "systematic" understanding of disease and social support. They write:

> It is suggested here that these two factors—group formation and system formation—which are as essential to psychic functioning as nourishment is to physical functioning, [as] the basic factors composing what is subjectively experienced as a feeling of "meaning," are invariably used in all successful interpersonal therapies, and are the necessary and sufficient components of the placebo effect (Adler and Hammett, 1973, p. 597).

Applied to clinical research design, this would suggest that the physician can maximize the beneficial effects of participation by organizing the medical intervention in a "symbolically effective" way to promote "group formation and system formation." These goals should therefore be coordinated with scientific objectives in experimental design. This requirement holds, incidentally, regardless of whether the trial aims to cure the patient or merely to contribute to knowledge.

THE SICK ROLE

The crisis over AIDS has dramatized two interconnected problems already painfully familiar to many neurological patients and their physicians: modern medicine is less and less able to treat patients with chronic incurable illnesses, and it is not designed to deliver experimental treatment. The poor fit between the social structure of the institution, the needs of the chronically ill, and the requirements of research accounts for the many problems in experimental medicine, such as poorly informed subjects, the consequent dubious validity of consent, the interruption of continuity of care on exit from experiments, recruiting difficulties, poor compliance, and so on. These problems can only worsen as the public comes to see the research mission less as a scientific activity than as a dimension of treatment. Ultimately, the survival of the scientific model of the controlled trial is at stake.

These problems suggest the urgent need for reforms in the social organization of medicine. The place to begin consideration of this complex question is the so-called "sick role," one of the foundations of the medical institution. The maladaptation of medicine to the new demands for experimental treatment is due in large part to the definition of the sick role in a form that makes "group formation and system formation" nearly impossible to achieve. This, in turn, explains why researchers have such problems recruiting participants for controlled trials once access to unproven drugs is eased.

Contrary to common usage, the sick role is not a state of pathological psychological withdrawal. The term was originally introduced by Talcott Parsons to define illness in its social aspect as a form of "deviance" involving legitimate temporary release from normal social responsibility in exchange for a sincere effort to recover.

> The sick role . . . channels deviance so that the two most dangerous potentialities, namely, group formation and successful establishment of the claim to legitimacy are avoided. The sick are tied up, not with other deviants to form a "sub-culture" of the sick, but each with a group of non-sick, his personal circle and, above all, physicians. The sick . . . are deprived of the possibility of forming a solidary collectivity (Parsons, 1951, p. 477).

While these conditions are not particularly onerous for individuals with brief acute illnesses, the isolation of medical "deviants" is undoubtedly bad for chronic patients. There is considerable evidence that the chronically ill benefit from contact with others who share the same disease. Renee Fox's classic study of clinical research on such patients shows the overwhelming importance of the shared experience of mission and risk in the experimental setting. Her observations are particularly interesting in the light of the role ascribed to meaning in the previous section. She writes:

> Seen in the broadest possible perspective, what we observed in the conference room, laboratory, and on the ward were two groups of men who were faced with common stresses of magnitude: great uncertainty, limitation, hazards, and death. Through a process of interaction with members of their own group and with one another, physicians and patients arrived at comparable ways of dealing with their stresses. . . . Each derived support and guidance from the tight-knit group to which they belonged, and also from their intimate contact and close identification with one another (Fox, 1959, p. 253).

While the Parsonian isolation is not always maintained, it remains the norm from which departures such as this only occasionally occur, sometimes against considerable medical resistance (Brossat and Pinell, 1989). Where social contacts among patients are encouraged, they are in the nature of ad hoc adaptations of "standard" care to the needs of "special" patients, usually with a psychotherapeutic alibi of some sort. But the crisis of experimental medicine suggests the usefulness of far more drastic and systematic changes than have so far occurred. The benefits Renee Fox attributes to the close-knit research group cannot otherwise be achieved, nor, isolated, can patients be properly educated for consent and joined in groups capable of supporting the pursuit of "meaning."

Studies of group activity by patients are rare, perhaps because physicians and researchers are not normally involved. But the application of group therapy to the chronically ill offers a favorable terrain for study. Interestingly, no matter how the therapists have conceived and designed such therapeutic groups, the results confirm the need for a fundamental revision in the sick role. I would like to look briefly at three studies that offer excellent reasons to end the social isolation of chronically ill patients. The full implications of this change for experimental treatment will be taken up in the conclusion to this chapter.

Chafetz and his collaborators noted, at the beginning of their group therapy program for victims of Parkinson's disease, that self-imposed isolation characterized all the patients, regardless of the severity of their illness, and sometimes beginning immediately on diagnosis (Chafetz et al., 1955, pp. 961–962). Here is the characteristic "sick role" phenomenon as it is frequently interpreted in the literature. Yet these patients quickly opened up in group therapy around the exchange of information about symptoms. They soon went on to share each other's complaints about being mistaken for drunks or blamed for slowness (Chafetz et al., 1955, p. 962). Hartings and his collaborators found that in their groups, MS patients forged a similar common bond through criticism of the medical profession, particularly its slowness in diagnosing their illness (Hartings et al., 1976, p. 68).

The groups were intended to reduce anxiety and depression through therapeutic intervention. In fact, discussion remained fairly superficial from a psychological standpoint and achieved the goal in ways the organizers had not always anticipated. For example, Chavetz had not planned to have his group leaders educate the patients about their condition, but education turned out to be one of the patients' chief demands (Chafetz et al., 1955, p. 963).

Similar experiences are reported by Hartings with MS patients and by Buchanan with kideny transplant patients. These latter groups were formally charged with an educational as well as a psychological mission. ''An attempt is made to impart a base of accurate information about MS, so that coupled with an ongoing relationship to the Center staff, a patient might more easily resist faddish cures, plan realistically, and feel more in control of his life'' (Hartings et al., 1976, p. 66). Buchanan had his group leaders answer questions and invited medical experts to address the groups (Buchanan, 1975, p. 529). These educational activities were very effective in reducing anxiety and fear.

These ''system'' forming consequences of group therapy were complemented by properly social effects. When patients form a ''subculture'' through voluntary association, they supply each other with social support, a more and more widely recognized factor in maintaining health (Nuckolls et al., 1972). That the benefits of the groups had less to do with psychological therapy in the usual sense of the term than with the reform of the sick role can be seen from the following descriptions of the typical course of discussions.

Minimization of the severity of symptoms of colleagues and reassurance that all were suffering similar impairments was one method of group self-support. Another was through identification with famous people who had continued to function successfully in spite of their illness. The emphasis on research in the clinic, which carried over as one of the purposes of the group, provided tangible proof of interest in them and in the course of their disease (Chafetz et al., 1955, p. 962).

Going still further, Hartings' groups formed an incipient voluntary health agency:

Patients have generated helpful activities of their own. They publish a Newsletter four times a year and disseminate information on financial resources, recreational and cultural opportunities, new equipment, tax benefits and insurance, helpful hints for day-to-day living, good books, etc. Staff have encouraged these individuals to experience and exercise their power and ability to change adverse situations in helping one another (Hartings et al., 1976, p. 73).

The patients made friends in all the groups and desired continued interaction, requesting further meetings even a year after the end of Chafetz's experiment, but the organizers concluded, for reasons they do not explain, that "the advantages of more protracted groups are questionable" (Chafetz et al., 1955, p. 963). Like Chafetz, Buchanan also favors a time-limited approach (Buchanan, 1978, p. 426). These researchers appear to want their patients to return to the conventional sick role as soon as possible despite the latters' interest in innovating new relationships.

Hartings was more accepting of patients' demands that the groups continue, an outcome that seems appropriate given the manifold functions they performed for their members. On the basis of these functions and the new sick role they define, we can build a collaborative model of care for the incurably ill. This model offers a favorable environment for responsible experimental participation.

THE COLLABORATIVE MODEL

From an ethical standpoint, the chief danger in the new regulations is the possibility that vast numbers of uncomprehending patients will be recruited into experiments they would never have joined had they understood the implications of participation and felt really free to refuse. Studies tend to support Ingelfinger's fear that "the process of obtaining informed consent with all its regulations and conditions is no more than an elaborate ritual, a device that, when the subject is uneducated and uncomprehending, confers no more than the semblance of propriety on human experimentation" (Ingelfinger, 1972, p. 466). The sad truth is that most "patients consent to trials simply because they trust their doctors" (Mackilopp and Johnston, 1986, p. 187).

There is some evidence that this pessimistic conclusion is less applicable to the chronic patients with whom we are concerned here. One study reports "striking differences" in the management of their own care by acute and chronic sufferers (Lidz et al., 1983, p. 542). The former tend to deliver themselves over to the physician unreservedly while the latter often participate actively in decision making, discussing options, and suggesting or rejecting treatment alternatives. The study relates these differences in behavior to the different attitudes of acute and chronic patients toward the conventional passive sick role. The authors conclude that "with certain types of chronic patients and in certain types of organization structures, an active patient role is feasible" (Lidz et al., 1983, p. 543). These conclusions concur with Szasz and Hollander's suggestion that chronic care involves "mutual participation" of patient and physician in the search for the best course of action (Szasz and Hollander, 1956).

Such mutual participation can be routinely observed in the symptomatic treatment of chronic illnesses and in the decisions about treatment during the final weeks or days of life. Physicians skilled in managing illnesses such as AI.S, MS, or Parkinson's disease learn to listen to patients' discoveries about how to live with their illness and often pass along suggestions from one patient to another. Relief of symptoms has implications not only for comfort, but also for life extension, and here too patients and physicians often work together to achieve results that could not be achieved in the conventional physician-patient relationship. Finally, patients who depend on such aids as respirators are increasingly involved in the timing of their own death.

It is in this context that one must evaluate the frequently expressed hope that experimental medicine be carried on in an atmosphere of collaboration between researchers and subjects. This hope, which appears quixotic with regard to the majority of acutely ill patients, may not be so inappropriate in the case of chronic care. Here, in any case, is the argument for the collaborative model.

Unlike cure, which is essentially an individual matter, experimental treatment involves joining a collective effort to solve a scientific problem (Parsons, 1969, pp. 350–351). Admission to that collective should properly be open only to those who share its spirit, whatever personal benefits they may also expect. In a powerful article on this theme, Hans Jonas argues that for the subject to rise above the proverbial "guinea pig" status in the experiment, more is required than voluntary submmission to being used.

Mere "consent" (mostly amounting to no more than permission) does not right this reification. The "wrong" of it can only be made "right" by such authentic identification with the cause that it is the subject's as well as the researcher's cause—whereby his role in its service is not just permitted by him, but *willed*. That sovereign will of his which embraces the end as his own restores his personhood to the otherwise depersonalizing context (Jonas, 1969, p. 236).

Perhaps a sense of these moral realities motivated the founders of the clinical research center at the NIH when, in 1953, they laid down the following principle for themselves: "The patient or subject of clinical study is considered a member of the research team . . ." (Curran, 1969, p. 575). Such identification is an ideal to which experimental medicine does not always aspire and which it rarely achieves. Conservative objections to widespread participation in experimentation draw force from the already noted deficiencies in the conset process. But one wonders why the response to these deficiencies is not to improve patient education, rather than demanding restrictions on experimental participation.

The collaborative model is not utopian. It was followed in the experimental ward studied by Renee Fox. Jean Dausset, discoverer of HLA typing, lived up to this ideal in the design of his experiments. He organized an elaborate series of informational meetings and conferences to ensure that the hundreds of volunteers he required would understand the enterprise in which they were engaged. Dausset's subjects have been called *"les heros instruits"*—educated heros—a term that ought someday to apply to all human subjects (Bernard, 1978, p. 197).

If such successes are possible, it is necessary to reevaluate the often expressed concern of ethicists that patients suffering from incurable ailments are "coerced" by their illness into agreeing to participate. This position is reasonable if patients are ignorant victims of an experimental process that is likely to yield only knowledge. But it is paternalistic if there are participant interests other than cure. As with ordinary treatment, only the informed patient is qualified to weigh the risks against these benefits to self involved in experimental participation. The ethical obligation of medicine is fulfilled not by prohibitions, but by ensuring that patients are well equipped to make such a judgment. More attention to patient education will also help overcome the recruiting problems now experienced or anticipated in controlled trials.

How can medical practice adapt itself to the new educational requirements of widespread experimental participation by the chronically ill? It can be done, but not in the context of the usual program of experimental therapy, carried out with little or no associated educational effort and no long-term commitment to the patients. If the enlargement of opportunities for experimental participation is to be a blessing rather than a curse, it will be necessary to be innovative in the delivery of chronic care and clinical trials. Fortunately, the chronically ill are uniquely qualified to contribute to the creation of a new framework. Given their active orientation toward care and their positive attitude toward group activities, educational programs can be established by and for these patients to prepare them for participation in research.

Two basic desiderata can be identified:

To remove all pressures to participate: implementing clinical trials in the context of a program of continuing symptomatic care and support for patients that is not tied to the duration or success of the experiment

To ensure adequate understanding: the systematic use of patient meetings to prepare patients to understand their disease, the role of human subjects in research, and the experimental options.

A trend in this direction has been slowly emerging. Perhaps the crisis brought on by AIDS will finally result in the institutionalization of an alternative system of care for chronically ill patients based on a redefinition of the sick role and recognition of the educational functions of medicine. From mere objects of medicine, awaiting cure, patients might then become active partners in a larger research enterprise.

ACKNOWLEDGMENTS

I would like to thank Richard Smith and Ilana Lowy for their help with this article.

REFERENCES

1. Adler HM, Hammett VBO. 1973. The doctor-patient relationship revisited: An analysis of the placebo effect. Ann Intern Med 1973; 78:595–598.
2. Avina R, Schneiderman L. Why patients choose homeopathy. West J Med 1978; 128(4):366–369.
3. Barinaga M. Placebos prompt new protocols for AIDS drug testing. Nature 1988; 335(6):485.
4. Bernard J. L'espérance ou le nouvel état de la médecine. Paris: Buchet/Chastel, 1978.
5. Brody H. Placebos and the philosophy of medicine. Chicago: University of Chicago Press, 1980.
6. Brossat S, Pinell P. Coping with parents. Scoiol Health Illness, 1992 (in press).
7. Buchanan D. Group therapy for kidney transplant patients. Int J Psychiatry Med 1975; 6(4):523–531.
8. Buchanan D. Group therapy for chronic physically ill patients. Psychosomatics 1978; 19(7):425–431.
9. Cassileth R, Lusk EJ, Miller DS, Hurwitz S. Attitudes toward clinical trials among patients and the public. JAMA 1982; 248(8):968–970.
10. Chafetz M, Bernstein N, Sharpe W, Schwab R. Short-term group therapy of patients with Parkinson's disease. N Engl J Med 1955; 253(22):961–963.
11. Curran W. Governmental regulation of the use of human subjects in medical research: The approach of two federal agencies. Ethical aspects of experimentation with human subjects. Daedalus: J Am Acad Arts Sci 1969, pp. 402–454.
12. Edsall G. A positive approach to the problem of human experimentation. Ethical aspects of experimentation with human subjects. Daedalus: J Am Acad Arts Sci 1969, pp.463–479.
13. Fletcher RH, O'Malley MS, Earp MS, Littleton BA, Fletcher SW, Greganti A, Davidson RA, Taylor J. Patients' priorities for medical care. Med Care 1983; 21(2):234–242.
14. Fox R. Experiment perilous. Philadelphia: University of Pennsylvania Press, 1959.
15. Freedman B. A moral theory of consent. Hastings Cent Repo 1975; 5(4):32–39.
16. Glaser B, Strauss A. Awareness of dying. In: Katz J. Experimentation with human beings. New York: Russell Sage, 1965, pp.1098–1101.
17. Goyan J. Drug regulation: Quo vadis? JAMA 1988; 260(20):3052–3053.
18. Hartings M, Pavlou M, Davis F. Group counseling of MS patients in a program of comprehensive care. J Chronic Dis 1976; 29:65–73.
19. Illich I. Medical nemesis. New York: Pantheon Press, 1976.
20. Ingelfinger FJ. Informed (but uneducated) consent. N Engl J Med 1972; 287(9):465–466.
21. Jonas H. Philosophical reflections on experimenting with human subjects. Ethical aspects of experimentation with human subjects. Daedalus: J Am Acad Arts Sci 1969, pp. 1–31.
22. Kane R, Olsen D, Leymaster C, Woolley F. Manipulating the patient: Comparison of the effectiveness of physician and chiropractor care. Lancet 1974; 1:1333–1336.
23. Kolata G. AIDS researcher seeks wide access to drugs in test. New York Times, June 26, 1989, p. 1.

24. Kuttner N. Medical students' orientation toward the chronically ill. J Med Educ 1978; 53:111–118.
25. Ladd J. Medical ethics: Who knows best? Lancet 1980; 2:1127–1129.
26. Levi-Strauss C. Structural anthropology. Trans by Jacobsen C, Schoepf BG. New York: McGraw-Hill, 1968.
27. Lidz C, Meisel JD, Osterweis M, Holden J, Marx J, Munetz M. Barriers to informed consent. Ann Intern Med 1983; 99(4):539–543.
28. Mackillop W, Johnston P. Ethical problems in clinical research: The need for empirical studies of the clinical trial process. J Chronic Dis 1986; 39(3):177–188.
29. Marwick C. Proposal to make investigational new drugs available without clinical trial participation in certain cases is receiving mixed responses. JAMA 1987; 257(22):3020.
30. Nuckolls K, Cassel J, Kaplan B. Pyschosocial assets, life crisis and the prognosis of pregnancy. Am J Epidemiol 1972; 95(5):431–441.
31. Parsons T. The social system. Glencoe, IL: Free Press, 1951.
32. Parsons T. Research and the professional complex. Ethical aspects of experimentation with human subjects. Daedalus: J Am Acad Arts Sci 1969 98(2):325–360.
33. Powles J. On the limitations of modern medicine. Sci Med Man 1973; 1:1–30.
34. Reidenberg M. Should unevaluated therapies by available for sale? Clin Pharmacolo Ther 1987; 42(6):599—600.
35. Shapiro A, Morris L. The placebo effect in medical and psychological therapies. In: Garfield SL, Bergin AE, eds. Handbook of psychotherapy and behavior change. New York: Wiley, 1978, pp. 369–410.
36. Szasz T, Hollander M. A contribution to the philosophy of medicine. AMA Arch Intern Med 1956; 97(5):585–592.

16

Toward a Cell Biology of Motor Neurons

Neil R. Cashman

McGill University and Montreal Neurological Institute
Montreal, Quebec, Canada

INTRODUCTION

Because of their large size and relatively accessible peripheral projection, motor neurons have been studied as a distinct neuronal population for over a century. Many essential concepts of neuronal function were first developed through study of motor neurons, their axons, and their terminals. However, as is the case for virtually any neuronal population, the cell and molecular biology that underlies the unique phenotypic characteritics of motor neurons is unclear. For human neurology, the problem of phenotypic distinctiveness is heightened by the existence of motor neuron–specific diseases. What pathological processes, genetic or acquired, could possibly select this neuronal population for degeneration, while sparing (at least relatively) all other neuronal systems? If we allow only familial syndromes to guide us, there appear to be a profusion of autosomal and X-linked genes, both dominant and recessive, which play a critical role in motor neuron survival. Yet, there is to date not a single confirmed report of a truly motor neuron–specific molecule. Perhaps the sum of unusual (but not unique) phenotypic characteristics defines the motor neuron; more likely, unique attributes have yet to be discovered and characterized.

This chapter will review some of the known phenotypic characteristics of spinal and brainstem motor neurons. Emphasis has been placed on functional attributes of motor neurons (particularly molecular mechanisms where known) as opposed to uncharacterized "markers." First, the various culture paradigms that have been developed to study the biology of motor neurons are briefly reviewed. Then, the motor neuron is considered from three perspectives: the extracellular matrix, the cell membrane, and the intracellular compartment (excluding nucleus; the molecular biology of motor neurons is discussed in elsewhere in this book). An effort was made to include the motor nerve terminal in this review, as a differentiated specialization of mature motor neurons.

MOTOR NEURON CULTURE

Differentiated characteristics of motor neurons have been studied in a wide variety of paradigms, each with special advantages and disadvantages. The spinal cord itself can be studied in situ in living animals (e.g., 1–4, reviewed in 5), or in tissue explant cultures (e.g., 6–10). In these systems, the immediate environment and connectivity of individual neurons are preserved, which is particularly advantageous for electrophysiological studies (see below). However, cells in situ are relatively inaccessible, and the heterogeneity of spinal cord cell populations places extreme limitations on biochemical and molecular studies. This is certainly a factor in the study of motor neurons, which constitute less than 1% of the cell bodies at a specific spinal level.

In part to surmount these problems, dissociated culture of primary embryonic tissue was developed (e.g., 11–15, reviewed in 16). In an ideal dissociated culture system, some of the in vivo complexity of neuronal populations is reduced (at the price of introducing unknown changes in their biology). Many neurons lie on top of a monolayer of supporting cells, freely accessible to pharmacological agents in the culture medium, and relatively easily identified for electrophysiological, immunohistochemical, or other experiments. Several strategies have been applied to increase the proportion of motor neurons in culture, including dissection of embryonic ventral horn (instead of whole spinal cord) (10,17) and density gradient centrifugation for large low-density cells (e.g., 18). Additionally, in the chick, ciliary ganglion neurons innervate striated muscle within the eye and thus constitute a source of motor neuron–like cells for culture (19). Some enrichment for motor neuron phenotypic characteristics is achieved with these methods, as assessed by choline acetyltransferase activity and the percentage of neurons forming synaptic contacts with cultured myotubes. However, as with explant culture, motor neurons are a distinct minority of the cells; studies dependent on bulk extraction of a purified cell population are severely restricted.

Motor neurons can be purified to homogeneity by fluorescence-activated cell sorting of dissociated spinal cord cells labeled by retrograde transport of fluorescent conjugates injected in limb muscle (20–22). Motor neurons thus derived do not survive in vitro without supporting cells, differ morphologically and electrophysiologically from unsorted cells, and are obtained in poor yield. However, freshly sorted motor neurons could provide a "gold standard" for some biochemical and molecular studies of motor neuron biology. Retrograde transport of fluorochromes or other marker molecules also provides a relatively unambiguous means with which to identify motor neurons in mixed cultures (23–25).

In principle, cell lines could provide an immortal and uniform reagent for bulk biochemical and molecular studies of motor neurons (reviewed in 16). Cell lines are also relatively hardy compared to primary cultures and are less likely to be adversely affected by media constituents, which may differ somewhat from laboratory to laboratory. Thus, cell lines have a potential to be standardized in a fashion impossible with primary cultures. However, there are many drawbacks to "freeing" a cell from the many constraints that apply to primary tissue. Cell lines may be "eternal," but the differentiated features they express may not be. Poorly differentiated cells within a culture often proliferate more rapidly than highly differentiated cells, producing overgrowth of "uninteresting" clones within a line. DNA loss, mutation, and gene silencing by changes in DNA methylation appear to occur at greater rates than in primary tissue (26–28). Thus, any data generated with cell lines must be viewed with caution until validated in a primary culture system.

Cell lines that display motor neuron attributes could in theory be derived from spontaneous or mutagen-induced transformation of primary tissue (neural tube or neural crest) (29), from retrovirally immortalized primary cells (30,31), or from cell fusion with neural tumor lines (27,32–37). However, the search for cell lines to serve as model motor neurons has not been entirely successful, in part due to a lack of definitions for what constitutes a motor neuron. Even the innervation of skeletal muscle cannot be regarded as a unique attribute of primary motor neurons, as indicated by the finding that many neurons of diverse lineage exhibit the ability to innervate myotubes in vitro, including retinal cells (38) and sympathetic ganglion cells (39).

No neural tube tumor cell line has been shown to constitutively innervate myotubes in vitro, but NS-26 (a clone of C-1300 mouse neuroblastoma; ref. 29) will form functional cholinergic synapses when treated with compounds that increase intracellular cAMP (34), and PC-12 (a rat pheochromocytoma) will also innervate myotubes when induced with nerve growth factor (NGF; ref. 40). Four reported hybrid cell lines will form abundant synapses when induced with db-cAMP, theophylline, or prostaglandin E, all maneuvers to increase intracellular cAMP (27,32–34): NG108-15 (N18TG2 × glioma C6BU-1), NBr-10 and NBr-20 (N18TG2 × BRL-30E rat liver cells), and NCB-20 (N18TG2 × Chinese hamster embryonic brain cells). Investigation of these lines has enabled Nirenberg and associates to clonally define some of the requirements for formation of functional neuromuscular synapses: synthesis of acetylcholine, voltage-gated calcium channels coupled to acetylcholine secretion, possession of 60-nm small

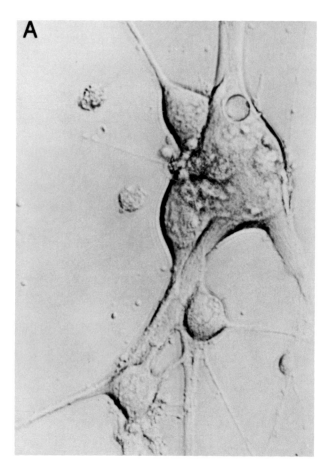

Figure 1 A clone of neuroblastoma-spinal cord hybrid cell line NSC-34 (A), which immortalizes many phenotypic attributes of motor neurons (see text). Large size and prominent process extension distinguish these cells from neuroblastoma parent line N18TG2 (B).

clear vesicles and 180-nm large dense-core vesicles, and secretion of an acetyl-choline-receptor aggregating protein (33,34). However, the synapses formed with the hybrid cell lines are defective in comparison with those formed by dissociated spinal cord cells (41).

The author's laboratory has attempted to produce immortal motor neuron hybrid cell lines by fusing embryonic mouse spinal cord cells (including motor neurons) with cells of the mouse neuroblastoma cell line N18TG2 (35–37).

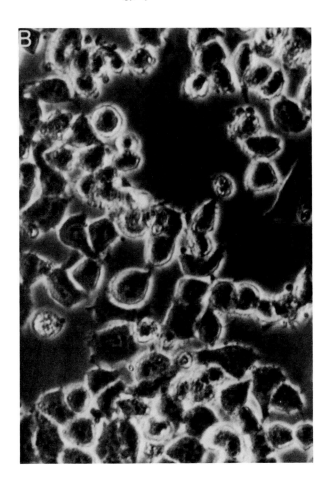

N18TG2 cells lack hypoxanthine-guanine phosphoribosyl transferase activity and hence cannot grow in hypoxanthine-aminopterin-thymidine (HAT) medium (26,27). Forty-three HAT-resistant cell lines have been obtained to date, and many have been characterized in terms of properties expected of motor neurons. One of the most promising lines from this point of view, NSC34, differs from the N18TG2 neuroblastoma parent in a variety of ways which suggest the possibility that the spinal cord parent cell (or cells) was (or included) a motor neuron. These properties are (a) extension of long neurites (Fig. 1); (b) formation of stable neurite:myotube connections; (c) capacity to support action potentials; (d) expression of choline acetyltransferase at levels similar to NG108 (27); (e) cell body/neurite staining with antibodies to neurofilament proteins L, M, and H; (f)

synthesis, storage, and evoked release of acetylcholine; (g) expression of unique immunological surface determinants also present on cultured motor neurons (37); and (h) receptors for S-laminin (41a), a neuromuscular junction-specific basal lamina protein (42). All these properties are expressed in the absence of cAMP agonists.

EXTRACELLULAR MATRIX AND BASAL LAMINA

Central nervous system (CNS) motor neurons, like virtually all other cells, are surrounded by a network of polysaccharides and proteins called the extracellular matrix (ECM). The motor neuron is unusual (compared with other CNS neurons) in that it also contacts basal lamina (an ECM specialization) at the neuromuscular junction. Basal lamina also comes in proximity to motor axons at nodes of Ranvier, where it is displaced from direct contact by intervening "gap substance." Clues regarding the distinct cell biology of motor neurons may be afforded by characterization of the molecules comprising their ECM. Some of the ECM surrounding motor neurons may be synthesized and secreted by these cells; some ECM molecules may have complementary motor neuron receptors mediating a variety of functions.

ECM of the Motor Neuron Soma

During neural development, the ECM of CNS contains a number of adhesive glycoproteins that participate in the regulation of neural proliferation, differentiation, migration, process extension, and synaptogenesis (reviewed in 43,44). In mature CNS, ECM is deficient in many of these adhesive glycoproteins, which may be one barrier to regeneration of injured neural tissue. Adult motor neuron ECM, similar to other central neurons, is predominantly composed of proteoglycans (reviewed in 45). Proteoglycans are extremely carbohydrate-rich molecules composed of glycosaminoglycan (GAG) side chains covalently linked to a core protein. GAGs are highly negatively charged, unbranched chains of repeating disaccharides, the first an amino sugar, and the second usually an uronic acid. Four major GAG families are described: (a) hyaluronic acid (which is not covalently linked with core proteins), (b) chondroitin sulfate and dermatan sulfate, (c) heparan sulfate, and (d) keratan sulfate. Heterogeneity of core protein sequence, type and number of attached GAGs, and type and extent of protein and GAG posttranslational modifications make the biology of proteoglycans extremely complex. Diverse functions are attributed to proteoglycans in different tissues, including their humble role as molecular stress elements in some connective tissues. More interestingly, proteoglycans participate in adhesive interactions [either inhibitory or facilitory for cell-cell (46) and cell-substrate (47,48) adhesion], as well as binding of growth factors (e.g., binding of Schwann cell mitogenic factors by a heparan sulfate proteoglycan; ref. 49). A small subpopulation of proteoglycans (usually heparan sulfate proteoglycans) are intrinsic membrane proteins, poised to mediate a link between extracellular and intracellular environments. Proteoglycans with unknown functions have also been detected in the cytoplasm and nucleus as well.

CNS neuron extracellular GAGs are predominantly chondroitin sulfate, hyaluronic acid, and heparan sulfate, in order of abundance (50). A chondroitin sulfate proteoglycan important in the biology of motor neurons was originally defined by the monoclonal antibody Cat-301 (51,52). This molecule has widespread expression on many neuronal subpopulations throughout the CNS, including spinal cord motor neurons. CNS expression is developmentally regulated in cats, hamsters, and primates, with immunoreactivity appearing late in development or early in postnatal life; spinal cord ventral horn exhibits immunoreactivity prior to dorsal cord neurons. Interestingly, in the cat lateral geniculate nucleus Y cells and corresponding visual cortex, Cat-301 immunoreactivity correlates with visual system activity, with marked suppression observed in visually deprived animals. Homologous experiments performed in hamster spinal cord reveal suppression of Cat-301 immunoreactivity of lumbar motor neurons in animals that have undergone sciatic nerve crush, cordotomy, or deafferentation during a critical period in development (53,54). Similar maneuvers in adult animals do not suppress Cat-301 immunoreactivity in visual or motor systems. Thus, Cat-301 defines a chondrotin sulfate proteoglycan in motor neuron extracellular matrix that is modulated by activity in development.

Motor Nerve Axon ECM

Nerve basal lamina participates in regeneration of motor axons after axotomy or crush. Normally, axons are ensheathed by Schwann cells, which are in turn ensheathed by a tube of Schwann cell–elaborated basal lamina. When a peripheral axon is severed, the regenerating axons advance *between* Schwann cells and the basal lamina (55). If Schwann cells are killed by freezing, axon extension still proceeds along the empty basal lamina tube (56), suggesting that the basal lamina alone can provide sufficient cues for axon growth. Laminin (reviewed in 57), a laminin-proteoglycan complex (58), and fibronectin (reviewed in 59) are among the molecules that have been implicated in this process.

Laminin, a major adhesive glycoprotein of basal lamina, has several isoforms, the best studied of which is a large (about 900 kDa) molecule composed of three disulfide bond–linked subunits (A, B1, and B2) coded by distinct genes. Several biologically active domains have been identified on laminin which mediate its interaction with other basal lamina constituents (e.g., collagen, GAGs) and with cells. In some cases the activity of these adhesive domains is mediated by relatively small sequences of amino acids. The sequence Tyr-Ile-Gly-Ser-Arg

(YIGSR) may comprise the major ligand for laminin cell adhesion (60); an Arg-Gly-Asp (RGD) sequence shared with fibronectin does not appear to function in cell attachment (61). The sequence Ile-Lys-Tyr-Ala-Tyr (IKVAV) has also been implicated in axon extension of NGF-primed PC12 cells (62). These distinct sites within laminin appear to function through distinct receptors on the neuron cell surface (ref. 63; see below).

Motor Nerve Terminals

Muscle basal lamina contains laminin, fibronectin, chondronectin, entactin, nidogen, and several species of collagen (reviewed in 64,65). Some of these proteins (e.g., collagen V) are absent from the neuromuscular junction, while others (e.g., laminin and fibronectin) are present in synaptic and extrasynaptic basal lamina. A third class of proteins including acetylcholinesterase, agrin, and S-laminin, are markedly concentrated in synaptic basal lamina (see below). The prominent role of the synaptic basal lamina in organizing the neuromuscular junction was shown in a series of experiments by Sanes and colleagues (66), in which regenerating motor axons were able to find and form contacts with synaptic basal lamina in the absence of postsynaptic muscle fibers (which had been crushed and not permitted to regenerate). Nerve terminals innervating these basal lamina "ghosts" appeared near-normal by morphological and physiological criteria (e.g., vesicle grouping in active zones, release and recycling of cholinergic vesicles; ref. 67), suggesting that the synaptic basal lamina was also capable of eliciting motor nerve terminal differentiation. The converse experiment, in which muscle fibers were damaged and allowed to regenerate in the absence of motor axons, also demonstrated that synaptic basal lamina has the ability to order and differentiate postsynaptic structures (68).

Agrin, first isolated from basal lamina of *Torpedo californica* electric organ, was originally defined by its ability to aggregate acetylcholine receptor and acetylcholinesterase on the surface of cultured myotubes (69). Although agrin is expressed in aneural muscle cultures (70) and is found by bioassay in many brain regions (71), it appears to be highly concentrated in spinal motor neurons (71) and at synaptic basal lamina (72). Ligation of motor axons demonstrate that agrin is indeed synthesized by motor neurons and transported in an anterograde fashion to nerve terminals (73). A representative from this group of molecules has recently been cloned from an electric ray expression library (74); molecular studies of regulation of this gene in motor neurons are forthcoming.

The high concentration of acetylcholine receptor in the postsynaptic junction is not only produced by aggregation of presynthesized receptor, but is also controlled by local synthesis of receptor subunits and insertion into membrane (75). A group of neuronal molecules displaying *a*cetylcholine *r*eceptor *i*nducing *a*ctivity (ARIA) has been studied by Fischbach and colleagues. A 42-kDa ARIA from chick brain, which is abundant in spinal motor neurons, was recently cloned and found to have striking homology with the scrapie prion protein (76,77), a host molecule that accumulates in protease-resistant amyloid deposits in scrapie-infected animals. Whether this ARIA represents the chicken prion protein or a related molecule should be resolved shortly. Interestingly, immunoreactivity of the normal cellular isoform of the scrapie agent protein is present in muscle, where it appears to be concentrated in the neuromuscular junction, although also observed on extrajunctional muscle cell membranes (78, and Cashman, unpublished).

Agrin and the ARIAs were defined as biological activities prior to their immunohistochemical characterization. Neuromuscular junction molecules have also been defined by immunological methods, and later by biological activity. Sanes and colleagues have raised polyclonal antisera and monoclonal antibodies against basal lamina from heterogeneous sources to identify at least three neuromuscular junction synapse-specific epitopes (64), including an epitope present on a protein originally named JS-1. After subsequent molecular cloning, JS-1 was named S-laminin (S for synapse) for its substantial homology to the B2 chain of laminin (42). S-laminin, in contradistinction to laminin, arrests axon elongation of ciliary ganglion neurons (which innervate striated muscle in the chick iris), suggesting that it may provide a "stop signal" for regenerating motor axons in vivo (42,79). Recently, an S-laminin adhesive sequence comprising the peptide Leu-Arg-Glu (LRE) was identified by inhibiting the adhesion of ciliary ganglion cells to an active fragment of the native protein (80). LRE-mediated S-laminin adhesion has also been observed with the NSC-34 neuroblastoma-spinal cord hybrid cell line (41a), but not with dorsal root ganglia neurons (80), suggesting the possibility of a motor neuron–specific receptor for this sequence. Interestingly, the same tripeptide is present in synaptic acetylcholinesterase (78), suggesting that this basal lamina enzyme may also participate in motor nerve terminal recognition of synaptic basal lamina.

Several proteoglycans concentrated at the neuromuscular junction in different species are also candidates for molecules that may mediate motor neuron–specific activities. Some resolution as to the identity or distinctness of this family of molecules should be forthcoming. Synapse-specific heparan sulfate proteoglycans have been shown to mediate aggregation of acetylcholine receptor in frogs (81), anchor "asymmetrical" (collagen-tailed) acetylcholinesterase in the electric ray (82), and accumulate at the neuromuscular junction in denervated rat muscle (83). A chondrotin sulfate proteoglycan in electric fish also localized to the motor neuron–electric organ junction (84), an enriched source of molecules that are often conserved at fish and mammalian neuromuscular junctions. Heparan sulfate proteoglycans have been previously shown to modulate adhesive activity of N-CAM (46) and laminin (47,58) but appear to inhibit axonal outgrowth when utilized as the only substrate molecule (85). Similar to heparan sulfate proteoglycan, chondroitin sulfate proteoglycans appear to associate with laminin and tenascin, adhesive glycoproteins of basal lamina (48).

CELL SURFACE MOLECULES AND MARKERS

Although most membrane molecules of motor neurons would be expected to subserve "housekeeping" functions in common with other neurons, it is likely that the unique developmental program and adult phenotypic characteristics of motor neurons must in part be mediated by interactions with the local environment. Some candidates for motor neuron–specific membrane molecules include: receptors (neurotransmitters, neuromodulators, trophic factors, viruses, and toxins); voltage-gated ion channels; adhesion molecules and adhesion molecule receptors; and glycolipids. Motor neuron neurotransmitters and neurotransmitter receptors, motor neuron trophic factors, and motor neuron virology (including viral receptors) are reviewed elsewhere in this book.

Motor Neuron Ion Channels

The gated flow of ions across cell membranes would require volumes for adequate review; this section will attempt to orient the reader toward this enormous mass of material as it may illuminate the cell physiology of motor neurons (reviewed in 5,16,86–89). Classically, the protein pores that mediate the flux of ions across a hydrophobic bilayer can be considered as comprising two general classes: the ligand-gated channels (such as nicotinic acetylcholine receptor of muscle) and the voltage-gated channels (such as the action potential Na^+ channel). More recent work suggests that some neurotransmitters (e.g., acetylcholine acting at the M-type K^+ channel) are able to modify voltage-dependent conductances. Ligand-gated ion channels (neurotransmitters and their receptors) are discussed elsewhere in this book; here, the behavior of channels not gated by external neurotransmitters will be considered.

Could the unique phenotype of motor neurons be due in part to a unique electrophysiology? At the level of single-cell recording, motor neuron passive electrical properties in vivo appear commensurate with cell size and dendritic tree when compared to other CNS neurons (1–6); in vitro, spinal cord cells and retrograde-dye-identified motor neurons display similar properties, depending on maturity, size, and "health" of cultures (10–16). Depolarization to threshold triggers an action potential, which can be followed by afterdepolarization (usually as a small shoulder on the repolarizing phase; refs. 6–8,12,90) and afterhyperpolarization (6–8,12–14,22,90). Motor neurons, unlike dorsal root ganglion cells, but similar to many other CNS neurons, display repetitive action potentials in vivo or in vitro on sustained current injection (12–14,91), and spontaneously in vitro from synaptic input (12–14).

The ion currents that mediate these phenomena are complex and still in the process of being elucidated. Classically, channels have been defined by kinetics, voltage dependence, effect of ion gradients, and pharmacological blockade; more recently, molecules that compose these membrane pores have been cloned and their structures analyzed. In motor neurons, as with virtually all neurons, depolarization during the action potential is predominantly due to an inward current of Na^+ through a fast-onset, high-threshold channel (reviewed in 88). The Na^+ channel in mammalian brain is a heterotrimeric complex. The major alpha-subunit has been molecularly cloned in several species, including rat, in which studies suggested at least three isoforms (92). Highly conserved among isoforms and species are four large homologous domains of at least six potential transmembrane regions each, some of which contribute to the charged environment lining the channel in its open configuration (88). The Na^+ channel alpha-subunit is similar in primary sequence to the $alpha_1$-subunit of the dihydropyridine-sensitive Ca^{2+} channel (93), to an A-current K^+ channel (94), and to subunits of the muscle nicotinic acetylcholine receptor (95,96), suggesting that these diverse channels may constitute a family diverged in evolution from an ancestral pore protein.

High-threshold and low-threshold voltage-dependent Ca^{2+} channels probably also contribute to the depolarization phase of the spinal and vagal motor neuron action potential (6–9), particularly in immature cells (6,25,89,97). Both Ca^{2+} currents were first observed in motor neurons (3,4), but are not unique to this neuron (87). High-threshold Ca^{2+} conductances are distributed predominantly at the dendrite and primarily responsible for afterdepolarization; the low-threshold Ca^{2+} conductance is distributed predominantly on the cell body (86). Ca^{2+} ions gated into the cell act not only as a carrier of charge across the membrane, but also as an important second messenger in the regulation of kinases, kinetics of other channels (see below), transmitter release, cytoskeleton integrity, activation of catalytic enzymes, and gene expression (98,99). Studies with patch clamping and other modern techniques at the presynaptic terminal at the neuromuscular junction suggest the existence of additional Ca^{2+} channel families that participate in Ca^{2+}-mediated vesicle fusion and acetylcholine release (100,101).

Voltage-dependent K^+ channels have been grouped into five families (reviewed in 102): (a) the channels carrying the delayed rectifier current, (b) the "A" current channels, (c) the K^+ channels responsible for anomolous rectification, (d) the Ca^{2+}-responsive K^+ channels, and (e) the neurotransmitter-gated K^+ channels. The delayed rectifier current, first identified by Hodgkin and Huxley as the major repolarizing current in squid axon, has recently been shown to display electrophysiological and pharmacological heterogeneity consistent with at least three molecular complexes (103–105). The fast transient current carried by "A" channels may contribute to repolarization, but also appears to regulate frequency of repetitive firing in many neuronal populations, including motor neurons (106). This channel family, several representatives of which were recently cloned by chromosome walking in mutant "shaker" drosophila (94,107,108), is extremely heterogeneous; at least two gene loci code for multiple alternately spliced transcripts. K^+ channels that participate in anomolous rectification [prominent in motor neurons (2), but also observed in other neurons (87)] are gated to pass more K^+ with hyperpolarization in relation to the resting potential. Ca^{2+}-activated K^+ channels, regulated by cytosolic Ca^{2+} (increased by activation of voltage- (or ligand-)sensitive ion channels, or from intracellular release of sequestered Ca^{2+}), contribute to afterhyperpolarization in motor neurons, which regulates firing frequency in repetitive trains (6,86,87). A Ca^{2+}-activated Cl^- channel has also been detected in motor neurons (109), but is not unique to this population.

As of this writing, no voltage-gated ion channel or ion channel isoform appears uniquely associated with motor neurons. It is probable that electrophysiologically defined currents which appear near-identical in kinetics and pharmacology may, indeed, be mediated by different proteins, coded for by different genes, arise from alternate mRNA transcripts, or have different posttranslational modifications. Some resolution from this welter of heterogeneity is to be expected in the near future, as the genes coding for these channels and their cell-specific regulation are increasingly elucidated.

Adhesion Molecules and Adhesion Molecule Receptors

Cell-cell and cell-substrate adherence play an important role in neural development, including the development and differentiation of motor neurons (reviewed in 110). Both calcium-dependent (L-cadherin, N-cadherin) and calcium-independent [neural cell adhesion molecule (N-CAM), cell-CAM (105)] "general" membrane adhesion molecules participate in the early cell aggregation that will define the boundaries of the developing neural tube. Committed motor neuron "neuroblasts" migrate from neuroepithelium to the ventral cord, possibly mediated by interactions with laminin (111,112). Motor neuron differentiation is accompanied by axon extension, which in chick ciliary ganglion cells is N-cadherin-dependent on astrocytes (113). Recent data suggests that purified N-cadherin displays comparable potency to laminin and L1 in axon extension of ciliary ganglion cells (114). Laminin and fibronectin are present in regions of motor neurite outgrowth in vivo (115), although the integrin receptor binding the RGD sequence may not be functioning (61). Axon outgrowth on muscle cell surfaces, as assayed by ciliary ganglion axon extension, involves N-CAM, N-cadherin, and integrin-class ECM receptors (116). In vitro, initial adhesive contact of spinal motor neuron terminals at developing muscle fibers is due in part to N-CAM and N-cadherin (117,118). Further discussion in this section will focus on data suggesting that motor neurons may participate in more restricted adhesive interactions, arising from studies of the prototypical ''general'' cell-cell adhesion molecule N-CAM, neuronal surface receptors for laminin and fibronectin, and several newly described developmentally regulated membrane glycoproteins.

N-CAM

N-CAM, first recognized by Edelman, is widely expressed in development (reviewed in 119,120), including some nonneural structures. It is abundantly expressed by developing myoblasts, myotubes, and motor axons, possibly participating in early motor axon-axon fasciculation and axon-myotube interactions (117,118). N-CAM muscle fiber surface expression is lost in maturity, except at the neuromuscular junction, where N-CAM is maintained on pre- and postsynaptic structures (including terminal axon and junctional Schwann cells; refs. 83,121,122). On denervation or tetrodotoxin-induced paralysis, N-CAM is again detectable over the entire muscle fiber membrane and accumulates in ECM of denuded synaptic areas (Fig. 2; refs. 83,121,122). If the muscle is reinnervated, N-CAM again becomes concentrated at the neuromuscular junction. Thus, the axon susceptibility of muscle appears to correlate with extrasynaptic N-CAM expression, and N-CAM may participate in reinnervation as a soluble, substrate-attached, or cell membrane-associated signal.

The biology of N-CAM is complex (reviewed in 119,120). Alternate transcripts from a single gene give rise to at least three polypeptide isoforms in muscle (155,145, and 125 kDa), only one of which (145 kDa) is a transmembrane protein. The 125- and 155-kDa isoforms are glycosylphosphatidylinositol-linked proteins in myotubes (123), anchored to the membrane outer leaflet by a novel glycan-lipid attachment. [This membrane anchorage is also observed with several other proteins concentrated at the neuromuscular junction, including Thy-1, one isoform of acetylcholinesterase, and the normal cellular isoform of the scrapie agent protein (124,125, and Cashman unpublished).] A secreted isoform of N-CAM has also been described in muscle and brain (126). Another level of N-CAM heterogeneity is provided by variable glycosylation of N-CAM isoforms, particularly by alpha-2-8-linked sialic acid chains (127). Regulation of sialic acid on N-CAM has been shown to alter adhesive properties of the molecule and also participates in the branching of motor axons in muscle (128).

Interestingly, a unique muscle-specific 37-residue insert has been described in the glycosylphosphatydlinositol-linked isoforms and the secreted isoform of muscle N-CAM (126,129,130). Is it possible that isoforms containing this unique region interact with motor axons? The insert is not present in the known homotropic receptor region of N-CAM, and muscle N-CAM at mature neuromuscular junction appears to be concentrated at the bases of the postsynaptic

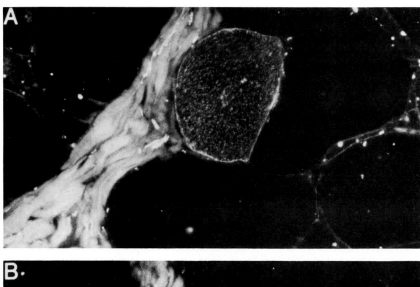

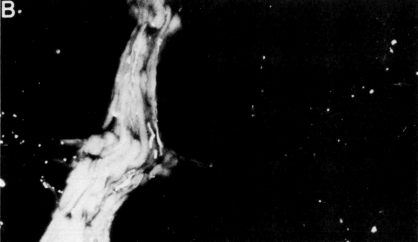

Figure 2 (A) Neural cell adhesion molecule (N-CAM) immunoreactivity in a denervated muscle fiber from patient with ALS. N-CAM expression appears prior to myofiber atrophy. (B) Same field in parallel section incubated with fluoresceinated second antibody alone (without anti-N-CAM primary antibody) demonstrating specificity of immunohistochemical reaction.

folds (118). However, release of soluble muscle N-CAM (by direct secretion or by endogenous phosphatidylinositol-specific phospholipase C) in development, reinnervation, or even stable maturity could interact with a previously unrecognized receptor present on motor terminals. Further characterization of the role of the muscle-specific domain is pending.

Basal Lamina Glycoprotein Receptors

Adhesive substrate molecules bind to cell membrane receptors, one major family of which are the integrins (reviewed in 44). The integrins are noncovalently associated heterodimers composed of alpha- and beta-subunits; at least 10 genes code for alpha-subunits, and three or more for beta-subunits. Antibodies to specific integrins can inhibit neuronal adhesion and process extension and, at the developing neuromuscular junction, may inhibit axonal interactions with muscle fiber basal lamina (116). Laminin receptor integrins $alpha_1beta_1$ and $alpha_3beta_1$ participate in NGF-induced neurite extension of PC12 cells (63), which are capable of innervating myotubes (40). Laminin also appears to be recognized by nonintegrin receptors (61,131,132), some of which may be partly restricted to motor neurons. A 67-kDa putative laminin receptor (133), functioning in neural adhesion but not process outgrowth, has been detected in retina and early motor neurons. The amino acid sequence YIGSR in laminin is also recognized by NG108 cells (60), which model certain aspects of motor neurons (see above).

New Developmentally Regulated Membrane Glycoproteins

More restricted glycoproteins can be found on subsets of neurons in development and are hypothesized to participate in directed axonal outgrowth and formation of specific synaptic contact (reviewed in 110). Dodd and Jessell found that surface glycoconjugates of the lactoseries are coexpressed with lectins recognizing this carbohydrate moiety in dorsal root ganglia; motor neurons express one of these lectins (134). Possibly, other nervous-system-restricted carbohydrate ligands and lectins may mediate specific cell-cell and early synaptic interactions. The axonal glycoprotein TAG-1 exhibits a developmental restriction limited to dorsal root ganglia, commissural spinocerebellar neurons, and motor neurons (135).

Glycolipids

Gangliosides (treated at greater length elsewhere in this book) have numerous functions, including regulation of affinity for receptors for neurotransmitters, growth factors, and cell adhesion; surface enzyme modulation; and neuritogenic activity (reviewed in 136). Motor neurons (perhaps due to size) may be uniquely susceptible to ganglioside storage diseases (137). Some gangliosides may be target antigens for gammopathy-associated motor neuropathy or neuronopathy. A cholinergic neuron–specific ganglioside has been described, but is not restricted to motor neurons (138). A synapse-specific carbohydrate epitope conserved on acetylcholinesterase and a glycolipid has been described (139), raising the possibility of a neuromuscular junction–specific glycosidase and/or lectin.

Uncharacterized surface epitopes

A motor neuron surface determinant in chicks is recognized by the monoclonal antibody SC-1, which also binds to spinal cord ventral epithelial cells, dorsal root ganglia, sympathetic ganglia, dorsal funiculus, and dorsal and ventral roots (140). In the CNS, the antigen is expressed maximally at stage 23–24 in the chick embryo, but declines thereafter. Although the surface staining is sensitive to protease treatment, no immunoblot activity is present, suggesting that the determinant is present on a protein but is destroyed by denaturation. A monoclonal antibody TOR 23, recognizing a determinant present on *Torpedo* presynaptic acetylcholinesterase (141), also stains a subset of neurons throughout the neuroaxis, including motor neurons in the spinal cord of rats (142) and humans (143). Shaw and colleagues described polyclonal antisera that may recognize motor neuron–specific determinants (37); monoclonal antibodies directed against these determinants are presently being characterized (Shaw and Cashman, unpublished).

INTRACELLULAR MARKERS OF MOTOR NEURONS

The intracellular compartment of neurons is the location of molecules that subserve a wide variety of neuron-specific functions, including neurotransmitter synthetic enzymes and the intracellular machinery for the synthesis, assembly, and transport of neurosecretory vesicles. Molecules essential for the expression of unique motor neuron phenotypic characteristics are likely to be present in this cellular compartment. A few examples are cytoskeletal proteins, cytosolic signal transduction components (such as unique protein kinases, or hormone receptors), and molecular determinants of the characteristic morphology of motor neurons. A possible hint toward the role of the intracellular compartment in motor neuron diseases is provided by the selective vulnerability of motor neurons in some viral diseases such as poliomyelitis; despite the fact that membrane receptors for this virus are not restricted to motor neurons, some characteristic of intracellular milieu confers selective vulnerability predominantly to motor neurons.

Intermediate Filaments

The subject of the motor neuron cytoskeleton is reviewed in depth elsewhere in this volume; this section will briefly note two recent advances in cell biology and development of intermediate filaments relevant to motor neurons.

The intermediate filaments are a family of structurally related proteins classically comprising five type families (reviewed in 144): the acidic and basic keratins of epithelial cells (types I and II); desmins of muscle, widely distributed vimentin, and glial fibrillary associated protein (GFAP) (type III); light-, medium-, and heavy-neurofilament proteins (type IV); and the nuclear lamins (type V). It is important to recall that neurofilament proteins are neither completely neuron-specific (145) nor are they the only intermediate-filament proteins expressed by neurons (e.g., 146). The latter is exemplified by the recent molecular cloning of two important new intermediate-filament proteins, peripherin and nestin.

Peripherin was originally identified as a protein (147) and mRNA (148) greatly up-regulated in PC-12 cells by NGF. Its sequence clearly displays significant homology with other intermediate-filament proteins, which is most marked with the type III family (later confirmed by intron mapping). Aside from the coexpression of vimentin and neurofilaments in the horizontal cells of the retina of some species (146), peripherin is the only nonneurofilament intermediate filament expressed by mature neurons (149). Peripherin is expressed by ganglia of the peripheral nervous system (autonomic and somatic) and selected neurons within the CNS, where it is notably associated with neurons that directly or indirectly subserve the somatic motor system: motor neurons of the spinal cord and brainstem, red nucleus, medial and lateral vestibular complex, and the dentate nucleus. However, some areas of peripherin expression do not apparently overlap with motor function, such as hippocampal pyramidal neurons. The potential participation of peripherin in cytoskeleton in neuronal health and disease is not clear; perhaps some important insights pertaining to genetic or acquired motor neuron disease may be obtained by further investigation of this molecule.

Nestin, a completely novel intermediate filament discovered by McKay and colleagues (150,151), is expressed by neuroepithelial cells prior to neuronal differentiation. Similar to all intermediate filaments, it has a conserved fibrillar "core domain" able to participate in coiled-coil interactions; however, greatly diverging N- and C-terminal domains, as well as intron placement, apparently place nestin in a new intermediate filament class. The discovery of nestin further complicates the pattern of intermediate-filament expression in neuronal development. Nestin expression is followed by vimentin (152), which in turn is followed by expression of mature neuronal intermediate filaments: neurofilaments and peripherin. The genetic and epigenetic signals orchestrating this sequence are unclear.

Enzymes and Peptides

Motor neuron neurotransmitters and their receptors are discussed elsewhere in this book. The major classical neurotransmitter of motor neurons, acetylcholine, is synthesized by the enzyme choline acetyltransferase. Even within the spinal cord, however, this enzyme is not unique to motor neurons (e.g., presympathetic ganglion cells; ref. 153). Several neuroactive peptides have recently been identified in motor neurons, which are presumably transported and released at the neuromuscular junction. The best studied is calcitonin gene–related peptide (CGRP), which participates in the regulation of transcription and phosphorylation of muscle acetylcholine receptor subunits (154–157). Other, less characterized motor neuron peptides include endothelin (158) and a number of other neuropeptides of unknown function.

Uncharacterized Motor Neuron Epitopes

Urakami and Chiu recently reported the generation of a monoclonal antibody (MO-1) that recognizes cell bodies and proximal axons of brainstem and spinal motor neurons in the rat (159). Virtually all somatic motor neurons were stained, but some immunoreactivity was observed in the red nucleus. Biochemical characterization of the molecule bearing the MO-1 epitope will be of great interest. Miller and colleagues have also reported internal epitopes of motor neurons shared with restricted subsets of other CNS neurons recognized by monoclonal antibodies directed against *Drosophilla* brain antigens (160). Antel and colleagues have also described restricted (but not motor-neuron-unique) patterns of immunoreactivity with a library of monoclonal antibodies (161).

CONCLUSIONS

In summary, although motor neurons in spinal cord and brainstem express the unique in vivo function of striated muscle innervation, the critical molecules that mediate their cell biology are still poorly understood. Little is known about the differentiation programs for neurons in general, arguably the most end-differentiated cells in the organism. The magnitude of the problem is conveyed by studies of RNA complexity in the CNS: fully one-third of all genes are expressed only in neural tissue (162). As such, this review must be considered an "essay" in the original sense of an uncompleted effort. The cell biology of motor neurons, or any neuronal population, will be written in the future.

On the other hand, progress on the elucidation of neuronal cell biology is being made at an ever-hastening rate. The exquisite tools of molecular biology have only recently been focused on the nervous system and are now added to increasingly sophisticated methodologies of physiology, biochemistry, and immunology. The accelerating accumulation of information regarding the normal cell biology of motor neurons should soon provide some insight into their abnormal biology in human motor neuron diseases.

ACKNOWLEDGMENTS

The author thanks Drs. K. Hastings, S. Carbonetto, M. Avoli, and J. Antel for their helpful comments and criticisms. L. Cetola and R. Cashman provided assistance in preparing the manuscript. The author's work was supported by Fonds de la recherche en santé de Québec, the Amyotrophic Lateral Sclerosis Association, the Amyotrophic Sclerosis Society of Canada, Association Français contre les myopathies, and the Musuclar Dystrophy Association. Heartfelt thanks to my wife, Rosemary.

REFERENCES

1. Brock LG, Coombs JS, Eccles JC. The recording of potentials from motoneurons with an intracellular electrode. J Physiol 1952;117:431–460.
2. Nelson PG, Frank K. Anomalous rectification in cat spinal motoneurons and effect of polarizing currents on excitatory postsynaptic potential. J Neurophysiol 1967; 30:1097–1113.
3. Schwindt PC, Crill WE. Effects of barium on cat spinal motoneurons studied by voltage clamp. J Neurophysiol 1980;44:827–846.
4. Schwindt PC, Crill WE. Properties of a persistent inward current in normal and TEA-injected motoneurons. J Neurophysiol 1980;43:1700–1724.
5. Burke RE, Rudomin P. Spinal neurons and synapses. In: Brookhart JM, Mountcastle VB, Kandel ER, Geiger SR, eds. Handbook of physiology—The nervous system. Bethesda MD: American Physiological Society, 1977:877–944.
6. Walton K, Fulton BP. Ionic mechanisms underlying the firing properties of rat neonatal motoneurons studied in vitro. Neuroscience 1986;19:669–683.
7. Harada Y, Takahashi T. The calcium component of the action potential in spinal motoneurons of the rat. J Physiol 1983;335:89–100.
8. Fulton BP, Walton K. Electrophysiological properties of neonatal rat motoneurones studied in vitro. J Physiol 1986;370:651–678.
9. Yarom Y, Sugimori M, Llinas R. Ionic currents and firing patterns of mammalian vagal motoneurons in vitro. Neurosci 1985;16:719–737.
10. Schmidt-Achert KM, Askanas V, Engel WK. Thyrotropin-releasing hormone enhances choline acetyltransferase and creatine kinase in cultured spinal ventral horn neurons. J Neurochem 1984;43:586–589.
11. Kim SU, Osborne DN, Kim MW, et al. Long-term culture of human fetal spinal cord neurons: Morphological, immunocytochemical and electrophysiological characteristics. Neuroscience 1988;25:659–670.
12. Fischbach GD, Dichter MA. Electrophysiologic and morphologic properties of neurons in dissociated chick spinal cord cell cultures. Dev Biol 1974;37:100–116.
13. Peacock JH, Nelson PG, Goldstone MW. Electrophysiologic study of cultured neurons dissociated from spinal cords and dorsal root ganglia of fetal mice. Dev Biol 1973;30:137–152.
14. Ransom BR, Neale E, Henkart M, Bullock PN, Nelson PG. Mouse spinal cord in

cell culture. I. Morphology and intrinsic neuronal electrophysiologic properties. J Neurophysiol 1977;40:1132–1150.

15. Kato AC, Touzeau G, Bertrand D, Bader CR. Human spinal cord neurons in dissociated monolayer cultures: Morphological, biochemical, and electrophysiological properties. J Neurosci 1985;5:2750–2761.

16. Fischbach GD, Nelson PG. Cell culture in neurobiology. In: Brookhart JM, Mountcastle VB, Kandel ER, Geiger SR, eds. Handbook of physiology: The nervous system. Bethesda MD: American Physiological Society, 1977;877–944.

17. Smith RG, Appel SH. Extracts of skeletal muscle increase neurite outgrowth and cholinergic activity of fetal rat spinal motor neurons. Science 1983;219:1079–1081.

18. Schnaar RL, Schaffner AE. Separation of cell types from embryonic chicken and rat spinal cord: Characterization of motoneuron-enriched fractions. J Neurosci 1981;1:204–217.

19. Hooisma J, Slaaf DW, Meeter E, Stevens WF. The innervation of chick striated muscle fibers by the chick ciliary ganglion in tissue culture. Brain Res 1975;85:79–85.

20. Schaffner AE, St. John PA, Barker JL. Purification of embryonic mouse motoneurons by flow cytometry. Soc Neurosci Abstr 1983;9:7.

21. Eagleson KL, Bennett MR. Survival of purified motor neurones in vitro: Effects of skeletal muscle-conditioned medium. Neurosci Lett 1983;38:187–192.

22. O'Brien RJ, Fischbach GD. Isolation of embryonic chick motoneurons and their survival in vitro. J Neurosci 1986;6:3265–3274.

23. Smith RG, Vaca K, McManaman J, Appel SH. Selective effects of skeletal muscle extract fractions on motoneuron development in vitro. J Neurosci 1986;6:439–447.

24. Fruns M, Krieger C, Sears TA. Identification and electrophysiologic investigations of embryonic mammalian motor neurons in culture. Neurosci Lett 1987;83:82–88.

25. McCobb DP, Best PM, Beam KG. Development alters the expression of calcium currents in chick limb motoneurons. Neuron 1989;2:1633–1643.

26. Minna JD, Yavelow J, Coon H. Expression of phenotypes in hybrid somatic cells derived from the nervous system. Genetics 1975;79(Suppl):373–383.

27. Hamprecht B. Structural, electrophysiological, biochemical, and pharmacological properties of neuroblastoma-glioma cell hybrids in cell culture. Int Rev Cytol 1977;149:99–170.

28. Antequera F, Boyes J, Bird A. High levels of de novo methylation and altered chromatin structure at CpG islands in cell lines. Cell 1990;62:503–514.

29. Augusti-Tocco, Sato G. Establishment of functional clonal lines of neurons from mouse neuroblastoma. Proc Natl Acad Sci USA 1969;64:311.

30. Frederiksen K, Jat PS, Valtz N, Levy D, McKay R. Immortalization of precursor cells from the mammalian CNS. Neuron 1988;1:439–448.

31. Cepko C. Retrovirus vectors and their applications in neurobiology. Neuron 1988;1:345–353.

32. Nelson PG, Christian CN, Nirenberg M. Synapse formation of between clonal

neuroblastoma x glioma hybrid cells and striated muscle cells. Proc Natl Acad Sci USA 1976;73:123–127.

33. Nirenberg M, Wilson S, Higashida H et al. Modulation of synapse formation by cyclic adenosine monophosphate. Science 1983;222:794–799.

34. Busis NA, Daniels MP, Bauer HC et al. Three cholinergic neuroblastoma hybrid cell lines that form few synapses on myotubes are deficient in acetylcholine receptor aggregation molecules and large dense core vesicles. Brain Res 1984;324: 201–210.

35. Cashman NR, Boulet S, Antel JP. Clonal cell lines from neuroblastoma–spinal cord cell hybridization. Soc Neurosci Abstr 1987;13:1511.

36. Pasternak S, Cashman NR, Hastings K. Motor neuron-specific genes: A hybrid cell cDNA cloning strategy. Soc Neurosci Abstr 1989;5:958.

37. Shaw IT, Boulet S, Wong E, Cashman NR. Unique immunological determinants of neuroblastoma-spinal cord (NSC) hybrid cells. Neurology 1989;40(Suppl 1): 183.

38. Puro DG, De Mello FG, Nirenberg M. Synapse turnover: The formation and termination of transient synapses. Proc Natl Acad Sci USA 1977;74:4977–4981.

39. Nurse CA, O'Lague PH. Formation of cholinergic synapses between dissociated sympathetic neurons and skeletal myotubes of the rat in cell culture. Proc Nat Acad Sci USA 1975;72:1955–1959.

40. Schubert D, Heinemann S, Kidokoro Y. Cholinergic metabolism and synapse formation by a rat nerve cell line. Proc Natl Acad Sci USA 1977;74:2579–2583.

41. Wilson S, Higashida H, Minna J, Nirenberg M. Defects in synapse formation and acetylcholine release by neuroblastoma and hybrid cell lines. Fed Proc 1978;37: 1784.

41a. Hunter DD, Cashman N, Morris-Valero R, Bulock JW, Adams SP, Sanes JR. An LRE (leucine-arginine-glutamate)-dependent mechanism for adhesion of neurons to S-laminin. J Neurosci (in press).

42. Hunter DD, Shah V, Merlie JP, Sanes JR. A laminin-like adhesive protein concentrated in the synaptic cleft of the neuromuscular junction. Nature 1989;338: 229–234.

43. Sanes JR. Extracellular matrix molecules that infuence neural development. Annu Rev Neurosci 1989;12:491–516.

44. Douville P, Carbonetto S. Extracellular matrix adhesive glycoproteins and their receptors in the nervous system. In: Margolis RU, Margolis RK, eds. Neurobiology of glycoconjugates. New York: Plenum Press, 1989:383–409.

45. Margolis RK, Margolis RU. Structure and localization of glycoproteins and proteoglycans. In: Margolis RU, Margolis RK, eds. Neurobiology of glycoconjugates. New York: Plenum Press, 1989:85–126.

46. Cole GJ, Loewy A, Glaser L. Neuronal cell-cell adhesion depends on interactions of N-CAM with heparin-like molecules. Nature 1986;320:445–447.

47. Lander AD, Fujii DK, Gospodarowicz D, Reichardt LF. Characterization of a factor that promotes neurite outgrowth: Evidence linking activity to a heparan sulfate proteoglycan. J Cell Biol 1982;94:574–585.

48. Chiquet M, Fambrough DM. Chick myotendinous antigen. II. A novel extracel-

lular glycoprotein complex consisting of large disulfide-linked subunits. J Cell Biol 1984;98:1937–1946.

49. Ratner N, Bunge RP, Glaser L. A neuronal cell surface heparan sulfate proteoglycan is required for dorsal root ganglion neuron stimulation of Schwann cell proliferation. J Cell Biol 1985;101:744–754.

50. Margolis RU, Margolis RK, Chang L, Preti C. Glycosaminoglycans of brain during development. Biochemistry 1975;14:85–88.

51. Hockfield S, McKay RD, Hendry SHC, Jones EG. A surface antigen that identifies ocular dominance columns in the visual cortex and laminar features of the lateral geniculate nucleus. Cold Spring Harbor Symp Quant Biol 1983;48:877–889.

52. Zaremba S, Guimaraes A, Kalb RG, Hockfield S. Characterization of an activity-dependent, neuronal surface proteoglycan identified with monoclonal antibody Cat-301. Neuron 1989;2:1207–1219.

53. Kalb RG, Hockfield S. Molecular evidence for early activity-dependent development of hamster motor neurons. J Neurosci 1988;8:2350–2360.

54. Kalb R, Hockfield S. Development of Cat-301 expression on motor neurons requires muscle afferents. Soc Neurosci Abstr 1988;14:769.

55. Scherer SS, Easter S, Jr. Degenerative and regenerative changes in the trochlear nerve of goldfish. J Neurocytol 1984;13:519–565.

56. Ide C. Nerve regeneration through the basal lamina scaffold of the skeletal muscle. Neurosci Res 1984;1:379–391.

57. Martin GR, Timpl R. Laminin and other basement membrane components. Annu Rev Cell Biol 1987;3:57–85.

58. Matthew WD, Patterson PH. The production of a monoclonal antibody that blocks the action of a neurite outgrowth-promoting factor. Cold Spring Harbor Symp Quant Biol 1983;48:625–631.

59. Ruoslahti E. Fibronectin and its receptors. Annu Rev Biochem 1988;57:375–413.

60. Graf J, Iwamoto Y, Sasaki M et al. Identification of an amino acid sequence in laminin mediating cell attachment, chemotaxis, and receptor binding. Cell 1987; 48:989–996.

61. Douville PJ, Harvey WJ, Carbonetto S. Isolation and characterization of high affinity laminin receptors in neural cells. J Biol Chem 1988;263:14964–14969.

62. Tashiro K, Sephel GC, Weeks B, et al. A synthetic peptide containing the IKVAV sequence from the A chain of laminin mediates cell attachment, migration, and neurite outgrowth. J Biol Chem 1989;264:16174–16182.

63. Tomaselli KJ, Hall DE, Flier LA, Gehlsen KR, Turner DC, Carbonetto S, Reichardt LF. A neuronal cell line (PC12) expresses two beta$_1$-class integrins—alpha$_1$beta$_1$ and alpha$_3$beta$_1$—that recognize different neurite outgrowth-promoting domains in laminin. Neuron 1990;5:651–662.

64. Sanes JR, Chiu AY. The basal lamina of the neuromuscular junction. Cold Spring Harbor Symp Quant Biol 1983;48:667–678.

65. Sanes JR. The extracellular matrix. In: Engel AG, Banker BQ, eds. Myology. New York: McGraw-Hill, 1986:155–175.

66. Sanes JR, Marshall LM, McMahan UJ. Reinnervation of muscle fiber basal lamina after removal of myofibers. Differentiation of regenerating axons at original synaptic sites. J Cell Biol 1978;78:176–198.
67. Glicksman M, Sanes JR. Development of motor nerve terminals formed in the absence of muscle fibers. J Neurocytol 1983;12:661–671.
68. Anglister L, McMahan UJ, Marshall RM. Basal lamina directs acetylcholinesterase accumulation at synaptic sites in regenerating muscle. J Cell Biol 1985;101: 735–743.
69. Nitkin RM, Smith MA, Magill C, et al. Identification of agrin, a synaptic organizing protein from torpedo electric organ. J Cell Biol 1987;105:2471–2478.
70. Leith E, Fallon JR. Cultured chick myotubes express agrin-related molecules. Soc Neurosci Abstr 1989;15:1352.
71. Magill-Sole C, McMahan UJ. Motor neurons contain agrin-like molecules. J Cell Biol 1988;107:1825–1833.
72. Reist NE, Magill C, McMahan UJ, Marshall RM. Agrin-like molecules at synaptic sites in normal, denervated, and damaged skeletal muscles. J Cell Biol 1987;105: 2457–2469.
73. Magill-Solc C, McMahan UJ. Agrin-like molecules are transported in an anterograde direction in motor axons. Soc Neurosci Abstr 1989;15:163.
74. Smith MA, Rupp F, Snow P, et al. Identification of an agrin cDNA. Soc Neurosci Abstr 1989;15:164.
75. Usdin TB, Fischbach GD. Purification and characterization of a polypeptide from chick brain that promotes the accumulation of acetylcholine receptors in chick myotubes. J Cell Biol 1986;103:493–507.
76. Harris DA, Falls DL, Walsh W, Fischbach GD. Molecular cloning of an acetylcholine receptor-inducing protein. Soc Neurosci Abstr 1989;15:164.
77. Falls DL, Harris DA, Johnson FA, Morgan MM, Corfas G, Fischbach GD. 42kD ARIA: A protein that may regulate the accumulation of acetylcholine receptors at developing chick neuromuscular junctions. Cold Spring Harbor Symp Quant Biol 1991;55 (in press).
78. Bendheim PE, Brown HR, Rudelli RD, et al. Nearly ubiquitous tissue distribution of the scrapie agent precursor protein. Neurology (in press).
79. Weis J, Hunter DD, Merlie JP, Sanes JR. S-Laminin inhibits neurite extension promoted by laminin. Soc Neurosci Abstr 1989;15:164.
80. Hunter DD, Porter BE, Bulock JW, Adams SP, Merlie JP, Sanes JR. Primary sequence of a motor neuron-selective adhesive site in the synaptic basal lamina protein S-laminin. Cell 1989;59:905–913.
81. Anderson MJ, Fambrough DM. Aggregates of acetylcholine receptors are associated with plaques of a basal lamina heparan sulfate proteoglycan on the surface of skeletal muscle fibers. J Cell Biol 1983;97:1396–1411.
82. Brandan E, Maldonado M, Garrido J, Inestrosa NC. Anchorage of collagen-tailed acetylcholinesterase to the extracellular matrix is mediated by heparan sulfate proteoglycans. J Cell Biol 1985;101:985–992.
83. Sanes JR, Schachner M, Covault J. Expression of several adhesive macromolecules (N-CAM, L1, J1, NILE, uvomorulin, laminin, fibronectin, and a heparan

sulfate proteoglycan) in embryonic, adult, and denervated adult skeletal muscle. J Cell Biol 1986;102:420–431.

84. Carlson SS, Wight TN. Nerve terminal anchorage protein 1 (TAP-1) is a chondroitin sulfate proteoglycan: Biochemical and electron microscopic characterization. J Cell Biol 1987;105:3075–3086.

85. Carbonetto S, Gruver MM, Turner DC. Nerve fiber growth in culture on fibronectin, collagen, and glycosaminoglycan substrates. J Neurosci 1983;3:2324–2335.

86. Crill WE, Schwindt PC. Active currents in mammalian central neurons. Trends Neurosci 1983;6:236–240.

87. Llinas RR. The intrinsic electrophysiological properties of mammalian neurons: Insights into central nervous system function. Science 1988;242:1654–1664.

88. Catterall WA. Structure and function of voltage-sensitive ion channels. Science 1988;242:50–61.

89. Spitzer NC. Ion channels in development. Annu Rev Neurosci 1979;2:363–397.

90. Nelson PG, Burke RE. Delayed depolarization in cat spinal motoneurons. Exp Neurol 1967;17:16–26.

91. Kernell D. High-frequency repetitive firing of cat lumbosacral motoneurones stimulated by long-lasting injected current. Acta Physiol Scand 1965;65:74–86.

92. Noda M, Ikeda T, Kayano T, et al. Existence of distinct sodium channel messenger RNAs in rat brain. Nature 1986;320:188–192.

93. Tanabe T, Takeshima H, Mikami A, et al. Primary structure of the receptor for calcium blockers from skeletal muscle. Nature 1987;328:313–318.

94. Papazian DM, Schwarz TL, Tempel BL, Jan YN, Jan LY. Cloning of genomic and complementary DNA from shaker, a putative potassium channel gene from *Drosophila*. Science 1987;237:749–753.

95. Noda M, Takashashi H, Tanabe T, et al. Primary structure of alpha-subunit precursor of *Torpedo californica* acetylcholine receptor deduced from cDNA sequence. Nature 1982;299:793–797.

96. Noda M, Takahashi H, Tanabe T, et al. Primary structures of beta and delta-subunit precursors of *Torpedo californica* acetylcholine receptor deduced from cDNA sequence. Nature 1982;299:793–797.

97. Ribera AB, Spitzer NC. A critical period of transcription required for differentiation of the action potential of spinal neurons. Neuron 1989;2:1055–1062.

98. Greenberg ME, Ziff EB, Greene LA. Stimulation of neuronal acetylcholine receptors induces rapid gene transcription. Science 1986;234:80–83.

99. Kennedy MB. Regulation of neuronal function by calcium. Trends Neurosci 1989;12:417–420.

100. Lemos JR, Nowycky MC. Two types of calcium channels coexist in peptide-releasing vertebrate nerve terminals. Neuron 1989;2:1419–1426.

101. Augustine GJ, Charlton MP, Smith SJ. Calcium action in synaptic transmitter release. Annu Rev Neurosci 1987;10:633–693.

102. Rudy B. Diversity and ubiquity of K channels. Neuroscience 1988;25:729–749.

103. Dubois JM. Evidence for the existence of three types of potassium channels in the frog Ranvier node membrane. J Physiol 1981;318:297–316.

104. Harris GL, Henderson LP, Spitzer NC. Changes in densities and kinetics of delayed rectifier potassium channels during neuronal differentiation. Neuron 1988;1: 739–750.
105. Frech GC, VanDongen AMJ, Schuster G, Brown AM, Joho RH. A novel potassium channel with delayed rectifier properties isolated from rat brain by expression cloning. Nature 1989;340:642–646.
106. Segal M, Rogawski MA, Barker JL. A transient potassium conductance regulates the excitability of cultured hippocampal and spinal neurons. J Neurosci 1984;4: 604–609.
107. Kamb A, Tseng-Crank J, Tanouye MA. Multiple products of the *Drosophila* shaker gene may contribute to potassium channel diversity. Neuron 1988;1:421–430.
108. Butler A, Wei A, Baker K, Salkoff L. A family of putative potassium channel genes in *Drosophila*. Science 1989;243:943–947.
109. Owen DG, Segal M, Barker JL, A Ca-dependent Cl⁻ conductance in cultured mouse spinal neurones. Nature 1984;311:567–570.
110. Jessell TM. Adhesion molecules and the hierarchy of neural development. Neuron 1988;1:3–13.
111. Liesi P. Do neurons in the vertebrate CNS migrate on laminin? EMBO J 1985;4: 1163–1170.
112. Carbonetto S, Evans D, Cochard P. Nerve fiber growth in culture on tissue substrata from central and peripheral nervous systems. J Neurosci 1987;7:610–620.
113. Tomaselli KJ, Neugebauer KM, Bixby JL, Lilien J, Reichardt LF. *N*-Cadherin and integrins: Two receptor systems that mediate neuronal process outgrowth on astrocyte surfaces. Neuron 1988;1:33–43.
114. Bixby JL, Zhang R. Purified *N*-cadherin is a potent substrate for the rapid induction of neurite outgrowth. J Cell Biol 1990;110:1253–1260.
115. Riggott MJ, Moody SA. Distribution of laminin and fibronectin along peripheral trigeminal axon pathways in the developing chick. J Comp Neurol 1987;258: 580–596.
116. Bixby JL, Pratt RS, Lilien J, Reichardt LF. Neurite outgrowth on muscle cell surfaces involves extracellular matrix receptors as well as Ca^{2+}-dependent and -independent cell adhesion molecules. Proc Natl Acad Sci USA 1987;84:2555–2559.
117. Rutishauser U, Grumet M, Edelman GM. N-CAM mediates initial interactions between spinal cord neurons and muscle cells in culture. J Cell Biol 1983;97: 145–152.
118. Landmesser L, Dahm L, Schultz K, Rutishauser U. Distinct roles for adhesion during innervation of embryonic chick muscle. Dev Biol 1988;130:645–670.
119. Rutishauser U. Developmental biology of a neural cell adhesion molecule. Nature 1984;310:549–554.
120. Edelman GM. Cell adhesion molecules in neural histogenesis. Annu Rev Physiol 1986;48:339–377.
121. Covault J, Sanes JR. Neural cell adhesion molecule (N-CAM) accumulates in

denervated and paralyzed skeletal muscles. Proc Natl Acad Sci USA 1985;82: 4544–4548.

122. Cashman NR, Covault J, Wollman RL, Sanes JR. Neural cell adhesion molecule in normal, denervated, and myopathic human muscle. Ann Neurol 1987;21:481–489.

123. Moore SE, Thompson J, Kirkness V, Dickson JG, Walsh FS. Skeletal muscle neural cell adhesion molecule (N-CAM): Changes in protein and mRNA species during myogenesis of muscle cell lines. J Cell Biol 1987;105:1377–1386.

124. Weber RJ, Hill JM, Pert CB. Regional distribution and density of Thy 1.1 in rat brain and its relation to subpopulations of neurons. J Neuroimmunol 1988;17: 137–145.

125. Low MG, Saltiel AR. Structural and functional roles of glycosylphosphatidylinositol in membranes. Science 1988;239:268–275.

126. Gower HJ, Barton CH, Elsom VL, et al. Alternative splicing generates a secreted form of N-CAM in muscle and brain. Cell 1988;55:955–964.

127. Rutishauser U. Polysialic acid as a regulator of cell interactions. In: Margolis RU, Margolis RK, eds. Neurobiology of glycoconjugates. New York: Plenum Press, 1989:367–382.

128. Landmesser L, Dahm L, Tang J, Rutishauser U. Polysialic acid as a regulator of intramuscular nerve branching during embryonic development. Neuron 1990;4: 655–667.

129. Barton CH, Dickson G, Gower HJ, et al. Complete sequence and in vitro expression of a tissue-specific phosphatidylinositol-linked N-CAM isoform from skeletal muscle. Development 1988;104:165–173.

130. Dickson G, Gower HJ, Barton CH, et al. Human muscle neural cell adhesion molecule (N-CAM): Identification of a muscle-specific sequence in the extracellular domain. Cell 1987;50:1119–1130.

131. Runyan RB, Maxwell GD, Shur BD. Evidence for a novel enzymatic mechanism of neural crest cell migration on extracellular glycoconjugate matrices. J Cell Biol 1986;102:432–441.

132. Smalheiser NR, Schwartz NB. Cranin: A laminin binding protein of cell membranes. Proc Natl Acad Sci USA 1987;84:6457–6461.

133. Drager UC, Rabacchi SA. A positional marker in the dorsal eye of the embryo. Soc Neurosci Abstr 1988;14:769.

134. Regan LJ, Dodd J, Barondes SH, Jessell TM. Selective expression of endogenous lactose-binding lectins and lactoseries glycoconjugates in subsets of rat sensory neurons. Proc Natl Acad Sci USA 1986;83:2248–2252.

135. Dodd J, Morton SB, Karagogeos D, Yamamoto M, Jessell TM. Spatial regulation of axonal glycoprotein expression on subsets of embryonic spinal neurons. Neuron 1988;1:105–116.

136. Ledeen RW. Biosynthesis, metabolism, and biological effects of gangliosides. In: Margolis RU, Margolis RK, eds. Neurobiology of glycoconjugates. New York: Plenum Press, 1989:43–83.

137. Cashman NR, Antel JP, Hancock LW, et al. *N*-acetyl-B-hexosaminidase B-locus defect and juvenile motor neuron disease: A case study. Ann Neurol 1986;19: 568–572.

138. Obrocki J, Borroni E. Immunocytochemical evaluation of a cholinergic-specific ganglioside antigen (Chol-1) in the central nervous system of the rat. Exp Brain Res 1988;72:71–82.

139. Scott LJC, Bacou F, Sanes JR. A synapse-specific carbohydrate at the neuromuscular junction: Association with both acetylcholinesterase and a glycolipid. J Neurosci 1988;8:932–944.

140. Tanaka H, Obata K. Developmental changes in unique cell surface antigens of chick embryo spinal motoneurons and ganglion cells. Dev. Biol 1984;106:26–37.

141. Kushner PD, Stephenson DT, Sternberg H, Weber R. Monoclonal antibody Tor 23 recognizes a determinant of a presynaptic acetylcholinesterase. J Neurochem 1987;48:1942–1953.

142. Stephenson DT, Kushner PD. An atlas of a rare neuronal surface antigen in the rat central nervous system. J Neurosci 1988;8:3035–3056.

143. Bjornskov EK, Stephenson DT, Kushner PD. Torpedo monoclonal antibodies react with components of the human peripheral nervous system. Muscle Nerve 1988;11:10–20.

144. Steinert PM, Roop DR. Molecular and cellular biology of intermediate filaments. Annu Rev Biochem 1988;57:593–625.

145. Trojanowski JQ, Lee VMY. Expression of neurofilament antigens by normal and neoplastic human adrenal chromaffin cells. N Engl J Med 1985;313:101–104.

146. Drager U. Coexistence of neurofilaments and vimentin in a neurone of adult mouse retina. Nature 1983;303:169–172.

147. Thompson MA, Ziff EB. Structure of the gene encoding peripherin, an NGF-regulated neuronal-specific type III intermediate filament protein. Neuron 1989;2:1043–1053.

148. Leonard GB, Gordham JD, Cole P, Greene LA, Ziff EB. A nerve growth factor-regulated messenger RNA encodes a new intermediate filament protein. J Cell Biol 1988;106:181–193.

149. Parysek LM, Chisholm RL, Ley CA, Goldman RD. A type III intermediate filament gene is expressed in mature neurons. Neuron 1988;1:395–401.

150. Hockfield S, McKay RDG. Identification of major cell classes in the developing mammalian nervous system. J Neurosci 1985;5:3310–3328.

151. Lendahl U, Zimmerman LB, McKay RDG. CNS stem cells express a new class of intermediate filament protein. Cell 1990;60:585–595.

152. Bignami A, Raju T, Dahl D. Localization of vimentin, the nonspecific intermediate filament protein in embryonal glia and early differentiating neurones. Dev Biol 1982;91:286–295.

153. Phelps PE, Barber RP, Houser CR, Crawford GD, Salvaterra PM, Vaughn JE. Postnatal development of neurons containing choline acetyltransferase in rat spinal cord: An immunocytochemical study. J Comp Neurol 1984;229:347–361.

154. Miles K, Greengard P, Huganir RL. Calcitonin gene-related peptide regulates phosphorylation of the nicotinic acetylcholine receptor in rat myotubes. Neuron 1989;2:1517–1524.

155. Takami K, Kawai Y, Uchida S, et al. Effect of calcitonin gene-related peptide on contraction of striated muscle in the mouse. Neurosci Lett 1985;60:227–230.

156. Mulle C, Benoit P, Pinset C, Roa M, Changeux JP. Calcitonin gene-related peptide

enhances the rate of desensitization of the nicotinic acetylcholine receptor in cultured mouse muscle cells. Proc Natl Acad Sci USA 1988;85:5728–5732.

157. Kirilovsky J, Duclert A, Fontaine B, Devillers-Thiery A, Osterlund M, Changeux, JP. Acetylcholine receptor expression in primary cultures of embryonic chick myotubes. II. Comparison between the effects of spinal cord cells and calcitonin gene-related peptide. Neuroscience 1989;32:289–296.

158. Shinmi O, Kimura S, Yoshizawa T, et al. Presence of endothelin-1 in porcine spinal cord: Isolation and sequence determination. Biochem Biophys Res Commun 1989;162:340–346.

159. Urakami H, Chiu AY. A monoclonal antibody that recognizes somatic motor neurons in the mature rat nervous system. J Neurosci 1990;10:620–630.

160. Hinton DR, Henderson VW, Blanks JC, Rudnicka M, Miller CA. Monoclonal antibodies react with neuronal subpopulations in the human nervous system. J Comp Neurol 1988;267:398–408.

161. Antel JP, Kuchibhotla J, Stefansson K. Generation of monoclonal antibodies (mAbs) recognizing neuronal elements in formalin-fixed paraffin-embedded human tissue. J Neuropathol Exp Neurol 1985;44:533–545.

162. Chikaraishi DM. Characteristics of brain messenger RNAs. In: Easter SS, Barald KF, Carlson BM, eds. From message to mind. Sinauer Sunderland, MA: Sinauer, 1988:52–65.

muscle declines proportional to the contribution of the affected motor unit. Subsequently, collateral sprouts of adjacent intact motor units grow out to reinnervate the denervated muscle fibers. If sufficient adjacent motor units are available, the entire set of denervated muscle fibers may eventually be reinnervated. The time necessary for reinnervation depends on the sprouting rate and the distance axonal outgrowths of intact neurons have to cross to reach the denervated muscle fibers (the time interval necessary for the initiation of axonal sprouting is omitted from the present discussion). With a higher sprouting rate and sufficient intact axons in their vicinity, less time will elapse until denervated muscle fibers regain innervation. Thus, sprouting efficiency will depend on the sprouting rate and the number of available intact motor units.

At the level of a single motor unit, the description of this process of de- and reinnervation is relatively straightforward. If, however, progressive degeneration is afflicting the entire set of motoneurons in a motor nucleus, a considerable complexity arises for two reasons: First, all motoneurons are not affected synchronously. With a certain decay rate, there is a sequential loss of motoneurons (which, of course, need not exclude the possibility of occasional coincidental cell death). Depending on their individual lifespan and the extent of denervation in their neighborhood, the surviving motor units will increase their size to different amounts. Therefore, each motor unit has its individual history, so that it cannot be considered representative of the behavior of the entire set of motor units during the denervation process. Second, the sprouting rate is not the only factor that determines the efficiency of reinnervation. Several other parameters may influence the reinnervation process: Given a specific sprouting rate, the rate of motoneuron loss and its entire time course determine the time available for axonal sprouts from intact motor units to reach denervated muscle fibers. The actual number of surviving motor neurons and the number of muscle fibers denervated and thus available for reinnervation will also influence sprouting efficiency. Their proportion continually changes during the entire disease process: hence, the influence these factors exert on the efficiency of reinnervation is not constant during the process. The spatial arrangement of motor units in the skeletal muscle is another factor that has to be considered. The territory that single motor units occupy determines the distance to and the number of muscle fibers of other units that may be reached by its outgrowing sprouts. As the number of intact motor units declines toward the end of the process, these distances increase, until a point is reached where a motoneuron dies before it can establish new axonal contacts with denervated fibers (25).

The previous considerations constitute a first qualitative concept of the process of de- and reinnervation in MND. At this level, an explanation can be given for the occurrence of reinnervation signs as detected by electromyography or muscle biopsy. However, difficulties arise if we look for quantitative data. For example, we may be interested in the effect a certain increase in the actual sprouting rate (for instance its doubling) has on the development of the denervation process in MND, and on the resultant clinical course. With regard to recent attempts to improve collateral reinnervation in MND patients (30,31), this question is obviously of some practical relevance for clinical research. It is, therefore, remarkable that available experimental data cannot offer a sufficient basis from which to derive a quantitative estimate for the effects of an increased sprouting rate. The reason for this deficiency is that no experimental conditions can be found that allow for a systematic analysis of the temporal relationship between motoneuron decay, the sprouting rate, and denervation of muscle fibers. In human patients as well as in animal models of the disease, exact values for some essential factors such as the sprouting rate remain undetermined (18). Furthermore, there is no possibility to manipulate single parameters, such as the decay rate of motoneurons, to observe the effects these alterations have on the course of denervation.

A COMPUTER MODEL OF MUSCLE FIBER DENERVATION

The inaccessability of realistic experimental conditions and the abstract nature of the problem are arguments for a theoretical analysis. Two distinct avenues may be followed:

The first may use mathematical equations to describe the behavior of the system. In principle, it is possible to describe the de- and reinnervation process by a set of equations that incorporate variables such as the sprouting rate and the number of innervated muscle fibers. This approach will lead to differential equations, with their solutions providing a quantitative description of the resultant denervation process. Although mathematical formulations have shown their power in many fields of scientific research, some disadvantages with regard to our problem cannot be overlooked: Usually, mathematical formalisms introduce constants the biological meaning of which may remain uncertain. Often, the description of complex systems leads to differential equations for which exact solutions are not known. In this case, simplifications are necessary, and approximations have to be made which may reduce the predictive value of the model for observation or experiments.

Modern computers help to cope successfully with some of these problems by using simulation models. The basic principle of these computer models is that the motor units are modeled according to available morphological and electrophysiological data. The rules for de- and reinnervation of a muscle fiber can then be incorporated into the program. As we saw in the previous description, these can be formulated in relatively simple terms at the level of a single motor unit. Then, an arbitrary time course and sequence of motoneuron loss can be chosen, and the program will apply the de- and reinnervation rules step by step for each muscle fiber. An essential advantage of this approach is that only the basic rules gov-

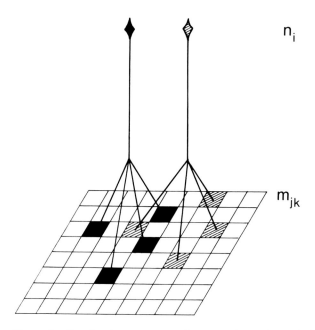

n_i

m_{jk}

Figure 1 Simulated arrangement of cross-sections of muscle fibers (m_{jk}) in a quadratic matrix and their assignment to peripheral motoneurons (n_i).

erning the behavior of single motor units have to be defined. The complexity arising from the large number of motor units with different sizes is then handled by the large storage capacity of the computer and its high calculation rate.

Based on these principles, computer simulations have recently been applied by Cohen et al. to analyze the changes found in skeletal muscle due to the rearrangement of motor units (32). The following discussion is confined to another aspect of chronic denervation, namely, the relation between the kinetics of motoneuron loss and the time course of fiber denervation. For this purpose, a computer program has been created that simulates a set of alpha-motoneurons and a set of muscle fibers innervated by it (33,34). The cross-sections of the simulated muscle fibers (which for simplicity are considered as quadratic with a diameter of 60 μm) are ordered in a square matrix (Fig. 1). Each motoneuron is assigned to a certain number of muscle fibers forming the motor unit. The size of the motor units, as well as their number and the territory they occupy inside the fiber matrix, can be varied. When a motoneuron has died, the fibers it innervated become denervated. Soon afterward, the program searches for inner-vated muscle fibers in their direct vicinity, which are considered possible sources for an outgrowing axonal ending of an intact motor unit. With a certain sprouting rate, this new axonal ending tries to reinnervate the denervated fiber. If there is more than one equidistant innervated muscle fiber in the vicinity, a random generator selects that fiber from which an axonal sprout will finally be sent out. For a detailed analysis, the sprouting rate, as well as the time course of motoneuron loss, can be varied by the experimenter to test their influence on the efficiency of reinnervation.

Figure 2 shows a program run with a linear motoneuron decay. The time course of motoneuron loss is shown in the upper diagram (Fig. 2A). Each step downward represents the death of a single neuron. The total number of muscle fibers innervated by intact motoneurons is given in curve a of the lower diagram (Fig. 2B). It describes the time course of muscle fiber denervation in response to the loss of motoneurons; hence, it is denominated as the denervation curve of the degenerative process. With each motoneuron lost, the number of innervated muscle fibers falls by an amount that corresponds to the size of the lost unit. Subsequently, collateral sprouts grow out to reinnervate the denervated fibers. When they establish new axonal contacts, the total number of innervated muscle fibers rises, and the size of the corresponding motor units increases. To have an estimate for the activity of reinnervation, the number of reinnervated muscle fibers is separately registered in curve b (Fig. 2B).

In the presented simulation experiment, a sprouting rate of 60 μm/month was assumed. As can be seen, the initial loss of motoneurons is well compensated by collateral sprouting until more than 50% of all motoneurons have been lost; these results are in good agreement with experimental findings (25,35,36). In this first phase of compensation, there is permanent denervation, but immediate reinnervation of almost all denervated fibers leads to their rapid connection to surviving motor units. The reinnervation of denervated muscle fibers causes these motor units to continuously increase their size. This has the consequence that with each subsequently lost neuron, the amount of denervated fibers increases. Hence, the steps downward in the denervation curve become larger, and an acceleration of fiber denervation develops toward the end of the process, even though the rate of motoneuron loss remains constant.

The simulation allows some important conclusions to be drawn about the temporal development of denervation: (a) With efficient reinnervation, the number of surviving motoneurons is not strictly correlated with the number of innervated muscle fibers; (b) a considerable portion of all initial neurons may be lost before persistent denervation develops; (c) even a change in the slope of the denervation curve cannot unequivocally indicate a change in the decay rate of motoneurons.

Two essential parameters influence the efficiency of reinnervation and the temporal development of denervation: the actual sprouting rate and the time course of motoneuron loss. An overview of the effects of both parameters on fiber denervation is depicted in Figure 3. Four time courses of neuron loss were

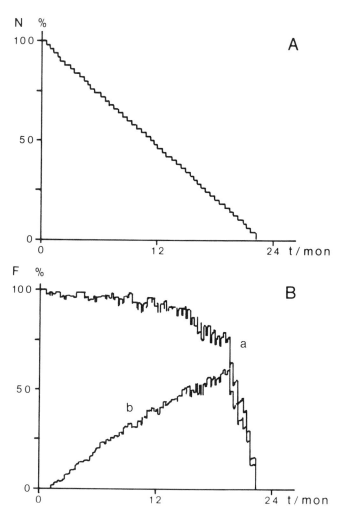

Figure 2 Time course of motoneuron loss and muscle fiber denervation. (A) Decline of the number (N) of intact motoneurons in percent. Each step downward represents the loss of a single neuron. (B, curve a) Denervation curve, showing the total number (F) of innervated muscle fibers (including all fibers that are reinnervated). (B, curve b) Total number of reinnervated muscle fibers. t, Time in months; assumed sprouting rate, 60 μm/month.

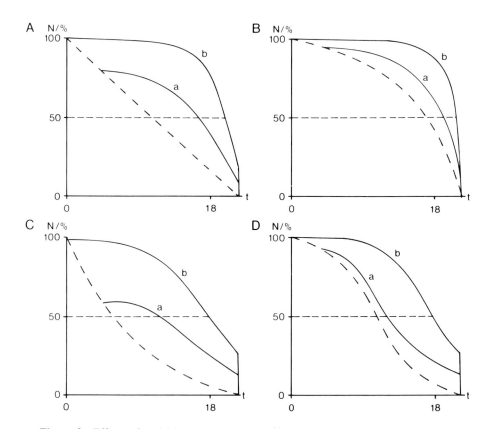

Figure 3   Effects of variable sprouting rates on the denervation curves in dependence from the time course of motoneuron loss. Four time courses of neuron loss are depicted in A–D by the broken lines with linear (A), accelerated (B), decelerated (C), and sigmoidal (D) neuron decay. Continuous lines a and b are the corresponding denervation curves of muscle fibers with sprouting rates of 12 μm/month (a) and 120 μm/month (b). N, Number of intact neurons or innervated muscle fibers, respectively; t, time in months. Depending on the time course of neuron loss, the efficiency of variable sprouting rates is quite different, and large discrepancies exist between the number of preserved neurons and the percentage of innervated muscle fibers.

considered: linear, accelerated, decelerated (exponential), and sigmoidal decay. In each of the four program runs identical sprouting rates were assumed. As can be seen, in all four cases an increase in the sprouting rate led to a distortion of the denervation curves toward the right side. This means that with a higher sprouting rate, more muscle fibers could be kept innervated for a longer time. The degree of distortion, however, was quite different, depending on the time course of motoneuron death. Relatively slight effects were observed with an accelerated decay, especially during the phase when more than 50% of all neurons were degenerated (Fig. 3B). In contrast, identical changes in the sprouting rate led to a much better preservation of innervation in the other three forms of neuron decay. The effects depended on the stage of the degenerative process and the type of neuron loss. For each decay curve, there was a different stage at which reinnervation exhibited its maximal efficiency. The most pronounced effects of reinnervation were observed with a decelerated decay, where even in advanced stages with less than 50% motoneurons left, sprouting was able to postpone the denervation for long periods (Fig. 3C).

Increasing the efficiency of reinnervation had an important effect on the slope of the denervation curves. The higher the sprouting rate, the longer the time during which a certain percentage of muscle fibers could be kept innervated. This higher efficiency increased the size of the surviving motor units, and at the end of the process, denervation rate was largest in those cases with the highest previous reinnervation activity. Hence, what may clinically or electromyographically be considered as a rapid deterioration need not always be due to a corresponding rate of motoneuron loss. Rather, it may also be caused by previous efficient sprouting. This finding has important clinical consequences: (a) Two diametrically opposed reasons are conceivable for the occurrence of extremely rapid progressive courses of the disease with massive denervation: Either there is such a dramatic loss of motoneurons that sprouting is unable to keep muscle fibers from being denervated, or motoneuron loss is moderate and previous reinnervation has been so efficient that the bulk of fibers becomes denervated with the loss of the last, markedly increased motor units. In both cases, the number of surviving neurons innervating a certain percentage of all muscle fibers is quite distinct: With rapid degeneration and sparse reinnervation, a closer relationship is to be found between the number of lost motoneurons and the amount of denervated fibers. In contrast, with extremely efficient previous reinnervation, only a few intact neurons will innervate a large number of muscle fibers, so that the degenerative process is much more advanced than may be expected from the severity of denervation. (b) Obviously, administration of therapeutic agents that improve the sprouting rate makes sense only if a marked shift in the denervation curve can be expected. This is impossible in those cases in which the final rapid denervation is due to efficient previous reinnervation, or in unfavorable forms of neuron loss such as accelerated decay (Fig. 3B).

The previous calculations show that with different time courses of neuron loss and different sprouting rates, various denervation curves can be obtained. On the other hand, identical denervation curves are conceivable with distinct types of neuron decay and a correspondingly different sprouting rate. For therapeutic trials it is necessary to separate these forms, as they provide quite distinct conditions for the action of a tested substance (37). Is it possible to achieve this

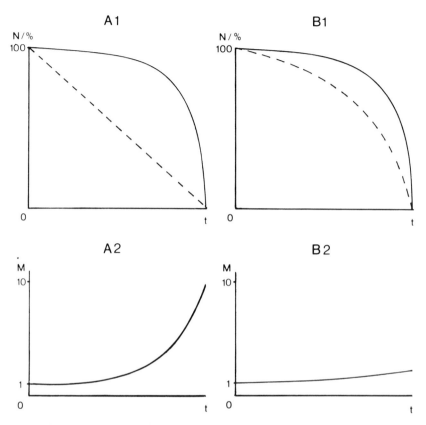

Figure 4 Identical denervation curves (continuous lines in A1 and B1) caused by different time courses of neuron loss (broken lines) due to different sprouting rates. N, Number of preserved motoneurons or innervated muscle fibers, respectively. The corresponding increases of motor unit size (M) with 1 = normal motor unit size are shown in A2 and B2. t, Time.

by clinical means? As the different types of neuron loss are characterized by a different efficiency of reinnervation, changes of the motor unit size should provide some information. An example is shown in Figure 4. A linear and an accelerated neuron decay led to identical denervation curves due to different sprouting rates. What distinguishes both forms is the efficiency of reinnervation. As can be seen, with a linear loss there is a larger increase of motor unit size due to more efficient sprouting. Hence, recordings of motor unit size (as can be clinically done by macro EMG recordings; 38) should help to separate both curves.

Linear Decay

Linear decay of motoneurons implies that the rate of neuron loss is constant during the entire process:

$$D(t) = \frac{dn}{dt} = -a \qquad (7)$$

with $a =$ constant. Integration of this differential equation leads to

$$N(t) = N_0 - a \cdot t \qquad (8)$$

which determines the actual number, $N(t)$, of surviving neurons at a time t, when $a \cdot t$ neurons have been lost. The constant a describes the rate of neuron loss; it can therefore be considered as the expression for the activity of the degenerative process.

An important consequence of linearity is that with the same process activity (as expressed by the same value of a) in motor nuclei with different initial numbers of nerve cells, the entire duration of the process (T) will be longer in cell assemblies containing a larger number of nerve cells (Fig. 6). The exact value can be derived from Eq. (8) with $N(T) = 0$, leading to

$$T = \frac{N_0}{a} \qquad (9)$$

which describes proportionality between disease duration and the initial number of nerve cells.

What conditions are conceivable for a degenerative process to exhibit a linear course? Considering a deterministic process in a homogeneous mixture of nerve cells, linearity can be caused by the action of a damaging agent which, without changing its amount and activity, starts in one or a few neurons and then captures the entire set cell by cell, thereby destroying the neurons it invades. Alternatively, if the process is of probabilistic nature and generalized from the beginning, a linear decline implies that the probability of subsequent cell death continuously increases during the process. For example, if we assume an initial pool of 100 neurons and a loss of one neuron per time interval, then at the beginning the probability of subsequent cell death is $1/100$ per interval. After half of all neurons have been lost, the probability of cell death has increased to $1/50$, because one further neuron will die within the next time interval. And at the end, when only one neuron is left, there is certainty ($p = 1.0$) for this neuron to die. Obviously, any deviation from these probability changes will lead to nonlinear forms of neuron loss.

N

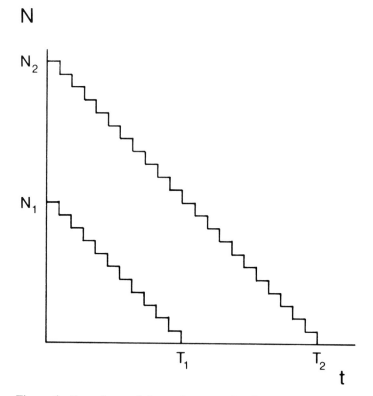

Figure 6 Dependence of the total process duration (T_1, T_2) on the initial number of available neurons (N_1, N_2). With identical decay rates, process duration is longer in the larger neuron pool.

Decelerated Decay

Decelerated decay of neurons implies that the decay rate continuously decreases during the entire process. Such a situation can be found in processes in which the decay rate at a certain time depends on the actual number, $N(t)$, of neurons that are alive. Then we obtain:

$$\frac{dN}{dt} = -b \cdot N(t) \tag{10}$$

with a constant b determining the fraction of all surviving neurons that will degenerate within the next time interval. The entire time course of motoneuron death can then be described by

$$N(t) = N_0 \cdot e^{-bt} \tag{11}$$

which assumes the course of an exponential or decelerated motoneuron loss. If we represent the activity of the degenerative process by the decay rate D at any time t, Eq. (10) indicates a continuous decline of the process activity.

An example for an exponential decay could be a process in which an infectious agent or toxin captures all neurons of the assembly before the outbreak of degeneration. The induced cellular alterations may increase the risk of individual cells to degenerate by equal amounts. If this risk does not change during the degenerative process, at any time t there will always be a constant fraction of all surviving neurons that will die within the subsequent time interval. The decay rate of neurons then depends on the actual number of surviving motoneurons as expressed by Eq. (10).

Accelerated Decay

The decay rate may depend not on the number of surviving neurons, but rather on the time that has elapsed. Then we obtain:

$$\frac{dN}{dt} = -c' \cdot t \tag{12}$$

Substitution of c' by $2c$ and integration of this equation leads to

$$N(t) = N_0 - ct^2 \tag{13}$$

which describes an accelerated decline of the number of intact neurons. With larger values of c, process activity is increased and the entire process duration T is reduced.

Characteristics of an accelerating decay may be found in generalized processes that lead to an accumulation of damage inside the affected cells and thus to an increased risk of degeneration. Then, with increasing process duration, more and more cells will be lost in subsequent intervals.

Sigmoidal Decay

We consider a pathological agent (for instance, a virus) which, after its invasion into intact cells, has to be multiplied and released in order to induce degeneration in other neurons. The number of neurons that will be damaged and lost then depends on the amount of released agents and thus on the number of cells already captured. This number of affected neurons at a time t is $N_0 - N(t)$. In addition, the decay rate also depends on the number, $N(t)$, of neurons that are intact and thus available for further degeneration. Hence we obtain:

$$\frac{dN}{dt} = -f \cdot N(t) \cdot [N_0 - N(t)] \tag{14}$$

with f = constant. If initially one neuron is captured by the infectious agent, integration of Eq. (14) leads to:

$$N(t) = \frac{N_0 \cdot (N_0 - 1)}{e^{f \cdot N_0 \cdot t} + N_0 - 1} \tag{15}$$

which describes a sigmoidal course of neuron loss. The characteristic feature of this kinetic is a continuous increase of cell loss at the beginning, which is followed by a short period of linearity with a final decline of process activity. The initial acceleration is explained by the fact that with an increasing number of affected nerve cells, there will be a corresponding increase in the amount of released damaging agents. At this stage, the number of intact cells outweighs the portion of affected cells, thereby allowing an unrestricted acceleration of cell death. Later in the course of the process, however, an increasing number of affected neurons finds a decreasing number of intact, susceptible cells. Hence, with further progression of the process, the number of susceptible cells is the limiting factor for the decay rate.

The action of an infectious agent limited to a single nucleus is not the only explanation for a sigmoidal decay. Similar characteristics of failure are found in aging processes in many biological systems (44,45). Mathematically, their behavior can be described by the Gompertz equation (46):

$$N(t) = N_0 \cdot \exp \left\{ \frac{h}{g} \, [1 - \exp (g \cdot t)] \right\} \tag{16}$$

where $\exp(x) = e^x$, and h and g are constants. To describe a pathological process of premature aging, the constants h and g in Eq. (16) have to be changed. This operation indicates only a quantitative change of the activity of basic mechanisms, but no qualitative alteration with the advent of new types of pathological processes.

The fundamental difference between these mechanisms and an infection is that with premature aging, all neurons can be assumed to contain the risk of premature death from the beginning of observation; i.e., no transmission of a damaging agent occurs during the disease. Instead, intracellular alterations may suffice to induce cell death. This may be due to an inherited defect in the cells' ability to maintain production of essential cellular proteins with advancing age; alternatively, exposure to exogenous agents may promote progressive intracellular alterations leading to the death of otherwise normal cells.

The similarity between kinetics of quite different natures is an important finding of the previous theoretical analysis, illustrating the caution that must be shown when interpreting the time courses of cell death in terms of possible pathological mechanisms. The reasons for this ambiguity of kinetic descriptions are: (a) in general, any observed curve may be fitted by a variety of analytical

A   B1   B2

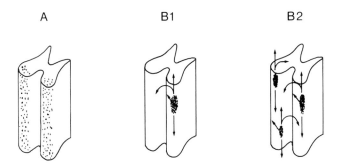

Figure 7   The different types of generalization of a degenerative process inside the anterior horns of the spinal cord. (A) Primary generalization with diffuse loss of motoneurons. (B1 and B2) Secondary generalization with a continuous spread around a focus. In B1, there is one initial focus; in B2, there is multifocal onset of degeneration.

expressions with distinct parameter combinations; (b) kinetics regard only one aspect of cell loss, namely, the numerical decline of intact cells in a limited neuron pool. It must, however, be recognized that the diminution of the number of intact cells is always accompanied by a spatial extension of lesions inside the affected cell assembly. The actual pattern of neuronal degeneration may or may not be essential for the further development of degeneration. Hence, two types of motor neuron loss can be distinguished:

1. Neuronal death develops independently from the actual anatomical and functional structure of the affected motor nucleus and the spatial distribution of the diseased neurons. This means that all neurons degenerate independently from each other solely due to internal pathological alterations. Such a situation may occur if all neurons are exposed simultaneously to a damaging agent before or during the degenerative process. Alternatively, the agent may have captured all neurons before the outbreak of degeneration so rapidly that the sequence in which the neurons have been invaded has no influence on the sequence of subsequent cell loss. Independent cell death will also occur in processes in which degeneration is solely due to internal alterations. Premature aging could be an example of this type of damage if no mutual interactions of the affected neurons contribute to their degeneration. The common feature of all these cases is that generalization of the underlying process or agent has taken place before the outbreak of degeneration (''primary generalization,'' Fig. 7A). The sequence of cell loss is then uninfluenced by the mode of their invasion, so that the kinetics of cell death solely reflect the essential formal features of the intracellular alterations leading to degeneration.

2. Alternatively, the development of degeneration may critically depend on the initial pattern and sequence of cell destruction and structural properties of the

involved motor nuclei. These factors are important if degeneration is caused by a damaging agent or process that has to be transmitted from affected cells to their intact neighbors. If only a few neurons are initially affected ("focal onset"), and if the spread of the agent parallels the development of degeneration, generalization will occur at the end of the process ("secondary generalization"). In this case, a continuous and systematic extension into adjacent areas can be expected (Fig. 7B). The activity of degeneration will then depend on the initial number of neurons captured (and thereby able to transmit the agent), their location inside the nucleus, and properties of the transmission process. In this situation, the kinetics of cell death reflect not only intracellular alterations, but also the mode of transmission of the damaging agent or process inside the cell assembly.

The term "transmissibility" may be considered equivalent to infectiousness, implying the propagation of viral or bacterial organisms. There is currently no experimental evidence for an infectious etiology of MND (47), and hence, the discussion of transmissible agents may seem rather theoretical. It should, however, be recognized that "transmissibility" may be used in a much broader sense. This notion covers the propagation of any damaging chemical or biological agent which in order to act must be transmitted from a source (which may be the bloodstream, the glia cells, the extracellular space, or affected neurons) to intact cells. The amount of damaging material may remain constant or it may increase due to its reproduction inside affected cells. Thus, transmission is not restricted to the propagation of infectious material such as virus particles; it also includes the spatial extension of toxic substances that invade the neurons from outside. Moreover, the term is also applicable to the development of degenerative processes that are induced not by the direct communication of an agent, but by a deficit of physiological factors necessary for the survival of intact neurons to which they are exposed. For instance, degeneration of an individual neuron may be due to its cut from trophic influences of adjacent degenerated cells to which it was connected (76,77). If this damaged neuron itself exerts a trophic activity on other cells, its loss may transmit degeneration to other neurons without a corresponding communication of damaging material.

As the mode of generalization of a damaging agent has important consequences for the interpretation of cell death kinetics, a more detailed discussion of the propagation of transmissible agents will be given in the following section.

SPATIAL EXTENSION OF DEGENERATION INSIDE A NEURON POOL

Considerations as to the spatial extension of a transmissible degenerative process introduce a remarkable complexity, as not only the structure of the affected cell assemblies but also the initial distribution of lesions and the mode of propagation of cell defects have to be incorporated into a theoretical concept. There are mathematical models available that are used in the theory of infectious diseases to describe the propagation of transmissible agents in two dimensions (48). In principle, they may be adapted to the description of neuronal degeneration inside a three-dimensional nucleus. However, a major drawback of this approach is that, even with two dimensions, rather complex formulations arise which present formidable difficulties in their handling, so that extreme simplifications are usually necessary to obtain concrete results.

An alternative way to attack the problem is the use of computer simulation models. This can be done in a way similar to that which has been described for analysis of the de- and reinnervation process in skeletal muscle. What is needed is a set of modeled motoneurons. Their interconnections, as well as the mode in which a damaging agent captures individual cells, have to be defined. The program user is free to change the structure of the neuron pool or the properties of the simulated degenerative process. According to the choice of parameters, the computer is able to calculate the temporal decline of the number of intact neurons (i.e., the kinetic curves), as well as the corresponding spatial pattern of degeneration inside the afflicted area and its further development.

The following section will provide some insight into such computer simulations. The calculations concentrate on the relation between the spatial extension of a transmissible agent and the resultant kinetics of cell loss. As an approximation, the neurons in the motor nucleus were considered to be arranged at equidistant positions in a three-dimensional grid comprising a column with a cross-section of $n \cdot m$ neurons and a height of k neurons. The total number of motoneurons is then given by $N_0 = n \cdot m \cdot k$. An example is given in Figure 8A, showing a cubic grid with $5 \cdot 5 \cdot 5$ neurons.

Our analysis will start with a deterministic transmissible process, first affecting a single neuron. It is assumed that a neuron inside the grid, once it has been captured by the damaging agent, transmits degeneration within one short time interval to its six nearest neighbors, i.e., four cells in the same plane, and one additional cell in the upper and lower adjacent layers, respectively (Fig. 8B). For those neurons located at the outer surfaces, edges, or corners of the grid, the number of direct neighbors is obviously lower (i.e., five, four, and three cells, respectively).

Figure 8, C and D, illustrates the influence of the site of onset of the lesion and the mode of transmission on the kinetics of neuron decay in the grid. With one neuron affected in the center, a rapid degeneration can be observed (Fig. 8, C1 and D). If the first affected cell is located at the grid's surface, a slowing of neuron decay occurs, although the elementary mechanisms of cell-to-cell transmission are unaltered (Fig. 8, C2 and D). This difference is obviously due to the fact that with a position inside the nucleus, more directions—and thus more cells—are available for the propagation of degeneration. If the process is trans-

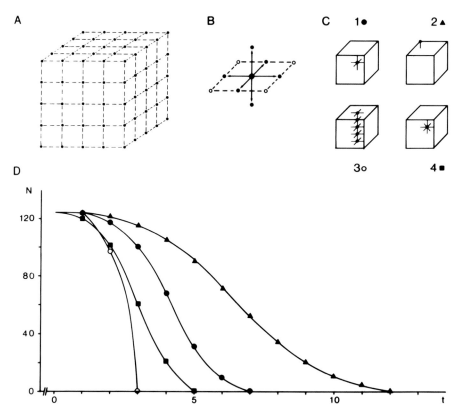

Figure 8 Simulation of the spread of a transmissible agent inside a motor nucleus. (A) 125 motoneurons are arranged in a cubic grid. (B) Each affected neuron transmits degeneration to its six neighboring cells. (C) Different sites of onset lead to different kinetics of cell death in D; in C1, degeneration starts in the center of the nucleus, in C2 in a neuron at the left posterior and upper corner of the grid. The sites of onset are symbolized by closed circles. N, Number of intact neurons; t, time in arbitrary units. In C3, transmission starts in five neurons with a corresponding rapid neuron loss in D (open circles). A rapid loss can also be observed if an affected neuron transmits degeneration more efficiently not to six, but to eight neighboring cells (C4 and D, closed squares).

mitted more efficiently not only to the six nearest cells, but to the entire shell of eight cells surrounding each neuron inside the grid, of course, a much more rapid progression develops (Fig. 8, C4 and D).

The anatomy of the affected nucleus is another important factor determining the time course of neuronal death, provided a transmissible agent is responsible for degeneration. In Figure 9, A1 and A2, degeneration develops in the same

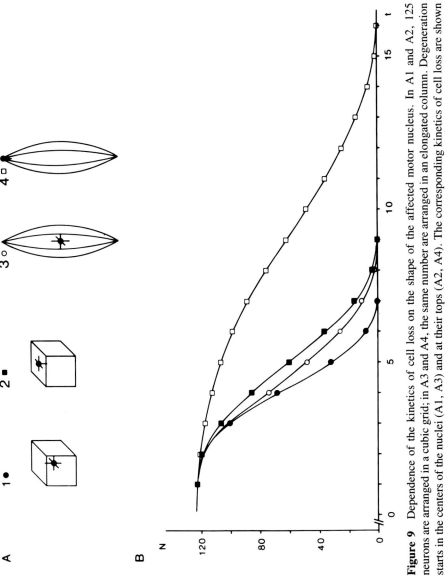

Figure 9 Dependence of the kinetics of cell loss on the shape of the affected motor nucleus. In A1 and A2, 125 neurons are arranged in a cubic grid; in A3 and A4, the same number are arranged in an elongated column. Degeneration starts in the centers of the nuclei (A1, A3) and at their tops (A2, A4). The corresponding kinetics of cell loss are shown in B. N, Number of intact cells; t, time in arbitrary units.

N / %

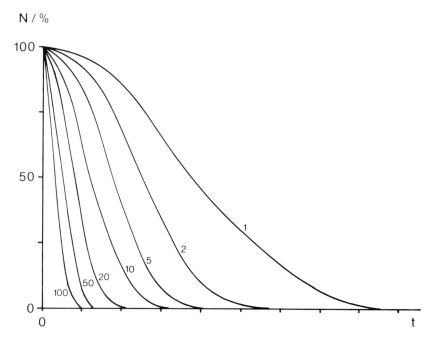

Figure 10 Dependence of the cell death kinetics on the number of initially affected neurons. Assumed is a transmissible agent, which continuously spreads inside a nucleus with 5·5·25 neurons. The initial number of affected cells is given with each curve. N, Number of intact neurons; t, time in arbitrary units.

cubic grid as in the previous simulations. In Figure 9, A3 and A4, an identical number of neurons are arranged in an elongated column with decreasing cross-sections at the ends. As can be seen, with cell death starting from corresponding positions in both cell assemblies, process duration is always extended in the elongated cell column. An extreme prolongation is observed when degeneration has to start from the top of this column (Fig. 9, A4, B). In this case, many more steps are necessary for the damaging process to traverse the entire nucleus.

Besides the distribution of primary lesions and the structure of the affected neuron pool, the number of initially affected neurons is an additional factor determining the rapidity of a transmissible form of degeneration. This is shown in Figure 10; as can be seen, the rate of neuron loss increases to a large extent when more neurons are initially involved.

It is important to note that irrespective of the initial conditions, in most instances, the kinetics of cell loss were sigmoidal. The reason for this behavior has already been given in the mathematical description of sigmoidal kinetics

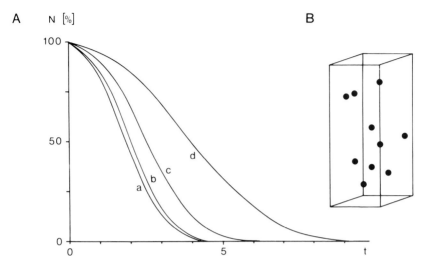

Figure 11 Kinetics of cell loss with transmission of degeneration inside a column of 5·5·25 cells. Ten neurons are initially affected (B). In A, different transmission probabilities (p) are assumed (a, $p = 1.00$; b, $p = 0.75$; c, $p = 0.5$; d, $p = 0.25$). N, Number of intact neurons; t, time in arbitrary units.

(p. 410). The rate of cell loss in a transmissible process depends not only on the number of affected neurons, but also on the number of intact neurons available for invasion. At the beginning, the number of surviving neurons is large enough to allow a progressive increase of cell loss. Toward the end of the process, the number of intact cells continuously decreases and thus the rate of neuron loss also declines.

Up to now, we considered the propagation of cell death as a deterministic phenomenon: With degeneration occurring in a certain neuron at time t, the death of its direct neighbors was certain to occur within the subsequent time interval. What happens if transmission of cell degeneration is probabilistic, so that there is only some likelihood for an affected neuron to communicate cell death to its neighborhood? In biological terms, this change corresponds to a variable time necessary for an agent to reach adjacent intact neurons due to different cell distances, tissue barriers, or resistances of individual neurons against their invasion. An example of stochastic calculations is shown in Figure 11, in which cell degeneration was calculated for a nucleus forming a column with 5·5·25 neurons. Ten neurons were randomly chosen as initially affected by the degenerative process (Fig. 11B). With a transmission probability $p = 1.0$, the propagation of cell death is deterministic as before, and rapid neuron loss characterized the corresponding kinetic (Fig. 11A,a). Then, p was reduced to values of

0.75, 0.5, and 0.25, respectively. This decrease means that only a fraction of all those neurons which in a deterministic process would be captured will degenerate within the next time interval. For instance, we may assume a transmission probability $p = 0.5$. In this case, only half of all neighbors will be lost in the subsequent interval, and with a further reduction of p, a corresponding lower number of neurons will die. Consequently, more time is needed for all neurons of the entire nucleus to be lost, so that the entire process is extended.

In conclusion, even these simplified models clearly demonstrate that with a transmissible agent, cell death kinetics depend not only on the particular mode of transmission, but also on circumstantial factors, such as the structure of the affected system or the initial distribution of lesions. When comparing the different time courses of cell death in the previous simulations, one could come to the conclusion that different process activities existed which may have been due either to distinct basic pathological mechanisms or to a variable resistance of individual cells in the different assemblies to an attack of the damaging agent. However, our simulations were based on identical elementary mechanisms governing the actual cell-to-cell transmission of the damaging agent. Hence, these examples clearly illustrate the limitations of pathophysiological interpretations solely based on kinetic descriptions. Sequential assessments of single muscles, even if done by sophisticated methods (such as quantitative strength measurements, electromyography of the corresponding muscles, or electrophysiological motor unit counting), can therefore provide only limited insight into the basic properties of the degenerative process.

SPATIAL DISTRIBUTION OF LESIONS— CLINICAL FINDINGS IN MND PATIENTS

Cell death kinetics are one aspect of the dynamics of motoneuron degeneration. Their second component is the spatial extension of the degenerative process in the entire motor system. As already pointed out, an essential feature of the degenerative process is the type of generalization of motoneuron loss. Whether there is a primary or secondary generalization in MND has major implications not only for the interpretation of cell death kinetics, but also for the evaluation of pathophysiological concepts.

Most current theories on the etiopathogenesis of MND favor defects that should affect all motoneurons more or less diffusely. This applies to the hypothesis of an exogenous intoxication as well as to concepts of disturbed calcium, glutamate, or DNA metabolism, or premature aging (49–54). Clinically, one would expect the occurrence of widespread degeneration of motoneurons from the onset of the disease, with a random involvement of individual muscle groups. Is such an irregular pattern found in MND patients?

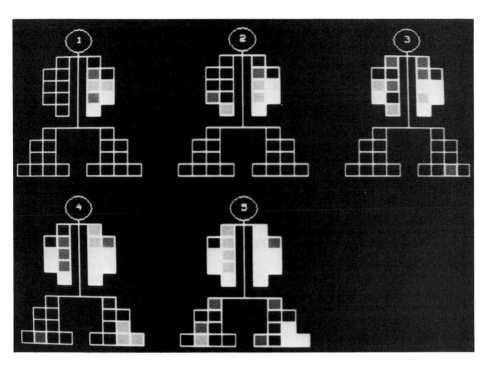

Figure 12 Development of muscular weakness in an ALS patient with focal onset in the left arm. Five consecutive examinations. Semianatomical scheme; each square represents a tested muscle group. Extensor muscle are located at the outside, flexor muscles at the inside of each extremity. Manual force testing with nine distinct grades encoded in nine gray-tone values, ranging from 0: brightest gray tone = complete paresis to grade 9: darkest gray tone = normal strength. There was a continuous spread of weakness with predominant involvement of the left side in arms and legs, which persisted until the end of observation. Details of the visualization method are described in Ref. 84.

In a recent clinical longitudinal study, the pattern of muscular weakness and atrophy and its temporal development has been assessed in detail in large groups of ALS patients (26). Focal onset of symptoms was a usual finding in patients who were examined in initial stages of their disease. Corroborating earlier observations (cf. 55), the site of onset was variable, with a slight preponderance for the cervical region. This finding seems to support the view of an irregular involvement of certain neuron pools. The further development, however, was remarkably systematic in two respects: (a) Confirming earlier observations of Munsat and co-workers, a linear decline of muscular strength was found in almost all patients (27). (b) Once weakness had started in a certain region (for instance, the hand muscles of one arm), there was continuous spread of paresis to other, previously intact regions. An example is shown in Figure 12. Adjacent muscles of the initially involved region were usually the next in which weakness developed irrespective of the site of onset. No patient was found in whom isolated paresis of one upper (or lower) extremity was directly followed by selective involvement of contralateral lower (or upper) extremity muscles. If both arms and legs were affected asymmetrically, there was always a concordant asymmetry in arm and leg muscles. Hence, no clinical evidence was found for a random involvement of different muscle groups. Instead, the development of muscular weakness in ALS was very systematic and seemed to follow the principle of secondary generalization with continuous spread into anatomically adjacent regions.

It must be recognized that the described clinical studies can provide only indirect evidence for the dynamics of the underlying degenerative process. Considering the discrepancies that may exist between motoneuron loss and fiber denervation, it is therefore premature to draw definitive conclusions about the pathophysiological features of motoneuron degeneration. However, it is rather unlikely that a generalized random process of neuron loss is so well matched with a variable degree of reinnervation and compensation in different muscles that the observed systematic pattern of muscle involvement is mimicked. Therefore, the obtained clinical findings create a rationale basis for the above-described theoretical considerations of transmissible damaging agents as a possible cause of neuron degeneration; the implications of this concept are obviously so important that additional investigations will be necessary to substantiate these data.

SIMULATING THE HISTOLOGICAL
PATTERN OF CELL LOSS

Clinical investigations, even if done carefully and with the use of additional methods such as EMG or muscle biopsies, can provide only indirect evidence for the mode of extension of neuronal degeneration inside the motor system. More information may be obtained by histological assessments of the spatial distribution of cell loss inside an affected motor nucleus. The microscopic pattern of degeneration should be influenced by the mode in which individual neurons are captured by the process. The simulation model also provides the means to examine the relation between the mode of transmission and the resultant spatial distribution of cell loss. The main features of the program are as follows: When the computer calculates the development of cell loss in a neuron pool, at each stage the distribution of lesions can be visualized at any cross-section of the assumed cell assembly. Thus, the spread of degeneration inside this section can be followed from its onset. As in the previous simulations, the program user is free to determine the shape of the considered assembly and the type of connections between individual neurons. In the above simulations, these contacts were extremely simplified, as one neuron was directly connected to its four nearest neighbors. Other arrangements are conceivable. For example, each neuron may have direct contacts not only to adjacent cells, but also to more distant neurons, possibly with a more or less random pattern due to direct or interneuronal connections. The intensity of these contacts may vary, which—of course—will influence the probability of transmission of an agent if it is communicated via these pathways.

If there is degeneration due to a primary generalization of the damaging agent, the particular structural properties of the affected cell assembly should have no influence on the development of degeneration. Each neuron bears its own risk for premature failure from the onset of degeneration, and it is purely intracellular alterations that lead to cell death. Hence, histological examinations will reveal a more or less random distribution of cell loss at any stage of the process. If there is a systematic transmission of a damaging agent from few initially affected cells with secondary generalization, the situation is much more complex: With one neuron initially captured, there may be a continuous spread around this source (Fig. 13A). This may be due to two distinct pathophysiological conditions: (a) The damaging agent is released from the first affected cell into the surrounding tissue, i.e, the mixture of glia cells and intercellular space. If this compartment is considered as homogeneous (which is, of course, a simplification), a diffusion-like process will spread around the source (a detailed discussion of this phenomenon is given in Ref. 56). (b) Alternatively, there may be a transmission of the damaging agent from neuron to neuron via dendritic, recurrent axonal or interneuronal cell contacts without any contribution of the surrounding extraneuronal space. In this case, a continuous spread around the source is conceivable only if we use our simple network in which each neuron is arranged on a grid with direct contacts only to neurons in its vicinity. If the neuronal contacts are not ordered so systematically, so that even remote cells have direct contacts with an affected neuron, a more or less random pattern of lesions appears although there is a systematic cell-to-cell transmission starting from a single source (Fig. 13B).

The situation becomes much more complex if more than one neuron is initially affected. If these cells are randomly distributed inside the nucleus, an arbitrary pattern develops which may conceal the further systematic transmission. The conclusion that can be drawn from these calculations is that the spatial extension of cell degeneration may be determined not only by properties of the agent, but also by the fine structure of the affected system. A homogeneous involvement of certain regions strongly suggests a systematic transmission of the damaging agent. On the other hand, a random pattern of cell loss does not exclude this possibility. As a consequence, the more or less widespread loss of

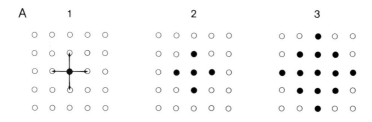

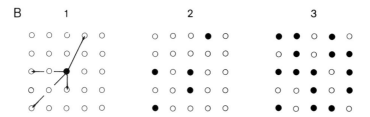

Figure 13   Cell-to-cell transmission of degeneration inside a quadratic motor nucleus. Open circles: intact neurons; closed circles: affected cells. In A, each affected cell transmits damage to its four neighbors with a resultant continuous spread of degeneration. In B, there is also a systematic cell-to-cell transmission. However, each neuron has direct contacts not always to the cells in its vicinity, but to more distant neurons. Hence, an irregular pattern of degeneration develops (1–3).

motoneurons with some cells well preserved, which is found in the anterior horns and lower brainstem nuclei (4), is not an unequivocal sign for a process generalized from the beginning; modes of a systematic cell-to-cell transmission are conceivable which lead to similar patterns.

CONCLUSIONS: THE ROLE OF SIMULATION STUDIES IN MND RESEARCH

In the previous sections, a theoretical approach to understanding the formal aspects of motoneuron degeneration with de- and reinnervation of skeletal muscle fibers has been outlined. Based on computer simulation studies and mathematical models, a quantitative description of the kinetics and dynamics of cell death was obtained. The calculations revealed a rather complex relationship between the time course of muscle fiber denervation and the kinetics of motoneuron death on the one hand, and between these kinetics and the properties of possible underlying pathological mechanisms on the other. The range of feasible parameter combinations was large, with a corresponding multiplicity of different outcomes. By itself, each of these models allows no decision to be made about whether it is realistic. From a purely mathematical point of view, this is not a major drawback, as it may seem interesting enough to create a general theory of neuron degeneration irrespective of its concrete realizations. However, from a clinical and pathophysiological viewpoint we have to explore the practical use of the theory and its applications in MND research.

In principle, the contribution made by the theoretical studies presented falls into two complementary components: First, the created models may help to provide insight into some general mechanisms of the degenerative process and their consequences for muscle fiber denervation. Second, with a sufficient degree of realism, predictions can be made as to the behavior of the real disease process, when certain parameters are varied.

To understand the principles governing a natural process, it is not always necessary to create a detailed model incorporating all aspects of the process. It is often helpful to first reduce the number of parameters used to those that seem most essential. The corresponding theoretical formulation implies a high level of abstraction and simplification. This may reduce the realism of the model, but at the same time the intelligibility of the complex interactions is increased. Occasionally, it is the case that, even with a high degree of simplification, natural phenomena can be described with remarkable exactness. In these instances, the factors that were not taken into account are presumably of minor significance.

If sufficient insight into the interactions of essential elements has been obtained, simulations can be improved by including additional factors that introduce more realistic features of the natural process. The model can then be used to make predictions as to the effects of parameter changes, which are not otherwise obtainable, either because single parameters cannot be directly observed or manipulated, or because the time scale of the process is too large or too small for the conduct of real experiments.

At the present stage of development, the simulations presented here can hardly be considered a realistic model of motoneuron degeneration and muscle fiber denervation in MND. The existence of different fiber types, as well as variabilities in the capability of individual motor units to send out axonal sprouts, has still not been taken into account. Only a tentative description of the temporal development of muscular weakness could be achieved by introduction of a force factor that related the denervation curves to the decline in force output. This parametrization is, of course, a crude approximation, as the generation of muscular force is determined by additional important factors, such as the recruitment pattern of single units, their discharge frequency, or fatiguability (12,57). The analysis of neuron degeneration inside the motor system was confined to pure lower motoneuron lesions, and only a simplified network of motoneurons was considered with rather oversimplified cell contacts. Hence, the model calculations provide a general framework of basic relations, which enable estimates to be done on the effects that factors such as the sprouting rate or the time course of neuron degeneration may exert on the innervation state of activated muscles and thus on the development of clinical deficits. These theoretical results have to be considered as fundamentals, which are necessary but not sufficient for an understanding of the disease process in human patients. There is no principal argument against the elaboration of more detailed programs, which assume more realistic features for improved predictions on the course of the disease process.

The simulations clearly illustrate the discrepancy that may exist between the development of muscle fiber denervation and the time course of motoneuron loss. Depending on the efficiency of reinnervation, similar types of motoneuron decay can lead to different denervation curves of muscle fibers. On the other hand, similar denervation curves may be generated by quite different time courses of motoneuron death; their essential difference is in the number of intact motoneurons available at the same stages of muscle fiber denervation and a variable intensity of reinnervation. These findings are of major importance for assessing the severity of the disease and its further prognosis. Obviously, pure strength measurements are insufficient to determine the stage of the disease and to analyze the kinetics of neuron loss. It is, therefore, necessary to combine these testings with electrophysiological assessments of the reinnervation intensity and the force output of individual motor units. Hence, quantitative EMG recordings as provided by single fiber- or macro EMG are useful tools for a more adequate evaluation of the course of the disease. More direct estimates of the time course of neuron degeneration are possible by using electrophysiological methods of motor unit counting (58–61). Recent investigations provide some evidence that an exponential loss of motor units is a characteristic of MND at least in advanced stages the disease (41–43). However, no sufficient information is as yet available on the initial phase of degeneration, and it cannot be ruled out that what appeared as an exponential loss was in fact the final phase of a sigmoidal decay of motoneurons. As discussed earlier, these differences in the kinetics would have major implications for the interpretation of the underlying pathological mechanisms, and further studies on initially intact muscles will be necessary to clarify this point.

Despite the available clinical and electrophysiological approaches to assess the time course of neuron loss in MND, it cannot be ignored that pathophysiological conclusions about to the properties of the underlying degenerative process are difficult to derive solely from kinetic descriptions of cell death in a single motor nucleus. Notwithstanding an additional involvement of central motoneurons (which reduces the significance of strength recordings for the determination of cell kinetics in a motor nucleus), a variety of circumstantial factors may influence the time course of cell death in a motor nucleus. Studies on the temporal development of neuron degeneration inside a motor nucleus therefore remain difficult to interpret in terms of the underlying pathological mechanisms.

The kinetics of cell death in a single nucleus are, however, not the only aspect of the dynamics of degeneration. A second component is the spatial spread of the process inside the entire motor system. Its study may offer interesting insights into fundamental properties of the underlying degenerative process, insights that are necessary for the interpretation of cell death kinetics. As already discussed, the type of generalization of the degenerative process is an essential formal aspect of MND. Clinically, its identification is possible by assessing the pattern of neuromuscular lesions and their further extension. Two general classes of processes must be distinguished: degeneration with primary and secondary generalization. Both types can be differentiated in human patients by using clinical and electrophysiological methods. The described recent clinical findings on MND patients are compatible with a focal onset of degeneration and a subsequent secondary generalization, thereby suggesting a continuous spread of a transmissible damaging agent or process inside the motor system (26). It is essential to realize that this concept of transmissibility is applied to an individual motor system with *motoneurons* as the elements captured by the etiological agent. This has strictly to be separated from transmissible (i.e., infectious) agents which are communicated between *individuals*; the failure of previous transmission experiments to induce MND in laboratory animals (47) therefore does not argue against this concept.

Cell-to-cell communication of a damaging agent or process, which has been analyzed in the previous simulations, could easily account for one unsolved problem of MND: the selectivity of neuronal death with preservation of surrounding neuronal and nonneuronal tissue, which is found even in advanced stages of the disease (4). According to this concept, once a damaging agent has entered the motor system in one region, its further propagation can only occur via motoneurons. The pathways may be direct dendritic or interneuronal contacts, which have been described for anterior horn cells (8,62). That some motoneurons are solely affected may be attributable to their peculiar location in the nervous system (63): Lower motoneurons are the only neurons that are connected to nonneuronal tissue; their peripheral endings are devoid of a blood-brain barrier and therefore exposed to noxious influences, which may be mediated by retrograde axoplasmic flow. Peripheral uptake by motor nerve endings and retrograde transport has been demonstrated experimentally for substances such as tetanus and cholera toxin (64,65), metals (66), immunoglobulins (67–70), and virus particles (71,72). A transsynaptic spread, which is essential for explaining the combined lesions in ALS, has been shown for toxins as well as viral particles (73–75). Alternatively, the loss of trophic influences from the periphery could also lead to a systematic loss of motoneurons (76,77). Hence, several conceivable mechanisms could account for the observed clinical phenomena, and current theories on the etiopathogenesis of MN that favor a primary more than the observed secondary generalization have to be reevaluated in light of this new concept.

In addition to these pathophysiological considerations, the planning and interpretation of therapeutic trials is another aspect that must be considered on the basis of the obtained theoretical results (37). It seems reasonable to assume that the opportunity to achieve and detect beneficial effects of a therapeutic agent will depend on the stage of the disease, i.e., the number of neurons available. Some time will be necessary for the agent to reach the neurons and to exert its beneficial effects. During this latency period (the actual duration of which remains currently unknown), further predamaged neurons will die. Even if all surviving neurons are simultaneously exposed to sufficient concentrations of the therapeutic agent, it seems unrealistic to assume that all of them can benefit; individual differences may vary the degree of their damage as well as their response to therapy. Hence, with a smaller number of available cells, there is less likelihood to exert protective effects. Thresholds for the stage of the disease are therefore conceivable below which no beneficial effects are detectable despite the principle efficiency of an administered agent. The identification of these clinical limits will be an issue for future theoretical and clinical investigations.

The studies presented in this chapter are not the only applications of computer simulations to neuromuscular problems. Willison created a computer program to analyze whether fiber-type distribution in skeletal muscles follows a random pattern (78). By comparing the results of stochastic calculations with histological findings, deviations from a random pattern could be found suggesting the existence of mechanisms that lower the adjacency of muscle fibers of the same unit. Computer simulations were also performed to analyze the relationship between the architecture of motor units and the motor unit action potentials recorded by EMG (79–83). In contrast to real experiments, these theoretical studies allowed estimates to be made of the contribution single muscle fibers of an activated motor unit make to the generation of the entire unit potential.

Cohen and co-workers recently described a computer program that modeled the spatial distribution of motor units with their corresponding fiber types in skeletal muscle (32). The de- and reinnervation process occurring in response to a progressive loss of motoneurons was simulated in a way similar to the calculations described in this chapter. In contrast to our studies, this model differentiated between distinct fiber types. Thus, attention could be devoted to the phenomenon of fiber-type grouping, which is found in chronic denervating diseases. By varying the fiber-type-specific death rates of the corresponding motoneurons, it could be shown that a preferential death of one type of motoneuron may account for the fiber-type predominance that is found in several neuromuscular disorders. In addition, the effects of collateral sprouting on the changes of the motor unit areas were tested. Confirming previous electrophysiological results (20), only a modest increase of the unit areas was found, indicating that axons in the vicinity of a denervated muscle fiber are responsible for reinnervation. In single-fiber EMG, an increase of the fiber density (FD) is used as an estimate of the intensity of reinnervation. The simulations made it possible to relate FD increases to the amount of motoneurons that had been lost; these results are therefore important to interpret clinical EMG findings with respect to the underlying degenerative process in the anterior horn cells.

All these different models clearly illustrate that besides direct observation, clinical investigation, and laboratory experiments, computer simulations may be used as an additional avenue for neuromuscular studies. As in any other field of scientific research in which computer modeling has found applications, this new approach should be considered a method which, in conjunction with experiments, offers new perspectives for the study of neuromuscular disorders. Obviously, the fitting of model calculations with direct observation and experimental results is no proof of the correctness of the assumptions on which the model was based. In addition, it cannot be expected that the molecular events that underlie cell destruction in MND will directly lead to observable clinical phenomena. Hence, dynamic studies and their theoretical fundamentals will not identify the etiology of MND. The mathematical models and computer simulations provide a guide for further experimental research and an interpretation of its results. Obtaining insight into complex phenomena, raising new questions for experimental research, and testing consequences of pathophysiological concepts are the main achievements of this new method; its ultimate aim is to better understand one of the most intriguing challenges in neurology.

ACKNOWLEDGMENT

These studies were supported by the Wilhelm-Sander-Stiftung and the Stifterverband für die Deutsche Wissenschaft.

REFERENCES

1. Tandan T, Bradley WG. Amyotrophic lateral sclerosis. Part 1. Clinical features, pathology, and ethical issues in management. Ann Neurol 1985;18:271–280.
2. Tandan, T, Bradley WG. Amyotrophic lateral sclerosis. Part 2. Etiopathogenesis. Ann Neurol 1985;18:419–431.
3. Mitsumoto H, Hanson MR, Chad DA. Amyotrophic lateral sclerosis. Recent advances in pathogenesis and therapeutic trials. Arch Neurol 1986;45:189–202.
4. Hirano A, Malamud N, Kurland LT, Zimmerman HM. A review of the pathological findings in amyotrophic lateral sclerosis. In: Norris FH, Kurland LT, eds. Motor neuron diseases. Research on amyotrophic lateral sclerosis and related disorders. New York: Grune & Stratton, 1969:51–60.

5. Iwata M, Hirano A. Current problems in the pathology of amyotrophic lateral sclerosis. In: Zimmerman HM, ed. Progress in neuropathology. New York: Raven Press, 1979:277–298.

6. Hughes JT. Pathology of amyotrophic lateral sclerosis. In: Rowland P, ed. Human motor neuron diseases. New York: Raven Press, 1982:61–73.

7. Burke RE. The physiology of alpha-motoneurons and their synaptic input in relation to the problem of amyotrophic lateral sclerosis. In: Andrews JM, Johnson RT, Brazier MAB, eds. Amyotrophic lateral sclerosis: Recent research trends. New York: Academic Press, 1974:119–133.

8. Burke RE. Motor units in cat muscles: Anatomical considerations in relation to motor unit types. In: Rowland P, ed. Human motor neuron diseases. New York: Raven Press, 1982:31–44.

9. Cullheim S. Relations between cell body size, axon diameter and axon conduction velocity of cat sciatic alpha-motoneurons stained with horseradish peroxidase. Neurosci Lett 1978;8:17–20.

10. Cullheim S, Kellerth JO. A morphological study of the axons and recurrent axon collaterals of cat alpha-motoneurones supplying different functional types of muscle unit. J Physiol 1978;281:301–313.

11. Harris DA, Henneman E. Identification of two species of alpha-motoneurons in cat's plantaris pool. J Neurophysiol 1977;40:16–25.

12. Henneman E, Mendell LM. Functional organization of motoneuron pool and its inputs. In: Brookhart JM, Mountcastle VB, Brooks VB, Geiger SR, eds. Handbook of physiology. Section 1. The nervous system. Vol. II. Motor control. Part 1. Bethesda, MD: American Physiological Society, 1981:423–507.

13. Kernell D, Zwaagstra B. Input conductance, axonal conduction velocity and cell size among hindlimb motoneurons of the cat. Brain Res 1981;204:311–326.

14. Andres PL, Hedlund W, Finison L, Conlon T, Felmus M, Munsat TL: Quantitative motor assessment in amyotrophic lateral sclerosis. Neurology 1986;36:936–941.

15. Beasley WC. Quantitative muscle testing: Principles and applications to research and clinical services. Arch Phys Med Rehabil 1961;42:398–425.

16. Brooks BR, Sufit RL, Clough JA, et al. Isokinetic and functional evaluation of muscle strength over time in amyotrophic lateral sclerosis. In: Munsat TL, ed. Quantification of neurologic deficit. Boston: Butterworth, 1989:143–154.

17. Kuether G, Struppler A, Lipinski H-G. Therapeutic trials in ALS—The design of a protocol. In: Cosi V, Kato AC, Parlette W, Pinelli P, Poloni M, eds. Adv Exp Med Biol 1987;209:265–276.

18. Bradley WG. Recent views on amyotrophic lateral sclerosis with emphasis on electrophysiological studies. Muscle Nerve 1987;10:490–502.

19. Lambert EH, Mulder DW. Electromyographic studies in amyotrophic lateral sclerosis. Mayo Clin Proc 1957;32:441–446.

20. Stalberg E. Electrophysiological studies of reinnervation in ALS. In: Rowland LP, ed. Human motor neuron disease. New York: Raven Press, 1982:47–57.

21. Tackmann W, Vogel P. Fibre density, amplitudes of macro-EMG motor unit potentials and conventional EMG recordings from anterior tibial muscle in patients with amyotrophic lateral sclerosis. J Neurol 1988;235:149–154.

22. Brooke MH, Engel WK. The histographic analysis of human muscle biopsies with regard to fiber types. 2. Diseases of the upper and lower motor neurons. Neurology 1969;19:378–393.

23. Dubowitz V. Muscle biopsy. A practical approach. London: Bailliere Tindall, 1985.

24. Patten BM, Zito G, Harati Y. Histologic findings in motor neuron disease: Relation to clinically determined activity, duration, and severity of disease. Arch Neurol 1979;36:560–564.

25. Hansen S, Ballantyne JP. A quantitative electro-physiological study of motor neuron disease. J Neurol Neurosurg Psychiatry 1978;41:773–783.

26. Kuether G, Struppler A. Dynamic aspects of the degenerative process in amyotrophic lateral sclerosis—A clinical and electromyographical study. In: Dengler R, ed. The motor unit, physiology, diseases, regeneration. Munich: Urban & Schwarzenberg, 1990:76–82.

27. Munsat TL, Andres PL, Finison L, Conlon T, Thibodeau L. The natural history of motoneuron loss in amyotrophic lateral sclerosis. Neurology 1988;38:409–411.

28. Swash M, Schwartz MS. A longitudinal study of changes in motor units in motor neuron disease. J Neurol Sci 1982;56:185–197.

29. Schwartz MS, Swash M. Pattern of involvement of the cervical segments in the early stage of motor neurone disease: A single fibre EMG study. Act Neurol Scand 1982;65:424–431.

30. Bradley WG, Hedlund W, Cooper C, et al. A double-blind trial of bovine brain gangliosides in amyotrophic lateral sclerosis. Neurology 1984;34:1079–1082.

31. Harrington H, Hallett M, Tyler R. Ganglioside therapy for amyotrophic lateral sclerosis: A double-blind controlled trial. Neurology 1984;34:1083–1085.

32. Cohen MH, Lester JM, Bradley WG, et al. A computer model of denervation-reinnervation in skeletal muscle. Muscle Nerve 1987;10:826–836.

33. Kuether G, Lipinski HG. Computer simulation of neuron degeneration in motor neuron disease. In: Tsubaki T, Yase Y, eds. Amyotrophic lateral sclerosis. Recent advances in research and treatment. Amsterdam: Excerpta Medica, 1988:131–138.

34. Kuether G, Lipinski HG. A computer model of neuron degeneration: Towards a better understanding of the clinical course of motor neuron disease. Lecture Notes Med Inform 1988;35:235–239.

35. Wohlfart G. Collateral reinnervation in partially denervated muscles. Neurology 1958;8:175–180.

36. Sharrad WJW. The distribution of the permanent paralysis in the lower limb in poliomyelitis: A clinical and pathological study. J Bone Joint Surg 1955;37B:540–558.

37. Kuether G, Lipinski HG. Computer simulation of motor neuron disease—Its implications for therapeutic trials. In: Rose FC, ed. Clinical trials in amyotrophic lateral sclerosis. New York: Demos, 1990:215–226.

38. Stalberg EV. Macro EMG, a new recording technique. J Neurol Neurosurg Psychiatry 1980;43:475–482.

39. Milner-Brown HS, Stein RB, Lee RG. Contractile and electrical properties of human motor units in neuropathies and motor neurone disease. J Neurol Neurosurg Psychiatry 1974;37:670–676.

40. Dengler R, Konstanzer A, Kuether G, Hesse S, Wolf W, Struppler A. Macro-EMG potentials and twitch forces of single motor units in amyotrophic lateral sclerosis. Muscle Nerve 1990;13:545–550.

41. Brown WF, Jaatoul N. Amyotrophic lateral sclerosis. Electrophysiological study (number of motor units and rate of decay of motor units). Arch Neurol 1974;30: 242–248.

42. McComas AJ. Neuromuscular function and disorders. London: Butterworths, 1977: 265–267.

43. Daube JR. Rates of anterior horn cell loss in amyotrophic lateral sclerosis (ALS). J Neurol Sci 1990;98 (Suppl):393.

44. Strehler, B. Time, cells, and aging. New York: Academic Press, 1977.

45. Hirsch HR, Peretz B. Survival and aging of a small laboratory population of marine mollusk, *Aplysia californica*. Mech Ageing Dev 1984;27:43.

46. Witten M. Reliability theoretic methods and aging: Critical elements, hierarchies and longevity-interpreting survival curves. In: Woodhead AD, Blackett AD, Hollaender A, eds. Molecular biology of aging. New York: Plenum Press; 1984:345–360.

47. Gibbs CJ, Gajdusek DC. An update on long-term in vivo and in vitro studies designed to identify a virus as the cause of amyotrophic lateral sclerosis, Parkinsonism-dementia and Parkinson's disease. In: Rowland LP, ed. Human motor neuron diseases. New York: Raven Press, 1982:343–353.

48. Bailey NTJ. The mathematical theory of infectious diseases and its applications. London, High Wycombe: Griffin, 1975.

49. Yase Y. The pathogenesis of amyotrophic lateral sclerosis. Lancet 1972;2:292–296.

50. McComas JA, Upton ARM, Sica REP. Motoneuron disease and ageing. Lancet 1973;2:1477–1480.

51. Bradley WG, Krasin F. A new hypothesis of the etiology of amyotrophic lateral sclerosis: The DNA-hypothesis. Arch Neurol 1982;39:677–680.

52. Calne DB, Eisen A, Mc Geer E, Spencer P. Alzheimer's disease, Parkinson's disease, and motoneurone disease: Abiotropic interaction between ageing and environment? Lancet 1986;2:1067–1070.

53. Spencer PS, Nunn PB, Hugon J, Ludolph AC, Ross SM, Roy DN, Robertson RC. Guam amyotrophic lateral sclerosis–Parkinsonism-dementia linked to a plant excitant neurotoxin. Science 1987;237:465–564.

54. Plaitakis A. Glutamate dysfunction and selective motor neuron degeneration in amyotrophic lateral sclerosis: A hypothesis. Ann Neurol 1990;28:3–8.

55. Munsat TL. Adult motor neuron disease. In: Rowland LP ed. Merrit's textbook of neurology. Philadelphia: Lea & Febiger, 1984:548–552.

56. Lipinski HG, Bingmann D. Diffusion in slice preparations bathed in unstirred solution. Brain Res 1987;437:26–34.

57. Burke RE. Motor units: anatomy, physiology, and functional organization. In: Brookhart JM, Mountcastle VB, Brooks VB,Geiger SR, eds. Handbook of physiology. Section 1. The nervous system. Vol. II. Motor control. Part 1. Bethesda, MD: American Physiological Society; 1981:345–422.

58. McComas AJ, Fawcett PRW, Campbell MJ, Sica REP: Electrophysiological esti-

mation of the number of motor units within a human muscle. J Neurol Neurosurg Psychiatry 1971;34:121–131.

59. Brown WF. A method for estimating the number of motor units in thenar muscle and the changes in motor unit count with age. J Neurol Neurosurg Psychiatry 1972;35:845–852.

60. Ballantyne JP, Hansen S. A new method for the estimation of the number of motor units in a muscle. I. Control subjects and patients with myasthenia gravis. J Neurol Neurosurg Psychiatry 1974;37:907–915.

61. Brown, WF, Strong MJ, Snow R. Methods for estimating numbers of motor units in biceps-brachialis muscles and losses of motor units with aging. Muscle Nerve 1988;11:423–432.

62. Cullheim S, Kellerth JO, Conradi S. Evidence for direct synaptic interconnections between cat spinal alpha-motoneurons via the recurrent axon collaterals: A morphological study using intracellular injection of horseradish peroxidase. Brain Res 1977;132:1–10.

63. Conradi S. Functional implications of structure and symptomatology of motor neurons in motor neuron disease. In: Struppler, A, Weindl A, eds. Clinical aspects of sensory motor integration. Berlin: Springer, 1987:86–90.

64. Price DL, Griffin J, Young A, et al. Tetanus toxin, direct evidence for retrograde intra-axonal transport. Science 1975;188:945–947.

65. Joseph KC, Kim SU, Stieber A, Gonatas NK. Endocytosis of cholera toxin into neuronal GERL. Proc Natl Acad Sci USA 1978;75:2815–2819.

66. Baruah JK, Rasool CG, Bradley WG, Munsat TL. Retrograde axonal transport of lead in rat sciatic nerve. Neurology 1981;31:612–616.

67. Fabian RH. Uptake of plasma IgG by CNS motoneurons: Comparison of antineuronal and normal IgG. Neurology 1988;38:1775–1780.

68. Schwab ME, Thoenen H. Retrograde axonal transport. In: Lajtha A, ed. Handbook of neurochemistry. Vol. 2. New York: Plenum Press, 1982:381–404.

69. Yamamoto T, Iwasaka Y, Konno H, et al. Retrograde transport and differential accumulation of serum proteins in motor neurons: Implications for motor neuron disease. Neurology 1987;37:843–846.

70. Drachman DB, Kuncl RW. Amyotrophic lateral sclerosis: An unconventional autoimmune disease? Ann Neurol 1989;26:269–274.

71. Murphy FA, Bauer SP, Harrison AK, Winn WC. Comparative pathogenesis of rabies and rabies-like viruses. Lab Invest 1973;28:361–376.

72. Kristensson K. Morphological studies of the neural spread of herpes simplex virus to the central nervous system. Acta Neuropathol 1970;16:54–63.

73. Schwab ME, Suda K, Thoenen H. Selective retrograde transsynaptic transfer of a protein, tetanus toxin, subsequent to its retrograde axonal transport. J Cell Biol 1979;82:798–810.

74. Ruda M, Coulter JD. Axonal and transneuronal transport of wheat germ agglutinin demonstrated by immunocytochemistry. Brain Res 1982;249:237–246.

75. Kristensson K, Nennesmo I, Persson L, Lycke E. Neuron to neuron transmission of herpes simplex virus: Transport from skin to brainstem nuclei. J Neurol Sci 1982;54:149–156.

76. Appel SH. A unifying hypothesis for the cause of amyotrophic lateral sclerosis, Parkinsonism, and Alzheimer disease. Ann Neurol 1981;10:499–505.

77. Norris FH, Bjornskov EK, Denys EH, et al. The hypothesis of a motor neurone growth factor and its role in amyotrophic lateral sclerosis, including generalisation to other system degenerations. In: Rose FC ed. Research progress in motor neurone disease. London: Pitman, 1984:255–262.

78. Willison RG. Arrangement of muscle fibers of a single motor unit in mammalian muscles. Muscle Nerve 1980;3:360–361.

79. Boyd DC, Lawrence PD, Bratty PJA. On modelling the single motor unit potential. IEEE Trans Biomed Eng 1978;BME-25:236–243.

80. Griep PAM, Boon KL, Stegeman DFA. A study of motor unit action potential by means of computer simulations. Biol Cybernet 1978;30:221–230.

81. Wani A, Guha S. Synthesising of a motor unit potential based on the sequential firing of muscle fibers. Med Biol Eng 1980;18:719–726.

82. Nandedkar S, Stalberg E. Simulation of macro EMG motor unit potentials. Electroenceph Clin Neurophysiol 1983;56:52–62.

83. Nandedkar S, Sanders DB, Stalberg EV. EMG of reinnervated motor units: A simulation study. Electroenceph Clin Neurophysiol 1988;70:177–184.

84. Lipinski HG, Kuether G. Graphical visualization of the pattern of muscular weakness in neuromuscular diseases. Comp Meth Prog Biomed 1991;34:69–73.

18

Animal Models of Amyotrophic Lateral Sclerosis

Anne Messer

Wadsworth Center for Laboratories and Research, New York State Department of Health, and State University of New York at Albany Albany, New York

INTRODUCTION

Human amyotrophic lateral sclerosis (ALS) is a progressive neurological disorder with an unknown, and probably heterogeneous, etiology. A fraction of the cases (5–10%) are hereditary, but even this designation does not give any real information about the pathogenic process (1,2). Fully involved ALS affects the lower motor neurons (including anterior horn cells and several of the cranial motor nerves) and upper motor neurons as evidenced in the corticospinal tracts. Major hypotheses that have been set forth to explain ALS are covered in other chapters in this volume. They include heavy-metal intoxication (particularly lead and aluminum), trace-element deficiency (calcium and magnesium), trophic-factor deficiency, defective DNA-repair enzymes, changes in proteases, immunological dysfunction, environmental neurotoxins, accelerated aging, defective axonal transport, and viral infection. Some of these overlap with, or may be the causes of, others (3–5).

Given the difficulty of studying the early stages of the pathological processes in ALS itself, a number of experimentally induced and naturally occurring animal models have been investigated. Thirty-eight of these have recently been covered in a comprehensive review by Sillevis Smitt and de Jong (5). Our recent studies of a late-onset semidominant mouse model of ALS have shown many neuropathological features shared with the human disease. In addition, recent genetic studies suggest the interaction of a second gene to control the timing of the onset and progression of symptoms in the syndrome. These have caused us to consider some previous animal model work from the perspective of a series of interacting systems over time. This chapter will first propose a framework for thinking about the general interaction of the hereditary background with potential disease inducers and the potential effects of genes on the timing of neuropathology and symptoms. It will then summarize several well-established animal models, with updates where available, within the context of the roles of inducing factors and genetic backgrounds on pathogenesis. Both published (6,7) and newer studies of the late-onset *motor neuron degeneration (Mnd)* mouse model will be included. Two recent examples where animal models of other neuromuscular diseases have helped to establish new avenues of investigation will then be cited.

Experimentally induced animal models are designed to test specific hypotheses of etiology or pathogenesis, while the natural models show phenotypic and (to varying degrees) pathological similarities to human disease, with mechanisms remaining to be investigated. The natural models are broader in scope than the induced models and may offer a source of reproducible perturbations that can be examined at many levels, from the initial abnormal event (which may be both temporally and physically removed from the motor neuron damage) to the final destruction of function at the neuromuscular synapse. This makes natural models more difficult to study, but offers the advantage that several hypotheses can be incorporated into a single natural animal model.

Theoretically, the motor neuron diseases of humans and their animal models can be divided into three broad categories:

1. Developmental—those which interfere with the proper development of the motor system
2. Degenerative—those in which fully mature, "normal" motor neurons appear to degenerate
3. Developmental/degenerative—those which show many signs of normal motor development, but carry a defect that will cause premature death or dysfunction later

One approach to the use of animal models, especially those which are experimentally induced, but potentially applicable to natural models, is to consider them the extreme end of the spectrum of causes and effects. Thus, if a toxin at high doses can cause a given pathology, similar chemicals at low doses may have slower, more chronic effects. A similar argument can be made for the study of gene products, where dose effects in homozygotes versus heterozygotes need to be examined. Such studies can be extended to include the possibility that the same abnormal gene product will have somewhat different effects in different species, or even on different genetic backgrounds within the same species. The advantage of doing many of these kinds of studies in an animal model is the potential to vary some of the modifying factors in a systematic way, thereby gaining insight into the actions of genes, toxins, viruses, and so forth in the genetically and environmentally diverse human population. The issue of timing is particularly critical. ALS is basically a disease of older individuals, which suggests that cumulative or aging effects of some kind are involved, either directly or as background modifiers of "acute" effectors. If a virus or toxin is the primary agent, it apparently does not usually have an immediate effect on young people. It therefore follows that an understanding of what causes the symptoms and pathology to develop in selected physiological systems relatively late in life (and much later in some cases than others) might allow postponement of the onset of debilitating symptoms to a time beyond the usual lifespan. Assuming that the development of the full-blown disease state requires several steps between the primary event and the dysfunctional nerve-muscle junction, animal models may be useful in defining a number of different steps, and, most important, in evaluating the interactions of "timing modifiers" on the basic process.

HEREDITARY MODELS

Naturally occurring, hereditary animal models allow examination of the early stages of the disease by yielding substantial numbers of individual cases that are essentially identical. A search of the literature yields 11 probable hereditary animal models for which studies are available (reviewed in ref. 5). With the exception of mouse *Mnd* and the heterozygous form of the *hereditary canine spinal muscular atrophy* (*HCSMA*), all these disorders show an early enough onset that a fundamental problem with the development or maturation of the motor system can be inferred. While these juvenile-onset models may offer valuable insights into the functional components of the motor neuron system and requirements for its integrity, they are probably better models of the early-onset human motor neuron diseases than of ALS. However, it is possible that both human ALS and those animal models which show adult onset still reflect a developmental defect that is manifest only after a number of months (in animals) or years (in humans).

Hereditary Canine Spinal Muscular Atrophy

HCSMA is a motor neuron disease of Brittany spaniels characterized clinically by weakness and muscle atrophy and pathologically by chromatolysis and abnormal accumulations of neurofilaments. Three phenotypes (accelerated, intermediate, and chronic) are distinguished on the basis of age of onset and rate of progression. The accelerated form affects pups, with full involvement by 6 months, the intermediate form delays full involvement until 3–4 years, and the chronic form develops nonprogressive weakness (8–10). Genetic studies, in-

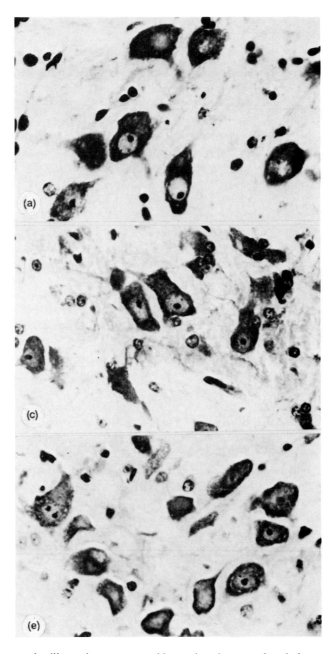

Figure 1 Photomicrographs illustrating neurons with varying degrees of pathology, including chromatolysis, eccentric nuclei, and distorted cell shapes among groups of brainstem lower motor neurons (a, d, f), preganglionic (b), and upper motor neurons (c, e); all are from severely affected mutants. (a) Hypoglossal nucleus; (b) dorsal motor nucleus of the vagus; (c) caudal pontine reticular formation; (d) facial nucleus; (e) red nucleus, caudal part; (f) motor trigeminal nucleus. Nissl stain; bar = 50 μm. (From Ref. 7.)

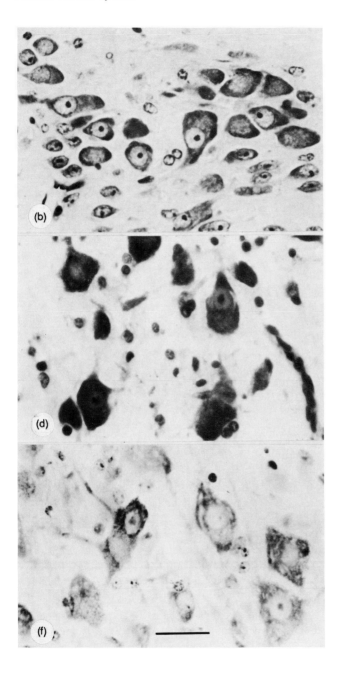

cluding outcrosses to beagle dogs, have shown that the disease is an autosomal dominant, with homozygotes showing the accelerated form and heterozygotes showing intermediate or chronic disease (11). Substantial progress has been made in studying the neuropathology; altered neurofilament transport or kinetics or reduced neurofilament synthesis could explain the similar pathologies seen at equivalent clinical stages of the various forms of the disease. Cork et al. (12) suggest that the underlying problem may be present quite early. This model combines the concepts of gene dosage and timing; the heterozygotes show what might be considered a degenerative disease, if studied in the absence of homozygote data (as would be the case in human studies). However, it is most likely that the abnormal primary gene product is present at or before birth, with the single dose simply manifest later and therefore developmental/degenerative.

HCSMA is a valuable model. There is a limit to the genetic studies that can be done in dogs, however, They are large, relatively slow to breed, and expensive to maintain. A mouse model has the advantage of small size and rapid generation time (e.g., we have been able to wean over 2300 *Mnd* mice and controls from our colony in the past 3 years). In addition, the extensive amount of genetics that has been done in mice, and the extent to which the mouse chromosomal map (13) has been correlated with the human map, allows a much more sophisticated analysis than is possible in any other vertebrate species.

The (*Mnd*) Mutation in the Mouse

Mnd was originally identified as a spontaneous, adult-onset neurological disease on the C57B16.KB2 background, where it was maintained owing to a double recombination in the mouse histocompatibility region. Careful investigation revealed that the neurological disorder was usually identifiable by 6–7 months of age, and that it progressed to total paralysis with premature death (6). All viral tests were negative; intracranial injections of *Mnd* spinal cord extracts into wild-type newborns did not transmit the disease to young mice of the same strain, and cross-fostering had no effect. Despite some variability in the ages of onset and speed of progression of symptoms in individual mice, the disease was clearly genetic. While many obligate +/*Mnd* mice from the original stocks showed clear neuropathology, with a similar age of onset and a milder disease course than *Mnd*/*Mnd* mice, current stocks held in a semisterile environment and bred over several years for a very consistent age of onset in *Mnd*/*Mnd* show greatly reduced penetrance in the heterozygous state. *Mnd* is therefore semidominant with variable penetrance, and work focuses mainly on *Mnd*/*Mnd*. Basic histopathology revealed substantial abnormalities of motor neurons in the spinal cords, more severe in lumbar than in cervical; in cranial nerves, especially 10 and 12; and in some upper motor neurons (Fig. 1 and Table 1; from ref. 7). The nature of the pathology was definitely not spongiform, and there were no obvious signs of

Table 1 Central Nervous System Pathology in *Mnd* Mutants

	Mildly affected	Severely affected
Spinal cord		
Lumbar	+ +	+ + + +
Thoracic	+	+ + +
Cervical	0	+ +
Medulla		
Reticular formation	0	+ +
Lateral reticular nucleus	0	+ +
Inferior olivary complex	0	+ / −
Hypoglossal nucleus	+	+ +
Dorsal motor nucleus of the vagus	+	+ +
Vestibular complex	0	+
Pons		
Facial nucleus	0	+
Motor trigeminal nucleus	0	+
Superior sensory trigeminal nucleus	0	+ / −
Abducens nucleus	0	+
Reticular formation	0	+ +
Cerebellum		
Cortex	0	+ / −
Deep nuclei	0	+
Midbrain		
Inferior collicull	0	0
Superior collicull	0	0
Red nucleus	0	+ +
Substantia nigra	0	0
Oculomotor complex	0	0
Perlaqueductal gray	0	+
Forebrain		
Striatum	0	0
Hippocampus	0	0
Hypothalamus	0	0
Cerebral cortex	0	+

inflammatory response. A statistically significant decease in the number of lumbar (L4) anterior horn neurons in moderately affected *Mnd/Mnd* versus age-matched controls has been found (7a).

At higher magnification, numerous inclusion bodies can be recognized in the affected soma (7). Affected neurons show a large increase in both mRNA and immunoreactivity for the lysosomal hydrolase B-glucuronidase, which may account for some of the material in the inclusion bodies (Messer, Plummer, and

Mazurkiewicz, in preparation). *Mnd* spinal cord motoneurons also have a very striking redistribution of all forms of neurofilament protein to the margins of the cell bodies (7a). This seems to be true even in the most mildly affected cases.

Similarities to human ALS include changes in the mouse model involving ubiquitin and TRH, as well as a failure to demonstrate immunopathology to date. Human ALS cases have been reported to show ubiquitin-containing deposits in the cytoplasm of motor neurons. Ubiquitin is a small cellular protein involved in selective proteolysis (14,15). *Mnd* mice also show these deposits, which are present in some lumbar motor neurons even before the onset of clinical symptoms (Mazurkiewicz et al., submitted). TRH levels in the spinal cords of *Mnd* mice are reduced (B. Brooks, personal communication), much as they seem to be in some cases of human ALS (16). Tests of spleen-cell responses to mitogens, levels of serum immunoglobulins, and serum antibodies to motor neurons yielded no statistically significant *Mnd*-specific changes. Weekly injections of cyclophosphamide (200 mg/kg) were done on a series of mutant and control mice to test two hypotheses: (a) immune suppression by the drug would delay the onset or lessen the severity of the motor symptoms, or (b) the drug would allow unrestricted replication of an endogenous retrovirus, similar to the effect of treatment of lactose dehydrogenase virus (LDV)–infected susceptible strains, causing rapid paralysis or recognizable exacerbation of the motor neuron disease (17,18). Mice were entered into the regimen at about 5 months of age, or shortly before the expected onset of mild symptoms. In two separate trials, using a total of 48 mice, the time course and severity of the disease appeared to be within normal limits in either direction (19).

In order to map the *Mnd* gene, F2 progeny from a B6 *Mnd/Mnd* outcross to AKR were scored for neurological symptoms and then assayed for strain- and chromosome-specific polymorphisms. Close linkage of *Mnd* to the endogenous xenotropic murine leukemia virus fragment *Xmv-26* on proximal chromosome 8 has been observed (Messer, Plummer, Maskin, Coffin, and Frankel, submitted).

In the course of examining the F2 mice from the AKR outcross, 8–12% showed a very early onset (<5 months) of disease symptoms, with much more rapid progression than B6 *Mnd/Mnd* mice. No such acceleration has been seen in outcrosses to five other strains, including C3H and BALB/c. Additional breeding experiments are consistent with the existence of a motor neuron timing (*mnt*) gene, unlinked to *Mnd* itself, which has an early allele on the AKR background. A second gene that can modify the timing of the main gene could also explain the variable presentation of symptoms seen in some human ALS family pedigrees (20).

Thus, the *Mnd* mouse should be useful in the investigation of many different aspects of human ALS. It appears to fall into the degenerative classification, although developmental/degenerative cannot be ruled out. Identification of the abnormal gene product, which is being approached through a combination of chromosomal localization, identification of the intrinsic site of the action of the gene, and cloning, is of obvious interest. Processes downstream in the chain of events leading from this gene change to motor dysfunction may mimic those seen in different sporadic forms of ALS, assuming that there are a certain number of final common pathways for pathogenesis. And the identification of an independent gene or mechanism that can slow the onset or course of the disease, such as that present in the intermediate and late forms of *Mnd*, has obvious therapeutic import.

Wobbler

Two early-onset autosomal recessive mouse mutants have been studied in detail. The *wobbler* (*wb*) mouse, first described in 1956 (21), is the subject of two recent reviews (3,5). It is an autosomal recessive mutation, showing signs of forelimb involvement by 3 weeks of age. Pathology is mainly vacuolar, affecting predominantly soma of the cervical motor neurons. Both the rate of axonal transport and the number of neurofilaments are greatly reduced in affected cells (22), and there is a selective reduction in the regenerative capacity of these cells as well (23). This disease is present very early; it clearly affects the development of the motor neurons, and many aspects of the pathology are rather different from those described for ALS. However, the mechanism of the differential vulnerability of the degenerating cells can be examined in such animals (24). It might also be interesting to examine aged and stressed heterozygotes for signs of a semidominant effect.

Wasted

Recently, another recessive mouse mutant, *wasted* (*wst*), has been reported to develop prominent vacuolar degeneration and accumulations of phosphorylated 200-kDa neurofilament immunoreactive protein in motor neurons in the anterior horn of the spinal cord and the brainstem cranial nuclei by 30 days of age (25). Tremor appears to involve all four limbs, although the paralysis was reported to affect mainly the hindlimbs. The disease is progressive, starting by 14–18 days, with wasting and death by day 31. No pathology was seen in young, unaffected littermates, some of which should have been heterozygotes, and the obligate heterozygote parents apparently did not show gross motor defects. No aged heterozygotes were examined. While, as with *wobbler*, the onset during development and the presence of vacuolar pathology suggest strong differences between this disease and ALS, some common targeting mechanism might again be at work. It is of particular interest that this mutant strain also develops reduced secretory immune responses and shows abnormal DNA repair mechanisms. An endogenous retrovirus has been postulated as a mechanism of action for both the immune and neurological defects, based on preliminary data (25).

IMMUNE ABNORMALITY MODELS

The possibilities of an autoimmune etiology for ALS have been considered for many years, since such a process could account for the late onset, progressive nature, and selectivity of the disease. In a recent review (26) Cashman and Antel conclude that, while there may not be an "immunology of classical ALS," immunology may contribute to the understanding of the disease. They point out that neither improvement with removal of serum antibodies nor passive transmission of symptoms to experimental animals has been demonstrated for ALS, although these do characterize more classical autoimmune diseases. Others feel that immune system abnormalities may still play some direct role in the pathogenic process. There have been no reproducible demonstrations of straightforward antibodies or cellular immune responses to motor neurons in patients [ie, reports seem to conflict (27)]. However, there are reports of increased autoimmune disorders (especially thyroid autoimmunity) in both ALS patients and their first-degree relatives (26,28). Also, a recent, testable hypothesis has been put forth that ALS may be an unconventional autoimmune disease involving antibodies directed against the carbohdyrate components of glycolipids (27). A direct test of the potential of autoimmunity to produce motor neuron disease has been done by inoculating guinea pigs with swine (29) or bovine (30) motor neurons. In the latter study, after 4 months, four of nine female and four of five male animals developed clinical weakness and degeneration of lower motor neurons in the spinal cord. However, *all* the animals, regardless of whether they developed symptoms and pathology, also developed high serum titers of antibodies against motor neurons, and IgG was found within their anterior horn cell bodies. There may have been differences in the panels of antibodies produced to the injections of whole motor neurons in different animals, either by chance or due to genetic heterogeneity in the outbred guinea pigs that were used, although many other explanations are possible. If a direct effect of the IgG is not responsible for the symptoms, some less obvious aspect of the long-term cellular immune response might be involved. Further attempts to elicit an antibody response to more specific epitopes (particularly gangliosides or thyroid antigens), as well as the use of more inbred animals, seem warranted.

More recently, guinea pigs immunized with whole bovine spinal cord homogenate have been shown to develop an experimental autoimmune gray-matter disease, which differs from the above in that IgG is found at the motor end-plate and around external membranes as well as within the cytoplasm (30a). Serum from both types of autoimmune disease appears to contain IgG that can be transported retrogradely from the periphery to motoneuron cell bodies (30b).

The interactions of the immune system with viruses could also play a role in the pathogenesis. This could be either of an autoimmune nature, via shared antigens, or a case of immune suppression (often due to age) allowing the replication of a hitherto repressed endogenous or endemic virus (see below).

VIRUSES

Murine Retrovirus

A wild mouse ecotropic murine leukemia virus (Cas-Br-E) induces a progressive hindlimb paralysis in susceptible mice over 6 months of age, due to degeneration of anterior horn cells in the lower spinal cord and brainstem (31). The basic pathology is spongiform, with evidence that the virus is actually replicating in glial cells adjacent to the affected neurons (32–34). Recently, studies using chimeric viruses have shown that a 372-base-pair fragment of the *env* gene, gp70 is both necessary and sufficient to produce neurological disease. Examination of the chimeric viruses in different mouse strains yields evidence for interaction of this domain with genetically determined cellular factors. This explains why only some mouse strains are susceptible. However, within susceptible strains, the specificity of the virus for anterior horn cells resides in a second viral gene, the long terminal repeat (LTR) (35). A mechanism whereby the *env* fragment (presumably from a virus with the correct LTR) binds to a receptor on the cell surface, which then interferes with the normal function of this receptor, is proposed. The Cas-Br-E virus animal model contains too many disparate elements to be a precise model of ALS; however, it does offer insights into factors that can affect the time of onset of disease, and possibly the interactions of endogenous and exogenous genomes. The immune system may also be part of this equation, since immunity could modulate the vigor of the virus, and lymphatic cells can themselves be affected by the same retrovirus.

Lactate Dehydrogenase–Elevating Virus

Lactate dehydrogenase–elevating virus (LDV) infection of aged or immunosuppressed young adult C58 or AKR mice leads to a rapidly progressive paralytic infection, which kills the mice in 2–3 weeks. The virus establishes a persistent, but apparently asymptomatic infection in other strains of mice, and in young, otherwise untreated mice of the two susceptible strains. The symptoms start in the hindlimbs and move up, although histological lesions can be found throughout the spinal cord and brainstem (36). The pathology shows severe inflammatory disease, leading to a marked spongiform appearance. Recent in situ hybridization evidence suggests that aging or immunosuppressive treatments induce substantial replication of an endogenous retrovirus in the affected neurons of C58 and AKR mice (37). This somehow, possibly through a new surface receptor, allows entry and pathological replication of the LDV, which correlates exactly with the symptoms (38). Thus, an endogenous virus (part of the genome) interacts with an exogenous virus and possibly the immune system to create a motor neuron disease. The timing element is also present, since "normal" aging will also render the mice of these strains susceptible. It is unclear whether the immunosuppressive treatments are actually inducing the endogenous retroviral genes via the immune system itself, or through an independent (although possibly related) mechanism. The cellular pathology does not correlate well with that described for ALS; however, the selective nature of the cells affected suggests that this model may point the way toward identifying properties of motor neurons that allow them to interact with endogenous and environmental factors in a unique way.

CHEMICAL MODELS

If heavy-metal or organic intoxication plays a significant role in the etiology of ALS, several factors need to be considered; animal models can help to sort out some of the variables. Both degenerative and developmental/degenerative classifications merit consideration. It is first necessary to distinguish between sporadic overexposure capable of swamping any metabolic system and supersensitivity to an otherwise innocuous or clearly subclinical level of a putative toxin. All are played out on a pattern of nervous system function that includes built-in levels of redundancies and/or limited regenerative capacities. Thus, the overexposure could be acute (immediate death of a small subset of neurons) or chronic (slow loss due to the stress of a mild, constant overload), with eventual dysfunction developing as normal aging reduces excess capacity (39). The supersensitivity could be due to changes in receptors, binding proteins, or second-messenger systems, leading to abnormal processing of the compound in question. Such changes may be part of the genetic constitution of a population and could even confer an advantage under other circumstances (similar to the inherited blood diseases that confer resistance to malaria). The possibility that a neurotoxin is produced endogenously in some individuals also falls in this category. In all cases, the adult onset and progressive nature of the human motor neuron diseases must be accounted for, although acute models may yield information on where to look for chronic effects.

The first use of experimentally induced models is therefore to screen potential inducer candidates by exposing them to an excess of the chemical in question and asking whether it is possible to elicit symptoms or pathology that resemble the human disease. The second phase, which requires both more control of the genetic substrate and better quantitation of the results, is to investigate what additional parameters can affect the severity of, and the sensitivity to, the response.

Toxins

Heavy Metals

Lead, aluminum, and mercury can all cause neuropathological changes and motor dysfunction after chronic exposure. Changes are invariably more widespread in the brain and spinal cords of these animals than in ALS, but there are definitely effects on motor neurons (5). Most studies have used guinea pigs, rabbits, or rats, which have only a modest degree of genetic homogeneity in experimental populations. There are not sufficient numbers to determine from the literature if any populations are especially sensitive or resistant; most do show neurofilamentous changes, with aluminum-induced effects the closest to those which have been reported for human ALS, although aluminum also induces neurofibrillary tangles, which do not appear in ALS (40).

Organic Toxins

There has been considerable interest in the possibility that either an ingested or an endogenous excitotoxin may be responsible for destruction of motor neurons (39). Sillevis Smitt and de Jong (5) review several of the papers on the feeding of the cycad amino acid L-BMAA, concluding that the slow toxin hypothesis is far from proven. The basic concept remains attractive, however. A recent report (41) has also shown that direct injection of kainic acid can produce neuropathological changes in rat spinal cord motor neurons, suggesting that excitoxicity is still a viable theory; it may be part of a larger picture of genetic vulnerability.

Trace Metal Deficiencies

Here again, the question of differences among populations in underlying metabolic properties, creating differing susceptibility to cumulative stress, looms large. Most deficiencies due to environmental causes can be considered developmental, since the population is presumably exposed in utero and during lactation; this may have very different effects than on a mature nervous system (see below). However, an interacting toxin or adult-onset induced inability (e.g., by virus infection or aging) to transport or utilize a trace element might give similar results. The swayback ataxia in lambs emerges during the first few months after birth, due to cooper deficiency (42). A similar disease in young goats showed many neuropathological similarities to ALS; both animal models have somatic accumulations of neurofilaments (43). Increased lysosomes and phosphorylated neurofilament immunoreactivity also characterized motor neurons of adult monkeys kept on low Ca/Mg diets for 1–4 years (5).

Thus, animal models with induced toxic exposures or trace element deficiencies show that this classification offers many possibilities for direct etiologies, and even more for interactions of predicating factors with the environment. Most of the measurements used to date on the models have of necessity been relatively nonspecific. In order to sharpen the rather broad category of possibilities, it will be necessary to continuously reconsider the material available in light of new human pathological findings. The study of Cork et al. (43) is an example of this approach. Hopefully, more specific parameters will soon be available to assess, at least for some subpopulations, what may be a heterogeneous set of causes.

LESSONS FROM ANIMAL MODELS OF OTHER NEUROLOGICAL DISEASES

As molecular genetics gets more sophisticated, new roles are emerging for the use of animal models to study neurological disease. The differences between the human and the animal cases can be pinpointed more precisely than in the past, and these differences can be used to investigate factors that can modify, and hopefully treat, the human disease. The first example of this is the cloning of the X-linked gene for Duchenne muscular dystrophy. Genetic methods to analyze the human DNA were combined with analyses of muscle transcripts from mice, on the grounds that an important gene should be conserved among species. Both the gene (44) and its protein product, dystrophin (45), were identified, and it was shown that the protein was abnormal or missing in patients with the disease (46). A mouse mutation producing very mild muscle changes was known to map to the homologous region of the mouse X chromosome; dystrophin was shown to be deficient in these animals as well, thus offering a genocopy of the human muscular dystrophy (45). However, despite having a very similar genetic defect, the mouse muscle does not atrophy as the human muscle does. There must be some other factor in the mouse muscle that can protect it even in the presence of a greatly reduced level of dystrophin. Thus, the mouse genocopy is not a perfect phenocopy, but the difference between the two could be extremely valuable therapeutically.

The second case concerns prion disease in human and mouse. These diseases have the (currently) unique property of infectious, sporadic, and genetic manifestations of a progressive, lethal spongiform encephalopathy within the same domain [reviewed in Westaway et al. (47)]. Experimental transmission of kuru or Creutzfeldt-Jakob disease from humans to animals requires frank inoculation, and some human disease has been traced to accidental inoculation from infected individuals. However, there are "sporadic" occurrences where no risk factors can be identified. The Gerstmann-Straussler syndrome is inherited as an adult-onset autosomal dominant neurodegeneration and yet can be transmitted to animals by inoculation of brain homogenates. One form has recently been shown to be a missense mutation of the endogenous prion gene (48). The equivalent disease in mice, scrapie, can be transmitted by intracerebral inoculation, with genetic control of the time from inoculation to death (49). This timing effect is due to two genes, the more important of which is tightly linked to the gene encoding the mouse prion gene. Thus, the combination of mouse and the human data illustrates the possibility that there are cellular genes that can be released to act as neural viruses, and that these genes contain intrinsic or linked timing components. While it is unlikely that ALS is directly linked to this unusual system, the concept that such interrelations of genes, viruses, and timing factors exist, and the role that animal models may play in elucidating other such mechanisms (e.g., the LDV story), is a broadening one.

CONCLUSIONS

As can be seen from the above discussions of selected animal models of ALS, there are many levels at which one can investigate the disease. There is evidence from both human and animal studies that it may require the interaction of a number of disparate factors to produce the final state. This seems reasonable for a late-onset disease that targets a specific cell population. In order to identify those processes which can contribute to late-onset disease, and, most important, to modify the pathogenic process, additional models that deal specifically with questions of timing and interactions of endogenous and environmental systems may be necessary.

Why is there such a relative paucity of inherited animal models of ALS, and late-onset hereditary diseases in general? It is probably *not* because these do not exist naturally. The problem in identifying animal models of late-onset diseases is that, by definition, they do not become severe enough to be readily apparent until after the optimal reproductive age of the animal. Very few commercial farm animals are kept this long, and even most research colonies for breeding are routinely replaced before breeding normally slows. Furthermore, if there is an effect of a neurological disease that interferes with breeding efficiency early in a disorder of gradual onset, it is most likely that the line in question will be sacrificed before the true nature of the severe disease can be recognized. For example, the accepted procedure in mouse husbandry is to euthanize any mouse that appears ill in a standard breeding colony, so as not to endanger the remainder of the colony. In an inbred mating scheme, this often includes sacrificing the mate as well. Therefore, it is only in research colonies that are specifically being screened for late-onset disease and/or are already being maintained (at substantial expense) to study problems of aging, or in companion animals that are kept for reasons other than procreation, that such disorders might be recognized. While anecdotal evidence for possible neurological disease in aging pet dogs and cats abounds, substantial logistic difficulties usually prevent these cases from being followed up. Since there is an increase in studies of aging, it may be valuable to remind investigators in that field that they are the most likely source of material for studies of late-onset neurological disorders, some of which may, in fact, represent acceleration of a normal aging process (50), and to educate funding agencies that the extra expense involved in maintaining animals long enough to study late-onset disease may have benefits in many areas.

This chapter has attempted to review a variety of induced, natural, and "naturally induced" models that target motor neurons, highlighting those aspects of the models which may have to do with interactions of genes, the immune system, viruses, and toxins. It is clear from recent studies of prion diseases (47) and oncogenes and tumor suppressors [reviewed by Martin (51)] that hidden within our genomes, as Shakespeare said, "there are more things in heaven and earth, Horatio, than are dreamt of in your philosophy."

ACKNOWLEDGMENTS

I thank Drs. Joseph E. Mazurkiewicz, Lorraine Flaherty, Norman Strominger, Benjamin Brooks, and Susan Lewis, and Esther Wylen, Linda Callahn, Bonnie Eisenberg, and Julie Plummer for their contributions to various parts of this work. The experiments in this laboratory were supported by grants from the ALS Association (AM), the Muscular Dystrophy Association (AM).

REFERENCES

1. Calne DB, Eisen A. The relationship between Alzheimer's disease, Parkinson's disease and motor neuron disease. Can J Neurol Sci 1989;16(Suppl):547–550.
2. Vassilopoulos D. The genetics of motor neurone disease. Prog Clin Biol Res 1989;306:91–104.
3. Mitsumoto H, Hanson MR, Chad DA. Amyotrophic lateral sclerosis. Recent advances in pathogenesis and therapeutic trials. Arch Neurol 1988;45:189–202.
4. Rowland LP. Motor neuron diseases and ALS: Research progress. Trends Neurosci 1987;10:393–398.
5. Sillevis Smitt PAE, de Jong JMBV. Animal models of amyotrophic lateral sclerosis and the spinal muscular atrophies. J Neurol Sci 1989;91:231–258.
6. Messer A, Flaherty L. Autosomal dominance in a late-onset motor neuron disease in the mouse. J Neurogenet 1986;3:345–355.
7. Messer A, Strominger NL, Mazurkiewicz JE. Histopathology of the late-onset motor neuron degeneration (Mnd) mutant in the mouse. J Neurogenet 1987;4: 201–213.
7a. Callhan LM, Wylen EL, Messer A, and Mazurkiewicz JE. Neurofilament distribution is altered in the *Mnd* (*motor neuron degeneration*) mouse. J Neuropathol Exp Neurol 1991 50:491–504.
8. Cork LC, Griffin JW, Munnell JF, Lorenz MD, Adams RJ, Price DM. Hereditary canine spinal muscular atrophy. J Neuropathol Exp Neurol 1979;28:209–221.

9. Cork LC, Griffin JW, Choy C, Padula CA, Price DL. Pathology of motor neurons in accelerated hereditary canine spinal muscular atrophy. Lab Invest 1982;46:89–99.

10. Cork LC, Troncoso JC, Price DL. Canine inherited ataxia. Ann Neurol 1981;9:492–499.

11. Sack GH, Cork LC, Morris M, Griffin JW, Price DL. Autosomal dominant inheritance of hereditary canine spinal muscular atrophy. Ann Neurol 1984;15:369–373.

12. Cork LC, Struble RG, Gold BG, et al. Changes in size and motor axons in hereditary canine spinal muscular atrophy. Lab Invest 1989;61:333–341.

13. Nadeau JH, Eppig JT, Reiner AH. Man on mouse homology map. Mouse News Lett 1989;84:52–54.

14. Leigh PN, Anderton BH, Dodson A, Gallo J-M, Swash M, Power DM, Ubiquitin deposits in anterior horn cells in motor neurone disease. Neurosci Lett 1988;93:197–203.

15. Lowe J, Aldridge F, Lennox G, et al. Inclusion bodies in motor cortex and brainstem of patients with motor neurone disease are detected by immunocytochemical localisation of ubiquitin. Neurosci Lett 1989;105:7–13.

16. Mitsuma T, Nogimori N, Adachi K, Mokoyama M, Ando K. Concentrations of immunoreactive thyrotropin-releasing hormone in spinal cord of patients with ALS. Am J Med Sci 1984;287:34–36.

17. Kozak C, Silver J. The transmission and activation of endogenous mouse retroviral genomes. Trends Genet 1985;331–334.

18. Murphy WH, Nawrocki JF Pease LR. Age-dependent paralytic viral infection in C58 mice: Possible implications in human neurological disease. Prog Brain Res 1983;59:291–303.

19. Messer A, Flaherty L. Immune function in the Motor neuron degeneration (Mnd) mutant. Mouse Newsl 1989;84:105.

20. Mulder DW, Kurland LT, Offord KP, Beard CM. Familial adult motor neuron disease: Amyotrophic lateral sclerosis. Neurology 1986;36:511–517.

21. Duchen LW, Strich SJ, Falconer DS. An hereditary motor neuron disease with progressive denervation of muscle in the mouse: The mutant "wobbler." J Neurol Neurosurg Psychiatry 1968;31:535–542.

22. Mitsumoto H. Axonal regeneration in wobbler motor neuron disease: Quantitative histologic and axonal transport studies. Muscle Nerve 1985;8:44–51.

23. Mitsumoto H, Bradley WG. Murine motor neuron disease (the wobbler mouse). Brain 1982;105:811–834.

24. Mitsumoto H, McQaurrie IG, Kurahashi K, Sunohara N. Histometric characteristics and regenerative capacity in wobbler mouse motor neuron disease. Brain 1990 (in press).

25. Lutsep HL, Rodriguez M. Ultrastructural, morphometric, and immunocytochemical study of anterior horn cells in mice with "wasted" mutation. J Neuropathol Exp Neurol 1989;48:519–533.

26. Cashman NR, Antel JP. Amyotrophic lateral sclerosis: An immunological perspective. Immunol Allergy Clin North Am 1988;8:331–342.

27. Drachman DB, Kuncl RW. Amyotrophic lateral sclerosis: An unconventional autoimmune disease. Ann Neurol 1989;26:269–274.
28. Appel SH, Stockton Appel V, Stewart SS, Kerman RH. Amyotrophic lateral sclerosis. Associated clinical disorders and immunological evaluations. Arch Neurol 1986;43:234–238.
29. Engelhardt JI, Joo F. An immune-mediated guinea pig model for lower motor neuron disease. J Neuroimmunol 1986;12:279–290.
30. Engelhardt JI, Appel SH, Killian JM. Experimental autoimmune motoneuron disease. Ann Neurol 1989;26:368–376.
30a. Engelhardt JI, Appel SH, Killian JM. Motor neuron destruction in guinea pigs immunized with bovine spinal cord ventral horn homogenate: Experimental autoimmune gray matter disease. J Neuroimmunol 1990;27:21–31.
30b. Engelhardt JI, Appel SH. Motor neuron reactivity of sera from animals with autoimmune models of motor neuron destruction. J Neurol Sci 1990;96:333–352.
31. Gardner MB. Type C viruses of wild mice: Characterization and natural history of amphotropic, ecotropic and xenotropic MuLV. Curr Top Microbiol Immunol 1978;79:215–139.
32. Brooks BR, Feussner GK, Lust WD. Spinal cord metabolic changes in murine retrovirus-induced motor neuron disease. Brain Res Bull 1983;11:681–686.
33. Brooks BR, Swarz JR, Narayan O, Johnson RT. Murine neurotropic retrovirus spongiform poliocephalomyelopathy: Acceleration of disease by virus inoculum concentration. Infect Immun 1979;23:540–544.
34. Brooks BR, Swarz JR, Johnson RT. Spongiform polioencephalomyelopathy caused by a murine retrovirus. Lab Invest 1980;43:480–486.
35. DesGroseillers L, Rassart E, Robitaille Y, Jolicouer P. Retrovirus-induced spongiform encephalopathy: The 3′-end long terminal repeat-containing viral sequences influence the incidence of the disease and the specificity of the neurological syndrome. Proc Natl Acad Sci USA 1985;82:8818–8822.
36. Stroop WG, Brinton MA. Mouse strain–specific central nervous system lesions associated with lactate dehydrogenase-elevating virus infection. Lab Invest 1983;49:334–345.
37. Contag CH, Plagemann PGW. Susceptibility of C58 mice to paralytic disease induced by lactate dehydrogenase–elevating virus correlates with the increased expression of endogenous retrovirus in motor neurons. Microb Pathog 1988;5:287–296.
38. Contag CH, Plagemann PGW. Age-dependent poliomyelitis of mice: Expression of endogenous retrovirus correlates with cytocidal replication of lactate dehydrogenase–elevating virus in motor neurons. J Virol 1989;63:4362–4369.
39. Calne DB, McGeer E, Eisen A, Spencer P. Alzheimer's disease, Parkinson's disease, and motoneurone disease: Abiotropic interaction between ageing and environment? Lancet 1986;1067–1070.
40. Troncosco JC, Sternberger NH, Sternberger LA, Hoffman PN, Price DL. Immunocytochemical studies of neurofibrillary pathology induced by aluminum. Brain Res 1986;364:295–300.
41. Hugon J, Vallat JM, Spencer PS, Leboutet MJ, Barthe D. Kainic acid induces early

and delayed degenerative neuronal changes in rat spinal cord. Neurosci Lett 1989;104:258–262.

42. Mills CF, Fell BF. Demyelination in lambs born of ewes maintained on high intakes of sulphate and molybdate. Nature 1960;185:20–22.

43. Cork LC, Troncoso JC, Klavano GG, et al. Neurofilamentous abnormalities in motor neurons in spontaneously occurring animal disorders. J Neuroapthol Exp Neurol 1988;47:420–431.

44. Koenig M, Hoffman EP, Bertelson CJ, Monaco AP, Feener C, Kunkel LM. Complete cloning of the Duchenne muscular dystrophy (DMD) cDNA and preliminary genomic organization of the DMD gene in normal and affected individuals. Cell 1987;50:509–517.

45. Hoffman EP, Brown Jr RH, Kunkel LM. Dystrophin: The protein product of the Duchenne Muscular Dystrophy locus. Cell 1987;51:919–928.

46. Hoffman EP, Fischbeck KH, Brown RH, et al. Characterization of dystrophin in muscle-biopsy specimens from patients with Duchenne's or Becker's muscular dystrophy. N Engl J Med 1988;318:1363–1368.

47. Westaway D, Carlson GA, Prusiner SB. Unraveling prion diseases through molecular genetics. Trends Neurosci 1989;12:221–227.

48. Hsiao K, Baker HF, Crow TJ, et al. Linkage of a prion protein missense variant to Gerstmann-Straussler syndrome. Nature 1989;338:342–345.

49. Carlson GA, Kingsbury DT, Goodman PA, et al. Linkage of prion protein and scrapie incubation time genes. Cell 1986;46:503–511.

50. Farrer LA. Genetic neurodegenerative disease models for human aging. Rev Biol Res Aging 1987;3:163–189.

51. Martin JB. Molecular genetic studies in the neuropsychiatric disorders. Trends Neurosci 1989;12:130–137.

19

Viruses and Amyotrophic Lateral Sclerosis

Edgar F. Salazar-Grueso and Raymond P. Roos

The University of Chicago
Chicago, Illinois

INTRODUCTION

Amyotrophic lateral sclerosis (ALS) is a disease of the motor system in which motor neurons of the spinal cord, brainstem, and brain degenerate. The etiology of ALS remains unknown. Possible causes include toxin-mediated injury, immune-mediated mechanisms, defective DNA repair, trophic factor abnormalities, and viral infection (reviewed in 1–3).

In this chapter, we review the evidence for a viral cause of ALS. We begin our discussion by evaluating the reported association of human motor neuron disease (MND) with viruses and unconventional agents. This is followed by a description of current investigations of naturally occurring and experimental animal models of virus-induced MND. In this latter section, we focus on the role these studies play in elucidating mechanisms of neural injury relevant to the understanding of ALS.

VIRUSES ASSOCIATED WITH HUMAN MND

The body of knowledge implicating a viral etiology in ALS is largely derived from reports related to virally caused human disease of the motor neuron, such as poliomyelitis, occasional case reports of MND in association with viruses and unconventional agents, as well as viral serological studies in MND. In this

Table 1   Amyotrophic Lateral Sclerosis (ALS) and Motor Neuron Disease (MND) Associated with RNA or DNA Viruses and Unconventional Agents

Agent	Associated clinical disease	Reference
RNA virus		
Picornaviruses		
poliovirus	Acute poliomyelitis	Reviewed in 50
	PPMA	7,10
	Associated with ALS	5,6,19,20,42
Coxsackie	Acute poliomyelitis	Reviewed in 50
Echovirus	Acute poliomyelitis	Reviewed in 50
Enterovirus 70, 71	Acute poliomyelitis	Reviewed in 50
Retrovirus		
HIV	ALS case report	27
HTLV-I	MND-like disease	30
Paramxyovirus		41
Mumps	Associated with ALS	
Flavivirus		
Schu virus	ALS-like case with CSF pleocytosis	44
Russian spring-summer encephalitis virus	Brachial amyotrophy	Reviewed in 43
DNA virus		
Adenovirus 26	ALS case report	45
Herpes virus		
Varicella zoster	ALS case report	46
Herpes simplex	Atypical MND case report	47
Unconventional agents		
Vilyuisk agent	Amyotrophic encephalitis	Reviewed in 48
SSE agent	Amyotrophic variant of CJD	25,38

PPMA, Postpolio progressive muscular atrophy; CJD, Creutzfeldt-Jakob disease; SSE, subacute spongiform encephalopathy.

section, we review the association of human cases of MND with poliovirus, retroviruses, spongiform encephalopathy agent, and other agents (see Table 1).

Poliovirus

The observation that poliomyelitis and ALS share certain clinicopathological abnormalities has led investigators to search for evidence of poliovirus involvement in ALS. Poliomyelitis is an acute paralytic illness caused by infection with poliovirus, a picornavirus with three different serological types (see later). Although poliovirus infection is said to cause a poliomyelitis, pathological studies have shown that infection is more widespread and actually results in a polioencephalomyelitis. Motor neurons bear the brunt of poliovirus infection, resulting in acute neuronal injury which often leads to cell death and subsequent paralysis. Similarly, motor neurons are the target of disease in ALS. Even though poliovirus infection and ALS share these important similarities, it is important to note that significant differences between these two illnesses exist. Poliomyelitis is an acute illness with intense inflammation, whereas ALS is an indolent disease in which scant, if any, inflammation is found.

Some investigators have found support for the role of poliomyelitis as the etiological agent of ALS by noting that survivors of paralytic poliomyelitis may be at increased risk for MND (4,5), while others have argued the contrary opinion (6–10). Much of the confusion in this area appears to arise from the recent observation that a motor system disease syndrome, known as postpolio muscular atrophy (PPMA) (34,35), may develop in patients 30–40 years after acute poliomyelitis. Although PPMA and ALS may resemble one another, the tempo of disease progression, frequency of upper motor neuron signs, and the electrodiagnostic findings of the two syndromes usually permit differentiation of the two entities (103).

Poliovirus can persist in cultured cells (28,29), immunosuppressed mice (11–13), and immunodeficient children (14,15). These observations have suggested the possibility that poliovirus may also persist in tissue from ALS patients. However, attempts to isolate poliovirus from the central nervous system (CNS) tissue of classical ALS patients (16–19) and of an ALS patient with antecedent poliomyelitis (19) have failed. In one instance (16), no virus could be isolated from ALS tissue even though it had been maintained in culture after repeated passages for a period of several months to a year.

In addition to the above unsuccessful attempts at virus isolation, nucleic acid hybridization experiments of CNS tissue from patients dying of ALS (20–23) and from a patient with an antecedent history of poliomyelitis and ALS (19) have failed to demonstrate poliovirus genome or have led to conflicting results. However, it is possible that the failure to detect poliovirus genome in ALS tissue by hybridization may have been the result of less than ideal experimental conditions. Positive hybridization may have been missed because of inadequate tissue preservation. Furthermore, the use of end-stage ALS autopsy tissue is unsatisfactory because few, if any, motor neurons remain to probe for the presence of putative genome. Finally, the probes that have been used for the hybridization experiments were obtained directly from random-primed viral RNA, rather than the more reliable and better characterized full-length or subgenomic poliovirus cDNA clones. Given the limitations just detailed, it is difficult to make any definite conclusions about the results of the above studies. Future studies using sensitive techniques such as amplification by polymerase chain reaction (PCR) and employing cloned poliovirus cDNA as a probe may be indicated to settle this issue. In this regard, the description of sequence similarity between human ribosomal RNA and poliovirus genome (104) is a potential complication of this experimental approach that may lead to spurious results.

The development and introduction of effective poliovirus vaccines in the late 1950s (Salk) and early 1960s (Sabin) led to successful eradication of poliomyelitis epidemics in the United States. Recent molecular studies have furthered our understanding of the pathogenesis of poliovirus infection, ushered in a foundation for the development of "perfect" vaccines, and clarified the molecular basis for viral neurovirulence. These studies are important to investigations of ALS and are reviewed in the next section.

Retroviruses

The discovery that infection with two retroviruses, human immunodeficiency virus (HIV) and human T-cell lymphocytic virus, type I (HTLV-I), can lead to neurological disease has revived interest in the viral etiology of ALS. The description of a similar neurological disease in mice infected with a neurotropic murine retrovirus has provided investigators with a natural animal model that can be used to study selected aspects of the human infection.

HIV infection leads to acquired immunodeficiency syndrome (AIDS) and allied immunodeficient states (e.g., AIDS-related complex) with opportunistic infections. Infection with HIV also causes meningitis, dementia, vacuolar myelopathy, myopathies, and inflammatory polyradiculoneuritis (reviewed in 26). Involvement of the motor system was suggested in a recent case report (27) of a homosexual man with HIV who developed ALS. This report was significant in that it raised concern that infection with HIV or a related retrovirus may be a cause of MND. However, the isolated nature of this case report suggests that the association was probably coincidental.

HTLV-I infection leads to the development of adult T-cell leukemia and lymphoma. Infection with HTLV-I also causes a chronic myelopathic disease, which is referred to as HTLV-I-associated myelopathy or tropical spastic paraparesis (HAM/TSP). More recently, HTLV-I infection has been associated with an inflammatory myopathy (85–89). At necropsy, cases of HAM/TSP demonstrate an inflammatory meningoencephalomyelitis and, on occasion, radiculoneuritis (30,31), findings dissimilar to those seen in ALS. Degeneration of the posterior and lateral columns with perivascular cuffing is usually present in HAM/TSP cases. There is also variable involvement of the anterior horn that ranges from normal-appearing anterior horn cells to chromatolytic and degenerating motor neurons (31). The anterior horn cell involvement and radiculoneuritis may explain the morphological and electrical evidence of muscle denervation observed in occasional patients.

In HAM/TSP, the presence of both upper motor neuron signs from myelopathy and lower motor neuron dysfunction from radicular and/or anterior horn cell involvement may cause diagnostic confusion with ALS. However, important findings present in HAM/TSP but not in ALS that help in their clinical distinction include: (a) the inflammatory nature of the cerebrospinal fluid; (b) the more chronic tempo of disease progression; (c) the presence of sensory symptoms; and (d) the involvement of sexual, bladder, and bowel function.

We have recently identified a familial upper MND syndrome associated with HTLV-I infection among members of three generations of a Paraguayan pedigree (89). Affected family members suffer from a clinical syndrome that resembles hereditary spastic paraplegia, an autosomal-dominantly inherited MND-like syndrome characterized by progressive degeneration of corticospinal tracts. Serological studies have demonstrated anti-HTLV-I antibody in sera and cerebrospinal fluid (CSF) of affected family members by enzyme-linked immunosorbent assay and Western blot. In addition, isolated peripheral blood mononuclear cells from affected family members have evidence of HTLV-I proteins by cocultivation and of HTLV-I gene sequences by amplification with the PCR method. This report is intriguing because it suggests that retrovirus infection may cause familial motor system disease.

In animals, murine neurotropic retroviruses cause motor system involvement as well as leukemia (32,33). The molecular mechanism for this viral-induced motor neuron cell death in mice is not well understood, but may be relevant to the pathogenesis and etiology of ALS (see later).

Spongiform Encephalopathy Agent

The subacute spongiform encephalopathies include scrapie in sheep and Creutzfeldt-Jakob disease (CJD) and kuru in humans. They are transmissible diseases with no evidence either clinically or pathologically of inflammation. The etiological agent is considered unconventional because the extreme chemical and physical resistance it manifests suggests that it does not contain nucleic acid. The diseased tissue is associated with a proteinase-resistant agent of 27–30 kDa [PrP 27–30 (36)], also referred to as "prion" protein (37), that may be a constituent of the infectious agent as suggested by recent transgeneic experiments (37a).

Studies of spongiform encephalopathies have proven of interest to investigations into the etiology of ALS. Lower motor neuron symptoms and signs are observed in over 10% of cases of transmissible CJD, but usually appear late in the course of the illness and are overshadowed by the plethora of other neurological abnormalities (38,100). On occasion, lower motor neuron involvement appears early and is a prominent feature of the so-called amyotrophic form of CJD. This variant tends to be of relatively long duration and, in contrast to the more typical cases, is usually not transmissible (38). More recently, Brown et al.

(25) called attention to cases of CJD in patients who received injections of cadaver-derived pituitary growth hormone for treatment of dwarfism. This report was of interest because one patient reportedly developed an atypical form of MND.

The relationship of these atypical cases of CJD with prominent motor neuron symptoms and signs to classical ALS remains unclear. Nevertheless, these observations have suggested the possibility that ALS is also caused by a transmissible unconventional agent. However, nonhuman primates inoculated with CNS tissue from ALS patients from mainland United States and Guam (24) have not, to date, developed disease (personal communication, D.C. Gajdusek).

Other Viruses and Unconventional Agents

A variety of other RNA- and DNA-containing viruses, as well as viral-like agents, cause diseases of the motor neuron or have been implicated in the pathogenesis of ALS (see Table 1). The details of some of the viral illnesses discussed are clearly distinct from classical ALS; however, it is of interest to note that they produce motor neuron damage. The link between ALS or MND with some of these agents is based on epidemiological associations or occasional case reports. With rare exceptions, the isolated and infrequent association of these reports makes it difficult to conclude that these agents are a cause of ALS.

Flaviviruses are small arthropod-borne RNA viruses that have an obligatory life-cycle in mosquito or tick vectors. Flaviviruses are reported to persist in experimental animal hosts. There is also evidence that flaviviruses may also persist in human disease. Russian spring-summer (RSS) encephalitis virus and the Schu virus are two flaviviruses that have been noted to be associated with motor system abnormalities (43,44,96).

Infection with RSS encephalitis virus usually leads to an acute meningoencephalitis with high fever, and occasionally focal seizures. This illness is of interest because a brachial amyotrophy syndrome that is restricted to cervical musculature and characterized by wasting and fasciculations ensues during infection (96). The motor deficit usually develops within 2–3 days after the onset of the acute illness. Pathological reports of the acute illness describe intense inflammation in meninges with prominent involvement of cervical spinal cord gray matter, especially anterior horn cells, medulla oblongata, pons, and cerebrum. Although the clinical and pathological features of RSS encephalitis may bear some faint resemblance to ALS, the abrupt onset of disease and the intense CNS inflammatory reaction make clear that these entities are separate and quite distinct.

Schu virus was isolated from various laboratory animals inoculated with CSF obtained from a German patient with a 7-year history of an ALS-like syndrome and CSF pleocytosis (44). Intracerebral inoculation of the isolated virus into cynomolgus monkeys led to seizures and paresis with pathological evidence of encephalitis and motor neuron damage. Although these findings were of interest, the isolation of virus from this case could not be confirmed (reviewed in 44).

Despite the involvement of the motor system in flavivirus infection just described, it is not likely that these viruses play a causative role in ALS. The seasonal and geographical restriction of flavivirus infection is not consistent with the generally uniform incidence and distribution (with minor exceptions) of MND throughout the world. In addition, serum antibody studies of arthropod-borne virus have not convincingly linked the etiology of ALS to infection with these viruses (94).

Of greater interest is the report of amyotrophy occurring not uncommonly in association with Vilyuisk (Viliuisk) encephalitis (VE) (48,97). VE is an infectious illness restricted to the inhabitants of the Yakut (Iakut) Republic (U.S.S.R.). An acute and chronic form of VE are recognized. The acute illness usually presents with fever, headaches, lethargy, and myalgia quickly evolving into a meningoencephalitis. Less commonly, the acute illness is manifest as encephalomyelitis, bulbospinomyelitis, or poliomyelitis. Cranial nerve dysfunction is apt to occur. During this phase, a moderate CSF pleocytosis is evident. About one-third of patients with acute disease evolve to one of several chronic forms within several weeks to a number of years.

Chronic variants of VE include, in order of decreasing frequency: (a) meningoencephalomyelitis (panencephalitis), (b) an amyotrophic syndrome, and (c) a dementing schizophrenia-like illness. In the chronic phase of illness, the CSF reveals a persistent pleocytosis with an elevated CSF protein. The amyotrophic variant of the chronic illness is of interest because this form clinically resembles classical ALS. However, the pathology of this variant is unlike that observed in ALS. It is characterized by inflammation in gray and white matter of the brain and spinal cord with areas of mild demyelination. Amyloid plaques and neurofibrillary tangles are found, and extensive scarring is widespread and evident (48). An RNA virus antigenically similar to Theiler's virus (see next section), a neurotropic picornavirus that naturally infects mice, was isolated from a case of VE (101,102); however, the isolate is likely to have been a containment.

Paramyxovirus infection (mumps) has been implicated in ALS. Quick (90) and Lehrich et al. (41) noted that as many as 20% of ALS patients reported a history of mumps occurring in adulthood. These studies were intriguing since the target of mumps virus, the salivary gland, is known to be a prominent source for nerve growth factor, an important CNS neurotrophic glycoprotein. However, serological studies failed to find any difference in anti–mumps antibody titers between controls and ALS patients (16,41,98). Other studies have also failed to find elevated levels of serum and CSF antibodies in ALS patients to a wide range of RNA and DNA viruses above levels found in controls (16,41,91–95). These results do not lend support to an immune-mediated etiology of ALS associated with viruses or viral antigens.

Finally, two reports of virus isolation/transmissions are included for historical interest; however, these studies have not been substantiated. In the first instance a viral-like agent etiologically related to subacute myeloopticoneuropathy (SMON) was reported to have been isolated from a few patients with ALS (49), but the claims could not be confirmed. Furthermore, the etiology of SMON is now linked to the toxic effects of halogenated 8-hydroxyquinolines (99). In the other case, Zil'ber et al. (39) reported transmission of ALS to rhesus monkeys following intracerebral inoculation. However, this report also could not be confirmed by others (reviewed in 40).

EXPERIMENTAL MODELS OF VIRUS-INDUCED MND

In the previous section, we reviewed the epidemiological findings, occasional case reports, and serological studies in association with virally caused human MND. In this section, we focus on natural and experimental animals models of viral-induced MND.

Rationale for the Study of Experimental Models

What can experimental virus-induced models of MND (as well as the occasional *naturally* occurring cases of viral-induced MND) teach us about MND in general? An example of the value of such investigations can be best gleaned from remembering the importance of the study of oncogenic viruses in our understanding of cancer. The identification of viral *onc* genes led to the recognition of cellular *proto-onc* genes normally present in the human genome that may become expressed and/or dysregulated to cause *nonviral* cancer. The study of experimental viral models of MND may similarly clarify nonviral genes and gene products important in *normal* motor neuron function as well as *nonviral-induced MND*—perhaps in two ways (50). First, we may be able to identify cellular counterparts—*"proto-virulence"* genes—to viral motor neuron *"virulence"* genes that could become expressed and/or dysregulated in nonviral MND. Such an event may not be unreasonable considering that the murine neurotropic retrovirus contains *"virulence"* genes that determine motor neuron damage (see later). Second, the study of viral virulence genes will be important in clarifying the selective vulnerability of motor neurons and the mechanisms by which motor neurons die.

Poliovirus

Poliovirus is probably the best-studied viral model of motor neuron selective death. The impetus for these studies relates to the need for developing a better vaccine. The pioneering studies of poliovirus are best understood after reviewing some basic concepts related to this virus.

Poliovirus types 1, 2, and 3 are members of the enterovirus genus of picornaviruses. The virus contains approximately 7450 nucleotides of single-stranded positive-sense RNA (see later) and four structural proteins. Poliovirus is classified into three serotypes; i.e., antibody raised against one of the three serotypes of poliovirus neutralizes that serotype of poliovirus, but not the other two serotypes. Presumably, the three serotypes of poliovirus have important antigenic differences despite an overall similarity of structure and biophysical properties. Following oral infection with poliovirus, there is a 1 in 1000 chance that paralytic disease will occur, with involvement of the motor neurons both in the spinal cord and in the brain; i.e., the disease is really a polioencephalomyelitis. Most cases of poliomyelitis are caused by poliovirus type 1. In contrast, the Sabin vaccine strains of the three poliovirus types are attenuated and very rarely cause paralytic disease. The reason for the attenuation of the Sabin strains was presumed to be related to the selection of an attenuated mutant to each of the poliovirus types during repeated passage of the strains in tissue culture. However, identification of the specific mutations and of the critical determinants of neurovirulence had to await the use of powerful new molecular techniques.

A key step in the delineation of neurovirulence determinants was the cloning and sequencing of the three parental (paralytic), vaccine (attenuated) poliovirus types and neurovirulent revertant strains. These studies demonstrated that there were a limited number of sequence changes between different strains of the same serotype. For example, there were only 10 nucleotide differences between the parental type 3 poliovirus and the Sabin vaccine strain, and only three of the differences resulted in an amino acid change (51). The minimal differences between these two strains may be responsible for the observation that poliovirus type 3 is the most common cause of vaccine-related poliomyelitis; i.e., the Sabin strain can easily revert to the neurovirulent phenotype. The sequence of the poliovirus type 3 neurovirulent back-mutant of the vaccine strain involves 10 nucleotide differences from the vaccine strain, and two of them involve reversion to a nucleotide present in the parental strain (51). One of the nucleotides that reverts in the vaccine strain is at position 472 in the 5' noncoding region of poliovirus type 3 RNA. This nucleotide appears to be critical in determining neurovirulence, as suggested from studies with infectious complementary DNA (cDNA) (51,52).

The use of infectious cDNA in poliovirus studies was key in the delineation of molecular determinants of the genome critical in neurovirulence. A knowledge of the replication scheme of poliovirus, and of positive-strand RNA viruses in general, is necessary to an understanding of the concept of infectious cDNA. Poliovirus and positive-strand RNA viruses have a single-stranded RNA genome that is in messenger RNA sense, with no DNA phase to the viral life-cycle; i.e.,

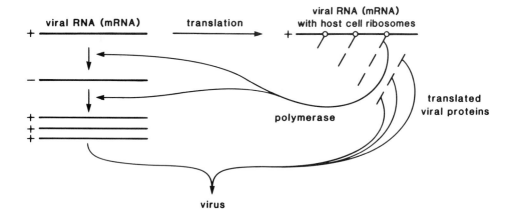

Figure 1 Diagram depicting the replication scheme of positive-strand viruses, such as poliovirus and Theiler's virus. The RNA genome is in the positive (+) or messenger-RNA (mRNA) sense and, therefore, can be directly translated by the ribosomal machinery of the host cell into viral proteins (ribosomes are indicated by small circles). One of the proteins produced is the enzyme (polymerase) that mediates replication of the viral genome into negative-strand RNA and the subsequent replication of this negative-strand RNA into positive-strand RNA. The positive-strand RNA can be packaged with the viral structural (capsid) proteins that were translated into a complete virion. The positive-strand RNA is considered infectious since its entry into a cell (via absorption of virus onto the cell surface or transfection of the RNA) leads to the production of infectious virus. [Reprinted from Ohara and Roos (50a), with permission from Little Brown and Company.]

the RNA genome contains codons that can be directly translated into viral proteins by the host cell ribosomes (Fig. 1). One of the viral proteins that can be translated from the viral RNA genome is an RNA polymerase important in the replication of the RNA. For this reason, the positive-strand RNA genome can be replicated into a minus RNA strand and then the minus strand can be replicated into more positive (genomic) strands. The positive strands can then be assembled into virions that contain viral proteins that were also translated. In other words, the entry of RNA into cells by virus infection (or artificially by transfection) leads to the production of infectious virus; i.e., viral RNA is infectious. We now know that poliovirus cDNA clones are also infectious (53). Full-length cDNA clones can be transcribed in vitro and the RNA produced can be transfected into cells to produce virus. Previously, manipulation of the poliovirus RNA genome was not possible since many of the enzymes necessary for such engineering do not work on RNA. The availability of poliovirus full-length infectious cDNA clones allowed these enzymes to be used to manipulate and mutate the poliovirus genome as a cDNA clone.

Poliovirus cDNA clones have been used in recombinant studies in which pieces of cDNA clones of the parental and vaccine strains have been "cut and pasted" to generate chimeric cDNAs. The chimeric cDNAs can be transcribed in vitro and the RNAs can then be transfected into cells to produce recombinant viruses. The recombinant viruses can be injected into animals to determine which gene segments are responsible for particular phenotypes, such as neurovirulence. Once the location of key areas is clarified, a particular nucleotide or segment can be changed by site-directed mutagenesis in order to provide a precise delineation of the determinants. Poliovirus infectious cDNA studies have implicated one nucleotide in the 5' noncoding region of the RNA as a key determinant of neurovirulence in all three poliovirus types (51,52,54); other areas of the genome [such as the region coding for amino acid 2034 in poliovirus type 3 VP3 capsid protein (51)] also contribute to the neurovirulent phenotype. The nucleotide in the 5' noncoding region is the same one that mutated during the attenuation of the parental strains into the Sabin strains. Of interest is the fact that this nucleotide rapidly and frequently reverts back to the parental sequence following oral administration of the vaccine (51). The reason for the high frequency of reversion may be because the mutated nucleotide (back to the sequence present in the paralytic strain) allows the virus to have enhanced growth in the gut. One might ask why there are not more vaccine-related poliomyelitis cases if the sequence of the vaccine strain frequently reverts to a neurovirulent phenotype. It may be that other viral determinants are important in the actual spread of the virus into the CNS. In addition, host factors such as the immune response may be able to prevent CNS infection because of the delay involving the generation of this mutation of the virus genome.

By what mechanism does this single nucleotide change affect neurovirulence? The 5' noncoding region is a relatively long stretch of the genome. It contains approximately 743 untranslated nucleotides and it is believed to play a role in the regulation of viral translation and replication. Current studies have identified a host factor(s), presumably a protein, that binds to the 5' noncoding region and may enhance translation (55,56). It may be that there are also motor neuron–specific factors that bind to the 5' noncoding region that influence the efficiency of translation of this RNA, and that the binding of these putative factors partly depends on the particular nucleotide at position 472. These cellular factors may influence the expression of other motor neuron mRNAs, especially mRNAs that do not have the typical 7-methyl guanosine "cap" on the 5' end of the RNA (which is not present on poliovirus RNA).

Are there other determinants of neurovirulence besides the single nucleotide in the 5' noncoding region? Although additional areas of the poliovirus genome appear to contribute to neurovirulence, they seem to have less of an impact on neurovirulence than this single nucleotide. Experiments related to the viral attachment protein on the virus as well as the poliovirus receptor on cells have elucidated other important regions of the genome. Studies with infectious poliovirus cDNA chimeras between mouse-adapted poliovirus and the wild-type poliovirus (which infects only primates) have identified a stretch of six to eight amino acids of a structural "capsid" protein, VP1, that appears to be important in the adaptation of the virus to mice (57,58). This amino acid sequence is believed to be important because it may directly or indirectly mediate binding to the mouse motor neuron. Interestingly, this segment constitutes a trypsin-sensitive major neutralization epitope of the virus.

The above studies interface well with ongoing investigations involving the cellular receptor for the virus. The poliovirus receptor that is present on susceptible tissue culture cells has recently been cloned (59), and the expression of this gene on neural cells is under investigation. Interestingly, the receptor appears to be an as yet unidentified member of the immunoglobulin superfamily; ICAM, another member of the immunoglobulin superfamily, is the receptor for another picornavirus, rhinovirus (60). Most recently, the human poliovirus receptor gene has been introduced into the mouse genome (60a,b). Investigations of these poliovirus-sensitive transgenic mice will be important in understanding poliovirus pathogenesis. The above studies will also be important in delineating motor neuron–specific proteins (such as the poliovirus receptor) as well as characterizing the binding of ligands (such as viral attachment proteins) to the receptor; i.e., these studies will teach us about normal motor neuron cell biology, an important foundation for beginning to understand motor neuron disease.

Theiler's Murine Encephalomyelitis Virus

Although poliovirus has been an excellent system for the study of genes and gene products critical in neurovirulence and motor neuron death, most animal experiments have involved a subhuman primate as the experimental host—unless mouse-adapted strains or transgenic mice were used. Our laboratory has investigated another picornavirus, Theiler's murine encephalomyelitis virus (TMEV). Studies with this virus have all the advantages of those performed with poliovirus (e.g., a simple virus that is well understood from a molecular and structural point of view; the availability of infectious cDNA), but some additional features make the TMEV system especially attractive. One important feature of TMEV is that the mouse is both the natural and experimental host for infection. In addition, TMEV strains are naturally divided into two subgroups that differ markedly with respect to their biological properties (61,62). GDVII strain and other members of the GDVII subgroup are highly neurovirulent and produce an acute fatal polioencephalomyelitis in weanling mice. In contrast, DA strain and other members of the TO subgroup produce a chronic, demyelinating, persistent infection with an apparently restricted virus expression (63). The "rich," diverse phenotype of TMEV strains provides the opportunity to explore genes critical for demyelination and virus persistence as well as neurovirulence.

Our strategy in exploring the molecular determinants for TMEV disease has

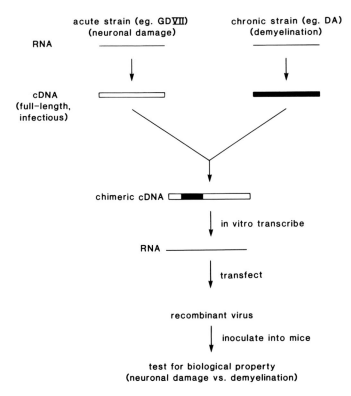

Figure 2 Diagram depicting the experimental plan for recombinant infections cDNA studies with strains of Theiler's murine encephalomyelitis viruses. GDVII strain produces an acute fatal neuronal infection in mice, while DA strain produces a chronic demyelinating disease. Full-length cDNAs in a transcription vector are generated from GDVII and DA viral RNAs. Segments of the cDNAs can be "cut and pasted" to make GDVII/DA chimeric cDNAs. The chimeric cDNAs are in vitro transcribed into full-length RNAs that are transfected into cells. The RNAs are infectious (see Fig. 1 and text) and virus is produced that can be inoculated into mice. The importance of a particular genome segment in neurovirulence or other strain-specific biological properties can be determined by evaluating the disease produced in animals inoculated with the various recombinant viruses.

been similar to that used with poliovirus (Fig. 2). As a key step, infectious cDNA clones of both GDVII and DA strains were produced (noted as pGDFL2 and pDAFL3, respectively) (64,65). Virus produced from these clones retained the phenotype of the parental wild-type virus. One plaque forming unit (pfu) of GDVII killed a 4-week-old mouse in less than 4 weeks. In contrast, greater than 10^6 pfus of DA did not kill a weanling mouse, but produced a chronic, demyelinating persistent infection.

A series of chimeric GDVII-DA cDNAs were generated (Fig. 3) (65). The

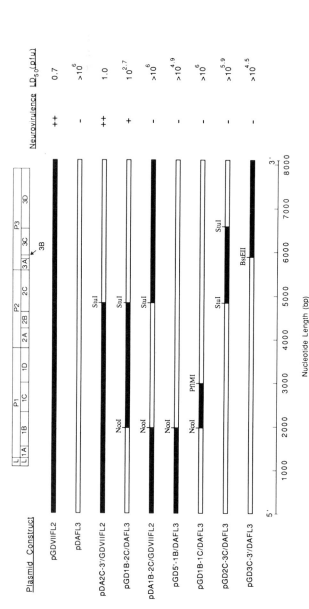

Figure 3 A series of TMEV chimeric cDNAs and their neurovirulence phenotype. The restriction sites used to generate the chimeric cDNAs are noted above the individual plasmid constructs. GDVII segments are shown as the dark, shaded areas, while DA segments are shown as the open, light areas of the genome. The TMEV coding area shown at the top of the figure, and the nucleotide position in the genome is shown at the bottom. The P1 area codes for the viral structural (capsid) proteins. Each of the chimeric cDNAs is transcribed in vitro, then the RNAs are transfected into tissue culture cells to generate virus, and finally the virus stock is inoculated into mice to determine neurovirulence. The neurovirulence phenotype is given as the number of plaque forming units (pfus) that kills 50% of mice (LD_{50}), as well as graded − (attenuated), + (somewhat neurovirulent), + (highly neurovirulent). The studies show that a major determinant of TMEV neurovirulence is within the GDVII 1B(VP2) to 2C coding region, most likely in the GDVII 1D(VP1) to 2A coding region. Genomic sequences 5′ to this region of GDVII RNA also contribute to expression of the full neurovirulence phenotype.

chimeras could be transcribed in vitro and the resultant RNAs transfected to produce recombinant viruses. These studies have identified a coding region from the capsid protein 1B (VP2) to the nonstructural protein 2C as critical for producing death of a weanling mouse (note recombinant DA1B-2C/GDFL2 virus in Fig. 3). An additional recombinant virus, DA1B-1C/GDFL2, is not neurovirulent, suggesting that the key determinant is within the 1D (VP1) to 2C coding region. This area has about 33 amino acid differences between the genomes of DA and GDVII strains. One might suspect that VP1, the only capsid protein coded for in this area, is the key area, especially considering that the poliovirus studies, noted above, identified a short amino acid stretch in VP1 as critical for mouse neuronal binding. It may be that efficient binding of TMEV to mouse neurons also requires a similar VP1 segment. For this reason, we are now involved in site-directed mutagenesis studies of the infectious DA cDNA clone to mutate sequences in an area aligned with the VP1 segment identified as important in the poliovirus studies. We are also mutating a trypsin-sensitive major neutralization site located at the carboxyl end of VP1C since this site appears to be important in disease pathogenesis (66), and since the poliovirus VP1 segment critical for mouse neuronal binding is also a trypsin-sensitive neutralization site. Although the GDVII 1B-2C coding area is critical in producing death of mice acutely, possession of this segment does not generate virus with the full neurovirulent phenotype of GDVII; i.e., the 50% lethal dose (LD_{50}) of GD1B-2C/DAFL3 virus is $10^{2.7}$, compared to the LD_{50} of 1 of GDFL2. The presence of the GDVII genome upstream from the 1B coding area to the GDVII 1B-2C coding area allows the virus to become fully neurovirulent. We are presently involved in more precisely defining the important determinants in this upstream area. The critical determinant may be localized in the 5' noncoding region, as is true with poliovirus.

The same recombinant viruses used for these studies of neurovirulence will clearly also be important in delineating important determinants of demyelination and virus persistence. For this reason, these investigations may be important in our understanding not only of MND, but of multiple sclerosis as well.

Murine Retrovirus

In the 1970s Gardner et al. described a colony of wild mice that developed leukemia and hind limb paralysis (reviewed in 67). The cause of this disease was identified as a murine neurotropic leukemia virus, also called Cas-B-E murine leukemia virus. The virus is a member of the oncovirus group of retroviruses, which are RNA viruses that replicate by means of reverse transcriptase to generate a DNA phase (prophase) in the virus life-cycle. It is now known that murine neurotropic retrovirus, as well as a temperature-sensitive (*ts*) mutant strain of Moloney murine leukemia virus (68) and "paralysis-inducing" murine leukemia viruses isolated from Friend virus (69), can experimentally produce paralysis when inoculated neonatally into certain strains of rodents. The pathology of the disease is of interest because of its noninflammatory nature, as is the case in ALS. There is spongiform degeneration of neurons with a marked proliferation of astroglial cells, primarily in the spinal cord. Basic questions related to these viruses include the following. What is the genetic determinant for paralysis in the particular virus? What is the pathogenesis for the motor neuron destruction; i.e., is there actual infection of the motor neuron or just of endothelial cells—as suggested by some experiments (70)? Answers to these questions may have important implications in our understanding of the pathogenesis of retroviral-induced human MND, such as those associated with HTLV-I and HIV.

In order to answer the questions raised above, Jolicoeur and colleagues cloned the murine neurotropic leukemia virus (71). Virus derived from the transfected neurotropic clone produced paralysis (as well as lymphoma) after inoculation of neonatal mice, confirming the importance of this virus in the development of the neurological disease. The availability of neurotropic murine leukemia virus–specific probes will make possible identification of the cells that harbor the virus. Chimeric DNAs between this clone and a cloned nonneurotropic retrovirus have been prepared. The chimeric DNAs were transfected into cells and the progeny virus then inoculated into mice to determine the phenotype. The chimeric studies demonstrated that a genome fragment from the neurotropic strain that comprises the *env* gene (which codes for the envelope glycoprotein, gp70) is sufficient to confer paralysis onto the recombinant virus (72). It is unclear how the gp70 could actually influence the neurotropism of the virus. One possibility is that this glycoprotein is important in binding to specific neural cells. Another possibility is that gp70 is somehow "toxic" to motor neurons. The latter hypothesis could be tested by observing the effect of gp70 on cultured motor neurons, or by carrying out transgenic studies. Additional chimeric DNAs and recombinant viruses demonstrated that the long terminal repeat (LTR) sequences also play a role (73). Jolicoeur and colleagues noted that the LTR can influence the incidence and clinical manifestations of the disease as well as the topographical distribution of the spongiform degeneration.

Wong and colleagues, on the other hand, have primarily investigated a *ts* mutant of Moloney leukemia virus. Interestingly, this virus produces not only a paralysis in BALB/c mice, but also body wasting, thymic atrophy, and lymphopenia due to T-lymphocyte destruction (74). The *ts* mutant has an abnormality in processing one of the precursor polyproteins of the envelope glycoproteins, Pr 80 (75). Chimeric DNAs generated from the genomes of the paralytogenic *ts* and nonparalytogenic wild-type strains have shown that the neurovirulence determinant lies within the *env* coding gene (76). It is believed that one amino acid in the *env* gene is responsible for the *ts* phenotype, the processing abnormality, as well as the neurovirulence of the *ts* mutant. This same mutant may be the key one in producing the immunosuppression syndrome since chimera studies have shown that this genetic determinant is also localized to the *env* gene.

Lactic Dehydrogenase–Elevating Virus

Lactic dehydrogenase–elevating virus (LDV) was discovered by Riley et al. (reviewed in 77,78). It is now believed to be a member of the Togaviridae family of RNA viruses in an as yet unnamed genus. The virus receives its name from the fact that it produces a lowering of lactic dehydrogenase (LDH) isoenzyme in mouse plasma. This lowering is thought to result from an infection of a subpopulation of macrophages of the mouse that is normally responsible for clearing the enzyme. A chronic asymptomatic persistent viremia ensues with circulating antibody complexes and a depressed humoral immune response.

On several occasions, inadvertent LDV contamination of transferred mouse tissue has confused investigators (79). The example most relevant to this chapter occurred in 1970 when Murphy noted that C58 mice aged over 6 months developed paralysis with neuronal destruction and gray matter perivascular cuffs 7–14 days after implantation of a leukemic cell line (80). The disease was initially called immune polioencephalomyelitis because it could be transferred by injection of serum from an affected mouse. The disease is now known to have been caused by a LDV strain (81).

Inoculation of different strains of purified LDV have been shown to produce polioencephalomyelitis or spongiform poliomyelopathy. The pathogenesis of this LDV-induced MND depends on the strain, age, and immune status of the mouse (82–84). Only C58 and AKR mice that are over 6 months of age are susceptible to the disease. However, susceptibility can be enhanced, or younger mice can be made susceptible, following immunosuppression with x-irradiation or drugs. Susceptibility is linked to the presence of multiple proviral copies of N-tropic endogenous murine leukemia viruses (MuLV) and Fv-$1^{n/n}$, the permissive allele for N-tropic, ecotropic virus replication. Immunosuppression produces a transient increase in ecotropic MuLV RNA levels in spinal cord motor neurons. Peripheral inoculation of LDV at this time leads to LDV infection of spinal cord motor neurons. LDV then spreads slowly throughout the spinal cord, producing cytolysis of neurons and progressive paralysis over the next 2–3 weeks (84).

A number of questions related to LDV-induced MND remain unanswered. (a) What is the origin of the MuLV that produces the motor neuron infection? (b) Does the MuLV result from induction of provirus in the motor neurons or from spread to motor neurons from MuLV produced in nonneural tissues? (c) What is the relationship of MuLV infection to the LDV infection—could a MuLV-induced surface protein act as an LDV receptor and what are the molecular determinants for paralytic disease in the genome of the MND-inducing strain of LDV?

The pathogenesis of LDV-induced MND is complicated. Its complexity reminds one that identification of a virus as the cause of a disease such as ALS may be extremely difficult. Multiple viruses could even be involved in the selective death of motor neurons. An understanding of the pathogenesis of non–viral-induced ALS may require a variety of experimental manipulations.

SUMMARY

We have reexamined the connection between human MND and infection with viruses and unconventional agents and have discussed current work on experimental models of animal MND. The link between poliovirus and ALS remains to be defined. The availability of better poliovirus probes and more sensitive molecular techniques, such as PCR, may help to determine whether poliovirus genome is also found in normal individuals and ALS patients.

From other accounts, occasional case reports of ALS or MND-like disease are found in association with different agents. Many of these findings, if not all, remain unconfirmed. Serological antiviral antibody studies fail to provide evidence for a viral etiology in ALS. Nevertheless, the increasing recognition of motor system disease with retrovirus infection in humans and animals is of interest to studies of ALS. The motor neuron involvement found in CJD indicates that noninflammatory disease, such as ALS, may be transmissible.

Experimental models of virus-induced MND in animals may clarify our understanding of ALS. Molecular studies of these viruses may identify genes and gene products that have a role in normal motor neuronal function, and that may become dysregulated in diseases of the motor neuron.

ACKNOWLEDGMENTS

The secretarial services of Lee Baksas in the preparation of this chapter are appreciated. This work was supported in part by Public Health Science Grant 1P01 NS21442 from the National Institutes of Health.

REFERENCES

1. Tandan R, Bradley WG. Amyotrophic lateral sclerosis. Part 2. Etiopathogenesis. Ann Neurol 1985;18:419–431.
2. Rowland L. Motor neuron disease and amyotrophic lateral sclerosis: Research progress. Trends Neurosci 1987;10:393–398.
3. Mitsumoto H, Hanson MR, Chad DA. Amyotrophic lateral sclerosis. Recent advances in pathogenesis and therapeutic trials. Arch Neurol 1988;45:189–202.

4. Zilkha KJ. Discussion on motor neurone disease. Proc R Soc Med 1962;55:1028–1029.
5. Martyn CN, Barker DJP, Osmond C. Motorneuron disease and past poliomyelitis in England and Wales. Lancet 1988;1:1319–1322.
6. Poskanzer DC, Cantor HM, Kaplan GS. The frequency of preceding poliomyelitis in amyotrophic lateral sclerosis. In: Norris FH Jr, Kurland LT, eds. Motor neuron disease: Research on amyotrophic lateral sclerosis and related disorders. New York: Grune & Stratton, 1969:286–290.
7. Alter M, Kurland LT, Molgaard CA. Late progressive muscular atrophy and antecedent poliomyelitis. In: Rowland L, ed. Human motor neuron diseases. New York: Raven Press, 1982:303–309.
8. Sood K, Nag D. Motorneuron disease and past poliomyelitis. Lancet 1988;2:393 (Letter).
9. Clements GB, Beghan WMH, Behan PO, et al. Relation between motorneuron disease and past poliomyelitis. Lancet 1988;2:1024–1025 (Letter).
10. Editorial. Late sequalae of poliomyelitis. Lancet 1986;2:1195–1196.
11. Miller JR. Prolonged intracerebral infection with poliovirus in asymptomatic mice. Ann Neurol 1981;9:590–596.
12. Jubelt B, Meagher JB. Poliovirus infection of cyclophosphamide-treated mice results in persistence and late paralysis. I. Clinical, pathologic, and immunologic studies. Neurology 1984;34:486–493.
13. Jubelt B, Meagher JB. Poliovirus infection of cyclophosphamide-treated mice results in persistence and late paralysis. II. Virologic studies. Neurology 1988: 494–499.
14. Wyatt HV. Poliomyelitis in hypogammaglobulinemia. J Infect Dis 1973;128:802–806.
15. Davis LE, Bodian D, Price D, et al. Chronic progressive poliomyelitis secondary to vaccination of an immunodeficient child. N Engl J Med 1977;297:241–245.
16. Cremer NE, Oshiro LS, Norris FH, et al. Culture of tissues from patients with amyotrophic lateral sclerosis. Arch Neurol 1973;29:331–333.
17. Weiner LP, Stohlman SA, Davis R. Attempts to demonstrate virus in amyotrophic lateral sclerosis. Neurology 1980;30:1319–1322.
18. Kascsak RT, Carp RI, Vilcek JT, et al. Virological studies in amyotrophic lateral sclerosis. Muscle Nerve 1982;5:93–101.
19. Roos RP, Viola M, Wollman R, et al. Amyotrophic lateral sclerosis with antecedent poliomyelitis. Arch Neurol 1980;37:312–331.
20. Brahic M, Smith RA, Gibbs CJ Jr, et al. Detection of picornavirus sequences in nervous tissue of amyotrophic lateral sclerosis. Ann Neurol 1985;18:337–343.
21. Kohne DE, Gibbs CJ Jr, White L, et al. Virus detection by nucleic acid hybridization: examination of normal and ALS tissues for the presence of poliovirus. J Gen Virol 1981;56:223–233.
22. Miller JR, Guntaka RM, Meyers J. Amyotrophic lateral sclerosis. Search for poliovirus by nucleic acid hybridization. Neurology 1980;30:884–886.
23. Viola M, Meyers J, Gramm K, et al. Failure to detect poliovirus genetic information in amyotrophic lateral sclerosis. Ann Neurol 1979;5:402–403.

24. Gibbs CJ Jr, Gajdusek DC. An update on long-term in vivo and in vitro studies designed to identify a virus as the cause of amyotrophic lateral sclerosis, parkinsonism-dementia, and Parkinson's disease. In: Rowland L, ed. Human motor neuron diseases. New York: Raven Press, 1982:343–353.

25. Brown P, Gajdusek DC, Gibbs CJ Jr, et al. Potential epidemic of Creutzfeldt-Jakob disease from human growth hormone therapy. N Engl J Med 1985;313: 728–731.

26. MacArthur JC. Neurologic manifestations of AIDS. Medicine 1987;66:407–437.

27. Hoffman PM, Festoff BW, Giron LT, et al. Isolation of LAV/HTLV-III from a patient with amyotrophic lateral sclerosis. N Engl J Med 1985;313:1493–1497 (Correspondence).

28. Miller JR, Britton CB, Kormer J. Persistent poliovirus infection in cell culture. Neurology 1984;34:237–238.

29. Colbere-Garapin F, Christodoulou C, Crainic R, et al. Persistent poliovirus infection of human neuroblastoma cells. Proc Natl Acad Sci USA 1989;86:7590–7594.

30. Vernant J-C, Buisson G, Bellance R, et al. Pseudo-amyotrophic lateral sclerosis, peripheral neuropathy and chronic polyradiculoneuritis in HTLV-I-associated paraplegias. In: Román GC, Vernant J-C, Osame M, eds., HTLV-I and the nervous system. New York: Alan R. Liss, 1989:361–365.

31. Iwasaki I. Neuropathology of HAM/TS: an overview. In: Iwasaki Y, ed., Neuropathology of HAM/TSP in Japan. Proceedings of the First Workshop on Neuropathology of Retrovirus Infections, Tokyo, Japan, Aug. 31, 1989:118–131.

32. Gardner MB, Henderson BE, Estes JD, et al. An unusually high incidence of spontaneous lymphoma in a population of wild house mice. J Natl Cancer Inst 1973;50:1571–1579.

33. Officer JE, Tecson N, Fontanilla E, et al. Isolation of a neurotropic type C virus. Science 1973;181:945–947.

34. Mulder DW, Rosenbaum RP, Layton DD Jr. Late motor neuron degeneration following poliomyelitis. Mayo Clin Proc 1972;47:756–761.

35. Brown S, Patten BM: Post-polio syndrome and amyotrophic lateral sclerosis: A relationship more apparent than real. In: Halstead LS, Wiechers DO, eds. Research and clinical aspects of the late effects of poliomyelitis. Birth Defects: Original article series 1987;23:83–98.

36. Bolton DC, Meyer RK, Prusiner SB. Scrapie PrP 27-30 is a sialoglycoprotein. J Virol 1985;53:596–606.

37. Prusiner SB. Novel proteinaceous infectious particles cause scrapie. Science 1982;216:136–144.

37a. Hsiao KK, Scott M, Foster D, et al. Spontaneous neurodegeneration in transgenic mice with mutant prion protein. Science 1990;250:1587–1590.

38. Salazar AM, Masters CL, Gajdusek DC, et al. Syndromes of amyotrophic lateral sclerosis and dementia: Relation to transmissable Creutzfeldt-Jakob disease. Ann Neurol 1983;14:17–26.

39. Zil'ber LA, Bajdakova ZL, Barababadze EM. Study of the etiology of amyotrophic lateral sclerosis. Bull WHO 1963;29:449–456.

40. Harter DH. Viruses other than poliovirus in human amyotrophic lateral sclerosis.

In: Rowland L, ed. Human motor neuron diseases. New York: Raven Press, 1982:339–342.

41. Lehrich J, Oger J, Arnason BGW. Neutralizing antibodies to poliovirus and mumps virus in amyotrophic lateral sclerosis. J Neurol Sci 1974;23:517–540.

42. Armon C, Daube JR, Windebank AJ, et al. How frequently does classic amyotrophic lateral sclerosis develop in survivors of poliomyelitis? Neurology 1990;40: 172–174.

43. Johnson RT, Brooks BR. Possible viral etiology of amyotrophic lateral sclerosis. In: Serratrice G, et al, eds. Neuromuscular diseases, New York: Raven Press, 1984:353–359.

44. Muller WK, Schaltenbrand G. Attempts to reproduce amyotrophic lateral sclerosis in laboratory animals by inoculation of Schu virus from a patient with apparent amyotrophic lateral sclerosis. Neurology 1979;220:1–19.

45. Delsedime M, Mutani R, Giuliani G. Un caso di sindrome tipo sclerosi laterale amiotrofica ad indagine virale positiva sul liquor. Acta Neurol (Napoli) 1974;29: 197–201.

46. Maida E, Kristoferitsch W. Amyotrophic lateral sclerosis following herpes zoster infection in a patient with immunodeficiency. Eur Neurol 1981;20:330–333.

47. Maida E, Traugott U, Eibl M. Transfer-fakyotitherapie bei einem fall von chronischer Herpes simplex myelitis. Nervenarzt 1978;671–673.

48. Gajdusek DC. Foci of motor neuron disease in high incidence in isolated populations of East Asia and the Western Pacific. In: Rowland L, ed. Human motor neuron diseases. New York: Raven Press, 1982:363–393.

49. Melnick JL, Seidel E, Inoue YK, et al. Isolation of virus from the spinal fluid of three patients with multiple sclerosis and one with amyotrophic lateral sclerosis. Lancet 1982;1:830–833.

50. Jubelt B, Lipton H. Enterovirus infection. In: Vinken PJ, Bruyn GW, Klawans HL, McKendall PR, eds., Viral disease. Handbook of clinical neurology. Amsterdam: Elsevier, 1989;12:307–347.

50a. Ohara Y, Roos RP. Viral infectious complementary-DNA studies may identify nonviral genes critical to central nervous system disease. Ann Neurol 1989;25: 305–309.

51. Minor PD, Dunn G, John A, Phillips A, Westrop GD, Wareham K, Almond JW. Attenuation and reversion of the Sabin type 3 vaccine strain. In: Semler BL, Ehrenfeld E, eds. Molecular aspects of picornavirus infection and detection. Vol. 18. Washington, DC: American Society for Microbiology, 1989:307–318.

52. Nomoto A, Kawamura N, Kohara M, Arita M. Expression of the attenuation phenotype of poliovirus type 1. In: Semler BL, Ehrenfeld E, eds. Molecular aspects of picornavirus infection and detection. Vol. 17. Washington, DC: American Society for Microbiology, 1989:297–306.

53. Racaniello VR, Baltimore D. Cloned poliovirus complementary DNA is infectious in mammalian cells. Science 1981;214:916–919.

54. Racaniello VR, La Monica N, Moss EG, O'Neill R. Genetic analysis of neurovirulence, using a mouse model for poliomyelitis. In: Semler BL, Ehrenfeld E, eds. Molecular aspects of picornavirus infection and detection. Vol. 17. Washington, DC: American Society for Microbiology, 1989:297–306.

55. Meerovitch K, Pelletier J, Sonenberg N. A cellular protein that binds to the 5'-noncoding region of poliovirus RNA: Implications for internal translation initiation. Genes Dev 1989;3:1026–1034.

56. Del Angel RN, Papavassiliou AG, Fernandez-Tomas C, Silverstein SJ, Racaniello VR. Cell proteins bind to multiple sites with the 5' untranslated region of polioviruse RNA. Proc Natl Acad Sci USA 1989;86:8299–8303.

57. Girard M, Martin A, Couderc T, Crainic R, Wychowski C. Modification of six amino acids in the VP1 capsid protein of poliovirus type 1, Mahoney strain, alters its host range and makes it neurovirulent for mice. In: Semler BL, Ehrenfeld E, eds., Molecular aspects of picornavirus infection and detection. Vol. 17. Washington, DC: American Society for Microbiology, 1989:265–280.

58. Murray MG, Bradley J, Yang X-F, et al. Poliovirus host range is determined by a short amino acid sequence in neutralization antigenic site I. Science 1988;241: 213–215.

59. Mendelsohn CL, Wimmer E, Racaniello VR. Cellular receptor for poliovirus: Molecular cloning, nucleotide sequence, and expression of a new number of the immunoglobulin superfamily. Cell 1989;56:855–865.

60. Greve J, Davis G, Meyer AM, et al. The major human rhinovirus receptor is ICAM-1. Cell 1989;56:839–847.

60a. Ren R, Costantini F, Gorgacz E, et al. Transgenic mice expressing a human poliovirus receptor; a new model for poliomyelitis. Cell 1990;63:353–362.

60b. Koike S, Taya C, Kurata T, et al. Transgenic mice susceptible to poliovirus. Proc Natl Acad Sci USA (in press).

61. Lipton H. Persistent Theiler's murine encephalomyelitis virus infection in mice depends on plaque size. J Gen Virol 1980;46:169–177.

62. Lorch Y, Friedman A, Lipton HL, Kotler M. Theiler's murine encephalomyelitis virus group includes two distinct subgroups that differ pathologically and biologically. J Virol 1981;40:560–567.

63. Cash E, Chamorro M, Brahic M. Theiler's virus RNA and protein synthesis in the central nervous system of demyelinating mice. Virology 1985;144:290–294.

64. Roos RP, Stein S, Ohara Y, Fu J, Semler BL. Infectious cDNA clones of DA strain of Theiler's murine encephalomyelitis virus. J Virol 1989;63:5492–5496.

65. Fu J, Stein S, Rosenstein L, Bodwell T, Routbort M, Semler BL, Roos RP. Neurovirulence determinants of genetically engineered Theiler's viruses. Proc Natl Acad Sci USA 1990;87:4125–4129.

66. Roos RP, Stein S, Routbort M, Senkowski A, Bodwell T, Wollmann R. Theiler's murine encephalomyelitis virus neutralization escape mutants have a change in disease phenotype. J Virol 1989;63:4469–4473.

67. Gardner MB. Retroviral spongiform polioencephalitis. Rev Infect Dis 1985;7: 99–110.

68. Wong PKY, Soong MM, Macleod R, Gallick GE, Yuen PH. A group of temperature-sensitive mutants of Moloney leukemia virus which is defective in cleavage of env precursor polypeptide in infected cells also induces hind-limb paralysis in newborn CFW/D mice. Virology 1983;125:513–518.

69. Kai K, Furuta T. Isolation of paralysis-inducing murine leukemia viruses from Friend virus passaged in rats. J Virol 1984;50:970–973.
70. Hoffman PM, Pitts OM, Bilello JA, Cimino EF. Retrovirus induced motor neuron degeneration. Rev Neurol 1988;144:676–679.
71. Jolicoeur P, Nicolaiew N, DesGroseillers L, Rassart E. Molecular cloning of infectious viral DNA from ecotropic neurotropic wild mouse retrovirus. J Virol 1983;45:1159–1163.
72. Paquette Y, Hanna Z, Savard P, Brousseau R, Robitaille Y, Jolicoeur P. Retrovirus-induced murine motor neuron disease: Mapping the determinant of spongiform degeneration within the envelope gene. Proc Natl Acad Sci USA 1989;86: 3896–3900.
73. DesGroseillers L, Rassart E, Robitaille Y, Jolicoeur P. Retrovirus-induced spongiform encephalopathy: The 3′-end long terminal repeat–containing viral sequences influence the incidence of the disease and the specificity of the neurological syndrome. Proc Natl Acad Sci USA 1985;82:8818–8822.
74. Wong PKY, Prasad G, Hansen J, Yuen PH. ts1, a mutant of Moloney murine leukemia virus-TB, causes both immunodeficiency and neurologic disorders in BALB/c mice. Virology 1989;170:450–459.
75. Yuen PH, Malehorn D, Knupp C, et al. A 1.6-kilobase-pair fragment in the genome of the ts1 mutant of Moloney murine leukemia virus TB that is associated with temperature sensitivity, nonprocessing of Pr80^{env}, and paralytogenesis. J Virol 1985;54:364–373.
76. Yeun PH, Szurek PF. The reduced virulence of the thymotropic Moloney murine leukemia virus derivative MoMuLV-TB is mapped to 11 mutations within the U3 region of the long terminal repeat. J Virol 1989;63:471–480.
77. Riley V. Persistence and other characteristics of the lactate dehydrogenase–elevating virus (LDH-virus). Prog Med Virol 1974;18:198–213.
78. Rowson KEK, Mahy BWJ. Lactate dehydrogenase–elevating virus. J Gen Virol 1985;66:2297–2312.
79. Riley V. Biological contaminants and scientific misinterpretations. Cancer Res 1974;34:1752–1754.
80. Murphy WH. Mouse model for motor neurone disease-immune polioencephalomyelitis. In: Behan PO, Rose RC, eds. Progress in neurological research. London: Pitman, 1979:175–193.
81. Martinez D, Brinton MA, Tachovsky TG, Phelps AH. Identification of lactate dehydrogenase–elevating virus as the etiological agent of genetically restricted, age-dependent polioencephalomyelitis of mice. Infect Immun 1980;27:979–987.
82. Pease LR, Abrams GD, Murphy WH. FV-1 restriction of age-dependent paralytic lactic dehydrogenase virus infection. Virology 1982;117:29–37.
83. Stroop WG, Brinton MA. Mouse strain–specific central nervous system lesions associated with lactate dehydrogenase–elevating virus infection. Lab Invest 1983;49:334–344.
84. Contag CH, Plagemann PGW. Age-dependent poliomyelitis of mice: Expression of endogenous retrovirus correlates with cytocidal replication of lactate dehydrogenase–elevating virus in motor neurons. J Virol 1989;63:4362–4369.

85. Piccardo P, Ceroni M, Rodgers-Johnson P, et al. Pathological and immunological observations on tropical spastic paraparesis in patients from Jamaica. Ann Neurol 1988;23(Suppl):S156–S160.

86. Wiley CA, Nerenberg M, Cros D, et al. HTLV-I polymyositis in a patient also infected with the human immunodeficiency virus. N Engl J Med 1989;320:992–995.

87. Tarras S, Sheremata WA, Snodgrass S, et al. Polymyositis and chronic myelopathy associated with presence of cerebrospinal fluid antibody to HTLV-I. In: Roman GC, Vernant J-C, Osame M, eds. HTLV-I and the nervous system. Vol. 51. New York: Alan R. Liss, 1989:435–441.

88. Evans BK, Gore I, Harrell LE, et al. HTLV-I-associated myelopathy and polymyositis in a US native. Neurology 1989;39:1572–1575.

89. Salazar-Greuso EF, Holzer TJ, Gutierrez RA, et al. Familial spastic paraparesis (FSP) syndrome associated with HTLV-I infection. N Engl J Med 1990;323:732–736.

90. Quick DT. Pancreatic dysfunction in amyotrophic lateral sclerosis. In: Norris FH, Kurland LT, eds. Motor neuron diseases. New York: Grune & Stratton, 1969:189–198.

91. Catalano LW Jr. Herpesvirus hominis antibody in multiple sclerosis and amyotrophic lateral sclerosis. Neurology 1972;22:473–478.

92. Cremer NE, Norris FH, Shinomoto T, et al. Antibody titers to coxsackieviruses in amyotrophic lateral sclerosis. N Engl J Med 1976;295:107–108 (Correspondence).

93. Kacsack RJ, Shope RE, Donnenfeld H, et al. Antibody response to arboviruses. Absence of increased response in amyotrophic lateral sclerosis. Arch Neurol 1978;35:440–442.

94. Kurent JE, Brooks BR, Madden DL, et al. CSF viral antibodies. Evaluation in amyotrophic lateral sclerosis and late-onset postpoliomyelitis progressive muscular atrophy. Arch Neurol 1979;36:269–273.

95. Provinciali L, Laurenzi MA, Vesprini L, et al. Immunity assessment in the early stages of amyotrophic lateral sclerosis: A study of virus antibodies and lymphocyte subsets. Acta Neurol Scand 1988;78:449–454.

96. Ogawa M, Okubo H, Tsuji T, et al. Chronic progressive encephalitis occurring 13 years after Russian spring-summer encephalitis. J Neurol Sci 1973;19:363–373.

97. Petrov PA. V. Vilyuisk encephalitis in the Yakut Republic (U.S.S.R.). Am J Trop Med 1970;19:146–150.

98. Provinciali L, Laurenzi MA, Vesprini L, et al. Immunity assessment in the early stages of amyotrophic lateral sclerosis: A study of virus antibodies and lymphocyte subsets. Acta Neurol Scand 1988;78:449–454.

99. Borg K, Tjalve H. Uptake of 63Ni2+ in the central and peripheral nervous system of mice after oral administration: Effects of treatments with halogenated 8-hydroxyquinolines. Toxicology 1989;54:59–68.

100. Brown P. The clinical neurology and epidemiology of Creutzfeldt-Jakob disease, with special reference to iatrogenic cases. Ciba Found Symp 135;1988:3–23.

101. Casals J. Immunological characterization of Vilyuisk encephalitis virus. In: Gajdusek DC, Gibbs CJ, Alpers M, eds. NINDB monograph No. 2. Slow, latent, and

temperate virus infections. Washington, DC: US Government Printing Office, 1965:115–118.

102. Rozhon EJ, Kratochvil JD, Lipton HL. Comparisons of structural and nonstructural proteins of virulent and less virulent Theiler's virus isolates using two-dimensional gel electrophoresis. Virus Res 1985;2:11–28.

103. Salazar-Grueso EF, Siegel I, Roos RP. The post-poliomyelitis syndrome: Evaluation and treatment. Comprehensive Ther 16(2):24–30, 1990.

104. McClure MA, Perrault J. Poliovirus genome hybridizes specifically to higher eukaryotic rRNAs. Nucleic Acids Res 1985;13:6797–6897.

20

Motor Neuron Disease and Autoimmunity

Florian Patrick Thomas

Montreal Neurological Institute, McGill University
Montreal, Quebec, Canada

Norman Latov

College of Physicians and Surgeons, Columbia University,
Neurological Institute, and Columbia-Presbyterian Medical Center
New York, New York

INTRODUCTION

Many hypotheses have been proposed for the cause of motor neuron disease (MND) since the first descriptions by Aran (1), Charcot and Joffroy (2), and Erb (3), but its cause in most patients remains obscure. Immunological abnormalities have been noted in a number of patients, and autoimmune mechanisms have been postulated for several motor neuron syndromes (4–7).

CLINICAL SPECTRUM OF MOTOR NEURON DISEASE

Within the spectrum of MND, autoimmunity has been considered for several syndromes. The most common form is amyotrophic lateral sclerosis (ALS), in which upper and lower motor neuron signs are combined. Lower motor neuron disease (LMND) is characterized by weakness and fasciculations with pathological changes of degeneration of lower motor neurons and sparing of corticospinal tracts and cortical motor neurons (8). In some cases where upper motor neuron signs are equivocal, ALS may be difficult to differentiate from LMND (9). Motor neuropathy is clinically similar to LMND, but there is histopathological and electrophysiological evidence for affection of motor nerves (10–14).

This chapter is dedicated to Dr. Betty Q. Banker and Dr. Maurice Victor.

In some cases, it is difficult to differentiate between motor neuropathy and lower motor neuron disease (15,16).

ASSOCIATED AUTOIMMUNE PHENOMENA

Autoimmune phenomena have been reported in a study by Appel et al. (7), who found clinical thyroid disease in 19% of a series of patients with ALS and their relatives; an additional 21% of family members had evidence of other autoimmune disorders. Twenty-three percent of another series of patients with ALS in the same study had increased levels of antibodies to thyroglobulin and microsomes.

Testing sera from patients with ALS, Denys et al. (17) found antinuclear staining at a much higher frequency than in neurological controls or in normal sera. IgM antibodies were more frequent than other isotypes. Conradi and Ronnevi (18) found increased cytotoxic activity in ALS plasma against normal erythrocytes.

ASSOCIATED NEOPLASTIC DISEASES

Several authors reported an unusually high incidence of cancer in patients with typical ALS (19–21). Case reports of such an association included cancers of the breast, lung, colon, pancreas, kidney, skin, and brain, and in some cases, there was improvement of the MND following resection of the tumor (22–26). However, this association has not been confirmed by other authors (27–33). Djib-Jalbut and Liwnicz (34) and Wong et al. (35) reported two patients with MND and small cell lung carcinoma; the patients' serum IgG selectively stained neurons in the anterior and intermediolateral horn and in the cerebellar and cerebral cortex. In addition to MND, Wong's patient also had limbic encephalopathy (35).

MND WITH MONOCLONAL GAMMOPATHY AND LYMPHOMA

Better evidence exists for a link between motor neuron syndromes and monoclonal gammopathies (9,36–38). Shy et al. (37) found paraproteins in 4.8% of all cases of MND, while Younger et al. (9), using the more sensitive method of immunofixation electrophoresis, found paraproteins in 9%; both figures were higher than expected in age-matched normal controls. While in most cases the monoclonal gammopathies are nonmalignant, in some they are associated with myeloma, Waldenstrom's macroglobulinemia, lymphoma, or chronic lymphocytic leukemia. MND with lymphoid malignancies without monoclonal gammopathy has also been described (39,40). The lymphoid disorders have been associated with classical ALS, as well as with LMND and motor neuropathy. Schold et al. (41) reported 10 cases of motor neuronopathy in association with lymphoma; seven of these improved spontaneously.

Lymphocytic neoplastic disorders could be associated with MND through a number of mechanisms: (a) Lymphocytes could secrete autoreactive antibodies that bind to neural tissue and cause disease. (b) Antibodies produced in response to tumor antigens may cross-react with motor neurons, thereby causing disease, a situation analogous to the mechanisms postulated for the Lambert-Eaton myasthenic syndrome (42,43). (c) Infiltration of the spinal cord, nerve roots, or peripheral nerves by lymphoid neoplasms can mimic MND (40,44). Or, (d) a retrovirus might cause both lymphoma and MND. In mice both MND and lymphoma can be caused by a neurotropic and lymphotropic murine leukemia virus (45,46), and HIV-1 infection can present with lymphoma and, rarely, motor neuron disease (47). Similarly, HTLV-I can lead to lymphoma and tropical spastic paraparesis (48). The mechanisms of the neurological disease associated with retroviral infections, however, are not yet understood.

LYMPHOCYTE FUNCTIONS IN MND

Total B-cell and T-cell counts were reported normal in patients with MND by several authors (7,49–51). However, Provinciali et al. (52) found B-cell and T-cell lymphopenia in ALS patients, compared with controls. Studying lymphocyte subsets, Appel et al. (7) found that in ALS patients 12.9% of the T cells were positive for the Ia antigen (a marker for T-cell activation), compared with 6.4% in non-ALS neurological disease patients and normal controls, but Bartfeld et al. (51) found no differences. Provinciali et al. (52) reported that ALS patients had reduced CD2-, CD8-, and Leu7-positive cells, and an increase of the CD4/CD8 ratio. Urbanek and James (53) found delayed migration of macrophages into an inflammatory field created by experimental skin abrasion in 10 cases of ALS, compared with controls, and a quantitative decrease in the cellular response in three. Hoffman et al. (54) found impaired cellular immunity in Guamanian ALS associated with HLA-Bw35 by skin-test response to common antigens, while Nemo et al. (55) found no difference between Guamanian ALS patients and normal controls in lymphocyte transformation following challenge with brain antigens.

SERUM AND CEREBROSPINAL FLUID IMMUNOGLOBULINS AND IMMUNE COMPLEXES

Ionasesco and Luca (56) reported elevated immunoglobulins in 29 MND patients. Provinciali et al. (52) found higher serum IgG in ALS patients compared with controls, and recently Younger et al. (9) reported a polyclonal increase in IgA or IgM in 18 of 120 patients with motor neuron syndromes, while no increase of IgG was found. Whitaker et al. (57) found significantly higher IgM levels in 5 of 13 patients with LMND, while they were normal in classical ALS and in controls; IgG, IgA, and C3 levels were normal in patients with motor neuron syndromes. Tavolato et al. (58) found increased immunoglobulins and white blood cell counts and decreased monocyte counts in ALS patients compared with normal controls, but no differences in comparison with disease controls. Other studies found no abnormalities in levels of immunoglobulin isotypes (50,59). Hoffman et al. (60) found higher IgA and IgG levels in Guamanian ALS patients than in normals, but the authors suggested that these differences were due to frequent intercurrent infections in their patients rather than to an autoimmune response. Pertschuk et al. (61) found increased numbers of jejunal mucosal cells with immunoglobulin and complement deposits in seven ALS patients; IgG deposits showed the largest increase.

Younger et al. (9) and Kostulas (62) detected oligoclonal bands in the CSF of 14 of 115 patients and in 2 of 14 patients, respectively. The oligoclonal bands were sometimes associated with lymphoma. Annunziata and Volpi (59) found increased C3c levels in CSF of 12 MND patients.

Increased levels of immune complexes have been observed in the serum (63), kidneys (63,64), and brains (65) of patients with MND, while Bartfeld et al. (50), Tachovsky et al. (66), and Noronha et al. (67) found no significant increase in serum immune complexes in ALS patients, and Behan and Behan (68) found no immune complexes in the kidneys.

IMMUNE SUSCEPTIBILITY GENES IN MND

Several HLA antigens have been reported to be overrepresented in MND patients. These included HLA A2, A3, A28, B40, and BW35 (69–72), while Bartfeld et al. (73) found a decrease of HLA-A9 in ALS patients. However, others found no abnormal frequencies in classical ALS (74,75) or in Guamanian ALS (76).

IMMUNE RESPONSE TO VIRAL ANTIGENS

Kott et al. (72,77) found cell-mediated immunity to poliovirus in 21 of 33 patients with ALS, while normal or disease controls did not show similar reactivity in their assays. Humoral response to poliovirus was similar in patients and controls. Bartfeld et al. (50) also found a significant in vitro cellular immune response to inactivated pooled poliovirus antigens in ALS, compared with normal or neurological controls. There was a greater response to types 2 and 3 than to type 1 poliovirus. Cunningham-Rundles et al. (78) found decreased lymphocyte transformation in patients with MND in response to polio antigen. The humoral response against a host of viral antigens, including polio, coxsackie, influenza A, measles, rubella, mumps, herpes simplex type 1 and 2, CMV, and varicella zoster, was the same in ALS and control sera (50,79–81).

MND AND POSTPOLIO MUSCULAR ATROPHY

A syndrome of increasing disability in postpolio patients [postpolio muscular atrophy (PPMA)] is being diagnosed with increasing frequency. Manifestations include new weakness, fasciculations, atrophy, and muscle pain. Standard electrophysiological studies and single-fiber EMG cannot distinguish new from old abnormalities, but recently Lange et al. (82) reported that low-amplitude recordings in macro EMG were specific for patients with PPMA, possibly indicating degeneration of terminal axonal branches. Dalakas et al. (83) found lymphocytic infiltrates and myopathic features in biopsied muscle of some PPMA patients, but Cashman et al. (84) found no specific alterations. Oligoclonal bands in the CSF and alterations in T-lymphocyte subsets have been reported in some patients with PPMA, but not in asymptomatic postpolio cases (83,85a). Recently an intrathecal antibody response to polio virus has been reported in these patients (85b). At this time, the cause of PPMA and its possible relation to poliovirus infection or ALS are still unclear.

AUTOANTIBODIES TO NEURAL TISSUE

Potential humoral factors have been investigated by incubating cultured tissue or cells with the serum from patients with MND, but findings remain controversial. Doherty et al. (86) reported toxic effects of MND sera on neurofilament expression in embryonic chick spinal cord cultures; however, this effect was not seen with an immunoglobulin preparation. Other groups have observed demyelination (87,88), toxic effects on cultured neonatal mouse spinal neurons (89,90), and impaired survival in dissociated chick embryo ciliary neurons (91) as an effect of MND sera. However, others failed to observe similar toxic effects in cultured motor neurons (92–94), cultured human neuroblastoma cells (95), cultured chick ciliary ganglion neurons (96), or cultured human embryonic spinal cord (97). Askanas et al. (98) found no effect of CSF from ALS patients on neuron-specific enolase of cultured embryonic rat motor neurons.

Several groups used indirect immunofluorescence to document binding of ALS sera to neural tissue or cell cultures (99–103). Harrison et al. (99) and Digby et al. (100) found binding of ALS immunoglobulin to human embryonic spinal cord cultures, but this could not be replicated by Cashman et al. (4). Bahmanyar et al. (101) found antineurofilament serum antibodies in 27% of all ALS cases and nonneurological disease controls, compared with 7% of normal controls. But they were present more commonly in some other neurological diseases. Edgington and Dalessio (102) and Lisak et al. (103) found increased titers of antimyelin antibodies in patients with ALS, multiple sclerosis, and Guillain-Barré syndrome compared with normal controls. Using a complement activation assay, Ionasesco and Luca (56) found serum autoantibodies reactive with brain and spinal cord tissue in 6 of 17 ALS patients.

Using the Western blot system, Ordoñez and Sotelo (104) found antibodies against fetal rat muscle proteins in ALS sera five times more frequently than in control sera, but did not identify any specific bands shared by all ALS sera. Gurney et al. (105–107) reported that 40% of ALS sera and experimental antisera blocked axonal sprouting induced by botulinum toxin. The serum antibodies bound to a 56-kDa protein from muscle, which they named neuroleukin. This protein was reported to induce axonal sprouting and neuronal survival, but later found to be identical to glucose phosphate isomerase, a ubiquitous intracellular housekeeping enzyme (108,109). Furthermore, the effect of ALS sera seen by Gurney was not reproduced by Donaghy and Duchen (110), and Hauser et al. (111) found reactivity against similar protein bands in many neurological and normal controls, while Ingvar-Maeder et al. (112) found no reactivity with muscle protein in 16 ALS sera.

Inuzuka et al. (113) found IgG reactive with several spinal cord protein bands in 6 of 44 ALS sera, two of seven LMND sera, and in 7 of 53 control sera from patients with other neurological diseases, but not in normal controls. Brown et al. (114) reported that antibodies to 52- and 70-kDa proteins in mouse spinal cord were more common in ALS than in control sera.

In electrophysiological studies Schauf et al. (115) found neuroelectric blocking activity in the sera of ALS patients, when applied to frog spinal cord and roots. However, greater effect was observed with MS sera. Uchitel et al. (116) recently demonstrated that serum immunoglobulins from ALS patients increased the resting release of acetylcholine from presynaptic nerve terminals at the neuromuscular junction.

In passive transfer experiments Denys et al. (117) found no effect of intraperitoneal injections of ALS immunoglobulins or plasma into mice.

IMMUNOGLOBULIN DEPOSITS IN MOTOR NEURONS

Donnenfeld et al. (65) reported deposits of IgG and the C3 component of complement within glial cells in the anterior horn cell area and in the motor cortex of more than a third of patients with ALS and other disease states associated with possible immune or infectious etiologies, but not in normal controls. Engelhardt and Appel (118) recently reported immunoglobulin deposits in motor neurons of the anterior horn in patients with ALS. Motor neurons have been shown to take up immunoglobulins from the serum, particularly those with antineuronal activity, possibly explaining the presence of the deposits in motor neurons of patients with ALS (119,120).

ANIMAL MODELS OF AUTOIMMUNE MOTOR NEURON DISEASE

Engelhardt et al. (121a,b), Garcia et al. (122a), and Appel et al. (122b) reported the induction of a motor neuron syndrome in guinea pigs by immunization with isolated swine or bovine motor neurons. Animals developed progressive weakness and wasting and signs of denervation by electrophysiological and morphological criteria. There was loss of motoneurons in the anterior horn without inflammatory changes. IgG deposits were detected in surviving spinal motoneurons and at the neuromuscular junction.

RESPONSE TO IMMUNE THERAPY

Norris et al. (123), Monstad et al. (124), Olarte et al. (125), Conomy et al. (126), and Silani et al. (127) found that plasmapheresis had no effect in patients with ALS. The combination of plasmapheresis with azathioprine was also without benefit (128). Corticosteroids and ACTH failed to alter the cause in a study by Baumann (129). The use of cyclosporine A by Appel et al. (130) and of cyclophosphamide by Brown et al. (131) was ineffective, although Appel found some benefit in men with recent onset of ALS. Patten (132) reported 18 patients with ALS and laboratory features of autoimmunity who responded to treatment that included steroids and cytoxan.

ASSOCIATION WITH AUTOANTIBODIES AGAINST KNOWN NEURAL ANTIGENS

Information regarding potential target antigens in patients with MND and autoantibodies came from the investigation of patients who also had monoclonal gammopathies. Monoclonal antibodies sometimes have the same specificities as polyclonal antibodies without gammopathy and investigation of the specificities of monoclonal antibodies can provide clues as to the identity of the autoantigens.

MOTOR SYNDROMES WITH ANTI-GM1 OR ANTI-GA1(B1-3)GA1NAC ANTIBODIES

Several related motor syndromes have been described in association with anti-GM1 or anti-Gal(B1-3)GalNAc antibodies. Two patients with LMND had lambda IgM M-proteins that reacted with GM1, asialo-GM1, and GD1b (133,134). They were found to react with the Gal(B1-3)GalNAc epitope on these gangliosides and to cross-react with Gal(B1-3)GlcNAc (135). Both patients had markedly elevated serum IgM levels. Electrophysiological studies revealed widespread fibrillations and fasciculations with essentially normal nerve conduction velocities. Similar patients with MND and IgM-kappa M-proteins were reported by Nobile-Orazio et al. (136) and Nardelli et al. (137). Nardelli's patient, in addition, had electrophysiological signs of a sensorimotor neuropathy.

Pestronk et al. (138) reported two cases of motor neuropathy associated with high-titer polyclonal anti-GM1 antibodies. Electrophysiological studies showed multifocal motor conduction block, sparing sensory fibers. While treatment with plasmapheresis and prednisone proved unsuccessful, both patients improved markedly upon cyclophosphamide administration. Patients with motor neuropathy and multifocal conduction block were also reported by Baba et al. (139), Kusunoki et al. (140), Krarup et al. (141), and Santoro et al. (142). The patient reported by Santoro et al. had IgM deposits at all nodes of Ranvier in a sural nerve biopsy. Baba et al. (139) reported three patients with multifocal motor neuropathy and anti-GM1 antibodies, which cross-reacted with the Gal(B1-3)GalNAc epitope (patient 1), with GM2, but not with GD1b (patient 2), and with asialo-GM1, but not with GM2 or GD1b (patient 3). These observations suggest that binding to GM1 itself rather than to other cross-reactive glycoconjugates may be responsible for the motor syndrome. Another patient with monoclonal Gal(B1-3)GalNAc IgM antibodies presented with a lower motor syndrome, but later developed sensorimotor peripheral neuropathy and a second monoclonal IgM of unknown specificity (143).

Sadiq et al. (144) compared anti-GM1 antibody levels in patients with various neurological diseases and in normal subjects and found increased titers (greater than 1:800) in patients with LMND, sensorimotor neuropathy, and motor neuropathy with or without conduction block. In other diseases, antibody levels were similar to those seen in normal subjects, indicating that the antibody levels do not increase nonspecifically after neural injury or as a consequence of inflammatory conditions. While in some reports anti-GM1 and anti-GD1a antibodies were found in up to 78% of patients with ALS (145), Sadiq et al. (144) and Shy et al. (146) found similar titers in patients with ALS and normal controls, indicating that anti-GM1 antibodies are not generally increased in ALS and that low-level anti-GM1 antibodies are part of the normal human antibody repertoire. Anti-GM1 antibodies may occur as polyclonal antibodies or as IgM monoclonal gammopathies, usually with lambda light-chain types.

EPITOPE AND TISSUE SPECIFICITIES OF ANTI-GM1 OR ANTI-GA1(B1-3)GA1NAC ANTIBODIES

The fine specificites of the anti-GM1 antibodies vary: Most antibodies react with the Gal(B1-3)GalNAc epitope, but in some patients they are more specific for GM1 or cross-react with other gangliosides (139,144).

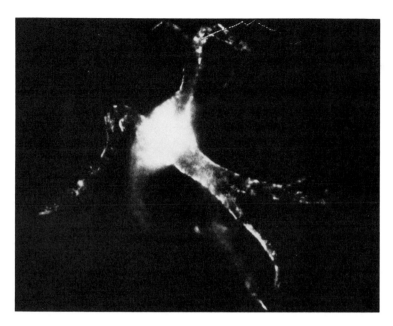

Figure 1   Isolated bovine motor neuron, unfixed, immunostained with serum from patient with anti-GM1 monoclonal IgM antibody and counterstained with a fluorescein isothiocyanate conjugated second antibody to human IgM. Immunofluorescence microscopy shows intense patchy or granular IgM deposits on cell surfaces. × 300. [Reproduced, with permission, from Thomas et al. (151).]

    In addition to gangliosides, the M-proteins with anti-Gal(B1-3)GalNAc activity also bind to neural glycoproteins (147). Of these, some are specific to the peripheral and central axonal and myelin protein fractions. In peripheral myelin, one protein band was sequenced and identified as the P0 glycoprotein (personal observation); another one may be identical to the 170-kDa protein identified by Shuman et al. (148).

    In tissue sections from human and different animals species, the anti-Gal(B1-3)GalNAc antibodies immunostain central and peripheral nervous system tissue from human, monkey, dog, and cat more strongly than tissue from rabbit, guinea pig, rat, and mouse (149). They stain gray matter more strongly than white matter and bind to terminal motor nerve fibers at the neuromuscular junction (149,150). While in tissue sections serum antibodies may bind to antigenic sites that are not normally accessible, in vivo injection studies into the extracellular space of the spinal cord showed that anti-Ga1(B1-3)GalNAc antibodies bind to the surface of neural cells (149). Binding to the surface of isolated intact bovine motor neurons was demonstrated for anti-GM1 antibodies (Fig. 1) (151). Using cholera toxin as a marker, GM1 has been localized to the surface of nodes of Ranvier in peripheral nerve, and it is not present on the surface of the internodal myelin sheath (152).

PATHOGENIC EFFECT OF ANTI-GM1 AND ANTI-GA1(B1-3)GA1NAC ANTIBODIES

The mechanism of action of these antibodies is unknown, but since GM1 and the Ga1(B1-3)GalNAc epitope are highly concentrated and widely distributed in both the central and peripheral nervous system (147,153–155), the resulting clinical syndrome might depend on the sites of action of the antibodies. This might, in turn, depend on the fine specificities and cross-reactivities of the antibodies, their size, conformation, and accessibility to the target tissue, and the topographical distribution of the target antigen.

In earlier studies the effects of anti-GM1 antibodies on the nervous system have been investigated in several experimental systems. Rabbits immunized with GM1 developed a noninflammatory neuropathy (156), and rabbit anti-GM1 antibodies induced demyelination in spinal roots and spinal cord after injection into the lumbosacral subarachnoid space of the rat (157). Also, the injection of anti-GM1 antibodies into the cisterna magna of neonatal rats interfered with development of pyramidal cell neurons and myelinization and impaired performance in learning tasks (158). In a goldfish model intraocular injections of anti-GM1 antibodies following crush injury to the optic nerve reduced sprouting in vitro (159) and axonal regeneration in vivo (160). In tissue culture systems, Schwartz and Spirman (161) found that rabbit anti-GM1 antibodies blocked the sprouting from dorsal root ganglia of chicken embryo induced by nerve growth factor. Doherty and Walsh (162) could not reproduce this effect, but did find specific binding of these antibodies and of B-cholera toxin, which is specific for GM1, to similar cultures. Antibodies raised against a ganglioside mixture containing mostly GM1 and GD1b were toxic for neonatal rat cerebellar cells in the presence of guinea pig complement (163). Anti-GM1 antibodies also induced myelin alterations in embryonic mouse spinal cord cultures (164). The autoantibodies might also have different effects in different experimental animal and culture systems, as there are significant differences in the concentration and distribution of the target glycoconjugates between species and probably at different stages of development (149,165).

The anti-Ga1(B1-3)GalNAc antibodies might cause LMND by binding to the surface of anterior horn cells in the spinal cord (149,151), and they might also

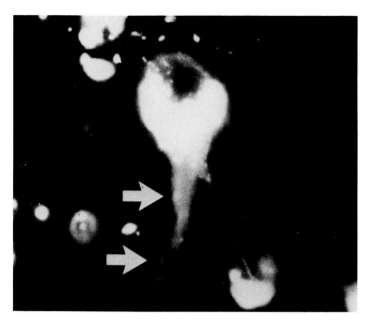

Figure 2 Lumbar ventral horn of patient who died with ALS and IgA monoclonal gammopathy, immunostained with fluorescein isothiocyanate conjugated antibody to human IgA. Immunofluorescence microscopy shows immune reactive IgA in perikaryon and dendrites (arrows) in addition to the more intense autofluorescent lipofuscin in the cell body. × 770. [Reproduced, with permission, from Hays et al. (180).]

cause motor neuropathy by binding at the nodes of Ranvier. In one patient with increased anti-GM1 antibodies and multifocal motor neuropathy with conduction block, IgM deposits were seen at the nodes of Ranvier and at the paranodal regions (142). This distribution is the same as previously reported for GM1 in peripheral nerve (152). Injection of this patient's serum into peripheral nerve resulted in conduction block at the injection site and in binding of IgM at the nodes of Ranvier, an effect that was abolished by preabsorbing the serum with GM1 (166). Rabbits immunized with GM1 or Gal(B1-3)GalNAc developed neuropathy and similar immunoglobulin deposits at the nodes of Ranvier (167). The reason for the preferential involvement of motor fibers is unknown, but the antigen might be more concentrated in motor fibers, or the motor fibers might be more susceptible to antibody-mediated injury, as there are important physiological and pharmacological differences between motor and sensory fibers (168–175).

Where they bind, anti-GM1 or anti-Gal(B1-3)GalNAc antibodies might cause disease through complement activation or disruption of nerve function. They might cause paranodal demyelination or interrupt conduction through direct or indirect interference with ion channels at the nodes of Ranvier (176–178). That anti-GM1 antibodies might have an effect on ion channels is supported by the finding that they induce epileptiform activity after injection into rat brain (179).

IGA MONOCLONAL ANTIBODIES AGAINST A NEURONAL SURFACE PROTEIN AND NEUROFILAMENT PROTEIN IN A PATIENT WITH AMYOTROPHIC LATERAL SCLEROSIS

Hays et al. (180) and Sadiq et al. (181) reported a patient with autopsy-proven typical ALS and an IgA lambda M protein, who had IgA deposits within surviving motor neurons (Fig. 2) and deposits of IgA and C3 within renal glomeruli. The IgA bound to axons and to the perikarya of nerve cells in the central and peripheral nervous system. In Western blots the IgA bound to the 200-kDa, high-molecular-weight neurofilament protein and cross-reacted with a 65-kDa protein on the surface of neuroblastoma cells and in spinal cord. This suggests that the IgA may have bound at the neuronal cell surface and accumulated in motor neurons, possibly causing the disease. The identity of the surface antigen and the role of the antibodies in the pathogenesis of ALS are under investigation.

FUTURE DIRECTIONS

There is increasing evidence that autoimmune mechanisms might be responsible for MND in a significant number of patients. Continued efforts to identify putative target antigens for autoantibodies in MND, to develop animal models of the disease, and to elucidate the mechanisms of action of the antibodies should result in the development of more reliable diagnostic tests for the various forms of MND, and of more specific and effective therapy for affected patients.

REFERENCES

1. Aran F. Recherches sur une maladie non encore décrite du systeme musculaire: Atrophie musculaire progressive. Arch Gen Med 1850;24:4–35.
2. Charcot JM, Joffroy A. Deux cas d'atrophie musculaire progressive avec lésions de la substance grise et des faisceaux antero-latéraux de la moelle épinière. Arch Physicol Neurol Pathol 1869;2:744–760.
3. Erb W. Ueber einen wenig bekannten spinalen Symptomen-complex. Klin Wochenschr 1875;12:357–359.
4. Cashman NR, Gurney M, Antel JP. Immunology of amyotrophic lateral sclerosis. Springer Semin Immunopathol 1985;8:141–152.

5. Cashman NR, Antel JP. Amyotrophic lateral sclerosis: An immunologic perspective. Immunol All Clin North Am 1988;8:331–342.

6. Drachman DB, Kuncl RW. Amyotrophic lateral sclerosis: An unconventional autoimmune disease. Ann Neurol 1989;26:269–274.

7. Appel SH, Stockton-Appel V, Steward SS, Kerman RH. Amyotrophic lateral sclerosis: Associated clinical disorders and immunological evaluations. Arch Neurol 1986;43:234–238.

8. Mills CK. The reclassification of some organic nervous diseases on the basis of the neuron. JAMA 1898;31:11–13.

9. Younger DS, Rowland LP, Latov N, et al. Motor neuron disease and amyotrophic lateral sclerosis: Relation of high CSF protein content to paraproteinemia and clinical syndromes. Neurology 1990;40:595–599.

10. Dyck PJ. Are motor neuropathies and motor neuron disease separable. In: Rowland LP, ed. Human motor neuron diseases. New York: Raven Press, 1982:105–114.

11. Parry GJ, Clarke S. Pure motor neuropathy with multifocal conduction block masquerading as motor neuron disease. Muscle Nerve 1985;8:617.

12. Parry GJ, Holtz SJ, Ben-Zeev D, Drori JB. Gammopathy with proximal motor axonopathy simulating motor neuron disease. Neurology 1986;36:273–276.

13. Rowland LP, Defendini R, Sherman W, et al. Macroglobulinemia with peripheral neuropathy simulating motor neuron disease. Ann Neurol 1982;11:532–536.

14. Hays AP. Separating motor neuron diseases from pure motor neuropathies: Pathology. In: Rowland LP, ed. Amyotrophic lateral sclerosis and other motor neuron diseases. New York: Raven Press, 1991:385–398.

15. Rowland LP. Peripheral neuropathy, motor neuron disease, or neuronopathy? In: Battistin L, Hashim G, Lajtha A, eds. Clinical and biological aspects of peripheral nerve diseases. New York: Alan R Liss, 1983:27–41.

16. Ghatak NR, Campbell WW, Lippman RH, Hadfield MG. Anterior horn changes of motor neuron disease associated with demyelinating radiculopathy. J Neuropathol Exp Neurol 1986;45:385–395.

17. Denys EH, Bjornskov EK, Jackson JE, Norris FH. Antinuclear antibodies in amyotrophic lateral sclerosis. In: Struppler A, Kuther G, eds. Trends in ALS research. München: Arwin Verlag, 1984:49–59.

18. Conradi S, Ronnevi L-O. Cytotoxic activity in the plasma of amyotrophic lateral sclerosis (ALS) patients against normal erythrocytes. Quantitative determinations. J Neurol Sci 1985;68:135–145.

19. Lord Brain R, Croft PB, Wilkinson M. Motor neurone disease as a manifestation of neoplasm. Brain 1965;88:479–500.

20. Norris FH, Engel WK. Carcinomatous amyotrophic lateral sclerosis. In: Lord Brain R, Norris FH, eds. The remote effects of cancer on the nervous system. New York: Grune & Stratton, 1965:24–41.

21. Gubbay SS, Kahana E, Zilber N, et al. Amyotrophic lateral sclerosis: A study of its presentation and prognosis. J Neurol 1985;232:295–300.

22. Stephens TW, Rousgas A, Ghose MK. Pure motor neuropathy complicating carcinoma of bronchus recovered after surgery. Br J Dis Chest 1966;60:107–109.

23. Buchanan DS, Malamud N. Motor neuron disease with renal cell carcinoma and postoperative neurologic remission. Neurology 1973;23:891–894.

24. Norris FH. Remote effects of cancer on the spinal cord. In: Vinken PJ, Bruyn GW, eds. Handbook of clinical neurology. Vol. 22. New York: American Elsevier, 1979:669–677.

25. Mitchell DM, Olczak A. Remission of a syndrome indistinguishable from motor neuron disease after resection of bronchial carcinoma. Br Med J 1979;2:176–177.

26. Peacock A, Dawkins K, Rushworth G. Motor neurone disease associated with bronchial carcinoma. Br Med J 1979;2:499–500.

27. Swank RL, Putnam TJ. Amyotrophic lateral sclerosis and related conditions. A clinical analysis. Arch Neurol 1943;49:151–177.

28. Wechsler IS, Sapirstein MR, Stein A. Primary and symptomatic amyotrophic lateral sclerosis: A clinical study of 81 cases. Am J Med Sci 1944;208:70–81.

29. Lawyer T, Netsky MG. Amyotrophic lateral sclerosis. A clinicoanatomic study of fifty-three cases. Arch Neurol Psychiatry 1953;69:171–192.

30. Shy GM, Silverstein I. A study of the effects upon the motor unit by remote malignancy. Brain 1965;88:515–528.

31. Vejjajiva A, Foster JB, Miller H. Motor neuron disease. A clinical study. J Neurol Sci 1967;4:299–314.

32. Jokelainen M. The epidemiology of amyotrophic lateral sclerosis in Finland. J Neurol Sci 1976;29:55–63.

33. Barron KD, Rodichok LD. Cancer and disorders of motor neurons. In: Rowland LP, ed. Human motor neuron diseases. New York: Raven Press, 1982:267–273.

34. Dhib-Jalbut S, Liwnicz BH. Immunocytochemical binding of serum IgG from a patient with oat cell tumor and paraneoplastic motoneuron disease to normal human cerebral cortex and molecular layer of the cerebellum. Acta Neuropathol 1986;69:96–102.

35. Wong MCW, Salanga VD, Chou S, Mitsumoto H, Kozachuk W, Liwnicz B. Immune-associated paraneoplastic motor neuron disease and limbic encephalopathy. Muscle Nerve 1987;10:661–662.

36. Latov N. Plasma cell dyscrasia and motor neuron disease. In: Rowland LP, ed. Human motor neuron diseases. New York: Raven Press, 1982:273–279.

37. Shy ME, Rowland LP, Smith T, et al. Motor neuron disease and plasma cell dyscrasia. Neurology 1986;36:1429–1436.

38. Bady B, Vial C, Brudon F, Lapras J, Kopp N, Trillet M. Neuropathies périphériques simulant une sclérose latérale amyotrophique au cours des gammapathies. Rev Neurol 1988;144:710–715.

39. Younger DS, Rowland LP, Sherman W, et al. Lymphoma, motor neuron disease, and amyotrophic lateral sclerosis. Ann Neurol 1991;29:78–86.

40. Rowland LP, Schneck SA. Neuromuscular disorders associated with malignant neoplastic disease. J Chronic Dis 1963;16:777–795.

41. Schold SC, Cho ES, Somasundaram M, Posner JB. Subacute motor neuropathy: A remote effect of lymphoma. Ann Neurol 1979;5:271–287.

42. Roberts A, Perera S, Lang B, Vincent A, Newsom-Davis J. Paraneoplastic myasthenic syndrome IgG inhibits 45Ca^{++} flux in a human small cell carcinoma line. Nature 1985;317:737–739.

43. Fukunaga H, Engel AG, Lang B, Newsom-Davis J, Vincent A. Passive transfer of

Lambert-Eaton myasthenic syndrome with IgG from man to mouse depletes the presynaptic membrane active zones. Proc Natl Acad Sci USA 1983;80:7636–7640.

44. Walton JN, Tomlinson BE, Pearce GW. Subacute "poliomyelitis" and Hodgkin's disease. J Neurol Sci 1968;6:435–445.

45. Gardner MB. Retroviral spongiform polioencephalomyelopathy. Rev Infect Dis 1985;7:99–110.

46. Paquette Y, Hanna Z, Savard P, Brousseau R, Robitaille Y, Jolicoeur P. Retrovirus-induced murine motor neuron disease: Mapping the determinant of spongiform degeneration within the envelope gene. Proc Natl Acad Sci USA 1989;86: 3896–3900.

47. Hoffman PM, Festoff BW, Giron LT, et al. Isolation of LAV/HTLV-III from a patient with amyotrophic lateral sclerosis. N Engl J Med 1985;313:324–325.

48. Roman GC, Vernant JC, Osame M. HTLV-1 and the nervous system. New York: Alan R Liss, 1989.

49. Antel JP, Noronha AB, Oger J, Arnason BGW. Immunology of amyotrophic lateral sclerosis. In: Rowland LP, ed. Human motor neuron diseases. New York: Raven Press, 1982:395–402.

50. Bartfeld H, Dham C, Donnenfeld H, et al. Immunological profile of amyotrophic lateral sclerosis patients and their cell-mediated immune responses to viral and CNS antigens. Clin Exp Immunol 1982;48:137–147.

51. Bartfeld H, Dham C, Donnenfeld H. Immunoregulatory and activated T cells in amyotrophic lateral sclerosis patients. J Neuroimmunol 1985;9:131–137.

52. Provinciali L, Laurenzi MA, Vesprini L, et al. Immunity assessment in the early stages of amyotrophic lateral sclerosis: A study of virus antibodies and lymphocyte subsets. Acta Neurol Scand 1988;78:449–454.

53. Urbanek K, Jansa P. Amyotrophic lateral sclerosis. Abnormal cellular inflammatory response. Arch Neurol 1974;30:186–187.

54. Hoffman PM, Robbins DS, Nolte MT, Gibbs CJ, Gajdusek DC. Cellular immunity in Guamanians with amyotrophic lateral sclerosis and Parkinsonism-dementia. N Engl J Med 1978;299:680–685.

55. Nemo GJ, Brody JA, Cruz M. Lymphocyte transformation study of Guamanian patients with amyotrophic lateral sclerosis and Parkinsonism-dementia. Neurology 1974;24:579–581.

56. Ionasesco V, Luca N. Recherches électrohorétiques sériques dans la sclérose latérale amyotrophique. Psychiatr Neurol 1961;142:31–43.

57. Whitaker JN, Sciabbarrasi J, Engel WK, Warmolts JR, Strober W. Serum immunoglobulin and complement (C3) levels. A study in adults with idiopathic, chronic polyneuropathies and motor neuron diseases. Neurology 1973;23:1164–1173.

58. Tavolato BF, Licandro AC, Saia A. Motor neurone disease: an immunological study. Eur Neurol 1975;13:433–440.

59. Annunziata P, Volpi N. High levels of C3c in the cerebrospinal fluid from amyotrophic lateral sclerosis patients. Acta Neurol Scand 1985;72:61–64.

60. Hoffman PM, Robbins DS, Oldstone MBA, Gibbs CJ, Gajdusek DC. Humoral

immunity in Guamanians with amyotrophic lateral sclerosis and Parkinsonism-dementia. Ann Neurol 1981;10:193–196.

61. Pertschuk LP, Cook AW, Gupta JK, et al. Jejunal immunopathology in amyotrophic lateral sclerosis and multiple sclerosis. Identification of viral antigens by immunofluorescence. Lancet 1977;1:119–1123.

62. Kostulas VK. Oligoclonal IgG bands in cerebrospinal fluid. Acta Neurol Scand 1985;72(Suppl 103):44–83.

63. Oldstone MBA, Perrin LH, Welsh RM. Potential pathogenic mechanisms of injury in amyotrophic lateral sclerosis. In: Andrews JM, Johnson RT, Brazier MAB, eds. Amyotrophic lateral sclerosis. New York: Academic Press, 1976: 251–262.

64. Palo J, Rissanen A, Jokinen E, Lähdevirta J, Salo O. Kidney and skin biopsy in amyotrophic lateral sclerosis. Lancet 1978;1:1270.

65. Donnenfeld H, Kascsak RJ, Bartfeld H. Deposits of IgG and C3 in the spinal cord and motor cortex of ALS patients. J Neuroimmunol 1984;6:51–57.

66. Tachovsky TG, Lisak RP, Koprowski H, Theofilopoulos AN, Dixon FJ. Circulating immune complexes in multiple sclerosis and other neurological diseases. Lancet 1976;2:997–999.

67. Noronha ABC, Antel JP, Roos RP, Medof ME. Circulating immune complexes in neurologic disease. Neurology 1981;31:1402–1407.

68. Behan PO, Behan WMH. Are immune factors involved in motor neurone disease? In: Clifford-Rose F, ed. Research progress in motor neurone disease. London: Pitman, 1984:405–411.

69. Antel JP, Arnason BGW, Fuller TC, et al. Histocompatibility typing in amyotrophic lateral sclerosis. Arch Neurol 1976;33:423–425.

70. Behan PO, Dick HM, Durward WF. Histocompatibility antigens associated with motor neurone disease. J Neurol Sci 1977;32:213–217.

71. Jokelainen M, Tiilikainen A, Lapinleimu K. Polio antibodies and HLA antigen in amyotrophic lateral sclerosis. Tissue Antigens 1977;10:259–266.

72. Kott E, Livni E, Zamir R, Kuritzky A. Neurology 1979;29:1040–1044.

73. Bartfeld H, Whitsett C, Donnenfeld H. HLA and disease. INSERM Internat Symp 1976;58:61–71.

74. Terasaki PI, Mickey MR. HLA haplotyping of 32 diseases. Transplant Rev 1975;22:105–119.

75. Pedersen L, Platz P, Jersild C, Thomsen M. HLA (SD and LD) in patients with amyotrophic lateral sclerosis (ALS). J Neurol Sci 1977;31:313–318.

76. Hoffman PM, Robbins DS, Gibbs CS, Gajdusek DC, Garruto RM, Terasaki PI. Histocompatibility antigens in amyotrophic lateral sclerosis and Parkinsonism-dementia on Guam. Lancet 1977;2:717.

77. Kott E, Livni E, Zamir R, Kuritzky A. Amyotrophic lateral sclerosis: Cell-mediated immunity to poliovirus and basic myelin protein in patients with high frequency of HLA-BW35. Neurology 1976;26(Suppl 1):376.

78. Cunningham-Rundles S, Dupont B, Posner JB, Hansen JA, Good RA. Cell-mediated-immune response to polio virus antigen in amyotrophic lateral sclerosis. Fed Proc 1977;36:1190A.

79. Cremer NE, Oshiro LS, Norris FH, Lennette EH. Cultures of tissues from patients with amyotrophic lateral sclerosis. Arch Neurol 1973;29:331–333.

80. Lehrich JR, Oger J, Arnason BGW. Neutralizing antibodies to poliovirus and mumps virus in amyotrophic lateral sclerosis. J Neurol Sci 1974;23:537–540.

81. Kurent JE, Brooks BR, Madden DL, Sever JL, Engel WK. CSF viral antibodies. Evaluation in amyotrophic lateral sclerosis and late-onset postpoliomyelitis progressive muscular atrophy. Arch Neurol 1979;36:269–273.

82. Lange DJ, Smith T, Lovelace RE. Postpolio muscular atrophy. Diagnostic utility of macroelectromyography. Arch Neurol 1989;46:502–506.

83. Dalakas MC, Elder G, Hallett M, Ravits J, Baker M, Papadopoulos N, Albrecht P, Sever J. A long-term follow-up study of patients with post-poliomyelitis neuromuscular symptoms. N Engl J Med 1986;314:959–963.

84. Cashman NR, Maselli R, Wollmann RL, Roos R, Simon R, Antel JP. Late denervation in patients with antecedent paralytic poliomyelitis. N Engl J Med 1987;317:7–12.

85a. Ginsberg AH, Gale MJ, Rose LM, Clark EA. T-cell alterations in late postpoliomyelitis. Arch Neurol 1989;46:497–501.

85b. Sharief MK, Hentges R, Ciardi M. Intrathecal immune response in patients with the post-polio syndrome. N Engl J Med 1991;325:749–755.

86. Doherty P, Dickson JG, Flanigan TP, Kennedy PGE, Walsh FS. Effects of amyotrophic lateral sclerosis serum on cultured chick spinal neurons. Neurology 1986;36:1330–1334.

87. Field EJ, Hughes D. Toxicity of motor neurone disease serum for myelin in tissue culture. Br Med J 1965;2:1399–1401.

88. Bornstein MB, Appel SH. Tissue culture studies of demyelination. Ann NY Acad Sci 1965;122:280–286.

89. Wolfgram F, Myers L. Amyotrophic lateral sclerosis: Effect of serum on anterior horn cells in tissue culture. Science 1973;179:579–580.

90. Roisen FJ, Bartfeld H, Donnenfeld H, Baxter J. Neuron specific in vitro cytotoxicity of sera from patients with amyotrophic lateral sclerosis. Muscle Nerve 1982;5:48–53.

91. Ebendal T, Askmark H, Aquilonius SM. Screening for neurotrophic disturbances in amyotrophic lateral sclerosis. Acta Neurol Scand 1989;79:188–193.

92. Horwich MS, Engel WK, Chauvin PB. Amyotrophic lateral sclerosis sera applied to cultured motor neurons. Arch Neurol 1974;30:332–333.

93. Liveson J, Frey H, Bornstein MB. The effect of serum from ALS patients on organotypic nerve and muscle tissue cultures. Acta Neuropathol 1975;32:127–131.

94. Ecob MS, Brown AE, Younger C, et al. Is there a circulating neurotoxic factor in motor neurone disease? In: Clifford-Rose CF, ed. Research progress in motor neurone disease. London: Pitman Press, 1984:249–254.

95. Lehrich JR, Couture J. Amyotrophic lateral sclerosis sera are not cytotoxic to neuroblastoma cells in tissue culture. Ann Neurol 1978;41:384.

96. Touzeau G, Kato AC. Effects of amyotrophic lateral sclerosis sera on cultured cholinergic neurons. Neurology 1983;33:317–322.

97. Touzeau G, Kato AC. ALS serum has no effect on three enzymatic activities in culture human spinal cord neurons. Neurology 1986;36:573–576.

98. Askanas V, Marangos PJ, Engel WK. CSF from amyotrophic lateral sclerosis patients applied to motor neurons in culture fails to alter neuron-specific enolase. Neurology 1981;31:1196–1197.

99. Harrison R, Jehanli A, Lunt GG, Behan PO. Serum immunoglobulins from patients with motor neurone disease bind to spinal cord neurones in culture. J Neuroimmunol 1982;3:S26.

100. Digby J, Harrison R, Jehanli A, Lunt GG, Clifford-Rose F. Cultured rat spinal cord neurons: Interaction with motor neuron disease immunoglobulins. Muscle Nerve 1985;8:595–605.

101. Bahmanyar S, Moreau-Dubois MC, Brown P, Cathala F, Gajdusek DC. Serum antibodies to neurofilament antigens in patients with neurological and other diseases and in healthy controls. J Neuroimmunol 1983;5:191–196.

102. Edgington TS, Dalessio DJ. The assessment by immunofluorescence methods of humoral anti-myelin antibodies in man. J Immunol 1970;105:248–255.

103. Lisak RP, Zwiman B, Norman M. Antimyelin Antibodies in neurologic diseases. Arch Neurol 1975;32:163–167.

104. Ordoñez G, Sotelo J. Antibodies against fetal muscle proteins in serum from patients with amyotrophic lateral sclerosis. Neurology 1989;39:683–686.

105. Gurney ME, Belton AC, Cashman N, Antel AP. Inhibition of terminal axonal sprouting by serum from patients with amyotrophic lateral sclerosis. N Engl J Med 1984;311:933–939.

106. Gurney ME, Heinrich SP, Lee MR, Yin H-S. Molecular cloning and expression of neuroleukin, a neurotrophic factor for spinal and sensory neurons. Science 1986;234:566–574.

107. Gurney KE, Apatoff BR, Spear GT, et al. Neuroleukin: A lymphokine product of lectin-stimulated T cells. Science 1986;234:574–581.

108. Chaput M, Claes V, Portetelle D, et al. The neurotrophic factor neuroleukin is 90% homologous with phosphohexose isomerase. Nature 1988;332:454–455.

109. Faik P, Walker JIH, Redmill AAM, Morgan MJ. Mouse glucose-6-phosphate isomerase and neuroleukin have identical 3′ sequences. Nature 1988;332:455–456.

110. Donaghy M, Duchen LW. Sera from patients with motor neuron disease and associated paraproteinemia fail to inhibit experimentally induced sprouting of motor nerve terminals. J Neurol Neurosurg Psychiatry 1986;49:817–819.

111. Hauser SL, Cazenave P-A, Lyon-Caen O, et al. Immunoblot analysis of circulating antibodies against muscle proteins in amyotrophic lateral sclerosis and other neurologic diseases. Neurology 1986;36:1614–1618.

112. Ingvar-Maeder M, Regli F, Steck AJ. Search for antibodies to skeletal muscle proteins in amyotrophic lateral sclerosis. Acta Neurol Scand 1986;74:218–223.

113. Inuzuka T, Sato S, Yanagisawa K, Miyatake T. Antibodies to human spinal cord proteins in sera from patients with motor neuron disease and other neurological diseases. Eur Neurol 1989;29:328–332.

114. Brown RH, Johnson D, Ogonowski M, Weiner HL. Antineural antibodies in the serum of patients with amyotrophic lateral sclerosis. Neurology 1987;37:152–155.
115. Schauf CL, Antel JP, Arnason BGW, Davis FA, Rooney MW. Neuroelectric blocking activity and plasmapheresis in amyotrophic lateral sclerosis. Neurology 1980;30:1011–1013.
116. Uchitel OD, Appel SH, Crawford F, Sczurpek L. Immunoglobulins from amyotrophic lateral sclerosis patients enhance spontaneous transmitter release at motornerve terminals. Proc Natl Acad Sci USA 1988;85:7371–7374.
117. Denys EH, Jackson JE, Aguilar MJ, Wilson AJ, Norris FH. Passive transfer experiments in amyotrophic lateral sclerosis. Arch Neurol 1984;41:161–163.
118. Engelhardt JI, Appel SH. IgG Reactivity in the spinal cord and motor cortex in amyotrophic lateral sclerosis. Arch Neurol 1990;47:1210–1216.
119. Yamamoto T, Iwasaki Y, Konno H, Iizuka H, Zhao J-X. Retrograde transport and differential accumulation of serum proteins in motor neurons: Implications for motor neuron diseases. Neurology 1987;37:843–846.
120. Fabian RH. Uptake of antineuronal IgM by CNS neurons. Comparison with antineuronal IgG. Neurology 1990;40:419–422.
121a. Engelhardt JI, Appel SH, Killian JM. Experimental autoimmune motoneuron disease. Ann Neurol 1989;26:368–376.
121b. Engelhardt JI, Appel SH, Killian JM. Motoneuron destruction in guinea pigs immunized with bovine ventral horn homogenate: experimental autoimmune gray matter disease. J Neuroimmunol 1990;27:21–31.
122a. Garcia J, Engelhardt JI, Appel SH, Stefani E. Increased mepp frequency as an early sign of experimental immune mediated motoneuron disease. Ann Neurol 1990;28:329–334.
122b. Appel SH, Engelhardt JI, Garcia J, Stefani E. Immunoglobulins from animal models of motor neuron disease and from human amyotrophic lateral sclerosis patients passively transfer physiological abnormalities to the neuromuscular junction. Proc Natl Acad Sci USA 1991;88:647–651.
123. Norris FH, Denys EH, Mielke CH. Plasmapheresis in amyotrophic lateral sclerosis. Muscle Nerve 1978;1:342A.
124. Monstad I, Dale I, Petlund CF, Sjaastad O. Plasma exchange in motor neuron disease. A controlled study. J Neurol 1979;221:59–66.
125. Olarte MR, Schoenfeldt RB, McKiernan G, Rowland LP: Plasmapheresis in amyotrophic lateral sclerosis. Ann Neurol 1980;8:644–645.
126. Conomy JP, Gerhard G, Goren H, et al. Plasmapheresis in the treatment of amyotrophic lateral sclerosis. Neurology 1980;30:356A.
127. Silani V, Scarlato G, Valli G, et al. Plasma exchange ineffective in amyotrophic lateral sclerosis. Arch Neurol 1980;37:511–513.
128. Kelemen J, Hedlund W, Orlin JB, et al. Plasmapheresis with immunosuppression in amyotrophic lateral sclerosis. Arch Neurol 1983;40:752–753.
129. Baumann J. Results of treatment of certain diseases of the central nervous system with ACTH and corticosteroids. Acta Neurol Scand 1965;41(Suppl 13):453–461.
130. Appel SH, Stewart SS, Appel V, et al. A double-blind study of the effectiveness of cyclosporine in amyotrophic lateral sclerosis. Arch Neurol 1988;45:381–386.

131. Brown RH, Hauser SL, Harrington H, Weiner HL. Failure of immunosuppression with a ten- to 14-day course of high-dose intravenous cyclophophamide to alter the progression of amyotrophic lateral sclerosis. Arch Neurol 1986;43:383–384.

132. Patten BM. ALS of autoimmune origin. Neurology 1985;35(Suppl 1):251.

133. Freddo L, Yu RK, Latov N, et al. Gangliosides GM1 and GD1b are antigens for IgM M-protein in a patient with motor neuron disease. Neurology 1986;36: 454–458.

134. Latov N, Hays AP, Donofrio PD et al. Monoclonal IgM with unique specificity to gangliosides GM1 and GD1b and to lacto-*N*-tetraose associated with human motor neuron disease. Neurology 1988;38:763–768.

135. Ito H, Latov N. Monoclonal IgM in two patients with motor neuron disease bind to the carbohydrate antigens Gal(B1-3)GalNAc and Gal(B1-3)GlcNAc. J Neuroimmunol 1988;19:245–453.

136. Nobile-Orazio E, Daverio R, Meucci N, et al. Monoclonal gammopathy and anti-glycolipid IgM antibodies in patients with motor neuron disease. J Neurol 1988;235:S63 (Abstract).

137. Nardelli E, Steck AJ, Barkas T, Schluep M, Jerusalem F. Motor neuron syndrome and monoclonal IgM with antibody activity against gangliosides GM1 and GD1b. Ann Neurol 1988;23:524–528.

138. Pestronk A, Cornblath DR, Ilyas AA, et al. A treatable multifocal motor neuropathy with antibodies to GM1 ganglioside. Ann Neurol 1988;24:73–78.

139. Baba H, Daune GC, Ilyas AA, et al. Anti-GM1 ganglioside antibodies with differing fine specificities in patient with multifocal motor neuropathy. J Neuroimmunol 1989;25:143–150.

140. Kusunoki S, Shimizu T, Matsumura K, Maemura K, Mannen T. Motor dominant neuropathy and IgM paraproteinemia: The IgM M-protein binds to specific gangliosides. J Neuroimmunol 1989;21:177–181.

141. Krarup C, Stewart JD, Sumner AJ, Pestronk A, Lipton SA. A syndrome of asymmetric limb weakness with motor conduction block. Neurology 1990;40: 118–127.

142. Santoro M, Thomas FP, Fink ME, Lange DJ, Uncini A, Wadia NH, Latov N, Hays AP. IgM deposits at nodes of Ranvier in a patient with amyotrophic lateral sclerosis, anti-GM1 antibodies and multifocal conduction block. Ann Neurol 1990;28:373–377.

143. Ilyas AA, Willison HJ, Dalakas MC, Whitaker JN, Quarles RH. Identification and characterization of gangliosides reacting with IgM paraproteins in three patients with neuropathy associated with biclonal gammopathy. J Neurochem 1988;51: 851–858.

144. Sadiq SA. Thomas FP, Kilidireas K, et al. The spectrum of neurological disease associated with anti-GM1 antibodies. Neurology 1990;40:1067–1072.

145. Pestronk A, Adams RN, Cornblath D, Kuncl RW, Drachman DB, Clawson L. Patterns of serum IgM antibodies to GM1 and GD1a gangliosides in amyotrophic lateral sclerosis. Ann Neurol 1989;25:98–102.

146. Shy ME, Evans VA, Lublin FD, et al. Antibodies to GM1 and GD1b in patients

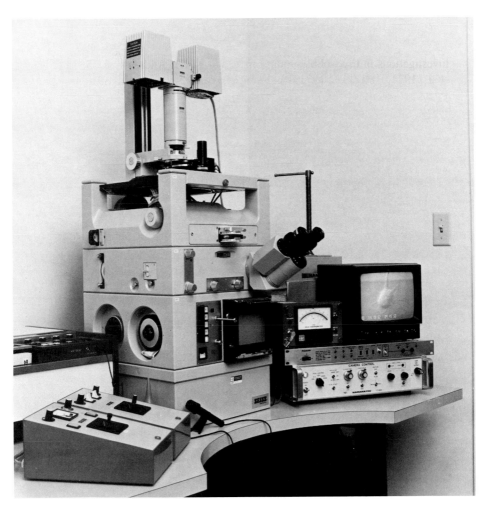

Figure 1 Equipment used for acquiring and storing fast axonal transport analog data in intact axons: Zeiss Axiomat microscope in the inverted configuration (center); video camera (out of view, mounted underneath the microscope); camera control unit, temperature and video monitors (right); video tape recorder and motorized stage control units (left). Not pictured are digital image enhancement and computer measuring systems.

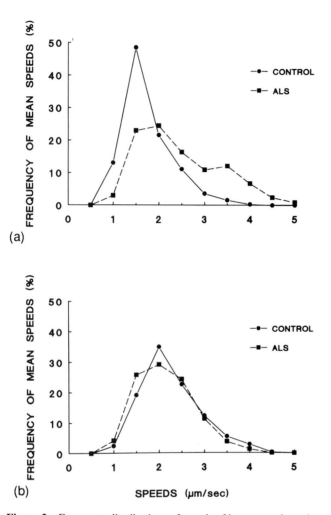

Figure 2 Frequency distributions of speeds of intra-axonal moving organelles in 17 ALS patients (data represent analysis of 1466 organelles in 33 axons in 13 nerves from ALS patients and 1455 organelles in 32 axons from nine nerves in control patients—data include information from additional patients studied and not previously published). These data show that there is a distribution of speeds of fast-moving organelles, not just one fast speed, and this distribution is shifted to a faster speed range in ALS in the anterograde direction (a) and to a slightly slower speed range in the retrograde direction (b) (see text).

Table 1 Organelle Traffic Density Analysis

	ALS	Controls
Total seconds	7225	6327
Anterograde density	4.2×10^{-2}	5.9×10^{-2}
Retrograde density	9.4×10^{-2}	29.8×10^{-2}
Total density	13.7×10^{-2}	35.6×10^{-2}

Amount of material fast transported in the anterograde and retrograde directions in ALS and control axons. Quantitative data on the amount of material transported is virtually nonexistent in the literature. These organelle traffic densities were obtained by counting the numbers of organelles moving in an optical plane per unit area of axoplasm per unit time in either the anterograde or retrograde direction (see text).

abnormalities in fast transport were found (Breuer et al., 1987): (a) an augmentation of mean fast organelle transport speed in the anterograde direction by 57% (statistically significant), (b) a reduction in the amount of anterograde moving material by 29% (statistically not significant), (c) a reduction of mean fast organelle speed in the retrograde direction by approximately 6% (statistically significant), and (d) a 68% reduction (statistically significant) in the amount of organelle traffic moving in the retrograde direction (Table 1).

The first finding, a faster *mean* anterograde speed in ALS axons, was not due to augmentation of speed of the fastest-moving organelles, but was due to the fact that more organelles were moving at faster speeds (the distribution of speeds was shifted to higher speed ranges). This finding is consistent with that in the wobbler mouse model, where no significant change was seen in the rate of advance of isotope, carried by the fastest-moving organelles (which define the leading edge of the advancing radioactive wave front). The finding that the distribution of organelle speeds behind this fastest-moving front is shifted to higher speed ranges, may be a compensation mechanism to offset diminished numbers of organelles moving in the anterograde direction (the second finding). Our interpretation of these findings is that, since more highly branched motor neurons and larger motor units are seen in the MND, remaining motor neurons have a greater amount of work to perform in maintaining a greater number of striated muscle cells. Thus, the finding of an augmented mean anterograde speed has given rise to the concept of modulation or regulation of transport to meet increasing demand. The abnormality seen in ALS has been interpreted as an "effort" on the part of the cell to meet this increased demand as a normal compensatory response. What effect such a compensatory effect might have if sustained over months or years in terms of metabolic exhaustion of the neuron remains to be explored.

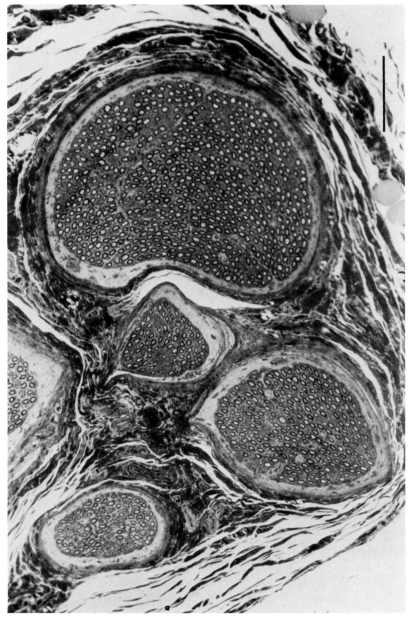

(a)

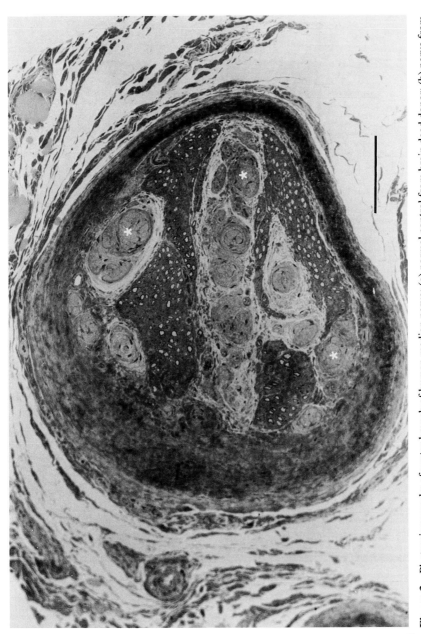

(b)

Figure 3 Photomicrographs of motor branch of human median nerve: (a) normal control from brain dead donor; (b) nerve from ALS patient showing marked loss of axons in fascicles and Renaut bodies (asterisks). Bars = 100 μm. (Reproduced with permission from Ref. 11.)

Table 2   Summary of Abnormalities in Axonal Transport

	Human ALS video-optical method[a]	Wobbler mouse model isotope method[b]
Fast anterograde	Fastest speeds unchanged Mean speed increased 57%* Amount decreased 29% (NS)	Fastest speeds unchanged Mean speed not evaluated Amount not evaluated
Fast retrograde	Mean speed decreased 6%* Amount decreased 68%*	Mean speed not evaluated Amount decreased
Slow (anterograde)	Speed not evaluated	Speed decreased Amount decreased

*$p < 0.001$. NS, Not significant.
[a]Breuer et al., 1987.
[b]Mitsumoto and Gambetti, 1986; Mitsumoto et al., 1990.

The third finding, the reduction of mean fast transport speed in the retrograde direction, while significant at the $p < 0.001$ level, is a small change, 6%, of undetermined biological significance. Hundreds of organelles are analyzed in each of these studies and thus small differences in speed are likely to attain statistical significance. No significant change in the rate of migration of retrograde label was found in the wobbler mouse model.

The fourth and most significant abnormality of the retrograde fast transport system was the 68% reduction in the *amount* of material transported back to the cell body. This is likely to be biologically significant, although the impact of such a reduction on neuronal function has yet to be determined. A significant reduction in the amount of retrogradely transported material was also found in the wobbler mouse model. Thus, consistent findings were made in both human ALS and the wobbler model of MND as ascertained by two different methods.

The changes in fast axonal transport described above are not seen in animal models of diabetic (Abbate et al., 1990) and alcoholic neuropathy (McLane et al., 1990), suggesting that they may be abnormalities specific for the motor neuron class of diseases. Presently, we are evaluating these observations further in an ongoing study of a denervation model, where fast transport is being studied in axons that have been made to sprout and reinnervate denervated muscle. In this experimental paradigm, motor units are larger and the neurons have a larger metabolic load. Fast transport function in this setting is being studied to see if all, some, or none of the abnormalities observed in ALS motor nerve are reproduced.

FAST AXONAL TRANSPORT CAN BE EXPERIMENTALLY MODULATED

In related work, it has been demonstrated that fast axonal transport speeds are reproducibly augmented in both anterograde and retrograde directions by the addition of parathyroid hormone (PTH fragment 1–34) or 50 mM potassium to the buffer bathing the axons under study (Breuer and Atkinson, 1988a). PTH is of interest because of a reversible ALS-like syndrome seen in some patients with hyperparathyroidism.

Experiments with PTH had the effect of stimulating fast axonal transport with both in vivo and in vitro application (Breuer and Atkinson, 1988b). Alzet osmotic minipumps for the chronic delivery of PTH (2.5 units/hr) were implanted subcutaneously in rats for up to a year. FAxT speeds were observed to be significantly increased in both the anterograde and retrograde directions throughout the study period. Speeds were highest early in the study (antero = + 30.0%, $p < 0.001$; retro = + 42.8%, $p < 0.001$), but there appeared to be some compensatory mechanism which lowered the speeds at 1 month (antero = + 15.0, NS; retro = + 16.0%, $p < 0.001$). Throughout these experiments the rats demonstrated no behavioral changes and no symptoms of disease.

The PTH effect on transport has dose-response characteristics (Breuer and Atkinson, 1988a) and these effects are abolished by prior incubation of axons in dihydropyridine calcium channel blockers (Breuer and Atkinson, 1988b), suggesting that calcium is playing a role in the augmentation of transport speed (in both the anterograde and retrograde directions).

The reversibility of the PTH effect was also tested. Alzet minipumps (delivery rate 2.5 units PTH per hour) were removed after 1 week and the transport speeds determined at different times following pump removal in different animals. The PTH-induced increases in transport speeds were reduced in both the antero (−46.9%) and retro (−68.0%) directions when analyzed 6 hr subsequent to pump removal (speeds in both directions were still significantly above normal). At 24 hr, transport speeds in both directions returned to normal (Breuer and Atkinson, 1988b). Thus, it appears from the rapid onset and rapid reversibility that the PTH effect is mediated through relatively short-term physiological events that do not lead to long-term molecular architectural changes of the transport mechanism. Changes in synthesis at the cell soma could not be involved when speed alterations are observed to occur rapidly in vivo and when axons are isolated from their cell bodies (in vitro experiments).

If the PTH effects are not mediated by long-term architectural changes or changes in cell synthesis, then the question arises "What is the site of FAxT speed alteration?" PTH effects are often mediated by intracellular Ca^{2+} changes. Calcium channel blockers (nitrendipine and nifedipine) were, therefore, applied to the in vitro PTH preparation and speeds were no longer significantly different from those of the control group (Breuer and Atkinson, 1988b).

Early evidence from other investigators (Ochs et al., 1977; Ochs, 1982; Lariviere and Lavoie, 1982) using isotopic tracers demonstrated that Ca^{2+} removal from the axonal buffer resulted in the complete blockade of FAxT over the several hours required for a tracer study. Using video microscopy techniques, the

Ca^{2+} effects were observed immediately (within minutes) with drastically reduced (but not completely halted) FAxT speeds. Ca^{2+} was still available to the axons primarily from the subaxolemmal reticulum stores, which are hypothesized to maintain FAxT at a reduced rate. After the Ca^{2+} stores are depleted, the FAxT stops. The mechanism of the Ca^{2+} action is currently unknown but is under investigation with a series of FAxT experiments manipulating Ca^{2+} at the extracellular and intracellular levels.

CONCLUSION

Significant alterations of axonal transport have been found in both human ALS and the wobbler mouse model. Further, the fast transport system, mediated by microtubules and motor proteins, is both up- and down-regulatable experimentally and calcium plays a role in this modulation. The cause of the transport abnormalities in the MND studied and the relationship of these abnormalities, if any, to the pathogenesis of these diseases remains unknown. Results thus far have generated testable hypotheses providing opportunities for further investigation along these lines.

ACKNOWLEDGMENT

Work reported here was supported by grants to ACB from NINCDS (NS 20384), the Whitaker Foundation, the Reinberger Foundation, the ALS Society, and the Cleveland Clinic Foundation.

REFERENCES

1. Abbate SL, Atkinson MB, Breuer AC. Amount and speed of fast axonal transport in diabetes. *Diabetes* 1991; 40(1):111–117.
2. Allen RD, Allen NS. Video-enhanced microscopy with a computer frame memory. J Microsc 1983; 129:3–17.
3. Allen RD, Allen NS, Travis JL. Video-enhanced contrast, differential interference contrast (AVEC-DIC) microscopy: A new method capable of analyzing microtubule related motility in the reticulopodial network of *Allogromia laticollaris*. 1981; Cell Motil 1:291–302, 1981.
4. Allen RD, Weiss DG, Hayden JH, Brown TD, Fujiwake H, Simpson M. Gliding movement of and bidirectional movement along single native microtubules from the squid axoplasm: Evidence of an active role of microtubules in cytoplasmic transport. 1985; J Cell Biol 100:1736–1752.
5. Andrews JM. The fine structure of the cervical spinal cord, ventral root and branchial nerves in the wobbler (wr) mouse. J Neuropathol Exp Neurol 1975; 34:12–27.
6. Andrews JM, Gardner MS, Wolfgram FJ, Ellison GW, Porter DD, Brandkamp

WW. Studies on a murine form of spontaneous lower motor neuron degeneration— The wobbler (WR) mouse. Am J Pathol 1974; 76:63–78.

7. Bird MT, Shuttleworth JR, Koestner A, Reinglass J. The wobbler mouse mutant: An animal model of hereditary motor system disease. Acta Neuropathol 1971; 19:39–50.

8. Bradley WG, Good P, Rasool CG, Adelman LS. Morphometric and biochemical studies of peripheral nerves in amyotrophic lateral sclerosis. Ann Neurol 1983; 14:267–277.

9. Breuer AC, Atkinson MB. Fast axonal transport alterations in amyotrophic lateral sclerosis (ALS) and in parathyroid hormone (PTH)-treated axons. Cell Motility Cytoskeleton 1988a; 10:320–321.

10. Breuer AC, Atkinson MB. Calcium dependent modulation of fast axonal transport. Cell Calcium 1988b; 9:293–301.

11. Breuer AC, Lynn MP, Atkinson MB, Chou SM, Wilbourn AJ, Marks KE, Culver JE, Fleegler EJ. Fast axonal transport in amyotrophic lateral sclerosis: An intra-axonal organelle traffic analysis. Neurology 1987; 37:738–748.

12. Brimijohn S. The role of axonal transport in nerve disease. In: Dyck PJ, Thomas PK, Lambert EH, Bunge R, eds. Peripheral neuropathy. Vol II, Chapter 22. 2nd ed. Philadelphia: Saunders, 1984.

13. Carpenter S. Proximal axonal enlargement in motor neuron disease. Neurology 1968; 18:841–851.

14. Chalfie M and Thomson JN. Organization of neuronal microtubules in the nematode *Caenorhabditis elegans*. J Cell Biol 1979; 82:278–289.

15. Chou SM. Pathognomy of intraneuronal inclusions in ALS. In Tsubaki T, Toyokura Y, eds. Amyotrophic lateral sclerosis. Tokyo: University of Tokyo Press, 1979: 135–176.

16. Chou SM, Kuzuhara S, Giggs CJ Jr, Gajdusek DC. Giant axonal spheroids along corticospinal tracts in a case of Guamaniam ALS. J Neuropathol Exp Neurol 1980; 39:345.

17. Duchen LW, Strich SJ, Falconer DS. An hereditary motor neuron disease with progressive denervation of muscle in the mouse. The mutant "wobbler." J Neurol Neurosrug Psychiatry 1968; 31:535–542.

18. Dustin P. Microtubules. 2nd ed. New York: Springer-Verlag, 1984.

19. Dyck PJ, Stevens JC, Mulder DW, Espinosa RE. Frequency of nerve fiber degeneration of peripheral motor and sensory neurons in amyotrophic lateral sclerosis: Morphometry of deep and superficial peroneal nerve. Neurology 1975; 25:781–785.

20. Griffin JW, Watson DF. Axonal transport in neurological disease. Ann Neurol 1988; 23:3–13.

21. Griffin JW, Price DL. Axonal transport in motor neuron pathology. In: Andrews JM, Johnson RT, Brazier MAB, eds. Amyotrophic lateral sclerosis. New York: Academic Pres, 1976:33–68.

22. Heidemann SR, Landus JM, Hamborg MA. Polarity orientation of axonal microtubules. J Cell Biol 1981; 91:661–665.

23. Iqbal Z, ed. Axoplasmic transport. Boca Raton, FL: CRC Press, 1986.

24. Kirschner MW. Implications of treadmilling for the stability and polarity of actin and tubulin polymers in vivo. J Cell Biol 1980; 86:330–334.

25. Lariviere L, Lavoie PA. Calcium requirement for fast axonal transport in frog motoneurons. J Neurochem 1982; 39(3):882–886.

26. Lasek RJ. Translocation of the neuronal cytoskeleton and axonal locomotion. Proc Trans R Soc Lond 1982; B299:313–327.

27. Leetsma JA, Sepsenwol S. Sperm tail axoneme alterations in the wobbler mouse. J Reprod Fertil 1980; 56:267–270.

28. Margolis RL, Wilson L. Microtubule treadmills: Possible molecular machinery. Nature 1981; 293:705–712.

29. Margolis RL, Job D, Pabion M, Rausch CT. Sliding of STOP proteins on microtubules: A model system for diffusion dependent microtubule motility. Ann NY Acad Sci 1986; 466:306–321.

30. Margolis RL, Whitten R, Rauch CT, Hassain H, Smith RA. Characterization of microtubule associated proteins in amyotrophic lateral sclerosis. In: Tsubaki and Yase, eds. Amyotrophic lateral sclerosis, research aspects. Amsterdam: Elsevier, 1988: 325–332.

31. McLane JA, Atkinson MB, McNulty JA, Breuer AC. Direct measurement of fast axonal transport in chronic ethanol-fed rats. J Alcohol Clin Exp Res 1991 (in press).

32. Mitsumoto H, Bradley WG. Murine motor neuron disease (the wobbler mouse). Degeneration and regeneration of the lower motor neurons. Brain 1982; 105:811–814.

33. Mitsumoto H, Gambetti P. Impaired slow axonal transport in wobbler mouse motor neuron disease. Ann Neurol 1986; 19:36–43.

34. Mitsumoto H, Ferut AL, Kurahashi K, McQuarrie I. Impairment of retrograde transport in wobbler mouse neuron disease. Muscle Nerve 1990; 13:121–126.

35. Norris FH. Moving axon particles of intercostal nerve terminals in benign and malignant ALS. In: Proceedings of the International Symposium on Amyotrophic Lateral Sclerosis. Tokyo: University of Tokyo Press, 1979: 375–385.

36. Ochs S. Calcium and the mechanism of axoplasmic transport. Fed Proc 1982; 41:2301–2306.

37. Ochs S. Basic properties of axoplasmic transport. In: Dyck PJ, Thomas PK, Lambert EH, Bunge R, eds. Peripheral neuropathy. Vol. II, Chapter 21. 2nd ed. Philadelphia: Saunders, 1984.

38. Ochs S, Worth RM, Chan S. Calcium requirements for axoplasmic transport in mammalian nerve. Nature 1977; 270:748–750.

39. Olmsted JB. Microtubule associated proteins. Annu Rev Cell Biol 1986; 2:421–457.

40. Pachter JS, Liem RKH, Shelanski ML. The neuronal cytoskeleton. Adv Cell Neurobiol 1984; 5:113–142.

41. Paschal BM, Shpetner HS, Vallee RB. MAPIC is a microtubule-activated ATPase which translocates microtubules in vitro and has dynein-like properties. J Cell Biol 1987; 105:1273–1282.

42. Pirollet F, Rauch CT, Job D, Margolis RL. Monoclonal antibody to microtubule

associated STOP protein: Affinity purification of neuronal STOP activity and comparison of antigen with activity in neuronal and non-neuronal cell extracts. Biochemistry 1989; 28:835–842.

43. Pollard TE, Cooper JA. Actin and actin-binding proteins. A critical evaluation of mechanisms and functions. Annu Rev Biochem 1986; 55:987–1035.
44. Schliwa M. The cytoskeleton. New York: Springer-Verlag, 1986.
45. Shpetner HS, Vallee RB. Identification of dynamin, a novel mechanochemical enzyme that mediates interactions between microtubules. Cell 1989; 59:421–432.
46. Steinert PM, Roop DR. Molecular and cellular biology of intermediate filaments. Am Rev Biochem 1988; 57:593–625.
47. Vale RD. Intracellular transport using microtubule based motors. Annu Rev Cell Biol 1987; 3:347–378.
48. Vale RD, Reese TS, Sheetz MP. Identification of a novel force generating protein, kinesin, involved in microtubule-based motility. Cell 1985a; 42:39–50.
49. Vale RD, Schnapp MP, Michison T, Steuer E, Reese TS, Sheetz MP. Different axoplasmic proteins generate movement in opposite directions along microtubules in vitro. Cell 1985b; 43:623–632.
50. Warner FD, McIntosh JR, eds. Cell movement. Vol. 2. Kinesin, dynein, and microtubule dynamics. New York: Alan R. Liss, 1989.
51. Weiss DG, ed. Axoplasmic transport. Berlin: Springer-Verlag, 1982.
52. Weiss DG, Gorio A, eds. Axoplasmic transport in physiology and pathology. Berlin: Springer-Verlag, 1982.

22

Growth Factors and Amyotrophic Lateral Sclerosis

Christopher E. Henderson

Centre de Recherche de Biochimie Macromoléculaire, CNRS-INSERM
Montpellier, France

INTRODUCTION

The mechanisms underlying the pathogenesis of sporadic amyotrophic lateral sclerosis (ALS) remain completely elusive, even after many years of sustained effort. It is symptomatic of current confusion that the editor of this volume should have chosen to include a chapter on a topic such as motoneuron growth factors, for which the hypotheses far exceed in number the reliable experimental results. However, a more reasonable point of view would be that, as we discover gradually more about the crucial role played by neurotrophic factors in the normal development of the nervous system, it seems more and more likely that a malfunction in this neuronal support system might underlie lesions of the central nervous system that we recognize as neurological diseases.

As will become immediately apparent, our knowledge of the molecules and mechanisms involved in keeping motoneurons alive is at best fragmentary. Our major task here will be to identify those rare instances in which an abnormality in growth factor action or metabolism has been convincingly described in ALS, and to pinpoint areas in which further progress must be made before the hypotheses presented can be seriously tested.

NEURONAL GROWTH FACTORS

Neuronal growth factors are molecules that regulate in situ the survival and development of certain neuronal populations (1). An exact definition is difficult because so few examples are actually known. In particular, the distinction between growth factors and nutrients is hard to make. Nevertheless, at our present state of knowledge, a candidate neurotrophic factor might be expected to be a polypeptide, synthesized and secreted locally at low levels by the target tissue (or other surrounding tissues) of the neuronal population under consideration. It should act by binding to specific receptors on the neuronal surface to promote cell survival and/or growth. It is possible to make one clear functional distinction between neurotrophic factors and other molecules also classified as growth factors, even if certain molecules may play both roles: in contrast to the mitogenic growth factors FGF, EGF, PDGF, etc., neuronal growth factors do not enhance cell proliferation, as their target neurons are postmitotic.

Before discussing the evidence for the existence of motoneuron growth factors, it will be helpful to summarize succinctly our present knowledge of the two neurotrophic molecules for which an in vivo role seems satisfactorily established.

Nerve Growth Factor

Nerve growth factor (NGF) is a basic polypeptide of molecular weight 13 kDa first discovered by Levi-Montalcini and colleagues (2). It can be easily purified from the submaxillary gland of male mice, in which it is found for unknown reasons at very high levels. In vitro, NGF is required for survival and enhances neurite outgrowth and neurotransmitter synthesis in cultures of most embryonic sensory and sympathetic neurons and also in cultures of cholinergic neurons of the forebrain. In vivo, NGF is synthesized by the peripheral target tissues of sensory and sympathetic neurons (3,4) and in the brain (5). NGF synthesis begins when the axons arrive in the target tissue; in parallel, expression of NGF receptors is initiated by the neurons, which transport the NGF in a retrograde fashion from the nerve terminals to the cell body (6). It is probable that a subsequent decrease in the levels of NGF production leads to a competition between neurons for a limited supply of growth factor, and that only those successful in this competition survive the phase of naturally occurring cell death. Subsequently, at least some of the neurons become less critically dependent on NGF. Nevertheless, NGF can play an important role in the life of the adult neuron, since after crushing a peripheral nerve, Schwann cells distal to the lesion express increased amounts of NGF and NGF receptor, presumably to enhance regeneration (7,8).

This outline of the mode of action of NGF may need to be adjusted as the powerful new techniques of molecular and cell biology allow more detailed study of even molecules expressed at very low levels. However, they provide a useful framework in which to interpret the far less complete data concerning hypothetical motoneuron growth factors. One further experimental result demonstrated early on the real importance of NGF in vivo, and it lies at the root of most hypotheses concerning growth factors and ALS. When antibodies to NGF are injected into neonatal rat pups, there is a dramatic and highly selective loss of sympathetic (but not of sensory) neurons (9); this phenomenon is referred to as immunosympathectomy. When a similar treatment is performed during embryonic development, in fact by immunizing the mother with NGF, then both sympathetic and sensory neurons are lost (10). Two conclusions may be drawn from these results. First, certain neuronal populations absolutely require a supply of endogenous NGF if they are to survive; this dependence can vary with the stage of development. Second, growth factor deprivation can give rise to extremely selective lesions of the nervous system, affecting a single class of neurons only. This latter observation is of clear potential interest for all degenerative diseases of the nervous system in which cell loss is restricted to certain neuronal populations.

Brain-Derived Neurotrophic Factor

The discovery of NGF, and of its relatively limited sphere of action, led to the idea that there might be other neuronal growth factors involved in the development of systems in which NGF was apparently without effect. Although much effort has been devoted to trying to identify such neurotrophic factors, the only new molecule for which one can predict with confidence a physiological role as a target-derived growth factor is the brain-derived neurotrophic factor (BDNF). Isolated originally from pig brain, it has a primary structure showing regions of high homology to that of NGF and indeed has a closely similar molecular weight and isoelectric point (11). In vitro and in vivo, however, it is clearly functionally distinct. It is synthesized mainly within the central nervous system and has known neurotrophic actions on both central (retinal ganglion cells) and peripheral (sensory) neurons (1). The latter, which represent the NGF-insensitive population of many sensory ganglia, presumably come into contact with BDNF via their central process, as the cell death resulting from section of this process may be prevented by local application of BDNF, but not NGF (12). As with NGF, BDNF is only produced by the target, and neurons only become BDNF-dependent, once the initial contacts have been formed (13). Although blocking antibodies are not available to perform the crucial equivalent of the immunosympathectomy experiment, this highly coherent body of evidence strongly suggests that BDNF can be included in the short list of molecules promoting neuronal survival in vivo.

Evidence for the Existence of Motoneuron Growth Factors

The neuromuscular system was in fact the first for which a target-dependent regulation of neuronal survival was demonstrated. In a series of classical experiments, Hamburger and colleagues showed that when motoneurons were deprived of their target muscle by early ablation of a limb bud, none of them survived the phase of naturally occurring cell death which normally leads to loss of only half the motoneurons in this population (14). Conversely, by grafting a supernumerary limb bud onto early embryos, they were able to save a fraction of the motoneurons that would normally have died (15). These results have been refined and extended, especially insofar as the role of electrical and contractile activity is concerned, by Oppenheim and colleagues (16,17).

Although the exact mechanisms of competition between motoneurons remain a subject of considerable controversy (18), most workers agree that muscle produces substances that are required for motoneuron survival at embryonic stages. These hypothetical factors are often referred to as motoneuron growth factors (MNGFs). We will use this abbreviation here for convenience, but it should be stressed that it refers only to the concept, and not to any identified member of the NGF family. A nice recent demonstration of the probable existence of such factors in muscle was provided by application of muscle extracts to chick embryos in ovo during the period of naturally occuring cell death: most of the motoneurons initially generated in the lumbar motor column were protected from cell death by this treatment (19).

It might be argued that cell death in the early embryonic period is only distantly related to the motoneuron loss observed in adult ALS patients. Although the body of evidence is less extensive, it is clear that neonatal motoneurons too are rapidly lost after nerve-muscle interactions are severed by axotomy (20–22). In humans, permanent axotomy by amputation results in loss of the corresponding motoneurons (23). However, it is clear that such phenomena will only be shown to be have a common mechanism once the factors involved have been defined on a molecular and cellular level.

In addition to their supposed role in regulating motoneuron survival, MNGFs have been implicated at other stages of motoneuron development, including formation of muscle nerve branches at embryonic stages, stabilization of synapses during the period of regression of polyneuronal innervation, and the response of motoneurons to injury (24). In the last instance, Brown and colleagues have elegantly demonstrated that the intramuscular nerve sprouting observed after partial denervation of adult muscle is caused by a "sprouting signal" (or MNGF) released by denervated muscle fibers, which can diffuse over limited distances through the muscle (25).

Attempts to Identify Candidate Motoneuron Growth Factors

No molecule involved in the regulation of motoneuron survival and development has yet been unequivocally identified (24). Our aim in this section is not to give an exhaustive review of the extensive but inconclusive literature on this subject, but to indicate a few examples of molecules (purified or nearly so) that at the time of writing seem of potential interest. None of the molecules described here has yet been directly tested in the context of ALS etiology; those which have are discussed below.

Most approaches to the identification of candidate MNGFs have employed cell cultures of embryonic motoneurons, either after purification or after enrichment with respect to other spinal cord cells. Muscle-derived preparations are tested for their effects on motoneuron survival, neurite outgrowth, or choline acetyltransferase activity.

Effects of Known Polypeptides
NGF itself has no known role in motoneuron development in vivo, although, curiously, motoneurons do express NGF receptors (26), and NGF can reportedly slightly enhance their neurite outgrowth on laminin in culture (27).

Other factors of known primary structure have been tested on purified motoneurons. Perhaps the most striking effect was obtained with transforming growth factor-beta (TGFβ), which markedly enhanced the survival of motoneurons purified by cell sorting and grown on living or killed astrocyte monolayers (28). Basic fibroblast growth factor (b-FGF) stimulated cell survival in mixed cultures of spinal neurons, though this effect was probably not limited to the motoneuron population (29).

Another interesting candidate is ciliary neuronotrophic factor (CNTF), which has neurotrophic actions on embryonic parasympathetic, sympathetic, and sensory neurons in vitro (30). No data have been published concerning its action on motoneurons, and it is not synthesized in adult muscle (31). However, one cannot at present exclude a role for CNTF in embryonic motoneuron development.

New Candidate Motoneuron Growth Factors
One promising candidate at the present time is the cholinergic development factor (CDF), which has been purified 5000-fold to apparent homogeneity from rat skeletal muscle (32). The purified factor has an apparent molecular weight of 20 kDa and a pI of 4.8 and within 2 days increases the level of choline acetyltransferase in spinal cord cultures approximately fivefold over control cultures. It is particularly interesting that highly purified preparations of this factor, when applied to chick embryos in ovo, are capable of considerably reducing the extent of naturally occurring cell death in the motoneuron population (33). The molecular properties of CDF are not dissimilar to those of CNTF. However, since the former is enriched in skeletal muscle at a stage (2 weeks postnatal) at which no CNTF mRNA is detectable, they are unlikely to be identical, but could be members of a new family of neurotrophic molecules.

Among the other molecules that affect cholinergic activity of purified motoneurons in vitro, one is probably identical to the cholinergic differentiation factor (34), which has now been shown to be identical to the leukemia inhibitory factor (LIF) (35), a protein that stimulates bone remodeling and acute-phase protein synthesis in hepatocytes. However, LIF does not apparently enhance motoneuron survival and can be separated from other survival-promoting and CAT-inducing activities in muscle-conditioned media (34).

HYPOTHESES CONCERNING GROWTH FACTORS AND MOTONEURON DISEASES

Over the years, several articles have presented hypotheses for the etiology of ALS based on a malfunction in the neuronal growth factor system (36–39). The starting point for all these hypotheses has been the idea that if, as we suppose, motoneurons are normally maintained alive by trophic support from their target muscle or other surrounding tissues, then motoneuron death in ALS (and other motoneuron diseases) could result from, or be accelerated by, inadequate nerve-muscle interactions. These hypotheses are essentially so similar that it seems best to state them here in a general form (Fig. 1).

Thus motoneuron death in ALS could be linked to: (a) a reduction in the production of a hypothetical MNGF by the muscle; (b) inhibition of the neurotrophic action of the MNGF on motoneurons; (c) loss of the ability of motoneurons to respond to the MNGF; or (d) (in familial forms) mutations in the MNGF gene.

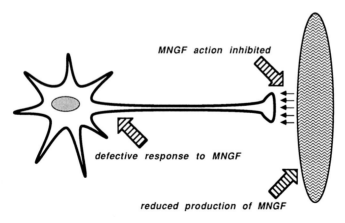

Figure 1 Possible mechanisms of ALS pathogenesis based on the hypothesis of a malfunction in the motoneuron growth factor (MNGF) system.

In the following sections, we will summarize the results of experiments directly designed to explore one of these hypotheses, and we will also review other growth factor anomalies in ALS not directly related to this model.

EXPERIMENTAL APPROACHES TO STUDYING A POSSIBLE NEUROTROPHIC DEFICIT IN ALS

From the preceding sections, it is clear that the major handicap facing those who wish to study a possible neurotrophic deficit in ALS is that no MNGF has been unequivocally identified. We will discuss here those attempts concerning candidate MNGFs and others involving other neuronal test systems or growth factors.

The "Neuroleukin" Episode

In 1984, considerable interest was aroused when Gurney et al. described the presence in ALS sera of antibodies that blocked sprouting at the neuromuscular junction paralyzed by botulinum toxin (40). These antibodies were reported to recognize a 56-kDa muscle protein, which was subsequently purified, cloned, and christened "neuroleukin" (41). In addition to promoting the survival of chick spinal and sensory neurons, "neuroleukin" was also a lymphokine. It thus seemed as if inhibition of a MNGF by circulating antibodies might indeed play a role in ALS pathology. However, several other experimental observations were in apparent contradiction with these results. First, in the hands of others, ALS antibodies did not inhibit sprouting (42) or neurite outgrowth (43,44) from spinal neurons. Indeed, some antibody preparations enhanced both neurite outgrowth in vitro (44) and survival of embryonic motoneurons in vivo (39). Second, antibodies to an apparently similar 56-kDa protein were found in sera from normal subjects and those with other neurological diseases (45) while ALS sera were found not to recognize recombinant "neuroleukin" (41). Finally, the deduced sequence of "neuroleukin" was shown to be identical to that of glucose-6-phosphate isomerase, a normally intracellular glycolytic enzyme, which is expressed at high levels in most embryonic tissues (46,47). These results do not exclude the possibility that glucose-6-phosphate isomerase may indeed have the biological activities reported for "neuroleukin," but the relevance of this enzyme to ALS pathology currently seems remote.

Other Studies Related to the Neurotrophic Hypothesis

Although examples are not numerous, different workers have looked either for a diminution of endogenous neurotrophic activity in ALS muscle and spinal cord or for inhibitory substances that might conceivably block neurotrophic activity.

Given that adult human motoneurons are virtually impossible to obtain in culture, cultures of embryonic neurons have usually been employed.

Using fetal human or rat spinal cord cultures, no convincing effects of ALS sera or CSF have been observed on enzymatic activities, neurofilament reactivity, or neurite outgrowth (48,49). However, it should be pointed out that none of the published studies have used identified (or purified) motoneurons. Furthermore, it may be that neurotrophic disturbances exist but are not detectable in serum. This might indeed be expected, as levels of bona fide neuronal growth factors are extremely low in serum, their action being essentially local (1).

Given the experimental problems encountered in culturing embryonic motoneurons, some workers have used other cholinergic (ciliary ganglion) or potentially cholinergic (sympathetic ganglia) neurons to screen for neurotrophic disturbances in ALS (50,51). Not surprisingly, perhaps, since these particular neurons are not affected in ALS, addition of serum or postmortem muscle or spinal cord from ALS patients did not inhibit neuronal survival, and ALS tissue extracts contained normal levels of survival-promoting activity.

One interesting result concerning hypothesis (c) is that the rate of retrograde organelle transport is slower in ALS peripheral nerve than in controls (52). This is not simply a rundown of the transport system in a sick neuron, since anterograde transport is considerably faster than in controls. It is likely that retrograde transport from the synapse to the cell body plays an important role in MNGF action. This phenomenon would thus be expected to result in a trophic deficit for the affected neuron.

Other Growth Factor Anomalies in ALS

It has been reported that levels of epidermal growth factor (EGF) are significantly reduced in cerebrospinal fluid from ALS patients compared to controls (53). In addition to its much studied mitogenic activity, EGF has been reported to enhance in vitro development of brain neurons, though not yet of motoneurons (54). This deficit could thus be imagined to play a role in ALS pathogenesis. Serum levels of insulin-like growth factor I, on the other hand, are normal in ALS (55).

Calcitonin gene–related peptide (CGRP) is coreleased from some motoneurons with acetylcholine and has been shown in culture to increase levels of acetylcholine receptor on embryonic myotubes (56,57). This peptide is normally present in a fraction of motoneurons in human spinal cord. In ALS, however, it is completely absent (58). Although it is difficult to rule out the possibility that this reflects simply the loss of those motoneurons which are usually CGRP-positive, the proposed role of CGRP as a muscle trophic factor means that its disappearance could have serious consequences for the muscle in ALS.

RESULTS WITH OTHER DISEASES OF THE ANTERIOR HORN

Aside from ALS, the motoneuron diseases that have been the most studied are the infantile spinal muscular atrophies (SMA), of which the most severe is Werdnig-Hoffmann disease (38). The questions concerning the mechanisms of motoneuron loss are strictly analogous to those already discussed for ALS, and there thus could be a common pathogenetic mechanism for the two. However, in SMA the neuronal loss is almost completely restricted to the anterior horn of the spinal cord, and the defect is heritable.

Using cultures of embryonic chicken spinal cord, Henderson and colleagues showed that neurite outgrowth could be enhanced by two probably distinct muscle-derived factors, termed "embryonic" and "neonatal" neurite-promoting activities (59). Whereas extracts of SMA muscle biopsies were without effect on the chick "embryonic" factor, the chick "neonatal" activity was strongly inhibited by the same muscle extracts (60). The effect was thus selective, and not simply cytotoxic. Control muscle extracts showed on average no inhibition of neurite outgrowth in the presence of "embryonic" or "neonatal" activities. Serum from SMA patients showed no inhibitory activity.

These preliminary results need to be confirmed using identified motoneurons before a trophic deficit can be considered to have been demonstrated. Even if that is the case, it will be necessary to rule out the possibility that the presence of inhibitors of growth factor action results simply from degeneration of the neuromuscular system, following a completely different primary insult.

CONCLUSION

The major conclusion of this brief review must be that, although the hypothesis of a neurotrophic malfunction in ALS seems potentially interesting for understanding the cause and/or the mechanism of progression of the disease, no solid experimental evidence has been provided in its support. Nevertheless, it is too early to reject the hypothesis, since the experimental methods for testing it completely do not as yet exist. In particular, we have no firm knowledge at all of the growth factor requirements of adult motoneurons and no unequivocally identified molecule that might play the role of an MNGF. In this field, basic research has to make considerable progress before the links with neuropathology can be other than suggestive.

As with many of the putative etiological factors in ALS discussed elsewhere in this book, it is theoretically possible that defects in the neuronal growth factor system may be involved either in initiating or in exacerbating the primary insult to the motoneurons and that, even if they are not, neurotrophic factors may provide a glimmer of (long-term) hope for slowing down neuronal death. However, our limited knowledge in this field means that it is premature to try to distinguish between primary and secondary effects and presumptuous even to discuss possible uses of growth factors as a basis for treatment.

To simplify the discussion, the neuronal deficit in ALS has been considered in this chapter mainly to be a problem of motoneuron survival in the spinal cord. Obviously, the well-documented lesions in the motor cortex and cranial motoneurons must also be taken into account. It is possible that their degeneration may be a secondary effect of the loss of spinal motoneurons; equally, a neurotrophic disturbance within the central nervous system could be imagined. However, our ignorance of neuron-target relationships within the spinal cord is such that hypotheses of this nature are bound to be extremely vague and thus of little use for suggesting experimental investigations.

In summary, therefore, deprivation of neuronal growth factors represents one of the very few known mechanisms for creating cell-type-specific lesions within the central nervous system and as such seems of considerable interest for degenerative diseases such as ALS. Our imagination of possible pathological mechanisms is often limited by what is already known. In this context, and whatever the differences between sporadic and familial forms of ALS, identification of the genetic loci affected in familial ALS and in spinal muscular atrophies, both currently under study, will have great importance.

NOTE ADDED IN PROOF

Since this chapter was written, ciliary neurotrophic factor (CNTF) has been shown to be active on survival of motoneurons in vivo (61–63) and in vitro (64). It has been proposed that it is involved in the protection of motoneurons after lesion of peripheral nerve.

ACKNOWLEDGMENTS

Work reported from the author's laboratory and was supported by the Association Française contre les Myopathies (AFM) and the Institut pour la Recherche sur la Moelle Epinière (IRME).

REFERENCES

1. Barde Y-A. Trophic factors and neuronal survival. Neuron 1989;2:1525–1534.
2. Levi-Montalcini R. The nerve growth factor: Thirty-five years later. EMBO J 1987;6:1145–1154.
3. Korsching S, Thoenen H. Nerve growth factor in sympathetic ganglia and corre-

sponding target organs of the rat: Correlation with density of sympathetic innervation. Proc Natl Acad Sci USA 1983;80:3513–3516.

4. Shelton DL, Reichardt LF. Expression of the beta-nerve growth factor gene correlates with the density of sympathetic innervation in effector organs. Proc Natl Acad Sci USA 1984;81:7951–7955.

5. Whittemore SR, Ebendal T, Lärkfors L, Olson L, Seiger A, Strömberg I, Persson H. Developmental and regional expression of beta-nerve growth factor messenger RNA and protein in the rat central nervous system. Proc Natl Acad Sci USA 1986;83:817–821.

6. Davies AM, Bandtlow C, Heumann R, Korsching S, Rohrer H, Thoenen H. Timing and site of nerve growth factor synthesis in developing skin in relation to innervation and expression of the receptor. Nature 1987;326:353–358.

7. Heumann R, Lindholm D, Bandtlow C, Meyer M, Radeke MJ, Misho TP, Shooter E, Thoenen H. Differential regulation of mRNA encoding nerve growth factor and its receptor in rat sciatic nerve during development, degeneration and regeneration: Role of macrophages. Proc Natl Acad Sci USA 1987;84:8735–8739.

8. Taniuchi M, Clarke HB, Johnson EM. Induction of nerve growth factor receptor in Schwann cells after axotomy. Proc Natl Acad Sci USA 1986;83:4094–4098.

9. Levi-Montalcini R, Booker B. Destruction of the sympathetic ganglia in mammals by an antiserum to a nerve growth protein. Proc Natl Acad Sci USA 1960;46: 384–391.

10. Gorin RD, Johnson EM. Experimental autoimmune model of nerve growth factor deprivation: Effects on developing peripheral sympathetic and sensory neurons. Proc Natl Acad Sci USA 1979;76:5382–5386.

11. Leibrock J, Lottspeich F, Hohn A, Hofer M, Hengerer B, Masiakowski PK, Thoenen H, Barde Y-A. Molecular cloning and expression of brain-derived neurotrophic factor. Nature 1989;341:149–152.

12. Kalcheim C, Barde Y-A, Thoenen H, Le Douarin N. In vivo effect of brain-derived neurotrophic factor on the survival of developing dorsal root ganglion cells. EMBO J 1987;6:2871–2873.

13. Rodriguez-Tébar A, Jeffrey PL, Thoenen H, Barde Y-A. The survival of chick retinal ganglion cells in response to brain-derived neurotrophic factor depends on their embryonic age. Dev Biol 1989;136:296–303.

14. Hamburger V. The developmental history of the motor neuron. Neurosci Res Progr Bull 1977;15S:1–37.

15. Hollyday M, Hamburger V. Reduction of naturally occurring motor neuron loss by enlargement of the periphery. J Comp Neurol 1976;170:311–320.

16. Pittmann R, Oppenheim RW. Cell death of motoneurons in the chick embryo spinal cord. IV. Evidence that a functional neuromuscular interaction is involved in the regulation of naturally occurring cell death and the stabilization of synapses. J Comp Neurol 1979;187:425–446.

17. Oppenheim RW, Haverkamp LJ. Neurotrophic interactions in the development of spinal cord motoneurons. In: Evered D, Whelan J, eds. Plasticity of the neuromuscular system, Ciba Foundation Symposium 138. Chichester: Wiley, 1988:152–171.

18. Oppenheim RW. The neurotrophic theory and naturally occurring cell death. Trends Neurosci 1989;12:252–255.

19. Oppenheim RW, Haverkamp LJ, Prevette D, McManaman JL, Appel SH. Reduction of naturally occurring motoneuron death in vivo by a target-derived neurotrophic factor. Science 1988;240:919–922.

20. Schmalbruch H. Motoneuron death after sciatic nerve section in newborn rats. J Comp Neurol 1984;224:252–258.

21. Lowrie MB, Krishnan S, Vrbovà G. Permanent changes in muscle and motoneurones induced by nerve injury during a critical period of development of the rat. Dev Brain Res 1987;31:91–101.

22. Kashihara Y, Kuno M, Miyata Y. Cell death of axotomized motoneurones in neonatal rats, and its prevention by peripheral reinnervation. J Physiol 1987;386: 135–148.

23. Kawamura Y, Dyck PJ. Permanent axotomy by amputation results in loss of motor neurons in man. J Neuropathol Exp Neurol 1981;40:658–666.

24. Henderson CE. The role of muscle in the development and differentiation of spinal motoneurons: In vivo studies. In: Evered D, Whelan J, eds. Plasticity of the neuromuscular system, Ciba Foundation Symposium 138. Chichester: Wiley, 1988: 172–191.

25. Brown M, Holland R, Hopkins W. Motor nerve sprouting. Annu Rev Neurosci 1981;4:17–42.

26. Raivich G, Zimmermann A, Sutter A. The spatial and temporal pattern of βNGF receptor expression in the developing chick embryo. EMBO J 1985;4:637–644.

27. Heaton MB. Influence of laminin on the responsiveness of early chick embryo neural tube neurons to nerve growth factor. J Neurosci Res 1989;22:390–396.

28. Martinou J-C, Le Van Thai A, Valette A, Weber M. Transforming growth factor-1 is a potent survival factor for rat embryonic motoneurons in culture. Dev Brain Res 1990;52:175–181.

29. Unsicker K, Reichert-Preibsch H, Schmidt R, Pettmann B, Labourdette G, Sensenbrenner M. Astroglial and fibroblast growth factor have neurotrophic functions for cultured peripheral and central nervous system neurons. Proc Natl Acad Sci USA 1987;84:5459–5463.

30. Lin L-FH, Mismer D, Lile JD, Armes LG, Butler ET, Vannice JL, Collins F. Purification, cloning and expression of ciliary neurotrophic factor (CNTF). Science 1989;246:1023–1025.

31. Stöckli KA, Lottspeich F, Sendtner M, Masiakowski P, Carroll P, Götz R, Lindholm D, Thoenen H. Molecular cloning, expression and regional distribution of rat ciliary neurotrophic factor. Nature 1989;342:920–923.

32. McManaman JL, Crawford FG, Stewart SS, Appel SH. Purification of a skeletal muscle polypeptide which stimulates choline acetyltransferase activity in cultured spinal cord neurons. J Biol Chem 1988;263:5890–5897.

33. Haverkamp LJ, Oppenheim RW, McManaman JL, Prevette D. The in vivo effects of muscle-derived neurotrophic factors on motoneuron death and differentiation. AFM Workshop on Spinal Muscular Atrophies, Les Embiez, France, Sept. 24–28, 1989 (Abstract).

The mechanism by which free radicals, such as the hydroxyl radical, degrade lipids has been the most extensively studied of these processes. Membrane polyunsaturated fatty acid (PUFA) molecules are primarily susceptible to this form of damage, which is termed nonenzymatic lipid peroxidation. In essence, the oxidizing free radical species is able to abstract a hydrogen atom from a carbon adjacent to a double bond in the PUFA, thus stabilizing its own structure and creating a lipid radical. This newly formed radical then avidly reacts with oxygen, resulting in the formation of a lipid peroxy radical. This derivative is deleterious to membrane conformation because it is polar with respect to other membrane lipids within the lipid bilayer and also highly reactive and able to abstract a hydrogen from a neighboring PUFA molecule, resulting in propagation of the chain reaction and accumulation of further polar peroxide groups within the membrane. Further decomposition of the lipid peroxide may also occur, leading to formation of various breakdown products of lipid peroxides within the cell.

DEFENSE MECHANISMS AGAINST FREE RADICALS

Enzymatic

The superoxide dismutases (SODs) appear to be the cell's primary defense against the superoxide radical, but the product of their action is hydrogen peroxide. Catalase is therefore required to further split this into water and molecular oxygen. Although high activities are present in liver, kidney, and erythrocytes, brain SOD levels are comparatively low. The selenium-containing enzyme glutathione peroxidase (GSHPX) is likely to be more important in the inactivation and breakdown of organic peroxides accumulating in the brain. This reaction hinges on the oxidation of reduced glutathione (GSH) to oxidized glutathione (GSSG). The reformation of GSH from GSSG is dependent on glutathione reductase, an enzyme also present in high concentrations in the brain (Reaction 5).

$$2GSH + LOOH \xrightarrow{\hspace{1cm}} GSSG + LOH + H_2O$$
$$\text{GSHPX}$$

glutathione reductase (5)

$$NADP^+ \qquad\qquad NADPH + H^+$$

Nonenzymatic

Ascorbic acid is an important antioxidant when present in high concentrations. The concentration is a critical factor as low levels can have a pro-oxidant effect by accelerating the dissociation of hydrogen peroxide. High concentrations of ascorbic acid are found in both the gray and white matter of the brain, and the choroid plexus has a specific transport mechanism that concentrates ascorbate in the cerebrospinal fluid (CSF) to a level approximately 10 times that in serum. Neurons have a further system which results in an even higher intraneuronal ascorbate content.

Vitamin E (α-tocopherol) is also an important antioxidant. Because it is fat soluble, it has a special role in preventing lipid peroxidation. Peroxidation is prevented by the donation of a hydrogen atom to the peroxy radical, thus leaving an unpaired electron on the tocopherol molecule. This tocopherol radical is innocuous, but is interestingly also converted back to the active vitamin by ascorbic acid, providing a further function for vitamin C in free radical defense mechanisms. The neurological sequelae of vitamin E deficiency are well recognized in humans. Patients with a-β-lipoproteinemia suffer from malabsorptive tocopherol deficiency and develop a neurological syndrome that clinically resembles spinocerebellar degeneration.

This discussion of antioxidants has so far centered on intracellular defense mechanisms against free radicals. Extracellular mechanisms must not be forgotten. Although human CSF contains very little GSHPX, SOD, catalase, ceruloplasmin, or transferrin, low-molecular-weight iron and copper complexes are present. These can act as powerful promoters of free radical formation. It seems clear that CSF must contain an effective antioxidant, the nature of which is not yet known (Halliwell and Gutteridge, 1985a).

DETECTION AND IDENTIFICATION OF FREE RADICALS

In order to demonstrate that increased free radical activity plays a crucial role in pathological processes, it is necessary to be able to provide evidence of increased activity of free radicals in the tissue to be studied. This is technically difficult since there is still no single accepted test for evidence of increased free radical activity in biological materials. In addition, the inherent inaccesibility of neural tissue imposes further restrictions on what is possible in patients with amyotrophic lateral sclerosis (ALS) and other neurodegenerative diseases. At present, it is generally accepted that a pathological process can be ascribed to a free-radical-mediated mechanism if there is evidence of increased free radical activity within the pathological material under study; if it can be prevented by the use of specific inhibitors of free radical activity (i.e., antioxidants or protective enzymes); and if the process can be mimicked by an exogenous source of free radicals. For ALS and other neurodegenerative disorders, there is some evidence that the first two of these may be true (see next section for details), but the last part does not appear to have been addressed.

FREE RADICALS AND NEURONAL CEROID LIPOFUSCINOSIS

The importance of free radical mechanisms in neurological disease was first suggested by studies of the neuronal ceroid lipofuscinoses (NCL). These disorders are characterized by the intra- and extraneuronal accumulation of lipofuscin, an "age pigment." Such age pigments had previously been found to be endproducts of the lipid peroxidation of membranes. Some NCL patients were found to have increased CSF levels of either aluminium or low-molecular-weight iron complexes. There is some evidence that Al(III) salts can accelerate Fe(II)-dependent membrane damage (Halliwell and Gutteridge, 1985b). These findings have led to trials of antioxidant therapy in patients suffering with NCL (Gutteridge et al., 1982).

FREE RADICALS AND PARKINSON'S DISEASE

The ease with which catecholamines produce free radical derivatives has been fundamental to ideas that the degenerative process in Parkinson's disease (PD) may depend at least partly on free-radical-mediated mechanisms. The neurological disease known as "locura manganica" has many features of PD and was related to occupational exposure to manganese in Chilean manganese miners in the classical work of Cotzias (Cotzias et al., 1968). It has since been suggested that this disease may have resulted from formation of catecholamine free radical derivatives triggered by manganese (Halliwell and Gutteridge, 1985a).

It must, however, be stressed that although similarities exist, locura manganica is clearly not the same disease as idiopathic PD and that studies of brain transition metal levels in PD have not shown any changes in the distribution of manganese, although increased iron and reduced copper levels have been found in the substantia nigra in PD (Jenner, 1989). Increased CSF copper concentrations have also been found in PD patients (Pall et al., 1987). Reduced nigral levels of PUFA and malondialdehyde have also been described in PD and raise the possibility that the increased nigral iron levels stimulate cell death through a pathway involving free radical formation and lipid peroxidation. Increased SOD levels have also been found in the substantia nigra. The evidence suggests that this increase is due to the manganese-containing, mitochondrial form of the enzyme. Recent work has suggested an impairment of complex I of the mitochondrial respiratory chain in PD (Jenner, 1989).

The discovery of MPTP PD [PD precipitated by exposure to 1-methyl-4-phenyl-1,2,3,6-tetrahydropyridine (MPTP)] has been of major importance in our efforts to understand the pathogenesis of neurodegenerative disease (Langston et al., 1982). It was suggested at an early stage that the toxic principle was not MPTP itself, but its metabolite MPP^+. The charged nature of this moiety, as well as its structural similarity to paraquat, led to suggestions that the pathogenesis of MPTP PD might depend on free radical mechanisms. It now seems unlikely that MPP$^+$ is sufficiently unstable to result in the formation of toxic oxyradicals, although the metabolism of MPTP itself has been shown to be associated with radical formation. This has been found to occur in aerobic mitochondrial preparations and may be prevented by the addition of SOD. The suggestion that mitochondria are important in the mediation of the toxic effects of MPTP is clearly of interest in relation to reports of an impairment of the mitochondrial respiratory chain in idiopathic PD (Jenner, 1989).

FREE RADICALS AND ALS

ALS is a neurodegenerative disorder in which the motor system is affected at all levels. Like PD, it is a systematized neuronal degeneration. Its ultimate cause remains unknown. Reduced RNA levels have been found in surviving motor neurons with preservation of DNA content (Davidson and Hartmann, 1981), which has been considered to suggest a defect of DNA transcription in ALS. Changes in trace element distribution have also been found in ALS. Increased selenium levels have been reported in erythrocytes (Nagata et al., 1985), cervical cord, liver, and bone (Mitchell, 1987; Mitchell et al., 1991). Increased spinal cord (Miyata et al., 1983; Mitchell et al., 1991; Mitchell, 1987, 1989) and reduced hepatic (Mitchell, 1989; Mitchell et al., 1991) manganese levels have also been found. These findings suggested that free-radical-mediated mechanisms might be implicated in the initiation of the degenerative process in ALS. As previously mentioned, free radicals are able to damage polynucleotides, and accumulation of radical species in the vicinity of DNA could thus disrupt transcription. In addition, the increased spinal cord selenium and manganese levels may be indicators of GSHPX and MnSOD activity increased in response to an increased free radical activity.

We have attempted to test this ''free radical hypothesis'' of ALS, examining CSF parameters of free radical activity and lipid peroxidation. Diene conjugates were measured as a reflection of the early stages of lipid peroxidation. Chloroform fluorescence was regarded as an index of the later stages of lipid peroxidation and methanol fluorescence as a measure of free radical damage to proteins. No differences in any of these parameters were found between ALS patients and controls (Mitchell et al., 1986, 1987). Although disappointing, this negative result was not necessarily surprising. The blood-brain barrier is intact in ALS, and correlates of abnormal free radical activity might not be found in CSF. It is to some extent surprising that the results of these studies were so unremarkable. Some changes might have been expected simply as a result of the degenerative process even if free radicals were not primarily involved in its initiation. Also, the indices considered in this work mainly related to free-radical-induced

Table 1 Tissue Glutathione Peroxidase
Activity in ALS

	Controls	ALS
Cervical white matter	35	21
	41	50
Cervical gray matter	44	4
	30	14
Thoracic white matter	30	24
	50	65
Thoracic gray matter	2	35
	23	45
Lumbar white matter[a]	45	5
	50	59
Lumbar grey matter[a]	11	4
	31	18
Liver	47	98
	127	60

[a]Lumbar enlargement of spinal cord.
All results given as units of GSHPX activity/mg protein.
Source: After Mitchell and Pentland (1990).

membrane damage. In view of the possibility that the fundamental trigger of ALS acts at an intracellular rather than a membranous level, it was considered important to try to make direct measurements of GSHPX activity in spinal cord and liver of patients dying of ALS. Although only a small number of results are so far available, the results show a wide variation, and some very low GSHPX activities have been found. In general, the activities seem higher in white than in gray matter. It is not possible to make a formal statistical analysis of these results, but a trend may be beginning to emerge. Any changes in the distribution of GSHPX resulting from disease activity in ALS might be expected to affect the gray rather than the white matter, and the cervical level and lumbar enlargement rather than the thoracic segment (a statement made solely on the basis of the distribution and density of anterior horn cells within the spinal cord) and the GSHPX activities appear to be lower in these regions in ALS patients than in controls. Results from two control subjects who died of nondegenerative neurological disease and two patients dying from ALS are shown in Table 1. These findings are, however, difficult to reconcile with the previously described high spinal cord, liver, and bone selenium levels.

There is a high level of suspicion that ALS is triggered by exposure to an environmental agent, probably of a chemical nature, in a manner similar to the model of MPTP PD. This model shows that a defined molecule can trigger a selective neuronal degeneration that mimics a recognized human neurological disease (Langston et al., 1982). The possibility that an analogous situation might obtain in ALS deserves further investigation.

REFERENCES

1. Braganza JM. Selenium deficiency, cystic fibrosis and pancreatic cancer. Lancet 1985;2:1238.
2. Cotzias GC, Horiuchi K, Fuenzalida S, et al. Chronic manganese poisoning. Clearance of tissue manganese concentrations with persistence of the neurological picture. Neurology 1968;18:376–382.
3. Davidson TJ, Hartmann HA. RNA content and volume of motor neurones in amyotrophic lateral sclerosis. J Neuropathol Exp Neurol 1981;40:187–192.
4. Dormandy TL. Free radical pathology and medicine. J Roy Coll Phys Lond 1989;23:221–227.
5. Gutteridge JMC, Rowley DA, Halliwell B, et al. Increased non-protein bound iron and decreased protection against superoxide radical damage in cerebrospinal fluid from patients with neuronal ceroid lipofuscinoses. Lancet 1982;2:459–461.
6. Halliwell B, Gutteridge JMC. Oxygen radicals and the nervous system. Trends Neurol Sci 1985a;8:22–26.
7. Halliwell B, Gutteridge JMC. The importance of free radicals and catalytic metal ions in human diseases. Mol Aspects Med 1985b;8:89–193.
8. Jenner P. Clues to the mechanism underlying dopamine cell death in Parkinson's disease. J Neurol Neurosurg Psychiatry 1989;(Suppl):22–28.
9. Joyce DA. Oxygen radicals in disease. Adverse Drug Reaction Bull 1987;(No. 127):476–479.
10. Langston JW, Ballard P, Tetrud JW, et al. Chronic Parkinsonism in humans due to a product of meperidine analog synthesis. Science 1982;219:979–980.
11. Mitchell JD. Heavy metals and trace elements in amyotrophic lateral sclerosis. In: Brooks BR, ed. Motor neurone disorders and amyotrophic lateral sclerosis. Philadelphia: Saunders, 1987;43–60.
12. Mitchell JD. Trace elements, neurological disease and amyotrophic lateral sclerosis. In: Chazot G, Arnaud P, Abdulla M, eds. Current trends in trace elements research. London: Smith-Gordon, 1989;116–124.
13. Mitchell JD, Pentland B. Trace elements and free radicals in ALS. In: Clifford Rose F, ed. The etiology of ALS. Epidemiological and neurotoxicological aspects. London: Smith-Gordon, (1990).
14. Mitchell JD, Jackson MJ, Pentland B. Indices of free radical activity in the cerebrospinal fluid in motor neurone disease. J Neurol Neurosurg Psychiatry 1987;50:919–922.
15. Mitchell JD, Pentland B, East BW, et al Trace elements and free radicals in motor neurone disease (amyotrophic lateral sclerosis). In: Rice-Evans C, ed. Free radicals, cell damage and disease. London: Richelieu Press, 1986:263–272.
16. Mitchell JD, East BW, Harris IA, et al. Manganese, selenium and other trace

elements in spinal cord, liver and bone in motor neurone disease. Eur Neurol 1991;31:7–11.

17. Miyata S, Nakamura S, Nagata H, et al. Increased manganese level in spinal cords of amyotrophic lateral sclerosis determined by radiochemical neutron activation analysis. J Neurol Sci 1983;61:283–293.

18. Nagata H, Miyata S, Nakamura S, et al. Heavy metal concentration in blood cells in patients with amyotrophic lateral sclerosis. J Neurol Sci 1985;67:173–178.

19. Pall HS, Williams AC, Blake DR, et al. Raised cerebrospinal fluid copper concentration in Parkinson's disease. Lancet 1987;2:238–241.

24

Neurotoxicology: Light Metals

Juan Cavieres Troncoso, Mark R. Gilbert,* and Nancy A. Muma

The Johns Hopkins University School of Medicine
Baltimore, Maryland

INTRODUCTION

Amyotrophic lateral sclerosis (ALS) was defined as a pathological entity by Charcot at the end of the last century (Schoene, 1985), yet its pathogenesis and etiology still elude us. Because of its progressive evolution and the involvement of a specific neuronal population, ALS has been categorized as a degenerative disorder, with the implication that an unknown metabolic derangement was restricted to the neuronal population at risk. However, the possibility of environmental agents as a cause or pathogenetic factor in motor neuron disease (MND) has also received wide attention (Johnson, 1982). The quest for an environmental factor in ALS was enhanced by the discovery of an infectious origin for kuru and Creutzfeldt-Jakob disease (CJD) (Gajdusek, 1977; Johnson, 1982), theretofore considered "degenerative disorders," and by the identification of an endemic form of MND in several regions of the western Pacific (Hirano et al., 1961). Moreover, many biological and chemical agents have been putatively implicated in the development of ALS (Garruto et al., 1984; Yase, 1972). In this chapter, we will first review the role of light metals as possible agents or contributing factors in ALS and MND and will then discuss the pathogenetic interactions of multivalent cations, aluminum in particular, with the

---

**Present affiliation*: University of Pittsburgh School of Medicine, Pittsburgh, Pennsylvania.

neuronal cytoskeleton. Throughout this chapter, MND will allude to a broad spectrum of disorders characterized by degeneration of lower or upper motor neurons, independently of their etiology or inheritance. The term ALS will refer to the sporadic form of the disease, whereas the term endemic MND will be applied to the degeneration of motor neurons, associated with Parkinsonism and dementia, that affects individuals who live in high-prevalence regions in the western Pacific.

COPPER

Copper (Cu), an essential element, is a component of several enzymes: ceruloplasmin; superoxide dismutase; cytochrome C oxidase; lysyl oxidase; and dopamine β-hydroxylase. Additionally, several oxidases are Cu dependent (Mason, 1979).

Several diseases are associated with abnormalities in Cu metabolism in humans and other animals. Swayback, a demyelinating disease of sheep, pigs, and goats, is thought to be due to a fetal lack of cytochrome C oxidase, which is a Cu-containing enzyme (Yanagihara, 1982). Similarly, Menkes' disease is a sex-linked recessive neurodegenerative human disorder in which there is a defect in Cu absorption (Menkes et al., 1962; Danks et al., 1972). In patients with Wilson's disease, an autosomal recessive disorder, excessive levels of Cu accumulate in liver, brain, kidney, and cornea, and pathological changes result in those organs (Goldfischer and Sternlieb, 1968; Mason, 1979).

Relatively few studies have examined the role of Cu in MND and, more specifically, in ALS. Cu levels were examined in studies of patients with MND: in muscle tissue, in the liver, and in spinal cord. Cu content in muscle was not significantly different from control levels; however, the correlation with age differed in patients with MND and controls. In control subjects, Cu levels were higher in aged individuals than young individuals, whereas in patients with MND, older patients had lower Cu levels than young individuals (Pierce-Ruhland and Patten, 1980). Cu content of cervical and lumbar enlargements of the spinal cord was higher in patients who died from MND (including ALS and progressive muscular atrophy) than in control patients (Kurlander and Patten, 1979). Furthermore, Cu levels correlated to zinc levels in patients with MND ($p < 0.05$; $r = 0.84$).

In another study, livers were examined in patients with MND. Abnormalities occurred in routine liver function tests in 23 of 44 patients with MND. Liver mitochondrial abnormalities included an increased incidence of intramitochondrial inclusions, lower cytoplasmic concentrations of mitochondria, and enlarged mitochondria (Masui et al., 1985). Cu was present in hepatic lysosomes of 8 of 13 MND patients examined; no Cu was found in six controls (Masui et al., 1985). Cu is also present in hepatic lysosomes of older patients with Wilson's disease (Goldfischer and Sterlieb, 1968). Physiological maintenance of Cu balance appears to depend on uptake by hepatic lysosomes and excretion into bile. Cu levels have been measured in serum and spinal cord in studies of patients with ALS (as opposed to grouping ALS patients with individuals with other MNDs). Serum Cu levels were lower in 1 of 14 patients with ALS and in 1 of 10 controls (Domzal and Radzikowska, 1983). There are conflicting results in reports concerning Cu levels in the spinal cords of patients with ALS; Yoshimasu et al. (1980) found no difference in Cu concentrations, whereas Yase et al. (1980) report elevated Cu concentrations in unfixed anterior horn and formalin-fixed spinal cord. Miyata et al. (1980) found elevated Cu levels in cervical and thoracic levels of spinal cord in an ALS patient compared to a control.

ZINC

Zinc is an essential element. Over 160 zinc metalloenzymes have been identified that are involved in nucleic acid, protein, carbohydrate, and lipid metabolism. These enzymes are essential for nucleic acid replication, transcription, and translation and play a role in regulating gene expression. Zinc is involved in polynucleotide conformation and in the winding and unwinding of DNA.

Zinc concentrations have been examined in several tissues in patients with MND, and no differences were found in comparison to controls in any of the tissues, including muscle (Pierce-Ruhland and Patten, 1980), cerebrospinal fluid (Mitchell et al., 1984), spinal cord, liver, and bone (Mitchell et al., 1986), and spinal cord enlargements (Kurlander and Patten, 1979).

In another study, ALS patients were examined separately from other MND patients. Erythrocyte concentrations of zinc in ALS patients were not significantly different from those in other neurological patients and controls (Nagata et al., 1985). Zinc was detected in the cervical, thoracic, and lumbar levels of the spinal cord of an ALS patient but not in a control (Miyata et al., 1980).

ALUMINUM

Aluminum and Endemic MND

A form of MND associated with Parkinsonism and dementia has an extraordinarily high prevalence in certain regions of the western Pacific, including Guam, New Guinea, and the Kii Peninsula in Japan (Hirano et al., 1961). This endemic MND is characterized pathologically by the classical changes of ALS but, in addition, shows widespread neurofibrillary degeneration (Hirano et al., 1966). Neurofibrillary tangles (NFT) in this disorder are composed primarily of paired helical filaments (PHF) and are identical to those present in Alzheimer's disease (Hirano et al., 1966). These neurofibrillary changes are also present at autopsy in clinically unaffected inhabitants of the endemic regions. Aluminum (Al), as well as other multivalent cations, has been implicated in the pathogenesis of endemic MND based on three sets of observations. First, high levels of Al and low concentrations of Cu and Mg are common environmental features in endemic regions in Guam, New Guinea, and the Kii Peninsula in Japan (Yase, 1972). Second, abnormally high levels of Al have been detected in patients with MND (Garruto et al., 1984; Yase, 1984; Perl and Pendlebury, 1986). Third, pathological changes of motor neurons have been induced in monkeys fed a low-Ca, high-Al, and high-Mn diet (Garruto et al., 1984, 1989).

Analyses of drinking water in regions of Guam where MND is endemic have shown a lack or an extremely low content of Cu and Mg and elevated levels of Mn compared to control regions (Yase, 1972). In soil samples of endemic areas, high levels of Al and Mn and low levels of Cu and Mg have been detected. Similar measurements were obtained from samples of rice plants and cattle hair in affected areas (Yase, 1972). The same type of environmental changes has been observed in villages with a high incidence of MND and Parkinsonian syndromes in West New Guinea and the Kii Peninsula, Japan (Yase, 1972).

A wide variety of methods have been employed to measure Al and other elements in tissues from individuals with MND and controls (for review, see chapter, this volume, by Kasarkis). Initial observations in tissues of the central nervous system of MND cases in Japan, using neutron activation analysis, have shown high levels of Cu (521 ± 288 ppm) compared to controls (251 ± 129 ppm). In Guam, values were also higher for affected individuals (446 ± 280 ppm) than controls (257 ± 39 ppm). X-ray microanalysis of metals in the cervical cord has demonstrated excessive deposition of Cu, Al, and Mn (Yase, 1984) in cases of MND. Subsequently, a study using scanning electron microscopy/x-ray spectroscopy demonstrated that Al selectively accumulates in NFT-bearing neurons of Guamanian natives affected with Parkinsonism-dementia and MND (Perl and Brody, 1980; Perl et al., 1982; Perl and Pendlebury, 1986). A third study, using a different x-ray spectrometry approach, also revealed increased levels of Al and Cu in NFG-bearing neurons of Guamanian (Chamorro) patients affected with MND. No prominent concentration of Cu or Al was found in non-NFT-containing regions within hippocampus of diseased cases or controls (Garruto et al., 1984). High levels of Al have also been found in NFT-bearing neurons of nonaffected individuals living in endemic regions (Perl et al., 1982).

In an attempt to reproduce environmental conditions present in foci of endemic MND, investigators have tried to develop animal models of this disorder. Both cynomolgus monkeys and *Macaca fuscata* (Japanese monkeys) have been used (Garruto et al., 1989). In both experiments, monkeys were treated chronically with a low-Ca, high-Al, and high-Mn diet. Experimental animals developed degeneration of motor neurons in the spinal cord associated with mild Ca and Al deposition. However, neurofibrillary degeneration of motor neurons in both studies was characterized mainly by aggregates of 10-nm neurofilaments and not by NFTs comprised of PHF (Garruto et al., 1989).

An environmental factor remains a compelling possibility as an etiological agent in the endemic form of MND. Altered equilibrium of multivalent cations in soil, water, and foodstuffs may lead to progressive neuronal degeneration, with the formation of PHF and NFT. However, two important caveats should temper enthusiasm for this hypothesis. First, animal models of acute or chronic Al intoxication do not recapitulate the development of NFT comprised of PHF, which are characteristic of neuronal degeneration in endemic MND. Second, high levels of Al in humans, as seen in patients with dialysis dementia (Savory et al., 1983), have been associated with degeneration of cortical nerve cells (Scholtz et al., 1987) but not of motor neurons.

Future directions of research in endemic MND include epidemiological, clinical, pathological, and experimental efforts. Considering the absence of information regarding Al concentration in motor neurons in MND (elevated Al levels have been reported only in NFT-bearing cerebral neurons), the results of an ongoing study of Al concentration in affected motor neurons (Perl, personal communication) in MND should be of great interest.

Effect of Aluminum on the Neuronal Cytoskeleton

The toxic effect of Al on the neuronal cytoskeleton was first noticed by Klatzo et al. (1965). In the course of experiments to induce antibodies by injecting antigens intracerebrally in rabbits, these investigators discovered that Al phosphate, present in the adjuvant medium, caused convulsions and striking neurofibrillary degeneration of cortical neurons. Ultrastructural observations of affected neurons revealed 10-nm filaments as components of NFT (Terry and Peña, 1965). Subsequently, it was demonstrated that the biochemical composition of filaments accumulating in neurons of Al-intoxicated animals was that of normal neurofilaments (NFs) (Selkoe et al., 1979). It is important to highlight that the nature of neurofibrillary degeneration in Al toxicity is characterized by the accumulation of NFs, which are normal nerve cell constituents, and, thus, are different from pathological changes of the cytoskeleton that occur in endemic MND or in Alzheimer's disease, characterized by PHF (Kidd, 1963).

Experimental Aluminum Encephalomyelopathy

The large majority of behavioral, physiological, and pathological studies of Al neurotoxicity have been conducted in the rabbit, as this species is particularly vulnerable to the development of accumulations of NFs (Klatzo et al., 1965; Troncoso et al., 1982; Ghetti et al., 1985). Other susceptible species include the cat, ferret, and monkey. The rat, for reasons that remain unknown, does not develop NF accumulation following in vivo Al salt administration and, therefore, cannot be used as animal model in this context.

Because most animal models of Al intoxication are of an acute nature, one must be cautious to compare clinical manifestations of these experimental animals to those of patients with endemic MND or ALS, both of which are chronic disorders. However, in rabbits injected intrathecally with Al powder (insoluble), the encephalomyelopathy that ensues is slowly progressive and is characterized clinically by weakness and pathologically by motor neuron degeneration, neuronophagia, muscle weakness, and neurogenic muscle atrophy (Bugiani and Ghetti, 1982).

Pathological Changes (Acute and Chronic)

Pathological changes in acute experimental Al neurotoxicity are dominated by neurofibrillary changes of multiple nerve cell populations, including motor neurons (Klatzo et al., 1965; Wisniewski et al., 1980; Troncoso et al., 1985a), without significant nerve cell death. After administration of $AlCl_3$ into the cisterna magna of 3-week-old rabbits, NF accumulations develop in proximal axons of spinal motor neurons within 1–2 days of injection. Subsequently, skeins of NFs appear in perikarya and dendrites; 8 weeks after injection, most spinal neurons are free of neurofibrillary degeneration, evidence of reversibility. No significant loss of motor neurons or axons (Kosik et al., 1983) takes place (Troncoso et al., 1982). In adult rabbits, 45 days after a high dose of aluminum salts (100-μl injections of 17% aluminum lactate on 2 consecutive days), neurofilament accumulations in cell bodies and proximal axons remain abundant (N.F. Muma, personal observation). When chronic intoxication schedules or insoluble Al is used, neuronal death is widespread throughout the CNS (Bugiani and Ghetti, 1982; Wisniewski et al., 1982; Ghetti et al., 1985). A comparison of the neurotoxic effects of Al on young versus old animals remains to be done.

Abnormality of Neurofilament Phosphorylation

Under normal circumstances, neurons express immunoreactivity for nonphosphorylated NF epitopes throughout the cell body, dendrites, and axon. In contrast, phosphorylated NF epitopes are restricted to axonal domains and are not evident in other neuronal compartments (Sternberger and Sternberger, 1983). Following intrathecal administration of aluminum salts to rabbits, the NF that accumulate in the perikaryon and dendrites of motor neurons contain both nonphosphorylated and phosphorylated epitopes (Troncoso et al., 1986). The presence of phosphorylated neurofilaments in the dendrites and perikaryon constitutes a distinct departure from normal and has been confirmed by several investigators (Munoz-Garcia et al., 1986; Bizzi and Gambetti, 1986).

Neurotransmitter/Enzyme Changes

Changes in the cholinergic system induced by Al toxicity are relevant to the dysfunction of motor neurons. Significant reductions in choline acetyltransferase (ChAT) and acetylcholinesterase (AChE) have been found in spinal and hypoglossal neurons of Al-intoxicated animals (Yates et al., 1980). However, another study failed to document decreased cholinergic activity in Al-induced neurofibrillary degeneration (Hetnarski et al., 1980). The activity of ChAT is decreased in the sciatic nerves of rabbits with Al-induced neurofibrillary degeneration of lumbosacral motor neurons (Kosik et al., 1983). In addition, a significant reduction in ChAT was found in entorhinal cortices and hippocampi of rabbits injected with Al intraventricularly (Beal et al., 1989). Studies in a neuroblastoma-gloma hybridoma have shown that exposure to 2 mM aluminum lactate, a concentration that does not supress cell growth, causes a 37% increase in ChAT and a 41% decrease in muscarinic receptors, measured by the binding of [3H] QNB. No changes were detected in activities of AChE to glutamate decarboxylase. In this experimental system, aluminum also raised the level of cyclic AMP by 20%, although adenylate cyclase activity was unchanged (Singer et al., 1990).

Mechanism of Cytoskeletal Disorganization

Despite the fact that Al does not have a radioactive isotope amenable for biological research, several groups of investigators, ours among them, have explored and begun to understand mechanisms leading to NF accumulation in motor neurons of Al-intoxicated rabbits. NFs are intermediate filaments of nerve cells and are composed of three polypeptide subunits—NF-L, 68 kDa; NF-M, 150–160 kDa; and NF-H, 190–210 kDa)—coded for by separate genes. The three subunits are synthesized and assembled into NFs in the neuronal perikarya and then transported anterogradely into the axon along with the SCa component of axonal transport (Hoffman and Lasek, 1975). Posttranslational modification of NFs, in the form of phosphorylation, occurs predominantly in the axon (Sternberger and Sternberger, 1983). Therefore, the observation that intrathecal injection of Al causes early accumulation of NFs in the proximal axonal region of motor neurons and is followed by involvement of the perikarya leads to four hypotheses in terms of pathogenetic mechanisms: increased synthesis of NFs; abnormal transport of NFs from the cell body into the axon; abnormal interactive among NF or between NF and other cytoskeletal constituents; and decreased degradation of NFs. The level of synthesis of NFs in Al neurotoxicity has been explored through measurements of mRNA for specific NF subunits in vivo (Muma et al., 1988; Parhad et al., 1989) and in vitro (Gilbert et al., 1989, submitted). Transport of NF has been explored with the labeling of motor neurons with radioactive amino acids, followed by monitoring of the movement of labeled NF along motor axons (Liwnicz et al., 1974; Bizzi et al., 1984; Troncoso et al., 1985b). The interaction of NF-NF has been explored by in vitro experiments with NF isolated from bovine spinal cord (Troncoso et al., 1990).

In Vivo Studies

One possible mechanism through which Al may cause NF accumulations might be an increase in NF synthesis. To determine whether alterations in NF synthesis are associated with Al-induced neurofibrillary pathology, levels of mRNA encoding cytoskeletal proteins (including NF subunits) were examined in the spinal cord and dorsal root ganglia of rabbits following intraventricular injections with Al lactate or saline (Muma et al., 1988). In spinal cord, levels of mRNA encoding NF-L and NF-H dropped to 29% and 50% of control, respectively, in Al-treated animals. β-Tubulin mRNA levels dropped to 37% of control; however, levels of mRNA coding for actin were not significantly different. Downregulation in NF mRNA levels is specific for cell populations in which Al-induced morphological changes are demonstrated. DRG cells do not display any morphological abnormalities following Al administration in vivo, and, correspondingly, in DRG, no change occurred in levels of mRNA coding for any of the cytoskeletal proteins examined (NF-L, NF-H, β-tubulin, actin). Parhad et al. (1989) found that levels of mRNA coding for several neuronal proteins (NF-L, -M, -H, neuronal-specific enolase, and amyloid precursor protein) transiently decreased in the spinal cord of Al-treated young rabbits, whereas the levels of GFAP mRNA (nonneuronal) were not affected. Moreover, the severity of the NF accumulations correlated with the decline in neuronal mRNA levels.

Tissue Culture Studies

In vivo studies of aluminum toxicity have been limited because of the difficulty in ensuring uniform exposure of the neuraxis with intrathecal injections, difficulty in evaluating recovery from exposure, and restricted evaluation of longitudinal changes in the nervous system. In order to circumvent these problems, which are inherent in an in vivo system, cultures of rabbit (Seil et al., 1969) and rat (Gilbert et al., 1989) sensory ganglion cells have been utilized to study Al toxicity. NF accumulations have been observed in cultures of dissociated sensory neurons as well as in ganglion explants following exposure to Al salts. Similar morphological changes have also been reported in some neuroblastoma cells lines (Miller and Levine, 1974; Cole et al., 1985; Nixon et al., 1989) after differentiation. Utilizing cultured DRG explants from fetal rats (Gilbert et al., 1989), the development of NF accumulations was studied over time. In this model, cultures were exposed to 1-mM concentrations of Al lactate for varied times. Regional increases in NF concentration were noted in the perikaryon after 1 day of exposure. After 3 days of exposure, a discrete NF mass was present in the perikaryon, and by 7 days, the NF mass was completely devoid of normal cellular organelles. At the later time points, the remainder of the perikaryon was almost completely devoid of NF. Measurements of mRNA levels for all three NF proteins over the course of exposure showed a marked decrease after only 1 day of exposure. NF mRNA was virtually undetectable at the later time points. Concurrent mRNA levels for class II β-tubulin showed a moderate decrease over the course of the experiment. Recovery from Al toxicity was assessed by examining cultures 1 week after Al was removed from the nutrient medium. There was morphological evidence of dissolution of the NF masses in the perikarya and NF mRNA levels were increased, indicating recovery from Al intoxication.

The development of neurofibrillary changes in cultured cells depends, among other factors, on the constitutive expression of NF by those cells. This is illustrated by the failure to induce NF accumulation or other cytoskeletal changes in a neuroblastoma-glioma cell line treated with aluminum lactate, although effects in neurotransmitter enzymes and receptors were detected (Singer et al., 1990). The neuroblastoma-glioma cells express phosphorylated and nonphosphorylated NF epitopes, but at a level that is, in our opinion, too low to allow any significant accumulation.

Aluminum and Axonal Transport of NFs

The hypothesis of impaired axonal transport in NFs in Al neurotoxicity has been explained by two groups of investigators and both have observed abnormal transport or NFs in motor neurons or the hypoglossal (Bizzi et al., 1984) and sciatic (Troncoso et al., 1985a) nerves. The abnormalities in NF transport consist of retention or newly synthesized NF proteins in the perikaryon and initial axon, decreased entry of NFs into the nerve fiber, and associated segmental axonal atrophy (Bizzi et al., 1984; Troncoso et al., 1985a). However, the rate of transport of these NFs that are able to get beyond the initial axonal segment appears normal. It has not been possible to disrupt axonal transport of NFs by application of Al to the sciatic nerve (J.C. Troncoso, unpublished observations) as has been accomplished with β,β'-iminodipropionitrile (Griffin et al., 1983). Axonal transport of other cytoskeletal proteins (i.e., tubulin and actin) is minimally or not altered in Al intoxication. Fast axoplasmic transport in rabbits with aluminum neurotoxicity is normal (Liwnicz et al., 1974). Taken in concert, these observations on NF transport suggest that Al interferes specifically with the entrance of NFs into the axon or perhaps with the incorporation of NFs onto the axonal transport system.

In terms of the pathogenesis of abnormal NF transport in Al neurotoxicity, abnormal phosphorylation or crosslinking of NF are the two leading hypotheses available. The first hypothesis arises from observations that NFs accumulate in perikarya of motor neurons and are inappropriately phosphorylated, as they contain phosphorylated epitopes that are normally present only in axonal domains (Bizzi and Gambetti, 1986; Munoz-Garcia et al., 1986; Troncoso et al., 1986). Thus, it is possible that Al induces the abnormal phosphorylation of NFs first and that this process, in turn, leads to impaired transport of NFs. However, the reverse sequence of events is also possible. The second hypothesis derives from experiments with NFs in vitro that demonstrate that Al, as well as other multivalent cations, can produce aggregation or crosslinking of NFs through an electrical charge effect (Troncoso et al., 1990).

Aluminum and NF Interactions In Vitro

Experimental evidence indicates that in vitro, multivalent cations cause lateral aggregation of epidermal keratins (Fukuyama et al., 1978) as well as the formation of paracrystalline arrays of glial acidic protein (Stewart et al., 1989) and desmin (Aebi, unpublished observation). This evidence led us to hypothesize that aluminum may have a similar effect on NF, as their subunits exhibit extensive sequence homology and share structural characteristics with other intermediate filaments (Weber et al., 1983; Geisler et al., 1985; Steinert and Parry, 1985; Aebi et al., 1988). To explore this hypothesis, we examined the effect of aluminum and other multivalent cations on NF in vitro. Interactions of these cations were investigated with bovine, rabbit, and rat spinal cord native NFs, and with filaments reconstituted from the 68-kDa subunit isolated from bovine spinal cord. Effects were assessed by electron microscopy of negatively stained samples. Our observations indicated that aluminum lactate causes lateral aggregation of native NF from the three different species as well as of the bovine-reconstituted NF. The aggregation of NF was also observed with other multivalent cations. Because aluminum causes a strong aggregation of NF in vitro, a similar phenomenon may occur in vivo, leading to accumulation of NFs in the neuronal perikarya of rabbits following aluminum administration (Troncoso et al., 1990).

Hypothesis for the Development of Neurofilament Changes in Animal Models of Aluminum Neurotoxicity

Although the exact mechanism of NF accumulation in Al neurotoxicity remains to be determined, available observations from animal, tissue culture, and in vitro experiments allow us to propose the following hypothesis. Following Al administration, the neuronal concentration of Al (possibly from Al^{3+}) reaches a critical level that leads to aggregation of adjacent NF on the basis of electrical charge effect. This phenomenon occurs only in neurons with high NF concentration and in that region of the nerve cell where NF-H is less abundant or less phosphorylated, such as perikarya and dendrites (NF-H may act as a spacer between NF) (Carden et al., 1987). Aggregated NFs form clusters that cannot be normally transported into the axon, thus accumulating first in the initial axon and then in the perikaryon. In this scenario, increased phosphorylation of NF in the parikaryon and down-regulation of NF mRNA would be secondary events. However, an alternative situation, in which Al interacts directly with nuclear proteins to cause a decrease in NF gene expression, cannot be totally ruled out.

The hypothesis of impaired degradation of NFs as the cause of their accumulation in Al neurotoxicity has received limited attention because the current consensus is that NFs are degraded in the distal axon. Thus, an impairment in NF degradation should lead to accumulation of NFs in distal axons and not in the initial portion of nerve fibers or in perikarya, as occurs following Al administration. However, emerging information on the processing and proteolysis of NFs in proximal axonal regions (Nixon et al., 1989) will force a thorough testing of this hypothesis.

Future efforts to unravel the mechanisms of Al neurotoxicity should encompass animal experimentation, as well as tissue culture and in vitro approaches. These efforts should explore interactions between Al and specific neuronal targets or proteins, taking into consideration the complex issue of speciation of Al in solution.

CONCLUSION

There is no substantial evidence to implicate light metals, in either excess or deficiency, as direct etiological agents in ALS. However, it remains a viable hypothesis that abnormal environmental levels of Al, Mn, and Cu may be responsible for, or contribute to, degeneration of nerve cells in endemic MND. Further testing of this hypothesis is necessary and will require the combined efforts of epidemiologists, clinicians, and pathologists.

ACKNOWLEDGMENTS

The authors are grateful to Drs. Donald L. Price, John W. Griffin, Paul N. Hoffman, and Zolton Annau for their encouragement and support and to Ms. Sharon Powell for her assistance with bibliographic searches. This work was supported by grants from the U.S. Public Health Service (NIM NS 15721, NS 10580, AG 03359, AG 05146) and funds from The Robert L. & Clara G. Patterson Trust. Dr. Muma is the recipient of a Leadership and Excellence in Alzheimer's Disease (LEAD) award (NIA AG 07914).

REFERENCES

1. Aebi U, Häner M, Troncoso J, Eichner R, Engel A. Unifying principles in intermediate filament (IF) structure and assembly. Protoplasma 1988;145:73–81.

2. Beal MF, Mazurek MF, Ellison DW, Kowall NW, Solomon PR, Pendlebury WW. Neurochemical characteristics of aluminum-induced neurofibrillary degeneration in rabbits. Neuroscience 1989;29:339–346.
3. Bizzi A, Gambetti P. Phosphorylation of neurofilaments is altered in aluminum intoxication. Acta Neuropathol (Berl) 1986;71:154–158.
4. Bizzi A, Crane RC, Autilio-Gambetti L, Gambetti P. Aluminum effect on slow axonal transport: A novel impairment of neurofilament transport. J Neurosci 1984;4: 722–731.
5. Bugiani O, Ghetti B. Progressing encephalomyelopathy with muscular atrophy, induced by aluminum powder. Neurobiol Aging 1982;3:209–222.
6. Carden MJ, Trojanowski JQ, Schlaepfer WW, Lee VM-Y. Two-stage expression of neurofilament polypeptides during rat neurogenesis with early establishment of adult phosphorylation patterns. J Neurosci 1987;7:3489–3504.
7. Cole GM, Wu K, Timiras PS. A culture model for age-related human neurofibrillary pathology. Int J Dev Neurosci 1985;3:23–32.
8. Danks DM, Campbell PE, Stevens BJ, Mayne V, Cartwright E. Menkes's kinky hair syndrome. An inherited defect in copper absorption with widespread effects. Pediatrics 1972;50:188–201.
9. DeBoni U, Crapper-McLachlan DR. Senile dementia and Alzheimer's disease. Life Sci 1980;27:1–14.
10. DeBoni U, Scott JW, Crapper DR. Intracellular aluminum binding: A histochemical study. Histochemistry 1974;40:31–37.
11. Domzal T, Radzikowska D. Ceruloplazmina i micdz wcurowicy chorych na stwardnienie zanikowe boczne (SZB). Neurol Neurochir Pol 1983;17:343–346.
12. Fukuyama K, Murozuka T, Caldwell R, Epstein WL. Divalent cation stimulation of in vitro fibre assembly from epidermal keratin protein. J Cell Sci 1978;33:255–263.
13. Gadjusek DC. Unconventional viruses and the origin and disappearance of kuru. Science 1977;197:943–960.
14. Garruto RM, Fukatsu R, Yanagihara R, Gajdusek DC, Hook G, Fiori CE. Imaging of calcium and aluminum in neurofibrillary tangle-bearing neurons in parkinsonism-dementia of Guam. Proc Natl Acad Sci USA 1984;81:1875–1879.
15. Garruto RM, Shankar SK, Yanagihara R, Salazar AM, Amyx HL, Gajdusek DC. Low-calcium, high-aluminum diet-induced motor neuron pathology in cynomolgus monkeys. Acta Neuropathol 1989;78:210–219.
16. Geisler N, Plessmann U, Weber K. The complete amino acid sequence of the major mammalian neurofilament protein (NF-L). FEBS Lett 1985;182:475–478.
17. Ghetti B, Musicco M, Norton J, Bugiani O. Nerve cell loss in the progressive encephalopathy induced by aluminum powder. A morphologic and semiquantitative study of the Purkinje cells. Neuropathol Appl Neurobiol 1985;11:31–53.
18. Gilbert MR, Harding BL, Hoffman PN, Griffin JW. Cytoskeletal changes during axonal growth and regeneration in cultured sensory neurons. Soc Neurosci Abstr 1989;15:879.
19. Gilbert MR, Harding BL, Hoffman PN, Griffin JW, Price DL, Troncoso JC. Aluminum-induced neurofilamentous changes in cultured rat dorsal root ganglia explants (submitted).

20. Goldfischer S, Sternlieb I. Changes in the distribution of hepatic copper in relation to the progression of Wilson's disease (hepatolenticular degeneration). Am J Pathol 1968;53:883–901.

21. Griffin JW, Fahnestock KC, Price DL, Cork LC: Cytoskeletal disorganization induced by local application of β,β'-iminodipropionitrile and 2,5-hexanedione. Ann Neurol 1983;14:55–61.

22. Hetnarski B, Wisniewski HM, Iqbal K, Dziedzic JD, Lajtha A. Central cholinergic activity in aluminum-induced neurofibrillary degeneration. Ann Neurol 1980;7: 489–490.

23. Hirano A, Malamud N, Kurland LT. Parkinsonism-dementia complex, an endemic disease on the island of Guam. II. Pathological features. Brain 1961;84:662–679.

24. Hirano A, Malamud N, Elizan TS, Kurland LT. Amyotrophic lateral sclerosis and Parkinsonism-dementia complex on Guam. Further pathological studies. Arch Neurol 1966;15:35–51.

25. Hoffman PN, Lasek RJ. The slow component of axonal transport. Identification of major structural polypeptides of the axon and their generality.

26. Johnson RT. Degenerative diseases. In: Viral infections of the nervous system. New York: Raven Press, 1982:271–293.

27. Karlik SJ, Eichhorn GL, Lewis PN, Crapper DR. Interaction of aluminum species with deoxyribonucleic acid. Biochemistry 1980;19:5991–5998.

28. Klatzo I, Wisniewski H, Streicher E. Experimental production of neurofibrillary degeneration. I. Light microscopic observations. J Neuropathol Exp Neurol 1965;24:187–199.

29. Kosik KS, Bradley WG, Good PF, Rasool CG, Selkoe DJ. Cholinergic function in lumbar aluminum myelopathy. J Neuropathol Exp Neurol 1983;42:365–375.

30. Kurlander HM, Patten BM. Metals in spinal cord tissue of patients dying of motor neuron disease. Ann Neurol 1979;6:21–24.

31. Liwnicz BH, Kristensson K, Wisniewski HM, Shelanski ML, Terry RD. Observations on axoplasmic transport in rabbits with aluminum-induced neurofibrillary tangles. Brain Res 1974;80:413–420.

32. Mason KE. A conspectus of research on copper metabolism and requirements of man. J Nutr 1979;109:1979–2066.

33. Masui Y, Mozai T, Kekehi K. Functional and morphometric study of the liver in motor neuron disease. J Neurol 1985;232:15–19.

34. Menkes JH, Alter M, Steigleder GK, Weakley DR, Sung JH. A sex-linked recessive disorder with retardation of growth, peculiar hair, and focal cerebral and cerebellar degeneration. Pediatrics 1962;19:764–779.

35. Miller CA, Levine EM. Effects of aluminum salts on cultured neuroblastoma cells. J Neurochem 1974;22:751–758.

36. Mitchell JD, Harris IA, East BW, Pentland B. Trace elements in cerebrospinal fluid in motor neurone disease. Br Med J 1984;288:1791–1792.

37. Mitchell JD, East BW, Harris IA, Prescott RJ, Pentland B. Trace elements in the spinal cord and other tissues in motor neuron disease. J Neurol Neurosurg Psychiatry 1986;49:211–215.

38. Miyata S, Nakamura S, Toyoshima M, Hirata Y, Saito M, Kameyama M, Mat-

sushita R, Koyama M. Determination of manganese in tissues by neutron activation analysis using an antimony pentoxide column. Clin Chim Acta 1980;106:235–242.

39. Muma NA, Troncoso JC, Hoffman PN, Koo EH, Price DL. Aluminum neurotoxicity: Altered expression of cytoskeletal genes. Mol Brain Res 1988;3:115–122.

40. Munoz-Garcia D, Pendlebury WW, Kessler JB, Perl DP. An immunocytochemical comparison of cytoskeletal proteins in aluminum-induced and Alzheimer-type neurofibrillary tangles. Acta Neuropathol (Berl) 1986;70:243–248.

41. Nagata H, Miyata S, Nakamura S, Kameyama M, Katsui Y. Heavy metal concentrations in blood cells in patients with amyotrophic lateral sclerosis. J Neurol Sci 1985;67:173–178.

42. Nixon RA, Lewis SE, Dahl D, Marotta CA, Drager UC. Early posttranslational modifications of the three neurofilament subunits in mouse retinal ganglion cells: Neuronal sites and time course in relation to subunit polymerization and axonal transport. Mol Brain Res 1989;5:93–108.

43. Parhad IM, Krekoski CA, Mathew A, Tran PM. Neuronal gene expression in aluminum myelopathy. Cell Mol Neurobiol 1989;9:123–138.

44. Perl DP, Brody AR. Detection of aluminum by SEM-x-ray spectrometry within neurofibrillary tangle-bearing neurons of Alzheimer's disease. Neurotoxicology 1980;1:133–137.

45. Perl DP, Pendlebury WW. Aluminum neurotoxicity—potential role in the pathogenesis of neurofibrillary tangle formation. Can J Neurol Sci 1986;13:441–445.

46. Perl DP, Gajdusek DC, Garruto RM, Yanagihara RT, Gibbs CJ Jr. Intraneuronal aluminum accumulation in amyotrophic lateral sclerosis and Parkinsonism-dementia of Guam. Science 1982;217:1053–1055.

47. Pierce-Ruhland R, Patten BM. Muscle metals in motor neuron disease. Ann Neurol 1980;8:193–195.

48. Savory J, Berlin A, Courtoux C, Yeoman B, Wills MR. Summary report of an international workshop on ''The Role of Biological Monitoring in the Prevention of Aluminum Toxicity in Man: Aluminum Analysis in Biological Fluids.'' Ann Clin Lab Sci 1983;13:444–451.

49. Schoene WC. Degenerative diseases of the central nervous system. In: Davis RL, Robertson DM, eds. Textbook of neuropathology. Baltimore: Williams & Wilkins, 1985:788–823.

50. Scholtz CL, Swash M, Gray A, Kogeorgos J, Marsh F. Neurofibrillary neuronal degeneration in dialysis dementia: A feature of aluminum toxicity. Clin Neuropathol 1987;6:93–97.

51. Seil FJ, Lampert PW, Klatzo I. Neurofibrillary spheroids induced by aluminum phosphate in dorsal root ganglia neurons in vitro. J Neuropathol Exp Neurol 1969;28:74–85.

52. Selkoe DJ, Liem RKH, Yen S-H, Shelanski ML. Biochemical and immunological characterization of neurofilaments in experimental neurofibrillary degeneration induced by aluminum. Brain Res 1979;163:235–252.

53. Singer HS, Searles CD, Hahn I-H, March JL, Troncoso JC. The effect of aluminum on markers for synaptic neurotransmission, cyclic AMP, and neurofilaments in a neuroblastoma x glioma hybridoma (NG108-15). Brain Res 1990;528:73–79.

54. Steinert PM, Parry DAD. Intermediate filaments: conformity and diversity of expression and structure. Annu Rev Cell Biol 1985;1:41–65.

55. Sternberger LA, Sternberger NH. Monoclonal antibodies distinguish phosphorylated and nonphosphorylated forms of neurofilaments in situ. Proc Natl Acad Sci USA 1983;80:6126–6130.

56. Stewart M, Quinlan RA, Moir RD. Molecular interactions in paracrystals of a fragment corresponding to the α-helical coiled-coil rod portion of glial fibrillary acidic protein: Evidence for an antiparallel packing of molecules and polymorphism related to intermediate filament structure. J Cell Biol 1989;109:225–234.

57. Terry RD, Peña C. Experimental production of neurofibrillary degeneration. 2. Electron microscopy, phosphatase histochemistry and electron probe analysis. J Neuropathol Exp Neurol 1965;24:200–210.

58. Troncoso JC, Price DL, Griffin JW, Parhad IM. Neurofibrillary axonal pathology in aluminum intoxication. Ann Neurol 1982;12:278–283.

59. Troncoso JC, Hoffman PN, Griffin JW, Hess-Kozlow KM, Price DL. Aluminum intoxication: A disorder of neurofilament transport in motor neurons. Brain Res 1985a;342:172–175.

60. Troncoso JC, Sternberger LA, Sternberger NH, Cork LC, Price DL. Phosphorylated neurofilaments in neurons in aluminum intoxication. Ann Neurol 1985b;18:149–150.

61. Troncoso JC, Sternberger NH, Sternberger LA, Hoffman PN, Price DL. Immunocytochemical studies of neurofilament antigens in the neurofibrillary pathology induced by aluminum. Brain Res 1986;364:295–300.

62. Troncoso JC, Glavaris EC, March JL, Häner M, Aebi U. Effect of aluminum and other multivalent cations on neurofilaments in vitro: An electron microscopic study. J Struct Biol 1990;103:2–12.

63. Troncoso JC, Häner M, March JL, Reichelt R, Engel A, Aebi U. Structure and assembly of neurofilaments: analysis of native neurofilaments and of various neurofilament subunit combinations (submitted).

64. Weber K, Shaw G, Osborn M, Debus E, Geisler N. Neurofilaments, a subclass of intermediate filaments: Structure and expression. Cold Spring Harbor Symp Quant Biol 1983;48:717–729.

65. Wen GY, Wisniewski HM. Histochemical localization of aluminum in the rabbit CNS. Acta Neuropathol (Berl) 1985;68:175–184.

66. Wisniewski H, Narkiewicz O, Wisniewska K. Topography and dynamics of neurofibrillar degeneration in aluminum encephalopathy. Acta Neuropathol 1967;9:127–133.

67. Wisniewski HM, Sturman JA, Shek JW. Aluminum chloride induced neurofibrillary changes in the developing rabbit: A chronic animal model. Ann Neurol 1980;8:479–480.

68. Wisniewski HM, Sturman JA, Shek JW. Chronic model of neurofibrillary changes induced in mature rabbits by metallic aluminum. Neurobiol Aging 1982;3:11–22.

69. Yanagihara R. Heavy metals and essential minerals in motor neuron disease. In: Rowland LP, ed. Human motor neuron diseases. Advances in neurology, Vol. 36. New York: Raven Press, 1982:233–248.

70. Yase Y. The pathogenesis of amyotrophic lateral sclerosis. Lancet 1972;2:292–295.
71. Yase Y. The role of aluminum in CNS degeneration with interaction of calcium. Neurotoxicology 1980;1:101–109.
72. Yase Y. Environmental contribution to the amyotrophic lateral sclerosis process. In: Serratrice G, et al, eds. Neuromuscular diseases. New York: Raven Press, 1984: 335–339.
73. Yates CM, Simpson J, Russell D, Gordon A. Cholinergic enzymes in neurofibrillary degeneration produced by aluminum. Brain Res 1980;197:269–274.
74. Yoshimasu F, Yasui M, Yase Y, Iwata S, Gajdusek DC, Gibbs CJ Jr, Chen K-M. Studies on amyotrophic lateral sclerosis by neutron activation analysis. 2. Comparative study of analytical results on Guam PD, Japanese ALS and Alzheimer disease cases. Folia Psychiatr Neurol Jpn 1980;34:75–82.

25

Neurotoxicology: Heavy Metals

Edward J. Kasarskis

University of Kentucky and Veterans Affairs Medical Center
Lexington, Kentucky

INTRODUCTION

The hypothetical involvement of toxic heavy metals in the pathogenesis of amyotrophic lateral sclerosis (ALS) dates back to the recognition of the entity itself by Aran in 1850, who noted an association of lead exposure and ALS (1). Since then, the concept that toxic metals may be related to ALS, albeit in a vague manner, has been nurtured by the continuing reports of ALS-like syndromes being linked to toxic metal exposures (2–7). Although these observations indicate the potential for these agents to more-or-less selectively affect motor neurons, it appears unlikely that a simple exposure to a toxic metal, such as lead or mercury, accounts for the induction of sporadic ALS in the typical patient (8). The toxicity of heavy metals is well known from industrial exposures and accidental poisonings, although the typical toxicity syndromes seem to bear little resemblance to classic ALS (9–11). As an example, Albers et al. have demonstrated the delayed development of peripheral neuropathies, but not of motor neuron disease, in workers exposed to elemental mercury in the workplace (12). On the other hand, some studies have disclosed a greater-than-anticipated prevalence of metal-related occupations, such as welding and painting, among ALS patients (4,13). Therefore, epidemiological considerations over the past 140 years have provided conflicting evidence in support of a role for toxic metals in the etiology of classic ALS.

A second source of support for the heavy metal hypothesis comes from the study of ALS in the endemic areas of the Western Pacific. Most authorities agree that ALS and ALS/Parkinsonism-dementia (PD) in Guam, the Kii Penisula in Japan, and among the Jakai and Auyui in New Guinea are related to an environmental factor (14–17). The studies of Yase, Garruto, and their colleagues have focused attention on a potential interaction between calcium/magnesium deficiency and augmented absorption of toxic trace metals such as manganese and aluminum in these patients (14,18–20). These data are extensively considered in the chapter by 'Troncoso, which should be consulted for a discussion of the evidence.

What is the enduring attraction to the toxic metal hypothesis of ALS? Several factors can be cited. Certainly part of the answer must be the manifest neurotoxicity of many trace elements (9–11,21), but this response is imprecise and circumlocutory. However toxic metals such as mercury and lead can clearly kill neurons (as well as other cells), and this fact confers legitimacy to the hypothesis. A second factor is that many metals can form both organic and inorganic compounds, which may have differing biological fates in regard to their penetration into the central nervous system (11,22). Third, elements such as lead and mercury are pervasive pollutants throughout the food chain, setting the stage for the possibility of a lifelong, low-level exposure to these substances (23). Finally, the biological half-lives of many metals within the human body are exceedingly long. Thus, the insidious chemical personalities of these substances are well matched to the enigmatic nature of ALS itself.

The crucial biological question regarding the toxic trace element hypothesis of ALS has not been clearly articulated and tested experimentally. Simply stated, it is this: Do motor neurons in the spinal cord and cortex selectively accumulate toxic metal(s) prior to their degeneration and death? Does heavy metal accumulation by motor neurons "mark" these cells for eventual ALS-type degeneration? Some evidence suggests that this may, in fact, be the case. As an example, the recent study of Møller-Madsen and Danscher indicates that mercury can accumulate in motor neurons of rats chronically exposed to low levels of inorganic mercury in the absence of overt neurotoxicity (24). They found that mercury was present in the motor neurons of the ventral spinal cord and within motor nuclei of the rhombencephalon. Moreover, mercury appeared to be enriched in the neuronal cytoplasm and was observed in lesser amounts in glial cells. While this study supports the notion that mercury accumulation might represent a precondition for selective neuronal death in ALS (25), the distribution of mercury sulfides (which were detected by their technique) does not parallel the distribution of pathological lesions in ALS in their entirety (26). The results of Møller-Madsen and Danscher do indicate, however, that motor neurons possess a selective affinity for exogenous inorganic mercury. Whether or not the same distribution of mercury exists in human spinal cord has not been reported to date.

Recent theories of pathogenesis have expanded to consider the possible interaction between two or more postulated insults, both of which must be present simultaneously to initiate and perpetuate selective degeneration of motor neurons (27). In the present context, the accumulation of toxic trace metals would represent a necessary, but not a sufficient, condition to initiate motor neuron degeneration. As one example among many, mercury could reside as a latent toxin within neurons by functioning as an enzymatic inhibitor. Under basal conditions, the mercury-induced "enzymatic lesion" (23) would be inconsequential. However, under conditions of increased demand for neuronal protein turnover (e.g., during sprouting/reinnervation) (21), protein synthesis by motor neurons would be insufficient and would result in the eventual death of the neuron.

If toxic trace elements are, in fact, an etiological factor in the pathogenesis of ALS, then one would predict that the presumed toxic metal would be unevenly distributed and would be present in excess within precisely those neurons that ultimately degenerate in ALS (28–30). That is, the putative toxic metal should be distributed among cells in normal individuals in the same pattern as the observed pathology in ALS. Second, in ALS spinal cord, histologically normal-appearing residual motor neurons should contain greater amounts of a toxic metal than controls, implying that metal enrichment is not an epiphenomenon or a nonspecific concomitant of degenerating neurons (31). As will be seen, these questions have not been adequately explored in any study to date, making the toxic metal hypothesis largely an untested one.

STUDIES OF TOXIC AND ESSENTIAL ELEMENTS IN ALS

Three excellent reviews of the subject have appeared since 1982 (8,23,32). Together they elaborate the historical development of the toxic metal hypothesis and summarize the pertinent aspects of basic toxicology of these elements for humans. These contributions should be consulted since this material will not be reiterated here.

The purpose of this review is threefold: first, to summarize and update the recent research progress in the field; second, to examine the results of these studies in regard to the discussion presented above; and third, to attempt to identify the needed future directions for research in this area.

The studies, which are summarized in Tables 1 and 2, were selected according to the following criteria. Each study had to have incorporated sufficient patients and controls in order to evaluate the data statistically. In the past, some reports were based on tissue analyses derived from a single patient. Although these efforts have been important historically and maintained interest in the field, they have been excluded from this review. Second, Tables 1 and 2 indicate that a number of different analytical techniques have been utilized for analysis of toxic and essential elements. Although every attempt was made to include studies that

Table 1 Studies of Heavy Metals in Western Pacific ALS

Author, year	Element concentration: ALS versus control		
	Increased	No sig. diff.	Reduced
Bone			
No studies reported			
Brain regions			
Yase(38),1978[a]	Al,Ca	Mn	—
Yoshimasu(43),1980[a]	Ca	Al,Mn	—
Yoshimasu(66),1982[a]	Al	Cu	Ca,Mn
Mizumoto(67),1984[a]	Al	—	—
Yase(20),1987[a,b]	Al,Fe	Ca,Cu,K,Mg,S,Si,Zn	—
Piccardo(68),1988[c]	Al	—	—
Yoshida(36),1988[d]	Al,Si	Ca,Cu,Fe,K,S	—
Cerebrospinal fluid			
No studies reported			
Erythrocytes			
Nagata(45),1985[a]	Se	Br,Fe,Rb,Zn	Mn
Liver			
No studies reported			
Muscle			
No studies reported			
Nails			
No studies reported			
Peripheral nerve			
No studies reported			
Plasma/serum			
Yanagihara(69),1984[e]	—	Ca,Mg	—
Spinal cord			
Yoshida(70),1977[f]	Al,Ca,Mn	—	—
Yoshida(71),1979[f]	Mn,Pb	Al,Ca	—
Mizumoto(72),1980[f]	Al,Ca,Fe,Mn,P,Si,Ti,V	Cl,Cu,K,S,Zn	—
Yoshimasu(43),1980[a]	Al,Ca	—	—
Yoshimasu(66),1982[a]	Al	Mn	Ca,Cu
Miyata(47),1983[a]	Mn	—	—
Kihira(73),1984[d]	—	Ca	—
Mizumoto(67),1984[a]	Al	—	—
Nagata(45),1985[a]	Mn	—	—
Yoshida(36),1988[d]	Al,Ca,Si,Ti,V	Cl,Cu,Fe,K,Mn,Pb,S,Zn	—
Urine			
Yanagihara(69),1984[e]	—	Ca,Mg	—
Whole blood			
No studies reported			

[a]Neutron activation analysis.
[b]Photon-excited x-ray fluorescence.
[c]Microprobe techniques.
[d]Emission spectrography.
[e]Atomic absorption spectrophotometry.
[f]Alpha-excited x-ray fluorescence.

Table 2 Studies of heavy metals in sporadic ALS

Author, year	Element concentration: ALS versus control		
	Increased	No sig. diff.	Reduced
Bone			
Campbell(13),1970[a]	—	Pb	—
Mitchell(74),1986[b]	—	Cl,Co,Cr,Cs,Fe,K,Mg, Mn,Na,Rb,Sb,Se,Zn	—
Brain regions			
Larsen(75),1981[b]	—	Mn,Se	As
Khare(76),1990[b]	Hg,K,Mn	Br,Co,Fe,Na,Se,Zn	Cl,Cs,Rb
Cerebrospinal fluid			
Kjellin(77),1967[a]	—	Fe	—
Conradi(78),1976[c]	Pb	—	—
Mallette(79),1977[a]	—	Ca,Cl,K,Mg,Na	—
House(80),1978[a,c]	—	Pb	—
Manton(81),1979[d]	—	Pb	—
Conradi(82),1980[e]	Pb	—	—
Stober(83),1983[c]	—	Pb	—
Cavalleri(84),1984[c]	—	Pb	—
Mitchell(85),1984[b]	—	Ag,Cl,Cr,Cs,Fe,K, Na,Rb,Se,Zn	Co
Kapaki(54),1989[c]	—	Pb	—
Erythrocytes			
Felmus(86),1982[c]	—	Ca	—
Stober(83),1983[c]	—	Pb	—
Khare(76),1990[b]	Cs,Hg	Br,Cl,Fe,K,Na, Rb,Zn	Se
Liver			
Mitchell(74),1986[b]	Se	Cl,Co,Cr,Cs,Fe,K, Mg,Mn,Na,Rb,Sb,Zn	—
Muscle			
Petkau(7),1974[f,g]	Pb	—	—
Conradi(87),1978[c]	—	Pb	—
Pierce-Ruhland(88),1980[h]	—	Al,As,Ba,Br,Cu,Fe, Hg,K,Mg,Mn,Ni,Pb, Rb,Zn	—
Mishra(89),1985[c]	—	Mg	Ca
Nails			
Khare(76),1990[b]	Zn	Br,Hg,Na,Se	Co,Cr,Fe,Sb,Sc
Peripheral nerve			
Petkau(7),1974[f,g]	Pb	—	—
Plasma/serum			
Kjellin(77),1967[a]	—	Fe	—
Conrdi(90),1978[e]	Pb	—	—

(*continued*)

Table 2   Continued

	Element concentration: ALS versus control		
Author, year	Increased	No sig. diff.	Reduced
Manton(81),1979[d]	—	Pb	—
Ronnevi(91),1982[c]	Pb	—	—
Domza(92),1983[a]	—	Cu	—
Stober(83),1983[c]	—	Pb	—
Cavalleri(84),1984[c]	—	Pb	—
Lu(93),1984[c]	Cd,Cu,Cr,Mn	Co,Ni	Au,Ca,Mn
Kapaki(54),1989[c]	—	Pb	—
Khare(76),1990[b]	Hg	Br,Cr,Cs,Fe,Na,Rb,Zn	Sc,Se
Spinal cord			
Petkau(7),1974[f,g]	Pb	—	—
Kurlander(64),1978[h]	Cu,Fe,Pb	Ca,Zn?Mn,?Se	—
Mitchell(74),1986[b]	Mn,Se	Cl,Co,Cr,Cs,Fe,K,	—
		Mg,Na,Rb,Sb,Zn	
Khare(76),1990[b]	Br	Cl,Co,Cs,Fe,Hg,Mn,	K,Zn
		Na,Rb,Sc,Se	
Urine			
Currier(4),1968[a]	—	As,Hg,Pb	—
Mallette(79),1977[a]	—	Ca,Cl	—
Norris(94),1978[a,c]	—	Se	—
Whole blood			
Campbell(13),1970[a]	—	Pb	—
Conradi(78),1976[c]	—	Pb	—
House(80),1978[a,c]	—	Pb	—
Manton(81),1979[d]	—	Pb	—
Stober(83),1983[c]	—	Pb	—
Cavalleri(84),1984[c]	—	Pb	—

[a]Fluorometric, spectrophotometric, or polarographic.
[b]Neutron activation analysis.
[c]Atomic absorption spectrophotometry.
[d]Isotope dilution.
[e]Flameless atomic absorption spectrophotometry.
[f]Microprobe techniques.
[g]Emission spectrography.
[h]Photon-excited x-ray fluorescence.

were methodologically sound, it is beyond the scope of this chapter to critique the precision and accuracy of the reported data. A few comments in this regard are in order, however, to assist the reader. In general, the more credible studies report their analytical results with Standard Reference Materials. The National Bureau of Standards (now the National Institute of Standards and Technology) certifies biological materials, such as bovine liver, as to the absolute amount of many elements. The analyses are typically performed by neutron activation analysis, which is a method free of interference from the biological matrix (33). The analysis of Standard Reference Materials is included in order to assure the investigator, and the reader, that the analytical data obtained are of high quality before any biological interpretation of the data is attempted. Many studies will also indicate the limits of detection for each element using their chosen method. Finally, attention to potential sample contamination is paramount inasmuch as many elements are present in low concentration in tissue such as brain and spinal cord. In this circumstance, the possibility of adulterating the sample prior to analysis is a real one. Sources of exogenous contamination are many and include ambient dust, rubber, metals, and reagents. Some studies report the elemental analysis of formalin-fixed tissue. Although the results may indeed be accurate for some elements, the possibility of contaminating the tissue by the formalin or, conversely, leaching some elements must be considered as a potential impediment to interpretation of these data. A full discussion of the problems of contamination when collecting clinical samples for trace element analysis has been given by Takeuchi (34) and by Ehmann et al. (35).

The literature regarding elemental analysis of ALS tissue has been divided according to source: Western Pacific (Table 1) versus sporadic (Table 2). Although one might challenge the aggregation of Guamanian and Japanese ALS cases, it appears to be a useful initial strategy in order to organize and evaluate the results of these studies (14). In several instances, only a single, more comprehensive report from a research group was cited if it included data or patient material that had been previously published or if it appeared in a less accessible journal. Specifically, Yoshida et al. (36) includes Ref. 37; Yase (38) summarizes Refs. 39–42; Yoshimasu et al. (43) includes Ref. 44; Nagata et al. (45) is cited in preference to Ref. 46; Miyata et al. (47) relates to Refs. 48 and 49.

Tables 1 and 2 are organized according to tissue type and, within each category, chronologically by first author. The analytical technique used by the investigators is also indicated. All the elements analyzed appear in the tables and are arranged according to the statistical deviation ($p < 0.05$ accepted as significant) of the ALS patient material from controls.

Table 1 summarizes the studies that evaluated ALS patients residing in the high-prevalence ALS foci of the Western Pacific. Most of these studies concern elemental analysis of spinal cord and brain regions and have concentrated on aluminum, calcium, and magnesium. Many of the investigations cited in Table 1 have been extended to include the cellular distribution of these elements using microprobe techniques (e.g., see 50,51). Troncoso's review in this volume evaluates the implications of these studies and should be consulted, especially in regard to aluminum. Among the other elements, manganese appears to be most consistently elevated in ALS tissue compared to controls, whereas other metals such as zinc and copper are unperturbed. In contrast to sporadic ALS, measurement of lead and mercury concentrations has been infrequently reported from this patient population. Similarly, a comprehensive evaluation of the elements in other tissues, such as bone, cerebrospinal fluid, liver, muscle, plasma, and urine, is lacking. These studies reflect an intense, sharply focused interest on the part of the cited investigators on the potential involvement of aluminum exposure, in association with calcium and magnesium deficiency, in the pathogenesis of ALS and ALS/PD in the endemic regions of the world (19,20). This fact, coupled with the dearth of aluminum analyses of tissue obtained from sporadic ALS cases, renders any meaningful comparisons between these patient groups virtually impossible.

Table 2 summarizes the studies of trace elements and toxic metals in classic sporadic ALS. A variety of tissues have been analyzed, including many non-neural tissues. In most cases, the majority of the elements are not perturbed in ALS tissues compared to controls. The elements that are increased in ALS appear to be those with the greatest inherent neurotoxicity, such as lead, mercury, and manganese. Unfortunately, there are no reports of aluminum analyses of ALs tissue taken from sporadic cases. Moreover, the cellular and regional distribution of any element in ALS brain or spinal cord using microprobe techniques has not been reported for sporadic ALS. Manganese appears to be elevated in some, but not all, studies of both sporadic and Western Pacific cases. The biological significance of this observation will require further study.

FUTURE DIRECTIONS FOR RESEARCH INTO THE TRACE ELEMENT HYPOTHESIS

I agree with Mitchell, who stated in his review of the subject, ''. . . attempts to demonstrate that ALS is the result of a simple trace element excess or deficiency seem unlikely to be rewarding'' (8). The operative word here is "simple," meaning that a toxic element is ingested or inhaled, which then directly and selectively kills motor neurons in the absence of any other contributing factor.

Circumstantial evidence, however, from both clinical observation and experimental studies, suggests that heavy metals could be coconspirators in the process of selective neuronal death in ALS. The studies outlined in Tables 1 and 2, as well as the clinical reports of ALS-like syndromes occurring in the setting of toxic metal exposures (2–7), support this notion and must be accounted for in any alternative hypothesis of pathogenesis. A particularly attractive formulation was advanced by Calne et al., who proposed that a remote environmental insult may be later expressed as "a consequence of age-related neuronal attrition" (27). Certainly the long biological half-lives make many toxic elements ideal candidates for such a mechanism. In fact, with respect to toxic metals, the environmental insult need not be remote but a chronic, ongoing one.

Other interpretations of the data are possible. For example, the presence of excess mercury, lead, or manganese in ALS tissue may not imply a pathogenetic role for these metals at all, but may merely be an epiphenomenon. However, the observations of Møller-Madsen and Danscher (24), if verified in human spinal cord, cannot be dismissed easily. It is conceivable that heavy metals such as mercury may selectively label specific membrane ligands of motor neurons. Investigating the biochemistry of this phenomenon may facilitate understanding the basic cell biology of motor neurons and which factors make them susceptible to degeneration in ALS.

What is needed in order to critically evaluate these ideas? First, additional analytical work is needed on bulk samples, especially in regard to aluminum for sporadic ALS. This will help define the chemical architecture of ALS brain and spinal cord and will facilitate comparisons between classic ALS and its variants from the Western Pacific. Next, examining the regional and cellular distribution of toxic and essential metals in control and ALS spinal cord will be important. This would be best accomplished using the microprobe techniques that have been employed in the investigation of the ALS/PD complex (50,51). Finally, further studies of the basic toxicology and biochemistry of heavy metals will be required to illuminate the interactions between toxic an essential elements both systemically and within the central nervous system.

PRACTICAL CONSIDERATIONS IN THE EVALUATION OF ALS PATIENTS

In the meantime, what/how much should a clinician do about heavy metals when evaluating and treating an ALS patient? The critical task is the identification of the *rare* patient with an ALS-like syndrome that is due to a toxic metal exposure, usually mercury or lead (2,4,5,7,52,53). These clinical reports are of interest because the physicians who cared for these patients identified them as individuals with motor neuron dysfunction in association with other signs/symptoms suggestive of a toxin exposure, rather than typical patients with ALS. The key to the recognition of these patients is a detailed history, focusing on their occupation, hobbies, habits, and environment (55–57). It is conceded that the diagnosis of lead or mercury toxicity is not trivial, in part because many of the screening tests such as blood and urine concentrations do not accurately reflect the total body burden of these elements. However, in patients with a strong history of exposure to heavy metals, screening tests are frequently abnormal and will identify patients with ongoing exposures (56,57). For example, measuring the concentration of lead and mercury in blood and in a 24-hr urine collection is useful in this regard. Patten has proposed upper limits for mercury, arsenic, and lead excretion in his normal population (58), which is in general accord with other recommendations (57).

The identification of persons with an excess body burden of toxic metals, acquired in the distant past, is more problematic because blood and urine concentrations may be within the normal range for the population. In this circumstance, changes reflecting a known biochemical effect of heavy metals are sought. For example, in the case of lead, urinary delta-aminolevulinic acid (ALA), zinc protoporphyrin (ZPP), and free erythrocyte protoporphyrin (FEP) are measured (56,57). However, similar biochemical indicators are not available to monitor the consequences of prior mercury exposure.

A second strategy to identify individuals with excessive body burdens of lead employs calcium disodium EDTA to chelate lead from the skeleton. The mobilized lead is excreted in the urine and quantitated (59). This approach, in conjunction with other measures of lead body burden, continues to be used to discover asymptomatic children with excessive skeletal lead (60). The data are more meager for adults, although this strategy has been generalized from the pediatric experience (55). Recently, a noninvasive technique to measure bone lead has been developed. The L-line x-ray fluorescence (LXRF) method successfully identified adults and children with abnormal EDTA mobilization tests and correlated well with other indices of chronic lead exposure (61,62). In the future, the LXRF technique will probably supplant the other methods for evaluation of patients with suspected lead toxicity.

Do typical ALS patients have excessive concentrations of lead, mercury, or other toxic heavy metal in their skeletons? Should the otherwise typical ALS patient be treated with chelation therapy? Patten reported that 9 of 38 ALS patients had abnormal EDTA lead mobilization tests (59,63), suggesting that a substantial group of ALS patients may be harboring inordinate body burdens of lead. However, Campbell et al. did not find any difference between ALS and controls in the concentration of lead in iliac crest bone biopsy specimens (13). This important question will need to be critically reexamined using the LXRF technique in the future before any firm conclusions can be drawn.

The efficacy of chelation therapy for the typical ALS patient (i.e., patients without evidence of excessive body burdens of lead or mercury) cannot be supported by the literature. To date, 53 ALS patients have been reported who were treated with either EDTA or penicillamine (3,23,64,65). The patients' progressive course was not substantially altered by chelation, and more importantly, in three patients (23,65), the deterioration actually appeared to accelerate during attempted therapy. Therefore, wholesale chelation of patients with idiopathic ALS cannot be endorsed. If, however, a patient with an "ALS-like syndrome" can be proved to have an excessive body burden of a toxic metal, then chelation therapy by an experienced physician would be indicated.

ACKNOWLEDGMENTS

The original research from our group cited in this review resulted from collaboration with Drs. William D. Ehmann, William R. Markesbery, and Subhash S. Khare and was supported by a grant from the Muscular Dystrophy Association and NIH Grant NS 25165. The author also thanks Dr. Huaichen Liu for her assistance.

REFERENCES

1. Aran FA. Recherches sur une maladie non encore decrite du systeme musculaire. Arch Gen Med 1850;24:1–35.
2. Adams CR, Ziegler DK, Lin JT. Mercury intoxication simulating amyotrophic lateral sclerosis. JAMA 1983;250:642–643.
3. Campbell AMG, Williams ER. Chronic lead intoxication mimicking motor neurone disease. Br Med J 1968;4:582.
4. Currier RD, Hearer AF. Amyotrophic lateral sclerosis and metallic toxins. Arch Environ Health 1968;17:712–719.
5. Kantarjian AD. A syndrome clinically resembling amyotrophic lateral sclerosis following chronic mercurialism. Neurology 1953;11:639.
6. Livesley B, Sissons CE. Chronic lead intoxication mimicking motor neurone disease. Br Med J 1968;4:387–388.
7. Petkau A, Sawatzky A, Hillier CR, Hoogstraten J. Lead content of neuromuscular tissue in amyotrophic lateral sclerosis: Case report and other considerations. Br J Indust Med 1974;31:275–287.
8. Mitchell JD. Heavy metals and trace elements in amyotrophic lateral sclerosis. Neurol Clin 1987;5:43–60.
9. Lansdown R, Yule W. Lead toxicity: History and environmental impact. Baltimore: Johns Hopkins University Press, 1986.
10. Singhal RL, Thomas JA. Lead toxicity. Baltimore: Urban & Schwarzenberg, 1980.
11. Bryson PD. Comprehensive review in toxicology. Rockville, MD: Aspen, 1989.
12. Albers JW, Kallenbach LR, Fine LJ, Langolf GD, Wolfe RA, Donofrio PD, Alessi AG, Stolp-Smith KA, Bromberg MB. Neurological abnormalities associated with remote occupational elemental mercury exposure. Ann Neurol 1988;24:651–659.
13. Campbell AMG, Williams ER, Barltrop D. Motor neurone disease and exposure to lead. J Neurol Neurosurg Psychiatry 1970;33:877–885.
14. Garruto R, Yase Y. Neurodegenerative disorders of the Western Pacific: The search for mechanisms of pathogenesis. Trends Neuro Sci 1986;9:368–374.
15. Garruto RM, Yanagihara R, Gajdusek DC. Disappearance of high-incidence amyotrophic lateral sclerosis and Parkinsonism-dementia on Guam. Neurology 1985;35:193–198.
16. Yase Y. The pathogenesis of amyotrophic lateral sclerosis. Lancet 1972;2:292–295.
17. Spencer PS, Nunn PB, Hugon J, Ludolph AC, Ross SM, Roy DN, Robertson RC. Guam amyotrophic lateral sclerosis–Parkinsonism-dementia linked to a plant excitant neurotoxin. Science 1987;237:517–522.

18. Garruto RM, Gajdusek DC. Factors provoking the high incidence of amyotrophic lateral sclerosis and Parkinsonism-dementia of Guam: Deposition and distribution of toxic metals and essential minerals in the central nervous system. In: Gottfries CG, ed. Normal aging, Alzheimer's disease and senile dementia aspects on etiology, pathogenesis, diagnosis and treatment. Brussels: Editions Univ Bruxelles, 1985: 69–82.

19. Garruto RM, Swyt C, Fiori CE, Yanagihara R, Gajdusek DC. Intraneuronal deposition of calcium and aluminium in amyotropic lateral sclerosis of Guam. Lancet 1985;2:1353.

20. Yase Y. The pathogenetic role of metals in motor neuron disease—The participation of aluminum. Adv Exp Med Biol 1987;209:89–96.

21. Chang LW. Neurotoxic effects of mercury-a review. Environ Res 1977;14:329–373.

22. Clarkson T. The pharmacology of mercury compounds. Annu Rev Pharmacol 1972;12:375–405.

23. Conradi S, Ronnevi L-O, Norris FH. Motor neuron disease and toxic metals. Adv Neurol 1982;36:201–231.

24. Møller-Madsen B, Danscher G. Localization of mercury in CNS of the rat. I. Mercuric chloride (HgCl₂) per os. Environ Res 1986;41:29–43.

25. Chang LW, Hartmann HA. Electron microscopic histochemical study on the localization and distribution of mercury in the nervous system after mercury intoxication. Exp Neurol 1972;35:122–137.

26. Hughes JT. Pathology of amyotrophic lateral sclerosis. Adv Neurol 1982;36:61–74.

27. Calne DB, McGeer E, Eisen A, Spencer P. Alzheimer's disease, Parkinson's disease, and motorneurone disease: Abiotrophic interaction between ageing and environment? Lancet 1986;2:1067–1070.

28. Hirano A, Donnefeld H, Sasaki S, Nakano I. Fine structural observations of neurofilamentous changes in amyotrophic lateral sclerosis. J Neuropathol Exp Neurol 1984;43:461–470.

29. Brownell B, Oppenheimer DR, Hughes JT. The central nervous system in motor neurone disease. J Neurol Neurosurg Psychiatry 1970;33:338–357.

30. Lawyer T, Netsky MG. Amyotrophic lateral sclerosis. A clinicoanatomic study of fifty-three cases. Arch Neurol Psychiatry 1953;69:171–192.

31. Mandybur TI, Cooper GP. Increased spinal cord lead content in amyotrophic lateral sclerosis—Possibly a secondary phenomenon. Med Hypotheses 1979;5:1313–1315.

32. Yanagihara R. Heavy metals and essential minerals in motor neuron disease. Adv Neurol 1982;36:233–247.

33. Ehmann WD, Vance DE. Advances in neutron activation analysis. CRC Crit Rev Anal Chem 1989;20:405–443.

34. Takeuchi T. Nuclear activation techniques in the life sciences. J Radioanal Chem 1980;59:545–569.

35. Ehmann WD, Markesbery WR, Kasarskis EJ, Vance DE, Khare SS, Hord JD, Thompson CM. Applications of neutron activation analysis to the study of age-related neurological diseases. Biol Trace Elem Res 1987;13:19–33.

36. Yoshida S, Yase Y, Iwata S, Mizumoto Y, Chen K-M, Gajdusek DC. Comparative trace-element study on amyotrophic latral sclerosis (ALS) and Parkinsonism-dementia (PD) in the Kii Peninsula of Japan and Guam. Wakayama Med Rep 1988;30: 41–53.

37. Yoshida S, Yase Y, Iwata S, Mizumoto Y, Gajdusek DC. Trace-elemental study on amyotrophic lateral sclerosis (ALS) and Parkinsonism-dementia (PD) in the Kii Peninsula of Japan and Guam. Clin Neurol 1987;27:79–87.

38. Yase Y The basic process of amyotrophic lateral sclerosis as reflected in Kii Peninsula and Guam. In: den Hartog Jager WA, Bruyn GW, Heijstee APJ, eds. Neurology, Proceedings of the 11th World Congress of Neurology. Amsterdam-Oxford: Excerpta Medica, 1978:413–427.

39. Yase Y. Amyotrophic lateral sclerosis. Brain Nerve 1982;24:7–15.

40. Iwata S. Study of the effects of environmental factors on the local incidence of amyotrophic lateral sclerosis. Ecotoxicol Environ Safety 1977;1:297–303.

41. Yase Y. Calcium, metals and nervous system in the elderly. J Nutr Sci Vitaminol 1985;31:S37–S40.

42. Yase Y, Yoshimasu F, Uebayashi Y, Iwata S, Sasajima K. Neutron activation analysis of calcium in central nervous system tissue of amyotrophic lateral sclerosis cases. Folia Psychiatr Neurol Jpn 1974;28:371–378.

43. Yoshimasu F, Yasui M, Yase Y, Iwata S, Gajdusek DC, Gibbs CJ, Chen K. Studies on amyotrophic lateral sclerosis by neutron activation analysis-2. Comparative study of analytical results on Gram PD, Japanese ALS and Alzheimer disease cases. Folia Psychiatr Neurol Jpn 1980;34:75–82.

44. Yoshimasu F, Uebayashi Y, Yase Y, Iwata S, Sasajima K. Studies on amyotrophic lateral sclerosis by neutron activation analysis. Folia Psychiatr Neurol Jpn 1976;30: 49–55.

45. Nagata H, Miyata S, Nakamura S, Kameyama M, Katsui Y. Heavy metal concentrations in blood cells in patients with amyotrophic lateral sclerosis. J Neurol Sci 1985;67:173–178.

46. Katsui Y, Nagata H, Miyata S, Nakamura S, Kameyama M. Heavy metal concentrations in blood cells of patients with amyotrophic lateral sclerosis—Study of five cases in Mie. Clin Neurol 1987;27:19–22.

47. Miyata S, Nakamura S, Nagata H, Kameyama M. Increased manganese level in spinal cords of amyotrophic lateral sclerosis determined by radiochemical neutron activation analysis. Neurol Sci 1983;61:283–293.

48. Miyata S, Nakamura S, Toyoshima M, Kameyama M, Koyama M. The distribution of manganese in the spinal cord of amyotrophic lateral sclerosis—Determination of manganese by neutron activation analysis. Clin Neurol 1980;20:917–923.

49. Miyata S, Nakamura S, Toyoshima M, Hirata Y, Saito M, Kameyama M, Matsushita M, Koyama M. Determination of manganese in tissues by neutron activation analysis using an antimony pentoxide column. Clin Chim Acta 1980;106:235–242.

50. Perl D, Gajdusek DC, Garruto RM, Yanagihara RT, Gibbs CJ. Intraneuronal aluminum accumulation in amyotrophic.lateral sclerosis and Parkinsonism-dementia of Guam. Science 1982;217:1053–1055.

51. Garruto RM, Fukatsu R, Yanagihara R, Gajdusek DC, Hook G, Fiori CE. Imaging

of calcium and aluminum in neurofibrillary tangle-bearing neurons in Parkinsonism-dementia of Guam. Proc Natl Acad Sci USA 1984;81:1875–1879.

52. Boothby JA, DeJesus PV, Rowland LP. Reversible forms of motor neuron disease. Lead "neuritis." Arch Neurol 1974;31:18–23.

53. Brown IA. Chronic mercurialism. A cause of the clinical syndrome of amyotrophic lateral sclerosis. Arch Neurol Psychiatry 1954;72:647–681.

54. Kapaki E, Segditsa J, Zournas C, Xenos D, Papageorgiou C. Determination of cerebrospinal fluid and serum lead levels in patients with amyotrophic lateral sclerosis and other neurological diseases. Experientia 1989;45:1108–1110.

55. Rempel D. The lead-exposed worker. JAMA 1989;262:532–534.

56. Friberg L, Nordberg GF, Vouk VB, eds. Handbook on the toxicology of metals. Amsterdam: Elsevier/North Holland Press, 1979.

57. Zenz C. Occupational medicine. Principles and practical applications. Chicago: Year Book Medical Publishers, 1988.

58. Patten BM. Mineral and metal metabolism in amyotrophic lateral sclerosis. In: Rose FC, ed. Research progress in motor neurone disease. Bath: Pitman Press, 1982: 189–227.

59. Emmerson BT. Chronic lead nephropathy: The diagnostic use of calcium EDTA and the association with gout. Aust Ann Med 1963;12:310–324.

60. Weinberger HL, Post EM, Schneider T, Helu B, Friedman J. An analysis of 248 initial mobilization tests performed on an ambulatory basis. Am J Dis Child 1987;141:1266–1270.

61. Rosen JF, Markowitz ME, Bijur PE, Jenks ST, Wielopolski L, Kalef-Ezra JA, Slatkin DN. L-line x-ray fluorescence of cortical bone lead compared with the $CaNa_2$ EDTA test in lead-toxic children: Public health implications. Proc Natl Acad Sci USA 1989;86:685–689.

62. Somervaille LJ, Chettle DR, Scott MC, Tennant DR, McKiernan MJ, Skilbeck A, Trethowan WN. In vivo tibia lead measurements as an index of cumulative exposure in occupationally exposed subjects. Br J Indust Med 1988;45:174–181.

63. Patten BM. Mobilization of lead in amyotrophic lateral sclerosis. Neurology 1983;33:239.

64. Kurlander HM, Patten BM. Metals in spinal cord tissue of patients dying of motor neuron disease. Ann Neurol 1979;6:21–24.

65. Conradi S, Ronnevi L-O, Nise G, Vesterberg O. Long term penicillamine treatment in amyotrophic lateral sclerosis with parallel determination of lead in blood, plasma and urine. Acta Neurol Scand 1982;65:203–211.

66. Yoshimasu F, Yasui M, Yase Y, Uebayashi Y, Tanaka S, Iwata S, Sasajima K, Gajdusek C, Gibbs CJ, Chen K-M. Studies on amyotrophic lateral sclerosis by neutron activation analysis-3. Systematic analysis of metals on guamanian ALS and PD cases. Folia Psychiatr Neurol Jpn 1982;36:173–179.

67. Mizumoto Y, Iwata S, Sasajima K, Yoshimasu F, Yase Y. Reactor neutron activation analysis for aluminium in the presence of phosphorus and silicon-contribution of ^{28}Al activities from $^{31}P(n,\alpha)^{28}Al$ and $^{28}Si(n,p)^{28}Al$ reactions. Radioisotopes 1983;33:8–14.

68. Piccardo P, Yanagihara R, Garruto RM, Gibbs CJ, Gajdusek DC. Histochemical

staining and x-ray microanalytical imaging of aluminum in amyotrophic lateral sclerosis and Parkinsonism-dementia of Guam. Acta Neuropathol 1986;77:1–4.

69. Yanagihara R, Garruto RM, Gajdusek C, Tomita A, Uchikawa T, Konagaya Y, Chen K-M, Sobue I, Plato CC, Gibbs CJ. Calcium and vitamin D metabolism in Guamanian chamorros with amyotrophic lateral sclerosis and parkinsonism-dementia. Ann Neurol 1984;15:42–48.

70. Yoshida S. X-ray microanalytic studies on amyotrophic lateral sclerosis. I. Metal distribution compared with neuropathological findings in cervical spinal cord. Clin Neurol 1977;17:299–309.

71. Yoshida S. X-ray microanalytic studies on amyotrophic lateral sclerosis. III. Relationship of clacification and degeneration found in cervical spinal cord of ALS. Clin Neurol 1979;19:641–652.

72. Mizumoto Y, Iwata S, Sasajima K, Yase Y, Yoshida S. Alpha particle excited x-ray fluorescence analysis for trace elements in cervical spinal cords of amyotrophic lateral sclerosis. Radioisotopes 1980;29:385–389.

73. Kihira T, Mukoyama M, Ando K, Yase Y. Quantitative analysis of Ca in CNS by inductively coupled plasma emission spectroscopy—a study of Ca contents in amyotrophic lateral sclerosis (ALS) spinal cord. Clin Neurol 1984;24:498–504.

74. Mitchell JD, East BW, Harris IA, Prescott RJ, Pentland B. Trace elements in the spinal cord and other tissues in motor neuron disease. J Neurol Neurosurg Psychiatry 1986;49:211–215.

75. Larsen NA, Pakkenberg H, Damsgaard E, Heydorn K, Wold S. Distribution of arsenic, manganese, and selenium in the human brain in chronic renal insufficiency, parkinson's disease, and amyotrophic lateral sclerosis. J Neurol Sci 1981;51:437–446.

76. Khare SS, Ehmann WD, Kasarskis EJ, Markesbery WR. Trace element imbalances in amyotrophic lateral sclerosis. Neurotoxicology 1990;11:521–532.

77. Kjellin KG. The CSF iron in patients with neurological diseases. Acta Neurol Scand 1967;43:299–313.

78. Conradi S, Ronnevi K, Vesterberg O. Abnormal tissue distribution of lead in amyotrophic lateral sclerosis. J Neurol Sci 1976;29:259–265.

79. Mallette LE, Patten B, Cook JD, Engel WK. Calcium metabolism in amyotrophic lateral sclerosis. Dis Nerv Syst 1977;38:457–461.

80. House AO, Abbott RJ, Davidson DLW, Ferguson IT, Lenman JAR. Response to penicillamine of lead concentrations in CSF and blood in patients with motor neurone disease. Br Med J 1978;2:1684.

81. Manton WI, Cook JD. Lead content of cerebrospinal fluid and other tissue in amyotrophic lateral sclerosis. Neurology 1979;29:611–612.

82. Conradi S, Ronnevi L, Nise G, Vesterberg O. Abnormal distribution of lead in amyotrophic lateral sclerosis. J Neurol Sci 1980;48:413–418.

83. Stober T, Stelte W, Kunze K. Lead concentrations in blood, plasma, erythrocytes, and cerebrospinal fluid in amyotrophic lateral sclerosis. J Neurol Sci 1983;61:21–26.

84. Cavalleri A, Minoia C, Ceroni M, Poloni M. Lead in cerebrospinal fluid and its relationship to plasma lead in humans. J Appl Toxicol 1984;4:63–65.

85. Mitchell JD, Harris IA, East BW, Pentland B. Trace elements in cerebrospinal fluid in motor neurone disease. Br Med J 1984;288:1791–1792.
86. Felmus MT, Rasool CG, Bradley WG. Calcium content of RBCs from patients with amyotrophic lateral sclerosis. Arch Neurol 1982;39:454.
87. Conradi S, Ronnevi L, Vesterberg O. Lead concentration in skeletal muscle in amyotrophic lateral sclerosis patients and control subjects. J Neurol Neurosurg Psychiatry 1978;41:1001–1004.
88. Pierce-Ruhland R, Patten BM. Muscle metals in motor neuron disease. Ann Neurol 1980;8:193–195.
89. Mishra SK, Kumar S. Muscle calcium, calmodulin levels in amyotrophic lateral sclerosis. Neurology 1985;35(Suppl 1):73.
90. Conradi S, Ronnevi L, Vesterberg O. Increased plasma levels of lead in patients with amyotrophic lateral sclerosis compared with control subjects as determined by flameless atomic absorption spectrophotometry. J Neurol Neurosurg Psychiatry 1978;41:389–393.
91. Ronnevi L-O, Canradi S, Nise G. Further studies on the erythrocyte uptake of lead in vitro in amyotrophic lateral sclerosis (ALS) patients and controls. J Neurol Sci 1982; 57:143–156.
92. Domzal T, Radzikowska B. Ceruloplasmin and copper in the serum of patients. Neurol I Neurochir Polska 1983;3:343–346.
93. Lu FH, Lui CZ, Cheng HB, Wu ZK, Qiao HY. Significance of serum trace elements in various neurological diseases. China J Neuropsychiatry (Chung-hua Shen Ching Ching Shen Ko Tsa Chih) 1984;17:166–169.
94. Norris FH, Sang K. Amyotrophic lateral sclerosis and low urinary selenium levels. JAMA 1978;239:404.

26

Slow Toxins and Western Pacific Amyotrophic Lateral Sclerosis

Peter S. Spencer and Glen Kisby

*Center for Research on Occupational and Environmental Toxicology,
Oregon Health Sciences University
Portland, Oregon*

CHEMICAL TRIGGERS OF NEUROLOGICAL DISEASE

The clinical consequences of chemical attack on the nervous system surface after varying periods of time. Important variables, such as the type, potency, dosage, and target of the agent, the duration of exposure, and the susceptibility of the subject, compress or expand the interval between chemical exposure and disease expression. The interval may be measured in minutes for potent anticholinesterases that disrupt cholinergic neurotransmission (1), while days, weeks, or months of repeated exposure may be required for some drugs (vincristine) and occupational (methyl *n*-butyl ketone) chemicals to induce clinically apparent axonal degeneration (2,3). For certain chemicals, periods of one or more weeks may intervene between chemical exposure and disease onset, as in the peripheral neuropathy triggered by organophosphates and the tardive dystonia attributed to 3-nitropropionic acid (4,5). Like other self-limiting neurotoxic disorders, these may evolve for a short period of time after cessation of exposure (a phenomenon known as coasting) and then recover or become static. Neurotoxic conditions that are stable for years, such as the upper-motor-neuron disorder lathyrism, may progress to some degree later in life presumably because the deleterious effects of advancing age gradually increase clinical dysfunction (6,7). However, for the present purpose, it is important to note that age-associated progression of neurological dysfunction is usually unassociated with the relatively rapid downhill course characteristic of amyotrophic lateral sclerosis (ALS). Despite the wide range of timing in the clinical expression of chemical exposure, there is no precedent in neurotoxicology for a chemical comparable to a DNA-reactive (i.e., genotoxic) carcinogen which, after single or multiple exposures (depending on potency), triggers a relentlessly progressive cellular disease that takes years or decades to appear clinically (8). Nevertheless, a neurotoxic agent with comparable characteristics is currently being sought to explain the etiology of the western Pacific form of ALS and its Parkinsonism-dementia (PD) clinical variant (L. Kurland, this volume). Moreover, one of the agents (cycasin) under detailed scrutiny exhibits the properties of both a neurotoxin and a genotoxic carcinogen. This chapter explores the hypothesis that certain chemicals— *slow toxins** (9) or *gerontogens** (10)—may be etiologically linked with fatal, long-latency neurodegenerative diseases such as Western Pacific ALS/PD.

EVIDENCE LINKING ALS WITH CYCAD EXPOSURE

Western Pacific ALS/PD, the neuropathological hallmark of which is Alzheimer-type neurofibrillary degeneration (11), has occurred in high incidence among the Chamorros of Guam and Japanese residents of the Kii Peninsula of Honshu Island (12). A clinically similar condition has also been remarkably common among the Auyu linguistic group of Irian Jaya, Indonesia (13). Since the prevalence of this nontransmissible disease has declined in all three hotspots, an environmental chemical factor that has diminished concurrently with the adaptation of the affected groups to modern ways is likely to be responsible (14). Natural toxins must be involved in the Irian Jaya epidemic because man-made chemicals have been introduced only recently. On Guam, preference for traditional food is the only one of 23 tested variables significantly linked to susceptibility for PD (15).

Suspicion has centered on cycad plants, the leaves and seed of which are a cause of a progressive neuromuscular disease (cycadism†) and death in ruminants

---

*Gerontogens and slow toxins are unproven concepts. Slow toxins are defined as chemicals that increase the rate at which relevant populations of neurons susceptible to the aging process undergo cell loss. Gerontogens are putative agents that accelerate the time of onset and/or the rate of progression of particular aging processes. Both could act at any stage of the life-cycle continuum.
†Cycadism is a little-studied "paralytic" disease of cattle and sheep that graze on leaves and other components of cycad plants in the tropics and subtropics, Initially, there is a staggering, weaving gait, with crossing of the hindlimbs, incoordination, and ataxia. More severe forms are characterized by posterior motor weakness, muscle wasting, and dragging of extended hindlimbs. Neuropathological examination reportedly shows degeneration of descending spinal tracts, readily observed in the lumbar region, with similar involvement of the fasciculus gracilis and dorsal spinocerebellar tracts,

(16,17). Raw cycad seed kernel has been widely used in Guam as a topical medicine, although the practice has declined as manufactured pharmaceuticals have become available. Recent studies have also demonstrated a disappearing medicinal usage of unprocessed cycad seed in the two other western Pacific foci of ALS/PD (18,19). In Japan (Hobara focus), a steepe prepared from the whole dried cycad seed has been used as a tonic and for treatment of diarrhea, dysmenorrhea, and tuberculosis (18). Among the Auyu of Irian Jaya, the fresh cycad seed kernel has been commonly used to poultice large open wounds (19), a procedure similar to that used by the Chamorros. Exposure to cycad seed, therefore, has been a common feature in all three high-incidence disease foci, and the onset of ALS in individual patients living in these areas has been linked to prior exposure to the raw seed. In addition, on Guam, cycad seed kernel has been processed (by soaking in water for 1–30 days) for use in food and beverages (16). Processed cycad seed kernel and trunk sago have also been consumed in the Japanese Ryukyu Islands, where high-incidence ALS/PD is not recognized. However, the Japanese cycad food products lack detectable concentrations of the principal cycad toxin (20), in marked contrast to its presence in varying concentrations in cycad flour prepared Chamorro style (21, unpublished data). The difference may be related to the Japanese use of fermentation, as well as washing, to remove the cycad toxins.

EVIDENCE FOR LONG-LATENCY DISEASE

There is little question that Western Pacific ALS/PD is a long-latency disease. Evidence from Guam shows that migrants leaving the island prior to the age of 18 have developed clinically apparent disease 1–35 years later (22). Similarly, adult Filipino migrants to Guam who adopt the Chamorro life-style have become ill after 17–26 years of residency (23). In Irian Jaya, one individual who left a village with high-incident disease to attend school succumbed to the disorder after an absence of 15 years (24). Similarly, in this region, ALS developed in an individual approximately 10 years after using the cycad poultice for periods up to 1 month (19). In the Kii Peninsula, where the disease has essentially disappeared, a teenager who was given a cycad seed tonic repeatedly as a baby developed ALS at the age of 18 (18). On Guam, ALS appeared up to 45 years after the last exposure to cycad as food (25). These observations suggest a relationship between cycad exposure and the subsequent onset of disease, although it must be cautioned that epidemiology is only able to demonstrate associations with human disease. Cause-and-effect relations are revealed by pro-

---

most prominent in the cervical region. The condition of upper and lower motor neurons in this disease is undescribed.

ducing an exact animal model of the human disease; for Western Pacific ALS/
PD, this has yet to be accomplished.

While the experience of Filipino migrants to Guam demonstrates that ALS/PD
may be acquired by adults, that of the Japanese girl and of others in Guam and
Irian Jaya who developed motor neuron disease prior to the age of 20 suggests
exposure to the culpable agent in the opening years of life. This view is supported by the presence in middle-aged Japanese and Guam cases of neuroanatomical abnormalities suggestive of a developmental perturbation timed close to
the birth period (12). In these subjects, ectopic and multinucleated neurons are
found in the cerebellum and elsewhere, abnormalities that indicate disruption late
in the developmental period of mitosis and migration of neurons in those regions
(12). Since comparable abnormalities are seen in developing rodents treated with
the cycad toxin cycasin (26), this phenomenon may represent an important
biological marker of cycad exposure close to birth—probably during the initial
postnatal period.

The Alzheimer-type neurofibrillary tangle is a prominent neuropathological
feature of Western Pacific ALS/PD (11,27). One study of 302 Chamorro brains
removed from individuals who died after the age of 35 with no known neurological disease demonstrated neurofibrillary tangles in an extraordinary 70%, and
15% of those with tangles were indistinguishable from definitive PD cases (28).
This remarkable observation strongly supports the proposal of a widespread
exposure to an environmental etiological agent and, at the time of the study,
demonstrated that the large majority of affected subjects in this cycad-exposed
population was subclinically affected with the disease. Such individuals may be
the least exposed, or the most resistant, members of the population. If they
together represent the submerged portion of an iceberg, the clinical cases above
the surface are relatively few. These include individuals who develop PD late in
life and those who succumb to ALS at an early age. Since ALS has also declined
as environmental conditions have changed, these may represent the very tip of
the iceberg, i.e., the most heavily exposed or most susceptible group, while PD
patients occupy an analogous position closer to the surface (9,29).

CYCAD CHEMICALS AS SLOW TOXINS/GERONTOGENS

While the presence of subclinical neurofibrillary disease narrows the gap in
timing between environmental exposure and disease onset, it does not alter the
incontrovertible fact that, once expressed, the disease is rapidly progressive and
fatal. This is the feature that separates long-latency neurodegenerative diseases
from other neurotoxic illnesses, which, with few exceptions (e.g., tardive neurological consequences of acute carbon monoxide poisoning), are self-limiting or
reversible. Chemical induction of a relentlessly progressive degenerative process
would require either (a) tissue storage and continual release of the culpable

neurotoxic agent, or (b) an irreversible modification of a critical regulatory site in affected neurons. The most likely target is neuronal DNA. Williams and Weisburger (8) note that chemicals (carcinogens) that react with DNA differ from most other kinds of toxins in that (a) their biological effect is persistent, cumulative, and delayed; (b) divided doses are in some cases more effective than an individual large dose; and (c) the underlying mechanisms, particularly with respect to interaction and alteration of genetic elements and other macromolecules, are distinct.

How does this concept fit with the cycad hypothesis? Two (and possibly other) chemicals in cycad seed—cycasin and beta-N-methylamino-L-alanine (BMAA)—exhibit neurotoxic potential. The minor component, BMAA (0.02% w/w), behaves as a weak excitotoxin in central nervous system (CNS) tissue (30–33), induces cerebellar damage in young rats (34), and primates given large daily oral doses of BMAA for several weeks develop behavioral, pyramidal, and extrapyramidal dysfunction (35). While the primate response to BMAA displays some of the features one would wish to see in a model of Western Pacific ALS/PD, the experimental disorder is nonprogressive and lacks Alzheimer-like neurofibrillary tangles. While this does not exclude a role for BMAA, there is reason to posit that cycasin may be the more important etiological agent.

Cycasin is the principal toxic seed component (4% w/w) of those species of cycad (*Cycas* spp.) linked to Western Pacific ALS/PD. Like BMAA (21,36), cycasin is present as a contaminant of Chamorro-style cycad flour, but neither compound was detected by sensitive analytical methods in cycad food products from the Japanese Ryukyu Islands where ALS/PD is undescribed (20, unpublished data). Cycasin behaves as a cerebellar toxin in subcutaneously injected postnatal mice (26); "unilateral hindlimb weakness and general slowness of movements" appear in young adult rats fed cycasin by gastric tube (37), and the agent elicits the incompletely defined neuromuscular disease of cycadism in orally dosed goats (38). Neurological disease has also been reported in rhesus monkeys fed *chapatis* prepared from washed cycad flour containing (by paper chromatography) "almost no cycasin" (39, personal communication). Weakness and wasting, especially of one upper limb, with neuropathological evidence of degeneration of anterior horn cells and of pyramidal cells of the motor cortex, developed in a young animal fed for 4–9 months. A second mature animal fed for 2 years showed "argyrophilic dystrophic plaques amongst the degenerating neurites (axons) of the cerebral white matter, without any amyloid or neurofibrillary tangles" (40). Additionally, one of two animals fed cycad seed boiled for 80 min (containing "clearly detectable amounts" of cycasin) showed "swelling and chromatolysis of anterior horn cells, as well as of the axons of the anterior nerve roots, with the accumulation of neurofilaments in both" (40). Both groups of animals displayed hepatocellular changes typical of cycasin toxicity, and these were severe in animals fed the poorly detoxified boiled cycad.

Although cycasin has neurotoxic potential in rodents, ungulates, and primates, the hepatotoxic and neoplastic properties of the compound have commanded much more scientific interest (41). Rodents appear to be more susceptible than primates (42). Single, large oral doses of cycasin result in a high incidence of nephroblastomas, colon, and liver tumors in rats (41,43) but not in cycasin-treated animals lacking intestinal bacteria (44). Rats given the drug intraperitoneally also fail to develop tumors (45). These negative observations led to the conclusion that cycasin was cleaved by the enzyme β-glucosidase in intestinal bacteria to form the aglycone and active toxin/carcinogen methylazoxymethanol (MAM) (46–48). Sieber and colleagues (42) assessed the carcinogenicity and hepatotoxicity of cycasin and MAM in rhesus, cynomolgus, and African green monkeys. Eight animals treated from birth for up to 11 years with various combinations of cycad meal, cycasin, and MAM acetate displayed at autopsy toxic hepatitis, centrilobular liver necrosis, hyperplastic nodules, and cirrhosis. Hepatic changes were said to be similar to those noted in rhesus monkeys with cycad-induced neurological disease (40,41), although Sieber and colleagues did not describe the neurological status and CNS morphology of their animals. One monkey showed a well-differentiated hepatocellular carcinoma, and a second had multiple malignant tumors. No histological evidence of liver damage was found in an additional animal fed cycad meal containing 3% cycasin for 8 months. Furthermore, there is no epidemiological evidence that human exposure to cycads is associated with high cancer rates (49,50).

Why is cycasin an attractive candidate for the putative long-latency neurotoxin responsible for Western Pacific ALS/PD? Structurally, cycasin consists of a glucose molecule attached to MAM. Thus, a priori, the compound might be able to enter the brain and its associated cells by transport systems designed to carry glucose. Indeed, the intact MAM-glycone has been detected in the brain of young adult rats treated with cycasin via a gastric tube (39). Apparently, therefore, some cycasin may escape the action of bacterial β-glucosidase, cross the intestinal wall, and enter the bloodstream as the intact, nonreactive glycone. If cycasin also traverses the blood-brain regulatory interface, as the rat studies suggest, the compound may be able to enter nerve cells. Recent tissue culture studies demonstrate a time-dependent increase in the concentration of cycasin both in treated mouse cortical explants and rat primary astrocyte cultures (21). Whereas astrocytes are morphologically unaffected by cycasin, low micromolar concentrations of the compound selectively induce neuronal degeneration in the CNS explants (21). This is associated with an increasing concentration of MAM, presumably from the intracellular cleavage of the cycasin molecule by cytoplasmic β-glucosidase (21). MAM is known to form an active free radical (methyldiazonium ion) that methylates amino acids, proteins, and nucleic acids. In particular, MAM forms adducts with guanine nucleotides (6-*O* and 7-methyl guanine) (51,52), and adduct formation is believed to underlie the hepatotoxic,

50. Hirono I, Kachi H, Kato T. A survey of acute toxicity of cycads and mortality rate from cancer in the Miyako islands. Acta Pathol Jpn 1970;20:327–337.

51. Shank RC, Magee PN. Similarities between the biochemical actions of cycasin and dimethylnitrosamine. Biochem J 1967;105:521–527.

52. Matsumoto H, Higa HH. Studies on methylazoxymethanol, the aglycone of cycasin: methylation of nucleic acids in vitro. Biochem J 1966;98:20C–22C.

53. Wogan GN, Busby WF Jr. Naturally occurring carcinogens. In: Liener IE, ed. Toxic constituents of plant foodstuffs. New York: Academic Press 1980:329–369.

54. Nagata Y, Matsumoto H. Studies on methylazoxymethanol: Methylation of nucleic acids in the fetal rat brain. Proc Soc Exp Biol Med 1969;132:383–383.

55. Haddad RK, Rabe A, Dumas R. Comparison of the effects of methylazoxymethanol on brain development in different species. Fed Proc 1972;31:1520–1523.

56. Neuroteratogenicity of methylazoxymethanol acetate: Behavioral deficits of ferrets with transplancentally induced lissencephaly. Neurotoxicology 1979;1:171–189.

57. Cedar H. DNA methylation and gene activity. Cell 1988;53:3–4.

58. Enver T, Zhang JW, Papayannopoulou T, Stamatoyannoupoulos. DNA methylation: A secondary event in globin gene switching? Genes Dev 1988;2:698–706.

59. Bird AP. CpG-rich islands and the function of DNA methylation. Nature 1986;321: 209–213.

60. Seyfert VL, McMahon SB, Glenn WD, Yellen AJ, Sukhatme VP, Cao X, Monroe JG. Methylation of an immediate-early inducible gene as a mechanism for B cell tolerance induction. Science 1990;250797–800.

61. Yisraeli J, Adeslstein RS, Melloul D, Nudel U, Yaffe D, Cedar H. Muscle-specific activation of a methylated chimeric actin gene. Cell 1986;46:409–416.

62. Busslinger M, Hurst J, Flavell RA. DNA methylation and the regulation of globin gene expression. Cell 1983;34:197–206.

63. Barrows LR, Shank RC, Magee PN. S-Adenosylmethionine metabolism and DNA methylation in hydrazine-treated rats. Carcinogenesis 1983;4:953–957.

64. Tan N-W, Li FL. Interaction of oligonucleotides containing 6-O-methylguanine with human DNA (cytosine-5-)-methyltransferase. Biochemistry 29:9234–9240, 1990.

65. Spencer PS, Allen RG, Kisby GE, Ludolph AC. Excitotoxic disorders. Science 1990;248:144.

66. Gajdusek DC. Cycad toxicity not the cause of high-incidence amyotrophic lateral sclerosis/Parkinsonism-dementia on Guam, Kii Peninsula of Japan, or in West New Guinea. In: Hudson AJ, ed. Amyotrophic lateral sclerosis: Concepts in pathogenesis and etiology. Toronto: University of Toronto Press, 1990:317–325.

27

Neurotransmitters and Second Messengers in Amyotrophic Lateral Sclerosis

Benjamin Rix Brooks

University of Wisconsin—Madison, School of Medicine, and William S. Middleton Memorial Veterans Affairs Hospital Madison, Wisconsin

INTRODUCTION

Amyotrophic lateral sclerosis (ALS) is a neurodegenerative disorder affecting the motor system, consisting of motor neurons in the motor cortex, brainstem, and spinal cord as well as interneurons within these regions. The motor system employs excitatory amino acids, such as glutamate (Glu), in corticofugal pathways to spinal cord neurons (1). Glu is a type I neurotransmitter that may gate Na and K channels and affect Ca uptake. The motor system also employs acetylcholine (ACh), which is released by motor neuron collaterals to act at nicotinic receptors on Renshaw cells in the spinal cord (2) or is released by motor neuron axons to act at nicotinic receptors of neuromuscular junctions (3). ACh is a type II neurotransmitter that may gate Na and K channels. The motor system also employs peptides such as calcitonin gene-related peptide (CGRP) as type III neurotransmitters (4). These neuropeptides modulate the action of neurotransmitters or mediate trophic effects. CGRP will enhance ACh-induced depolarization at the neuromuscular junction (5) and increase synthesis of nictonic acetylcholine receptors (AChR) in striated muscle (6).

The pathological changes that occur in ALS suggest more widespread involvement of other neuronal systems (7). The neurotransmitter changes that occur in ALS include alterations in central nervous system (CNS) tissue content of excitatory and inhibitory amino acids (type I neurotransmitters), acetylcholine and biogenic amines (type II neurotransmitters), peptides (type III neurotransmitters), and neurotransmitter receptors. In addition, ALS patients also have changes in the cerebrospinal fluid (CSF) content of amino acids (type I neurotransmitters), amines (type II neurotransmitters), peptides (type III neurotransmitters), and cyclic nucleotides, calcium-calcium binding protein, or polyphosphoinositides (second messengers). These neurochemical changes may provide insight concerning the pathogenetic mechanisms of the underlying degenerative processes that occur in ALS.

TYPE I NEUROTRANSMITTERS—AMINO ACIDS

Evidence for Neurotransmitter Role of Amino Acids

The putative amino acid neurotransmitters occur in the highest (micromolar) concentration in the CNS (8). The excitatory dicarboxylic amino acids are aspartate (Asp) and Glu (9). Inhibitory amino acids are glycine (Gly), gamma-aminobutyric acid (GABA), and taurine (10). The types of evidence for the role of amino acids in a particular synaptic pathway include (a) immunocytochemical localization of the amino acid to particular regions and pathways, (b) reduction in the endogenous concentration of the amino acid in a particular CNS region following lesions of the pathway to that region, (c) reduction in high-affinity uptake of the amino acid following lesions of the pathway to that region, and (d) release of amino acid on stimulation either in vivo or in vitro (11).

These forms of evidence provide the basis for the putative assignments of the anatomical localization and function for type I amino acid neurotransmitters in the spinal cord (Table 1). Some evidence is consistent with Glu being an excitatory transmitter on motor neurons and interneurons for the corticospinal tract and involved in input to the dorsal horn from the dorsal root ganglion (12). Asp is an excitatory transmitter for interneurons and possibly for dorsal root ganglion cells (13). While Glu is more abundant throughout the CNS, proportionately more Asp than Glu is present in the ventral horn compared with the dorsal horn (14). There is evidence that Gly is a inhibitory transmitter on motor neurons, interneurons, and 1a interneurons for Renshaw cells and 1a inhibitory interneurons in the spinal cord (15). GABA is an inhibitory neurotransmitter of interneurons on 1a afferents and motor neurons (16).

Excitatory Amino Acids

Glu and Asp occur in micromolar concentrations in the CNS. Glu and Asp are nonessential amino acids synthesized from glucose via (a) alpha-ketoglutarate through transamination in mitochondria in nerve endings or glia, (b) alpha-ketoglutarate through reversal of glutamate dehydrogenase, (c) glutamine through glutaminase activity in nerve endings (Fig. 1), and (d) ornithine through transamination and dehydrogenation (17). The metabolic pools and transmitter

Table 1 Neurotransmitters in the Ventral Horn of the Spinal Cord

Transmitter	Cells of origin	Site of action	Direct action	References
•Type I neurotransmitter				
Asparate	Interneurons	Motor neurons	Excitation	1,11,13,29
(Asp)	DRG neurons	Interneurons	Excitation	
		Motor neurons	Excitation	
Glutamate	Corticospinal	Motor neurons	Excitation	1,9,11
(Glu)	neurons	Interneurons	Excitation	
	DRG (la afferent) neurons	Motor neurons	Excitation	
Gamma-amino butyric	Interneurons	la afferents	Presynaptic inhibition	16,21,24
acid		Motor neurons	Postsynaptic	
(GABA)			inhibition	
	Bulbospinal neurons	Motor neurons	Inhibition	
Glycine	Renshaw neurons	Motor neurons	Inhibition	1,2,22
(Gly)		la interneurons	Inhibition	
		Renshaw neurons	Inhibition	
	la inhibitory interneurons	Motor neurons	Inhibition	
•Type II neurotransmitter				
Acetylcholine	Motor neurons	Muscle (nicotinic)	Excitation	56,57,59, 62,63
(ACh)		Motor neurons (recurrent collateral)	Presynaptic Inhibition	
		Renshaw neurons (nicotinic)	Excitation	
	Propriospinal neurons	Motor neurons (muscarinic)	Excitation	
	Supraspinal neurons	Interneurons (muscarinic)	Excitation	
		Motor neurons (muscarinic)	Excitation	
Norepineph- rine (NE)	Locus ceruleus neurons	Inhibitory Interneurons	Inhibition	72,78–80
		Motor neurons	Facilitation/ inhibition	
Serotonin (5HT)	Raphe obscuris/ palidus neurons	Interneurons	Facilitation	77,121–123
		Motor neurons	Facilitation/ inhibition	
	Intrinsic neurons	?	?	

Table 1 Continued.

Transmitter	Cells of origin	Site of action	Direct action	References
• Type III neurotransmitter				
Colocalized with cholinergic neurons				
Calcitonin	Motor neurons	Muscle (nicotinic)	Facilitation	5,162
gene-related	DRG neurons	Interneurons	Facilitation	
peptide (CGRP)				
Colocalized with catecholaminergic neurons				
Neuropeptide	Locus ceruleus	Interneurons	Inhibition/	170
Y (NPY)	neurons		facilitation	
		Motor neurons	Inhibition/	
			facilitation	
	Intrinsic neurons	?	?	
Colocalized with serotoninergic neurons				
Enkephalin	Raphe obscuris/			
(ENK)	palidus neurons	Motor neurons	Inhibition	162,174
	Intrinsic neurons	?	?	
Galanin	Raphe obscuris/			
(GAL)	palidus neurons	Interneurons	Inhibition	179,180
		Motor neurons	Inhibition	
Substance P	Raphe obscuris/			
(Sub P)	palidus neurons	Interneurons	Facilitation	148,183
		Motor neurons	Facilitation	
	DRG neurons	Motor neurons	Facilitation	
	Intrinsic neurons	?	?	
Thyrotropin-	Raphe obscuris/			
releasing	palidus neurons	Interneurons	Facilitation/	148,183,197
hormone			inhibition	
(TRH)		Motor neurons	Facilitation/	
			inhibition	
	Intrinsic neurons	Interneurons	?	
Hypothalamic and other peptides				
Arginine	Parvocellular			
vasopres-	paraventricular	Interneurons	Variable	230
sin (AVP)	hypothalamic			
	neurons			
Cholecysto-	Supraspinal	Interneurons	Facilitation	236
kinin	neurons	Motor neurons	Facilitation	
(CCK)				
	DRG neurons	Interneurons	Facilitation	
	Intrinsic neurons	?	?	
Somatostatin	DRG neurons	Interneurons	Inhibition	257
(SOM)	Intrinsic neurons	?	?	
Vasoactive	DRG neurons	Interneurons	Facilitation	269
intestinal				
polypeptide (VIP)				

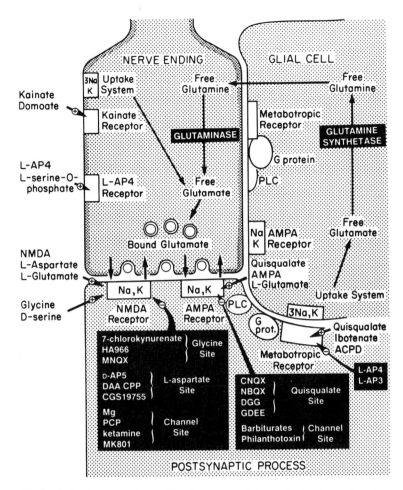

Figure 1 Excitatory amino acidergic neuron. Schematic drawing of excitatory amino acidergic neuron showing relationship of presynaptic nerve ending to glial cell and postsynaptic process. Four types of ionotropic excitatory amino acid receptor [NMDA (*N*-methyl-D-aspartate), AMPA (alpha-amino-3-hydroxy-5-methyl-4-isoxazoepropionate), L-AP4 (2-amino-4-phosphonobutyrate), kainate] are demonstrated with the appropriate agonists or positive modulators defined by positive (+) arrows. The metabotropic receptor is linked to a G protein and phospholipase C (PLC). The uptake of glutamate as well as its shunting through glutamine in glial cells and the presynaptic nerve endings is due to glutamine synthetase in glial cells and glutaminase in the presynaptic nerve ending. The inhibitors or negative modulators of the NMDA, AMPA, and metabotropic receptors are represented by white type in the black boxes designated with negative (−) arrows: HA996, 1-hydroxy-3-aminopyrrolidin-2-one; D-AP5, 2-amino-5-phosphopentanoate; CPP, 3-(2-carobypeperazin-4-yl)-propyl-1-phosphonate; CGS19755, 2-phosphono-methyl-2-piperidine carboxylate; PCP, phencyclidine; CNQX, 6-cyano-7-nitroquinoxoline2,3-dione; NBQX, 2,3-dihydroxy-6-nitro-7-sulfamoylbenzoquinoxaline; DGG, gamma-D-glutamylglycine; GDEE, glutamic acid diethylester; L-AP3-2-amino-3-phosphonopropionate.

pools are not distinguished, but some evidence supports vesicle localization of Glu and Asp. Glu is more concentrated than Asp, but Glu is nearly twice as concentrated in the intermediate horn (lamina VII) and ventral horn (laminar VIII and IX) than the dorsal horn (Fig. 2), while Asp is seven times more concentrated in the intermediate horn and four times more concentrated in the ventral horn than the dorsal horn.

Actions of Excitatory Amino Acids

Glu and Asp mediate, sometimes at subpicomolar concentrations, excitation depolarization potentials with effects on sodium and calcium influx as well as potassium efflux (11). These rapid–onset/offset "ionotropic" effects are mediated through at least four classes of receptors (18). These receptors are more commonly present on cell soma and major dendrites rather than secondary dendrites. The N-methyl-D-aspartate (NMDA) receptor is activated by Asp slightly better than Glu in some species. Three other receptor types are defined by their affinity for quisqualate (QA), kainate (KA), and 2-amino-4-phosphonobutyrate (L-AP4). They are all present in the spinal cord, though more abundantly in the dorsal horn. The effective concentrations for excitation by Glu or Asp may be femtomolar to nanomolar with instantaneous onset and rapid offset of action (19). The excitation potentials are not blocked by tetrodotoxin, indicating that the sodium ionic conductance is not involved. Both high-affinity (nanomolar), easily saturated, low-capacity uptake systems which are associated with glial and neuronal elements of synapses and moderate-affinity (micromolar), high-capacity uptake systems associated with glia are involved in rapidly removing synaptically active amino acids (20).

Inhibitory Amino Acids

Gly, GABA, and taurine are inhibitory amino acids present in micromolar concentrations in the CNS (21). Gly is a nonessential amino acid derived from glucose via serine. While Gly is less concentrated than Glu in the CNS, Gly is more concentrated in the spinal cord than in other CNS regions. Moreover, Gly is six times more concentrated in the intermediate horn and eight times more concentrated in the ventral horn (Fig. 2) relative to its concentration in the dorsal horn (14).

Actions of Inhibitory Amino Acids

Gly is associated with flat vesicles, and the effective concentration for inhibition by Gly is micromolar at a receptor that binds strychnine at nanomolar concentrations (22). Gly-induced inhibition is mediated through modulation of chloride permeability. This inhibition has a shorter ontime when glycine is released near

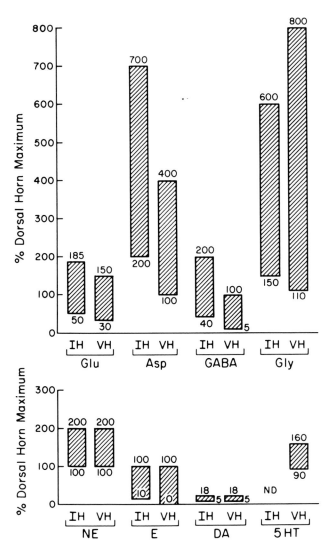

Figure 2 Spinal cord content of type I and type II neurotransmitters. Spinal cord content of type I (amino acid) neurotransmitters, glutamate (Glu), aspartate (Asp), gamma-aminobutyric acid (GABA), glycine (Gly), and type III (biogenic amine) neurotransmitters, norepinephrine (NE), epinephrine (E), dopamine (DA), serotonin (5HT), are expressed as the 95% confidence limit of the concentration (micromoles or picomoles/wet weight) for each transmitter in the Rexed lamina VII intermediate horn (IH) or Rexed lamina VIII and IX ventral horn (VH) of mammalian spinal cord. The concentrations are presented as a percent of the maximum observed Rexed laminae I–V dorsal horn concentration as adapted and recalculated from several sources (14,75,112–115). Intermediate horn concentrations for serotonin were not done (ND).

the cell soma than on distal dendrites, while Glu excitation has a shorter ontime following dendritic application. Therefore, Gly neurons are more likely to provide axosomatic synapses. Moderate (micromolar)-affinity Gly uptake systems are located synaptically (neurons and glia) and are responsible for inactivation (23).

While Gly is more concentrated in the spinal cord compared with other regions of the CNS, GABA and taurine play a role in a number of areas throughout the CNS (22). In the spinal cord, GABA and taurine are inhibitory amino acids concentrated primarily in lamina II of the dorsal horn, where they play a role in presynaptic inhibition of primary afferent terminals. GABA in some parts of the intermediate horn (lamina VII) is more concentrated (Fig. 2) than in the ventral horn (lamina VIII, IX). GABA in the neuronal pool is present primarily in interneurons, but there is a projection of GABAergic neurons to spinal cord motor neurons from neurons in the brainstem (24). GABA is a nonessential amino acid derived from glucose via Glu formed by transamination of alpha-ketoglutarate (Fig. 3). Glu is decarboxylated to GABA by glutamic acid decarboxylase [GAD] present in neurons and in axoaxonal, axodendritic, and axosomatic terminals (16). The GABA shunt involves uptake of released GABA by glial cells and transamination by mitochondrial GABA transaminase to give succininic semialdehyde. This same enzyme will form Glu from alpha-ketoglutarate. The resultant Glu is subsequently changed to $GluNH_2$ by glutamine synthetase in glial cells because GAD is absent from these cells. In the other parts of the CNS, GABA is removed from the extracellular space by moderate (micromolar)-affinity, temperature- and sodium-dependent GABA uptake systems. The uptake system in neurons is specifically blocked by 2,4-diaminobutyric acid or nipecotic acid, while the uptake system in glia is blocked by beta-alanine. In the spinal cord, this distinction of neuronal and glial uptake systems by specific blockers is lacking (25). GABA receptors are identified pharmacologically and by binding studies. Care must be taken in binding studies that very high-affinity (nanomolar) enzymes are distinguished from other binding sites. The $GABA_A$ receptor is sensitive to bicuculline and muscimol and insensitive to baclofen. It is located at the spinal level extrasynaptically on root fibers and reacts to micromolar amounts of GABA by inhibiting further release of GABA. The $GABA_B$ receptor is insensitive to bicuculline, slightly sensitive to muscimol, and sensitive to baclofen. It is located presynaptically in the dorsal horn and responds to millimolar amounts of GABA by modulating influx of calcium via changes in membrane conductance to chloride ions. The $GABA_B$ receptor mediates GABA-induced decreases in Glu, NE, DA, and 5-HT release (21). The GABA-induced chloride channel opening is nearly four times the Gly-induced chloride channel opening (22).

Much less is known about taurine other than it is synthesized from cysteine via the decarboxylation of cysteinsulfinic acid to hypotaurine, which is subsequently

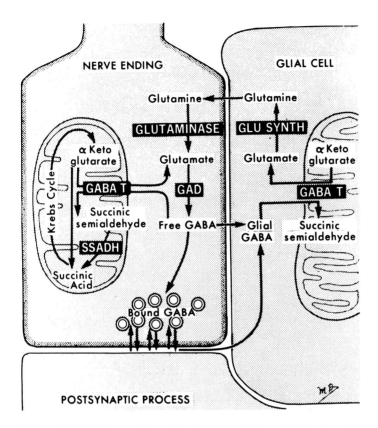

Figure 3 Inhibitory amino acidergic neuron. Schematic drawing of inhibitory amino acidergic neuron showing relationship of presynaptic nerve ending to glial cell and postsynaptic process. Released GABA is taken up by glia and metabolically linked to glutamine production via GABA transaminase (GABA T) and glutamine synthetase (GLU SYNTH). Free glutamine from the glial cell may move to the nerve ending, where it can be changed to glutamate by glutaminase and GABA by glutamic acid decarboxylase (GAD). Enzymes are printed as white type in black boxes and substrates as black type against white background. [Reproduced with permission (21).]

transformed to taurine. The effective inhibitory concentration on motor neurons is in the millimolar range and is mediated through chloride permeability changes. Uptake systems exist in brain tissue to concentrate taurine, but the slow turnover of this substance suggests that the bulk of the taurine pool is not related to a transmitter function (26).

Effect of Toxins or Injuries on Amino Acid
Type I Neurotransmitters

Neurochemical changes (Table 2) in the spinal cord are unique for particular types of injuries and may provide insight into the pathogenesis of ALS (27). Peripheral nerve lesions or rhizotomies will decrease Glu and Asp in both the dorsal horn and ventral horn (14,16,28). Such lesions will increase Gly and decrease GABA in the dorsal horn, with no changes in these amino acids in the ventral horn. Cordotomies or transections will decrease Glu and Asp in both dorsal and ventral horns below the lesion (14,16,29). Gly and GABA will be decreased in both ventral horns by such lesions without any change in the dorsal horn concentrations.

Effect of ALS on Amino Acid Type I Neurotransmitters

Changes in the amino acid content of CNS tissue in ALS have been extensively studied with various techniques (30–32). In several brain and spinal cord regions, tissue levels of Glu, Asp, and GABA, as well as N-acetyl-aspartyl glutamate (NAAG) and N-acetyl-aspartate (NAA), have been shown to be decreased (33,34). The decrease in tissue amino acids is consistent with both descending tract and peripheral lesions (Table 2) but could also be consistent with an excitotoxic mechanism. The difficulty is that the decrease in Glu is seen in multiple CNS regions in ALS patients. Thus the observed neurochemical changes cannot be due to descending tract or peripheral lesions. Taurine, an inhibitory amino acid, has been reported to be increased in ALS frontal cortex, thalamus, and spinal cord, compared with controls (30).

In only some studies have the synthetic or catabolic enzymes been studied in ALS tissue (34,35). Glutamate dehydrogenase (GDH) activity is normal in the ventral horn and increased in the dorsal horn (35). These findings may reflect induction of enzyme activity in response to decreased tissue levels of glutamate or increased activity of glutaminergic pathways to the dorsal horn. GAD activity is normal in ALS spinal cord as is the activity of N-acetylated-alpha-linked acidic dipeptidase, which catabolizes NAAG to Glu and NAA (34).

Amino acid receptors have been studied in ALS (36–38). Gly receptors have been shown to be decreased in ALS patients throughout several spinal cord areas compared to controls in two studies (36,37). Moreover, in association with the general decrease in Gly receptors, there is no significant decrease in the ventral horn over the dorsal horn (Fig. 2). Benzodiazepine receptors were also decreased in one patient but specifically in the ventral horn (37,38). Further studies are required. In particular, the distribution of NMDA receptors and specific GABA receptors must be studied in ALS.

The CSF concentrations of Glu, Asp, NAAG, and NAA (Fig. 4) are reported

Table 2 Effect of Peripheral and Descending Tract Injuries and ALS on Neurotransmitters in the Ventral Horn of the Spinal Cord

Transmitter		Peripheral lesion	Central lesion	ALS	References
Type I neurotransmitter					
Asparate (Asp)	Dorsal horn	Decrease	Decrease	Decrease	30–34,
	Ventral horn	Decrease	Decrease	Decrease	39–42
Glutamate	Dorsal horn	Decrease	Decrease	Decrease	30–34,
(Glu)	Ventral horn	Decrease	Decrease	Decrease	39–42
				Increase in CSF	
Gamma-amino	Dorsal horn	Decrease	No change	?/No change	30,36,
butyric acid	Ventral horn	No change	Decrease	?/No change	39–42,
(GABA)				No change/	44,45
				Decrease in CSF	
Glycine (Gly)	Dorsal horn	Increase	No change	?/No change	30,36,
	Ventral horn	No change	Decrease	?/No change	39–42,
				No change/	44,45
				increase in CSF	
Type II neurotransmitter					
Acetylcholine	Dorsal horn	No change	Decrease	Decrease	68,71
(ACh)	Ventral horn	No change	No change	Decrease	
				Decrease in thiamine	
				pyrophosphate in CSF	
Norepinephrine	Dorsal horn	Decrease	Decrease	?/No change	42,98,
(NE)	Ventral horn	?	Decrease	?/No change	102,103
				Increase in NE in	
				CSF	
Serotonin	Dorsal horn	Decrease	Decrease	?	108,110
(5HT)	Ventral horn	?	Decrease	?	
				No change in	
				5HIAA in CSF	
Type III neurotransmitter					
Colocalized with cholinergic neurons					
Calcitonin gene-	Dorsal horn	Decrease	No change	?	156
related peptide	Ventral horn	No change	No change	Decrease	
(CGRP)					
Colocalized with serotoninergic neurons					
Enkephalin	Dorsal horn	Increase	No change	?	156
(ENK)	Ventral horn	No change	No change	?/Decreased fibers	
Substance P	Dorsal horn	Decrease	No change	No change	189–192,
(Sub P)	Ventral horn	No change	Decrease	?/Decrease and	194,195
				decreased fibers	
				No change in CSF	

Table 2 Continued

Transmitter		Peripheral lesion	Central lesion	ALS	References
Thyrotropin-	Dorsal horn	No change	Decrease	No change	156,215–
releasing	Ventral horn	?/No change	Decrease	?/Decrease and	217,223
hormone				decreased fibers	
(TRH)				No change/decrease in CSF	
Hypothalamic and other peptides					
Arginine	Dorsal horn	No change	Decrease	?	232–234
vasopressin	Ventral horn	No change	Decrease	?	
(AVP)				Increase/decrease in CSF	
Cholecystokinin	Dorsal horn	Decrease	No change	No change	238
(CCK)	Ventral horn	No change	No change	No change	
				No change in CSF	
Oxytocin (OXY)	Dorsal horn	No change	Decrease	?	233
	Ventral horn	No change	Decrease	?	
				No change in CSF	
Somatostatin	Dorsal horn	Decrease	No change	?	195
(SOM)	Ventral horn	No change	Decrease	?	
				No change in CSF	
Vasoactive	Dorsal horn	Increase	No change	?	238
intestinal	Ventral horn	No change	No change	?	
polypeptide				Decrease in CSF	
(VIP)					

to be increased in some studies (34) and not increased in other studies (39–42). The techniques being applied are changing with more precision afforded by the use of high-pressure liquid chromatography (43). In several studies, however, lysine elevations (41,42) are confirmed in ALS, while increases in glycine have been seen in only one study (44). CSF GABA in ALS patients is normal (42) or decreased slightly in severe cases (45).

Role of Excitotoxic Amino Acids in the Pathogenesis of ALS

Injection of millimolar amounts of kainic acid into the ventral horn will produce a specific motor neuron cell death and loss with gliosis (46). The neurochemistry of this specific lesion has not yet been studied in spinal cord, but in the hippocampus, micromolar amounts of Glu will induce dendritic atrophy (47), which is an important early feature of the pathology of ALS (48). In motor neurons cultured with interneurons, Glu-activated NMDA receptors are nearly twice as

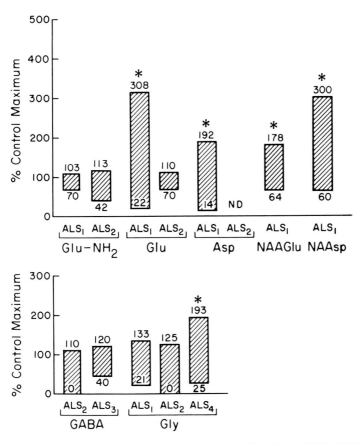

Figure 4 Amino acid neurotransmitters (excitotoxic amino acids) in CSF. Amino acids, glutamine (Glu-NH2), glutamate (Glu), aspartate (Asp), gamma-aminobutyric acid (GABA), glycine (Gly), and peptides, *N*-acetyl-aspartyl-glutamate (NAAGlu), *N*-acetyl-aspartate (NAAsp), in the cerebrospinal fluid (CSF) adapted and recalculated from several studies [ALS$_1$ (34); ALS$_2$ (42); ALS$_3$ (45); ALS$_4$ (44)] are presented as the 95% confidence limit of the CSF concentration calculated as a percent of the maximum observed in the control CSF. Glutamate and aspartate were significantly ($p < 0.05$; *) elevated in one study (ALS$_1$) but not in a second study (ALS$_2$). These differences may depend on the preparation of the samples and the methods employed (43). CSF NAAGlu and NAAsp were significantly elevated (34) but CSF Gly was elevated in only one study (44).

common as Glu-activated kainate receptors, but the channel opening time is longer with the latter receptor. However, when grown in the absence of interneurons, motor neurons display only the kainate receptor, potentially making them more susceptible to this excitotoxic amino acid (49). These findings suggest that interneurons may play a role in whether motor neurons are susceptible to excitotoxic effects of amino acid neurotransmitters at different times in the disease (50).

Kainic acid injections in the olfactory bulb will result in depletion of Glu and thyrotropin-releasing hormone (TRH) as well as muscarinic ACh receptors, TRH receptors, and benzodiazepine receptors. These neurochemical findings are similar to those observed in ALS (30,37,51). Moreover, excitotoxic lesions in the cerebral cortex that decrease cortical Glu result in an increase of neuropeptide Y without a change in norepinephrine (52). Although excitotoxic amino acids may produce some neurochemical abnormalities such as seen in ALS, the current working hypotheses are focused on (a) presumed elevated synaptic levels of Glu which have not been demonstrated, (b) putative potentiation by Gly of Glu-mediated neurotoxicity through enhanced recovery from Glu-induced desensitization, and (c) a possible decrease in GDH activity that has not been found in the spinal cord of ALS patients (53). Despite some inconsistencies with the excitotoxic pathogenesis theories of ALS, the possible role of environmental excitotoxic amino acids which may be exogenously administered through dietary intake is coming under increasing scrutiny and the neurochemistry of the lesions induced by these substances administered orally should be studied (54). More research is required to characterize the neurochemical changes in experimentally induced excitotoxic amino acid motor neuron degeneration. Special attention should be paid to other endogenous excitotoxic amino acids, such as quinolinic acid, and endogenous antagonists, such as kynurenic acid, in ALS (55).

TYPE II NEUROTRANSMITTERS—ACETYLCHOLINE, CATECHOLAMINES, AND SEROTONIN

Evidence for Neurotransmitter Role of Acetylcholine and Biogenic Amines

Acetylcholine (ACh), norepinephrine (NE), epinephrine (E), dopamine (DA), and serotonin (5-HT) are present in the CNS in nanomolar concentrations. Historically, these transmitters were recognized prior to the amino acid neurotransmitters. ACh and biogenic amines may have "ionotropic" effects following synaptic release by opening ion channels and affecting membrane potential. However, the principal changes induced by these neurotransmitters are "metabotropic" effects with slower onset/offset that may require second messengers to change postsynaptic membranes and potentials as well as biochemical and metabolic events (56). The types of evidence for the role of these chemicals in a particular synaptic pathway include (a) immunocytochemical localization of the neurotransmitter or its synthetic enzymes to particular regions and pathways, (b) reduction in the endogenous concentration of the neurotransmitter following lesions of the pathway to that region, (c) increment in the receptors for the neurotransmitter or decrement in the high-affinity uptake of the neurotransmitter following lesions of the pathway to that region, and (d) release of neurotransmitter on stimulation either in vivo or in vitro (56).

Acetylcholine

Multiple cholinergic neuronal systems occur in the CNS (Fig. 5). The motor system includes large pyramidal Betz cells in the motor cortex projecting to the spinal cord via the corticospinal tract and large pyramidal anterior horn cells in the spinal cord projecting to muscles in the periphery. However, local spinal cord neuronal circuits, such as the Renshaw cells, have provided the strongest evidence to date of the type described above for ACh as a neurotransmitter.

Actions of ACh

ACh is a type II neurotransmitter that may gate Na and K channels. Nearly 85% of motor neurons are depolarized by ACh with prolonged depolarization (57). ACh is released by motor neuron collaterals to act at nicotinic receptors on Renshaw cells in the spinal cord (2) or is released by motor neuron axons to act at nicotinic receptors of neuromuscular junctions (3). These effects are not reproduced by intracellular injection of cyclic guanosine monophosphate (cGMP) by iontophoresis (58). Renshaw cells comprise an inhibitory feedback circuit which includes a cholinergic axon collateral from alpha-motoneurons to depolarize the Renshaw cell, which in turn hyperpolarizes with Gly the alpha-motoneuron. Only 30% of interneurons are activated by iontophoretic Ach at concentrations higher than required to activate Renshaw cells by axon collaterals from motoneurons. Therefore, other transmitter mechanisms are probably involved in presynaptic inhibition (59).

ACh is synthesized by choline acetyltransferase (ChAT) from choline and acetyl coenzyme A. ChAT is present as a cytoplasmic enzyme and a membrane-bound enzyme that may be associated with ACh in the synaptosomal fraction (60). It has a micromolar K_m for acetyl coenzyme A and a millimolar K_m for choline. Spinal cord ChAT is higher in the ventral horn than the dorsal horn. The proportion of ChAT in the ventral horn is higher in the cervical than the lumbar spinal cord (61). Synthesis is limited by the access to acetyl coenzyme A synthesized via thiamine pyrophosphate–dependent pyruvate dehydrogenase in the mitochondria and to choline which is taken up into the nerve endings. Many tissues have a low-affinity (10–100 micromolar) uptake system while neurons

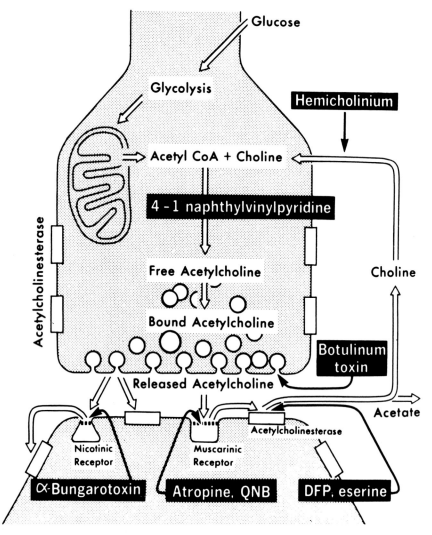

Figure 5 Cholinergic neuron. Schematic drawing of cholinergic neuron showing relationship of presynaptic nerve ending to postsynaptic process. Production of acetylcholine by choline acetyltransferase is inhibited by 4-1 napththylvinylpyridine. Uptake of choline is inhibited by hemicholinium. Vesicle release is inhibited by botulinum toxin. Either predominantly nicotinic receptors or muscarinic receptors are present postsynaptically. Nicotinic receptors are inhibited by alpha-bungarotoxin while muscarinic receptors are inhibited by atropine or quinuclidinylbenzilate (QNB). Acetylcholine esterase is inhibited by eserine or diisopropyl fluorophosphate (DFP). Inhibitors are printed as white type in black boxes. [Reproduced with permission (62).]

have a moderate-affinity (1–5 micromolar) uptake system. Free choline in the brain is 25–45 micromolar (62). Acetylcholine esterase (AChE) is primarilly a membrane-bound enzyme that breaks down ACh to choline and acetate. Half the choline used for ACh synthesis is derived from reuptake of choline derived from enzymatically cleaved ACh. Phosphatidylcholine is also a potential source for choline (63).

Both nicotinic and muscarinic cholinergic receptors are present in the spinal cord but only muscarinic receptors have been mapped. Muscarinic receptors measured by N-methyl scopolamine (NMS) or quinuclidinyl benzilate (QNB) are more concentrated in the ventral horn than the intermediate horn of the spinal cord from control subjects (37,64). These findings are not explained by the postmortem changes that may occur (65).

Effect of Toxins or Injuries on Cholinergic Type II Neurotransmitters

Chronic motor neuron loss following subacute or chronic nonreversible AChE inhibitor toxins has been demonstrated with consequent decrease in ChAT and AChE (66). Peripheral nerve lesions or rhizotomies will only minimally affect AChE activity in the dorsal or ventral horns. Very proximal ventral rhizotomies will cause loss of neurons in lamina VIII and IX with resultant loss of ChAT (63). Transections of the spinal cord will lead to accumumlation of AChE on the side of the transection proximal to the cell body of AChE-positive neurons (67).

Effect of ALS on Cholinergic Type II Neurotransmitters

The cholinergic neuronal enzyme for ACh synthesis (ChAT) in ALS spinal cord is significantly decreased in the ventral horn of the spinal cord (Fig. 6) measured biochemically (68). ChAT activity is near normal or slightly decreased in individual surviving neurons measured biochemically compared with controls (69). However, lactic dehydrogenase (LDH) activity is slightly increased (70). This finding suggests that motor neurons with increased LDH activity may be more resistant to ALS. Muscarinic receptors measured by the two different ligands, QNB and NMS, are also decreased in the spinal cords of ALS patients (64,65). These changes are more evident in the ventral horn in lamina VIII and IX than in the intermediate horn in lamina VII (Fig. 7). Choline uptake systems are not changed overall but are increased in lamina IX in the sacral spinal cord in some patients (Fig. 8). AChE activity in the ventral horn of the spinal cord of ALS patients is also decreased (68).

CSF thiamine pyrophosphate, a cofactor for mitochondrial pyruvate dehydrogenase synthesis of coenzyme A, is decreased in ALS patients compared with

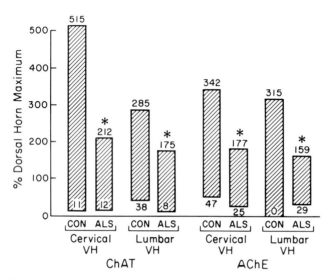

Figure 6 Neuronal cholinergic enzymes in ALS. Choline acetyltransferase (ChAT) and acetylcholine esterase (ChE) enzyme activities are presented as the 95% confidence limits relative to the maximum value measured in the dorsal horn in control (CON) and amyotrophic lateral sclerosis (ALS) patient spinal cords obtained at autopsy (61). ChAT activity is higher in the cervical than lumbar spinal cord ventral horn (VH). AChE is comparable in both the cervical and lumbar VH. Both ChAT and AChE activity is significantly ($P < 0.05$; *) decreased in the cervical and lumbar VH of ALS patients compared with controls.

controls (71). It is not clear, however, whether this might be due to decreased ChAT activity as a result of neuronal loss.

Catecholamines

Norepinephrine (NE) is the most prominent catecholamine in the spinal cord (72) compared with epinephrine (E) and dopamine (DA). The catecholamines in the spinal cord originate primarilly from projections of locus ceruleus in the lateral pons to the spinal cord ventral horn via the ventral and lateral funiculi of the spinal cord (73). These neurons (Fig. 9) may contain neuropeptide Y or as yet unidentified neuropeptides that can localize with either NE, E, or DA in terminal varicosities on the target neurons (74). NE is increased nearly twofold in the ventral horn compared with the dorsal horn (75). Moreover, NE is increased caudally in the spinal cord compared with more rostral segments (76).

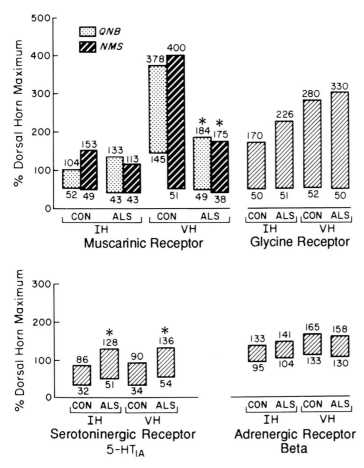

Figure 7 Spinal cord receptors in ALS. Receptors were measured by tissue autoradiography of bound radioactive ligands and quantitative densitometry. Muscarinic cholinergeric receptors were measured by binding of quinuclidinyl benzilate (QNB) and *N*-methyl scopolamine (NMS) in two different studies (37,64). Glycine receptors were measured by binding of strychnine (37). Serotoninergic receptors were measured by binding of 8-hydroxy-*N*,*N*-dipropyl-2-aminotetralin to define 5-HT$_{1A}$ receptors (64). Beta-adrenergic receptors were measured with pindolol (64). Receptor density is presented as the 95% confidence limits relative to the maximum value in Rexed laminae I–V in control (CON) subjects and amyotrophic lateral sclerosis (ALS) patients in Rexed lamnia VII intermediate horn (IH) and in Rexed lamina VIII and IX ventral horn (VH). Muscarinic cholinergic receptors are significantly ($p < 0.05$; *) reduced in the ventral horn but not the intermediate horn in two separate studies (37,64). Glycine receptor binding is significantly reduced throughout the CNS in ALS patients, but there is not a specific relative decrease in the ventral horn. 5-HT$_{1A}$ receptors, but not beta-adrenergic receptors, are significantly increased in both the intermediate and ventral horn of ALS patients.

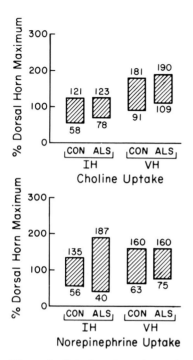

Figure 8 Spinal cord uptake mechanisms in ALS. Uptake into spinal cord tissue was measured by tissue autoradiography and quantitative densitometry (64). Choline uptake was measured with hemicholinium. Norepinephrine uptake was measured with desmethylimipramine. Uptake is presented as the 95% confidence limit relative to the maximum value in Rexed lamina I–V in control (CON) subjects and amyotrophic lateral sclerosis (ALS) patients in Rexed lamina VII intermediate horn (IH) and in Rexed laminae VIII and IX ventral horn (VH).

Actions of Catecholamines

Iontophoretic application of NE will cause primarilly depression of activity of motor neurons in only 50% of studied neurons, but may facillitate the action of Glu, which is directly excitatory (77). Stimulation of the locus ceruleus will cause facillitation of motor neurons and fusimotor neurons that can be blocked by phenoxybenzamine (78).

Dihydroxyphenylalanine (DOPA) is formed from tyrosine by soluble tyrosine hydroxylase, which is the limiting step in NA synthesis ln neuronal cytoplasm. The enzyme has a micromolar K_m for tyrosine similar to the tissue amino acid content and requires molecular oxygen and tetrahydrobiopterin as cofactors. It is present immunocytochemically in all catecholaminergic neurons but not sero-

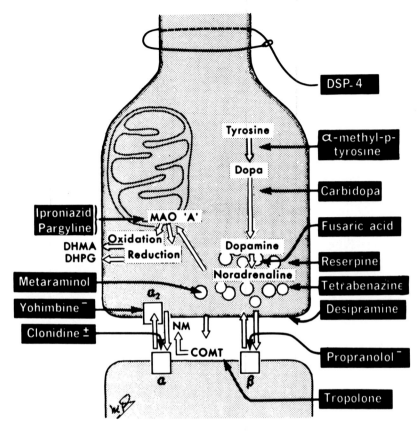

Figure 9 Noradrenergic neuron. Schematic drawing of noradrenergic neuron showing relationship of presynaptic nerve ending to postsynaptic process. Substrates as black type against white background. Inhibitors or pharmacological antagonists are represented by white type against black background: DSP-4, *N*-(chloroethyl)-*N*-ethyl-2-bromobenyla-mine. [Reproduced with permission (79).]

toninergic neurons (79). DOPA decarboyxlase is an aromatic amino acid decar-boxylase that requires pyridoxal phosphate as a cofactor to form DA (80). This aromatic amino acid decarboxylase is immunocytochemically present in both catecholaminergic and serotoninergic neurons. DA is the terminal product in dopaminergic neurons but the substrate for dopamine beta hydroxylase, a copper and ascorbic acid requiring enzyme present in storage vesicles of noradrenergic and adrenergic neurons that form NE or E (Fig. 10). DBH is immunocytochem-ically localized in noradrenergic and adrenergic neurons. E is formed from NE by phenylethanolamine-*N*-methyltransferase (PMNT), a *S*-adenosylmethionine-

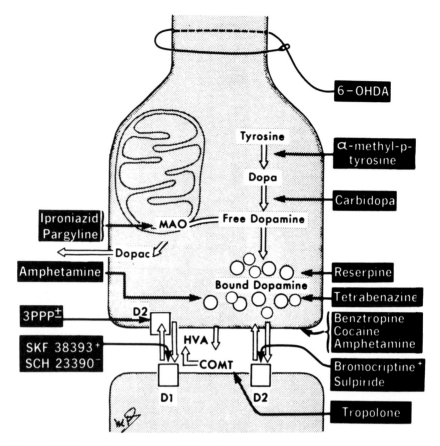

Figure 10   Dopaminergic neuron. Schematic drawing of dopaminergic neuron showing relationship of presynaptic nerve ending to postsynaptic process. Substrates as black type against white background. Inhibitors or pharmacological antagonists ($-$) and pharmacological agonists ($+$) are represented by white type against black background: 6-OHDA, 6-hydroxydopamine. [Reproduced with permission (79).]

requiring enzyme that is not localized in storage vesicles of adrenergic neurons (81).

Catabolism of these catacholamines occur via two forms of monoamine oxidases (MAO) localized primarilly in mitochondria (79). MAO-A catabolism of 5HT is 100% inhibited by clorgyline at concentrations that cause less than 30% inhibition of catecholamine breakdown (82). MAO-A is localized primarilly in noradrenergic, adrenergic, and dopaminergic neurons. MAO-B catabolism of catecholamines is 70% inhibited by deprenyl at concentrations that do not inhibit

5HT catabolism by this enzyme. MAO-B is primarilly localized in serotoninergic neurons and glia (83). Both membrane-bound and soluble catechol-*O*-methyl transferase (COMT) activities exists in the CNS, primarilly in glia, and result in methylation of catecholamines and their catabolites. The *O*-methylation of these substances is particularly effective in reducing their pharmacological activity. MAO catabolism proceeds initially to the aldehyde form of the monoamine with further oxidation to the acid under the control of the aldehyde oxidase or further reduction to the alcohol by alcohol dehydrogenase. NE in the brain and spinal cord is catabolized to primarilly dihydroxyphenylethylene glycol (DHPG) and 3-methoxy-4-hydroxyphenylethylene glycol (MHPG) via reduction (84). DA in brain and spinal cord is catabolized primarilly via oxidation to homovanillic acid (HVA).

Compared with cholinergic neurons where ACh is broken down by AChE and choline is taken up into the nerve terminals by an energy-dependent, moderate affinity (1–5 micromolar) uptake system, catecholaminergic neurons take up the active biogenic amine neurotransmitter via an energy-dependent slightly more efficient moderate affinity (0.2–1 micromolar) uptake system. Specificity to the type of neurotransmitter is shown by the differential capacity of desipramine to efficiently block NE uptake, while benztropine efficiently blocks DA uptake (79).

Biogenic amine receptors are membrane-bound proteins that uniquely bind agonist ligands and may be differentially linked to second-messenger systems. There are presynaptic autoreceptors in addition to postsynaptic receptors (85). Adrenergic receptors for NE differentially bind 2-[(2′,6′-dimethoxy) phenoxy-ethalolamino-] methylbenzodioxan (alpha-1) or clonidine (alpha-2). Alpha-1 receptors are antagonized by prazosin, are diffusely localized, and specific alpha-1 agonist binding is insensitive to guanine nucleotides, while alpha-2 receptors are antagonized by yohimbine, are present primarilly presynaptically, and specific alpha-2 agonist binding is decreased by guanine nucleotides. Alpha-2, but not alpha-1, adrenergic receptors inibit specific forms of adenylate cyclase (86). Adrenergic receptors for E differentially bind dihydroalprenol (beta-1) and iodohydroxybenzylpindol (beta-2). Beta-1 receptors are antagonized by practolol and are localized primarilly postsynaptically, while beta-2 receptors are antagonized by butoxamine and are present on glia and endothelial cells. Both types of beta-adrenergic receptors stimulate specific forms of postsynaptic adenylate cyclase in neurons or glia (87). Dopaminergic receptors for DA differentially bind 2,3,4,5-tetrahydro-7,8-dihydroxy-1-phenyl-1H-benzapine (D-1) or *N*-propyl(pyrazolo-3′,4′)-6,7-hexahydroquinoline (D-2). D-1 receptors are present postsynaptically, require micromolar concentrations of agonists for activation, and are antagonized specifically by SCH 23390, while D-2 receptors are localized both pre- and postsynaptically, require nanomolar concentrations of agonists, and are antagonized by sulpiride (88). Binding affinity of both receptor types is inhibited by guanine nucleotides. D-1 receptors are linked to postsynaptic adenylate cyclase, and agonists increase cyclic AMP production (89). D-2 receptors may be linked to inositol phospholipid second-messenger systems and may have no effect on adenylate cyclase or inhibit adenylate cyclase activity.

Effect of Toxins or Injuries on Catecholamine Type II Neurotransmitters

Nearly 90% depletion of ventral horn NE occurs following administration of 6-hydroxydopamine (90). Iminodipropionitrile (IDPN)-induced axonal neuropathy will increase NE transiently with minimal change in DA and a slight decrease in HVA (91). Methylmercury will increase cortical, caudate-putamen, and spinal cord NE and MHPG. DA is slightly increased but HVA is unchanged, while DOPAC is slightly decreased (92). Transection of the spinal cord results in a decrease in ventral horn NE and MHPG below the level of transection, as will chemical transection with calcium-induced spinal paralysis (93). Catecholamines in the intermediolateral column are not decreased by locus ceruleus lesions which decrease ventral horn NE but are decreased by lesions to the ventrolateral medulla (94). Local spinal cord NE-containing terminals survive chronic spinal cord transection but their origin is unclear (95). Dorsal rhizotomy will decrease ipsilateral DA before NE (96). Direct spinal cord trauma may transiently increase DA but NE is not increased (97).

Effect of ALS on Catecholaminergic Type II Neurotransmitters

NE measured in the CNS of patients with Parkinsonism and ALS was normal or slightly increased (98). DA is decreased in certain CNS regions (99). Spinal cord $beta_2$-adrenergic receptor binding measured with pindolol is similar in both the intermediate and ventral horns (Fig. 7) of controls and ALS patients (65,100). NE uptake in the spinal cord intermediate horn or ventral horn measured with desmethylimipramine does not change significantly (65). Deprenyl binding sites, however, are increased, particularly in the corticospinal tract of ALS patients (101).

Both plasma and CSF NE may be increased in ALS patients (45,102,103). Plasma NE release is significantly increased following transition from the supine to standing position in bulbar ALS patients compared with nonbulbar ALS patients and control subjects (104). CSF NE is increased particularly in more severely affected patients (102). In addition, 3-methoxy-4-hydroxyphenylethylene glycol (MHPG) and dihydroxyphenylacetic acid (DOPAC) are increased in the CSF, confirming not only increased NE production but also parallel increased catabolism (Fig. 11). E is not increased in the CSF of ALS patients compared with normal subjects (42).

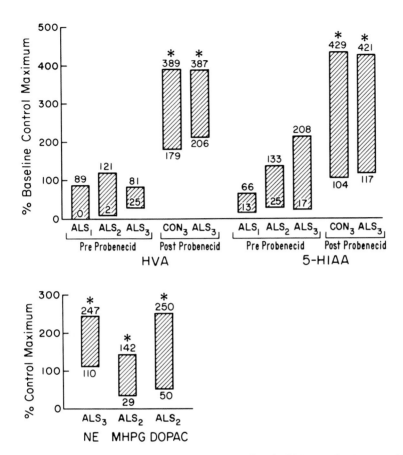

Figure 11 Amine neurotransmitters and metabolites in CSF. Baseline homovanillic acid (HVA), 5-hydroxyindole acetic acid (5-HIAA), norepinephrine (NE), 3-methoxy-4-hydroxyphenylethylene glycol (MHPG), and dihydroxyphenylacetic acid (DOPAC) were measured in the cerebrospinal fluid of control subjects (102,110) with other neurological and neuromuscular diseases (CON3) and amyotrophic lateral sclerosis patients from three studies [ALS₁ (108); ALS₂ (42); ALS₃ (102,110)]. Amine neurotransmitter and metabolite concentrations are presented as the 95% confidence limits relative to the baseline control maximum preprobenecid or the control maximum in patients who did not receive probenecid. Postprobenecid concentrations of HVA and 5-HIAA were significantly ($p <$ 0.05; *) increased in both CON3 and ALS3 patients, but there was no significant difference in baseline or postprobenecid values between control and ALS patients. NE, MHPG, and DOPAC were significantly increased in ALS patients compared with controls.

In contrast to changes in NE metabolism that have been confirmed in at least three laboratories (42,102,103), there is controversy concerning DA metabolism and accumulations of HVA. In earlier studies of ALS-Parkinsonism-dementia complex of Guam and occidental sporadic ALS, baseline and oral probenecid-augmented CSF HVA concentrations were reported to be decreased compared with control subjects with other neurological diseases (105–107). While HVA increased with L-dopa treatment, ALS symptoms persist (107). Recent studies of baseline CSF HVA concentrations have shown no difference from control subjects, although a gender effect on concentration was demonstrated (108). Intravenous probenecid administration, which produces a more rapid blockade of HVA transport from the CSF compartment that is a function of the CSF probenecid concentration, does not differentiate early sporadic ALS patients from neuromuscular disease control subjects of matched age, gender, and disability in terms of HVA turnover and DA metabolism (109,110). The earlier findings in ALS-Parkinsonism-dementia complex of Guam may have been contaminated with Parkinsonism patients, who definitely may show decreased DA and HVA CNS tissue concentrations and decreased HVA accumulation in the CSF (105,106). Indeed, ALS patients with signs of Parkinsonism may show decreased binding of fluorodopa in the globus pallidum bilaterally (111). The ALS patients reported in our study with intravenous probenecid did not manifest major or minor signs of Parkinsonism.

Serotonin

5-Hydroxytryptamine or serotonin [5HT] is increased nearly twofold in the ventral (laminar VIII and IX) horn compared with the dorsal (lamina I–V) horn (112–115). The origin of the dorsal horn serotonin is from bulbospinal neurons (Fig. 13) which originate in the raphe magnus of the midventral medulla and descend via tracts containing small myelinated and unmyelinated axons in the dorsolateral funiculus (116). Ventral horn serotonin results from bulbospinal neurons that originate in the raphe pontis of the inferior middorsal pons and the raphe obscurus of the inferior middorsal medulla. These neurons may also contain one or more neuropeptides that immunocytochemically colocalize with 5HT (117). Target motor neurons for 5HT terminals are more ventrolateral in the distribution of the extensor motor neuron pools (118). Contacts are preferentially axodendritic (>80%) rather than axosomatic (<20%) and can occur in the neuropil distant from the cell body (119).

Actions of 5HT

Stimulation of the medullary raphe nuclei will facilitate the segmentally evoked monosynaptic reflex. This effect had delayed onset consistent with slow conduction velocity of this small fiber system (120). This facillitation can be de-

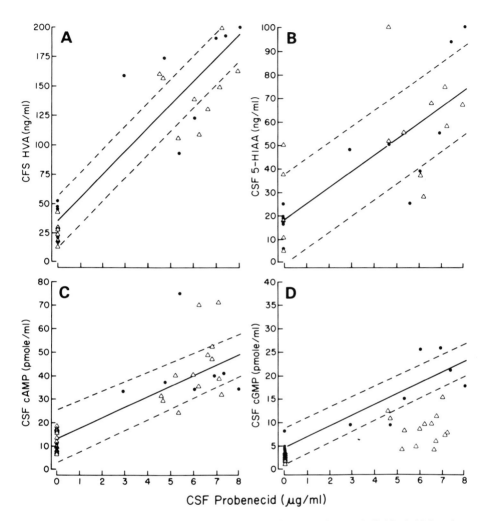

Figure 12 CSF monoamine metabolites and cyclic nucleotides in individual ALS and control neuromuscular disease patients. Homovanillic acid (HVA), 5-hydroxyindole acetic acid (5-HIAA), cyclic adenosine monophosphate (cAMP), cyclic guanosine monophosphate (cGMP), and probenecid were measured in seven control subjects (●) with other nonneuropathic neuromuscular disease and 14 patients with ALS (△) before and after intravenous probenecid (40 mg/kg) to block the egress of these substances from the cerebrospinal fluid compartment (109,110). CSF HVA and 5HIAA increased comparably in seven controls and nine ALS patients with sufficient sampling following probenecid. CSF cAMP increased comparably in seven controls and 13 ALS patients with sufficient sampling following probenecid. CSF cGMP did not increase comparably in 14 ALS patients compared with seven control patients.

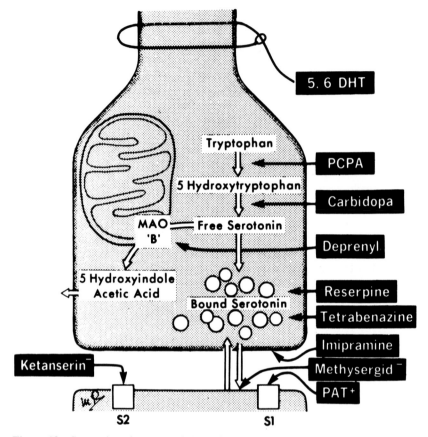

Figure 13 Serotoninergic neuron. Schematic drawing of serotoninergic neuron showing relationship of presynaptic nerve ending to postsynaptic process. Substrates as black type against white background. Inhibitors or pharmacological anatgonists ($-$) and pharmacological agonists ($+$) are represented by white type against black background: 5,6 DHT, 5,6-dihydroxytryptamine. [Reproduced with permission (124).]

creased by systemically administered 5HT antagonists, such as methysergide (121). Locally ionotrophoresed 5HT causes minimum effects directly on motor neurons but can definitely enhance the effects of Glu or Asp on motor neurons (77,122). These effects can be inhibited by $5HT_2$ receptor antagonists (123).

The first step in serotonin synthesis is the conversion of tryptophan to 5-hydroxytryptophan by the tryptophan 5-monooxygenase (tryptophan hydroxylase) in the presence of molecular oxygen and tetrahydrobiopterin as a cofactor.

The cytoplasmic enzyme has a micromolar K_m for tryptophan that is slightly higher than the average tryptophan concentration in the brain (124). Neuronal L-aromatic amino acid decarboxylase is a cytoplasmic pyridoxal-dependent enzyme that decarboxylates 5-hydroxytryptophan to 5HT. Catabolism of 5HT via mitochondrial MAO-B immunocytochemically localized in serotoninergic neurons and glia occurs with a millimolar K_m but the micromolar K_m of MAO-A for 5HT suggests that this enzyme may be more active in vivo in producing 5-hydroxy indoleacetic acid (125).

Serotonin uptake occurs via a moderate (micromolar)-affinity, sodium-dependent pathway present in neurons and glia (126). Imipramine and other heterocyclic antidepressants, as well as fluoxetine, are efficient uptake inhibitors (127). In addition, imipramine binding may be used to demonstrate uptakes sites in a similar distribution to the very-high-affinity (nanomolar) binding sites defined by 5HT. Two major classes of 5HT binding sites are currently defined. First, high (nanomolar)-affinity 5HT binding sites with either high (nanomolar-$5HT_{1A}$) or moderate (micromolar-$5HT_{1A}$) affinity spiperone binding are widely distributed in the CNS as putative inhibitory receptors. Second, moderate (micromolar) affinity 5HT binding sites with high (nanomolar) affinity for spiperone are more localized in cortical, hippocampal, and basal ganglia regions as putative excitatory receptors (128).

Effect of Toxins or Injuries on Serotoninergic Type II Neurotransmitters

5HT is reduced nearly 80% in the ventral horn by serotoninergic-specific neurotoxins such as 5,6- or 5,7-dihydroxytryptamine without much change in the dorsal horn concentration (129). Transection of the spinal cord or cordotomy will reduce both dorsal and ventral horn 5HT (130). Dorsal rhizotomy will decrease 5HT in the dorsal horn ipsilaterally to the lesion with mild increases caudal to the lesion. Ventral rhizotomy will not materially effect 5HT in the ventral or dorsal horn (131).

Effect of ALS on Serotoninergic Type II Neurotransmitters

Spinal cord $5HT_{1A}$ serotoninergic receptors are normally similarly distributed within the dorsal (laminae I–V), intermediate (lamina VII), and ventral (laminae VIII–IX) horns. In ALS spinal cord, $5HT_{1A}$ receptor binding (Fig. 7) is increased in the intermediate and ventral horns (65). This upregulation of $5HT_{1A}$ receptors is unique and suggests 5HT depletion that is known to up-regulate $5HT_{1A}$ receptors (132). However, rhizotomy decreases $5HT_{1A}$ receptors (133) while chronic exposure to TRH may up-regulate spinal cord $5HT_{1A}$ receptors (134).

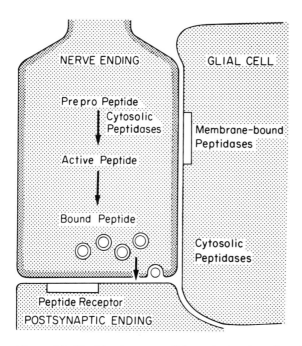

Figure 14 Peptidergic neuron. Schematic drawing of peptidergric neuron showing relationship of presynaptic nerve ending to postsynaptic process and glia. Substrates as black type against white background.

Platelet MAO activity in ALS patients is elevated compared with controls in one study (135), but not in another study (108). Baseline CSF 5HIAA in several studies is not significantly different in ALS patients than controls (108). CSF 5HIAA following intravenous probenecid (Fig. 12) is similarly increased in both non-ALS and ALS patients, indicating that 5HIAA turnover is not affected in ALS (109,110).

TYPE III NEUROTRANSMITTERS—PEPTIDES

Evidence for Neurotransmitter Role of Peptides

The putative peptide transmitters are present in the CNS in the lowest (picomolar) concentration of the three groups of neurotransmitters (136). Some peptidergric neurons (Fig. 14) are neurosecretory and can release peptides directly into the bloodstream or CSF, not just at synapses. Peptidergic neurons in the hypothalamus may send diffuse projections to many CNS regions, while peptidergic neurons in other CNS regions may send only specific projections to restricted CNS regions (raphe obscurus et pallidus/TRH/spinal cord ventral horn). Many peptidergic neurons are actually neurons that contain type II biogenic amine neurotransmitters as well as one or more type III peptide neurotransmitters. These neurons have varicose axons permitting release of type II and/or type III neurotransmitters at multiple sites throughout the neuropil. Type III peptide neurotransmitter–induced ''metabotropic'' effects may have even slower onset and more prolonged duration than type II biogenic amine neurotransmitter–induced ''metabotropic'' effects. These neurotransmitters may have ''metabotropic'' effects not only on neurons but on glia (56,136).

The evidence for a neurotransmitter role of peptides in the CNS is similar in many aspects to that required to establish amino acid and amine neurotransmitters (137): (a) Peptides that are neurotransmitters are present in specific CNS regions at concentrations that are sufficient for physiological function (138). (b) The peptide should be concentrated under appropriate conditions in synaptic fractions of homogenates from CNS regions in which the peptide is active and in which the peptide is preferentially located (139). (c) If the pathway in which the peptide is active can be interrupted by surgical or toxic ablation, the peptide content should decrease (140). (d) Developmental changes such as axonal growth and synaptic development should be paralleled by increments in the peptide (141). (e) The peptide, its precursors, their messenger ribonucleic acids (mRNAs), and the enzymes required for synthesis and posttranslational modification should be present by biochemical assay, radioimmunoassay, immunohistocytochemical analysis, or in situ hybridization in the neuronal cell soma (142). (f) The peptide should be releasable from the appropriate regional CNS tissue slice in vitro via a potassium-stimulated, calcium-dependent mechanism (143). (g) The peptide should be bound to presynaptic vesicles (144). (h) The peptide and its precursors should move from the cell soma to the nerve terminal by axoplasmic flow. Amine neurotransmitter synthetic enzymes are also compartmentalized, as are peptide neurotransmitter synthetic enzymes, but some amine neurotransmitter synthetic enzymes also travel from cell soma to nerve terminals via axonal transport (145). (i) The enzymes required to inactivate the peptide should be present in the CNS region where the peptide is active. These are localizable to the axons and nerve endings in peptidergic neurons but may also be present in dendrites and glia (146). (j) Uptake mechanisms that remove peptides from the extracellular space have not been demonstrated presynaptically in peptidergic neurons or in glia (Fig. 14). This feature is the major difference between amino acid and aminergic neurotransmitter systems (136). (k) High-affinity binding sites for the peptide should be present on postsynaptic membranes by binding studies on isolated membranes or by autoradiography with appropriately labeled ligand. Interpretation of binding studies must account for the possibility of membrane-bound enzymes which may specifically or nonspecifically degrade the pertinent neuropeptide (147). (l) Local application of the peptide by iontophoresis should mimic electrical stimulation of the pathway in which the peptide is a putative neurotransmitter. When available, specific antagonists to the peptide function should, when locally applied, mitigate the peptide effects (148). These criteria are particularly difficult to fulfill because the peptide effect may be to modulate other neurotransmitters rather than directly excite or inhibit neurons, and specific antagonists for some peptide actions may not yet be available (136,137).

Origin of Spinal Cord Peptides

Peptides in the spinal cord result from the presence of (a) intrinsic peptidergic neurons that may have segmental, rostral, and/or caudal projections, (b) afferent projections to the spinal cord from dorsal root ganglia, or (c) various supraspinal projections to the spinal cord from cortex, basal ganglia, hypothalamus, or brainstem (74). The concentration of each peptide in the ventral horn relative to the dorsal horn concentration (Fig. 15) is unique to each peptide and a function of the position of the spinal cord segment (149). Spinal cord content in the dorsal horn and ventral horn (Fig. 16) of several peptides increases caudally (150).

Peptides Colocalized in Cholinergic Motor Neurons

Calcitonin-Gene-Related Peptide [CGRP]

CGRP is a 37-amino-acid peptide that is encoded by alternative messenger RNA transcripts of the calcitonin gene peptide family (4,151). There are two forms of CGRP, alpha and beta (142). Both forms are present in all neurons, but alpha-CGRP is preferentially expressed in capsaicin-sensitive sensory neurons while beta CGRP is preferentially expressed in motor neurons. CGRP-containing neurons are present in the ventral horn but not the dorsal horn of the spinal cord. CGRP colocalizes with ChAT in large ventral horn motor neurons but not in other cholinergic neurons, such as the basal forebrain nucleus of Meynert or cholinergic neurons in the autonomic nervous system (152). In the dorsal root ganglia, three CGRP-containing neuronal systems occur which project to the dorsal horn: large and medium-sized neurons containing CGRP without

---

Figure 15 Spinal cord content of type III neurotransmitters. Substance P (Sub P), thyrotropin-releasing hormone (TRH), calcitonin gene–related peptide (CGRP), somatostatin (SOM), methionine-enkephalin (ENK), cholecystokinin (CCK), peptide histidine isoleucine (PHI), and vasoactive intestinal polypeptide (VIP) concentrations (pmoles/ gram wet weight tissue) in Rexed lamina VII and IX ventral horn (VH) of the mammalian spinal cord are presented as 95% confidence limits relative to the maximum value in Rexed laminae I–V of the dorsal horn (4,114,115,148,149). Only TRH is dramatically increased in the VH compared with the dorsal horn. VIP and PHI are relatively increased in the cervical spinal cord VH compared with lumbar spinal cord VH.

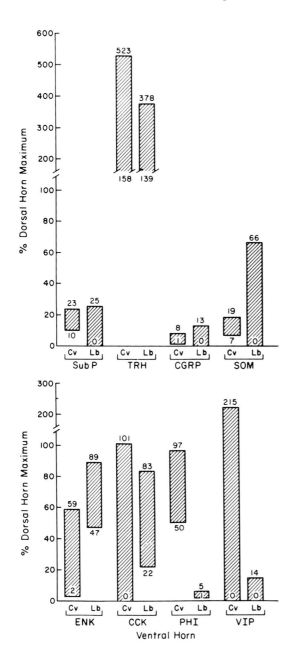

colocalized substance P (sub P) send fibers to laminae I and II in the dorsal horn; small to medium-sized neurons containing both CGRP and sub P also project to the same area. It is possible that there is a supraspinal CGRP system projecting to laminae IV–VI and X but its cells of origin and purpose are unknown (74).

The sexually dimorphic (different in males compared with females) motor neurons in the cremasteric nuclei, dorsomedial nuclei, or spinal nuclei for bulbocavernosus and dorsolateral nuclei differ in their CGRP content in males and females (153). While nearly all motor neurons that are not sexually dimorphic in the lumbosacral spinal cord contain CGRP, the dorsomedial nuclei contain more CGRP-positive neurons in females than in males. The proportion of CGRP-positive neurons increases in castrated males and is decreased in castrated males by testosterone administration (154). Spinal cord NE, 5HT, and 5HIAA are also increased in castrated males but return to normal with testosterone treatment (155). Males compared with females have an increased proportion of CGRP-positive fibers around motor neurons in the cremasteric nuclei and increased somatostatin (SOM)-positive neurons and fibers throughout all the sexually dimorphic motor neuron nuclei. The SOM innervation to these nuclei is similar to that seen for Onuf's nuclei in humans, where there are also increased CPON, ENK, galanin (GAL), and neurokinin (NK) immunoreactive fibers (156).

Actions of CGRP.   The function of CGRP in motor neurons includes regulation of the synthesis of postsynaptic ACh receptors in muscle (6,157), increasing the pharmacological effects of ACh (158) and directly augmenting the contraction of striated muscle (5). In the dorsal horn, CGRP potentiates the release of sub P from primary afferent terminals (159) and inhibits breakdown of sub P by sub P endopeptidase (160). Iontophoretic application of CGRP produces slow-onset, prolonged neuronal excitation (161). CGRP enhances Glu and Asp release from spinal cord slices (162).

Effects of Toxins or Injuries on CGRP.   The observation that capsaicin will reduce dorsal horn CGRP by 85% while dorsal rhizotomy will decrease dorsal horn CGRP by only 60% is consistent with the fact that both alpha- and beta-CGRP are expressed in the dorsal root ganglia and only a subpopulation of these neurons is capsaicin sensitive (163). Both treatments will reduce CGRP- and sub P–containing fibers in the dorsal horn. Proximal ventral rhizotomy will decrease CGRP-containing neurons in the ventral horn. Spinal cord transection also decreases CGRP in the ventral horn motor neurons; however, dorsal rhizotomy prevents this transection-induced decrease in CGRP (164).

Effect of ALS on CGRP.   CGRP-containing motor neurons decrease in the cranial motor nuclei of the brainstem and the ventral horn of the spinal cord in ALS patients (156). Motor neurons in the sexually dimorphic (Onuf's) nuclei are preserved in ALS (165). It is possible that the elevated CSF NE in ALS patients

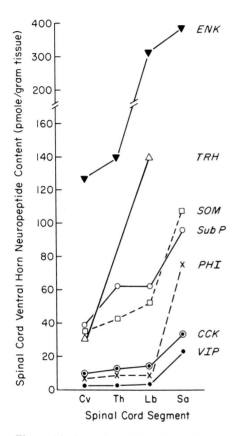

Figure 16 Rostral caudal gradient of spinal cord content of type III neurotransmitters. Enkephalin (ENK), thyrotropin-releasing hormone (TRH), somatostatin (SOM), substance P (Sub P), peptide histidine isoleucine (PHI), cholecystokinin (CCK), and vasoactive intestinal polypeptide (VIP) concentrations in spinal cord ventral horn (pmole/gram wet weight tissue) are plotted according to spinal cord segment: cervical (Cv), thoracic (Th), lumbar (Lb), or sacral (Sa). Most peptides increase caudally, with the most dramatic and statistically significant ($p < 0.05$) differences between cervical and sacral segments (140,149,177).

may be related to the stimulatory effect of CGRP on noradrenergic sympathetic outflow (166).

Peptides Colocalized in Catecholaminergic Neurons

Neuropeptide Y (NPY)

NPY is a 36-amino-acid peptide derived from a 97-amino-acid precursor polyprotein of the pancreatic polypeptide, neuropeptide Y, and peptide YY gene family (167). NPY and the C-flanking peptide of NPY (CPON) are colocalized with NE in locus ceruleus neurons that project to the spinal cord (168). Intrinsic NPY-containing spinal cord interneurons are localized in the dorsal horn (169). In the intermediolateral horn, NPY is colocalized with ENK in neurons that project to the periphery. NPY-containing fibers are located in laminae, I, II, V, VI, VII, and X (74). CPON-containing fibers as well as ENK-containing fibers project to the sexually dimorphic nuclei in animals and Onuf's nuclei in humans (156).

Actions of NPY. NPY administered alone increases the inward K current through activation of a G protein, decreases the discharge of action potential by locus ceruleus neurons, inhibits the release of NE, but may potentiate the hyperpolarizing effects of NE and other alpha-2 agonists, but not opoid mu-agonists (170).

Effect of Toxins or Injuries on NPY. NE and NYP are depleted by 6-hydroxydopamine. Transection of the spinal cord will decrease NPY fibers caudal to the transection (74).

Effect of ALS on NPY. NE is increased in the CSF of ALS patients. NPY is increased in the cortex following excitotoxic amio acid–induced pathology (52), but tissue content of NE or NPY has not been adequately studied in ALS patients.

Peptides Colocalized in Serotoninergic Neurons

Enkephalin (ENK)

Enkephalins are five-amino-acid pentapeptides derived from the preproenkephalin A (ENKA) gene group of the endogenous opioid gene peptide family, which includes the preopiomelanocortin (POMC) gene group and the preproenkephalin B or preprodynorphin (DYN) gene group (136). The ENKA and DYN gene groups are expressed more widely in a number of tissues than the POMC gene group. ENK is present as two pentapeptides with either a terminal methionine (met-ENK) or leucine (leu-ENK) amide that are derived from a 267-amino-acid precursor, preproenkephalin A, that contains six copies of met-ENK and one copy of leu-ENK. Various breakdown products of this precursor polypeptide are found in the different regions of the CNS (171). ENK is present in the spinal cord in a very high concentration, which increases caudally (150). Intrinsic spinal cord ENK-containing neurons are located particularly in lamina II but are also present throughout laminae III–VII of the dorsal and intermediate horns as well as the sacral parasympathetic preganglionic neurons (172). These parasympathetic preganglionic neurons containing both ACh and ENK, ENK and pancreatic polypeptide, or ENK and NPY are in the intermediate horn of the spinal cord projecting to the periphery. ENK fibers present in the spinal cord originate from endogenous ENK neurons in the dorsal raphe nuclei and reticular formation of the brainstem that contain ENK alone or ENK colocalized with 5HT (173). These neurons project primarilly to the dorsal horn, while intrinsic spinal cord neurons in lamina VII that contain ENK alone send fibers to the ventral horn, where they contact almost exclusively CGRP-negative, ChAT-positive, AChE-positive neurons (152). Axodendritic contacts are most prominent, with occasional axoaxonal contacts and exceedingly rare axosomatic contacts.

Actions of ENK. ENK applied iontophoretically has many effects, including decreasing Glu-induced depolarization of spinal cord neurons, inhibiting ACh and NE release from CNS neurons, and inhibiting sub P and CGRP release by primary dorsal horn afferents (162,174–176).

Effects of Toxins or Injuries on ENK. Dorsal rhizotomy will result in an increase in met-ENK in the dorsal horn of the spinal cord (163). Reserpine will increase ventral horn met-ENK (177).

Effect of ALS on ENK. ENK immunoreactive fibers in the ventral horn are relatively decreased in ALS, possibly due to loss of target motor neurons, but tissue levels of met-ENK by radioimmunoassay have not been investigated (156).

Galanin (GAL)

GAL is a 29-amino-acid peptide that is colocalized with 5HT in some bulbo-spinal descending systems (74). Very few GAL/5HT fibers project to the ventral horn of the spinal cord.

Actions of GAL. GAL will decrease the release of ACh and DA from neurons (179,180).

Effects of Toxins or Injuries on GAL. Sciatic neurectomy increases dorsal horn Gal (181).

Effects of ALS on GAL. Ventral horn GAL immunoreactive fibers are not significantly altered in ALS spinal cord (156).

Substance P (Sub P)

Sub P is an 11-amino-acid peptide in the tachykinin gene peptide family which is derived from the alpha-preprotachykinin 112-amino-acid precursor polyprotein that contains only sub P copies, while the 130-amino-acid precursor polyprotein beta-preprotachykinin contains copies of sub P, substance K, and alpha-neurokinin (136). Sub P–containing neurons are present in lamina II more than lamina I. Sub P–containing fibers are present in lamina I, II, IV–VI, VII, VIII–IX, and X (74). Sub P–containing neurons are present in the dorsal root ganglia with and without CGRP (163). In addition, sub P is present in neurons from the caudal raphe nuclei that contain either TRH, 5HT, or TRH and 5HT (182). Sub P is associated with larger granular vesicles in synapses that are axodendritic and axosomatic rather than axoaxonic.

Actions of Sub P. Sub P alone will increase the excitatory effect of Glu and Asp on motor neurons but not directly depolarize motor neurons (148). Application of sub P and 5HT together will enhance Glu and Asp responses more reliably than sub P alone (183). Sub P is released by a sodium-and-calcium-dependent process (137). Sub P release is decreased by opiates, NE, GABA, and 5HT (175).

Effect of Toxins or Injuries on Sub P. Capsaicin causes loss of sub P as well as sub P/CGRP–containing neurons in dorsal root ganglia and dorsal horn laminae and loss of sub P–containing fibers in the dorsal horn from the dorsal root ganglia. 5,7-DHT depletes sub P more from the ventral horn than the dorsal horn of the spinal cord (140). 6OHDA has no effect, while reserpine and tetrabenazine deplete sub P from the ventral horn of the spinal cord (177).

Dorsal rhizotomy and peripheral nerve section will produce more of a decrease in dorsal horn sub P but little change in ventral horn sub P (181,184). Sub P increases caudal to spinal cord transection (185). Capsaicin treatment as well as dorsal rhizotomy will increase postsynaptic high-affinity (nanomolar) sub P receptors (186,187). The neurotoxins 5,7-DHT and 6OHDA have no effect on sub P receptors (188).

Effect of ALS on Sub P. Sub P immunoreactive fibers have been described as decreased in lamina IX of the ventral horn of ALS spinal cords without an apparent decrease in dorsal horn sub P immunoreactive fibers (189,190). Neurokinin is another member of the tachykinin peptide family. Neurokinin immunoreactive fibers to the ventral horn are also relatively decreased in ALS patients (156). Sub P measured by radioimmunoassay in several studies in the dorsal, intermediate, and ventral horn of the spinal cord suggests a decrease in all these areas in ALS patients compared with control subjects (191,192). However, compared with controls, the ventral horn content of sub P as a proportion of the dorsal horn content actually increases in autopsied spinal cord tissue in ALS patients (Fig. 17). Consistent with the loss of postsynaptic receptors, possibly on motor neurons, sub P receptors are decreased in the ventral horn but not the intermediate horn of ALS spinal cords compared with controls (193). Sub P in the CSF is significantly decreased in some neuropathies but not in ALS (194,195).

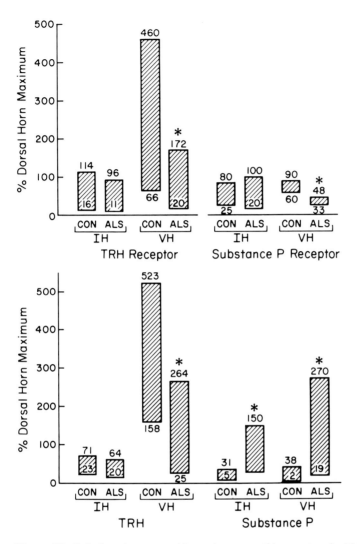

Figure 17 Spinal cord neuropeptides and neuropeptide receptors in ALS. Thyrotropin-releasing hormone (TRH) receptor (64) and substance P receptor (193) were measured in spinal cord of control subjects and ALS patients by tissue autoradiography and quantitative densitometry. TRH (216,217) and substance P (191,192) were measured in punch biopsies by radioimmunoassay of Rexed lamina VII intermediate horn (IH) and Rexed laminae VIII and IX ventral horn (VH). Receptor densities and neuropeptide content are presented as 95% confidence limits relative to the maximum in Rexed laminae I–V of the dorsal horn. TRH and substance P receptor densities are significantly ($p < 0.05$; *) reduced in the VH but not the IH in ALS patients compared with controls. TRH content in punch biopsies is significantly reduced in the VH but not the IH in ALS patients compared with controls. While several studies suggest that substance P content may decrease in the spinal cord of ALS patients, the proportion of substance P in the VH relative to the DH may actually increase significantly in the VH but not IH region of the spinal cord in ALS patients compared with controls (191,192).

Thyrotropin Releasing Hormone (TRH)

TRH is a three-amino-acid tripeptide derived from cleavage of a 255-amino-acid precursor polypeptide, prepro TRH, that contains five TRH copies (196). Posttranslational cyclization of the N-terminal Glu to pyroGlu occurs in the last stages of TRH, neurotensin (NT), and luteinizing hormone–releasing hormone (LHRH) processing (136). TRH immunoreactive neurons are present in the dorsal horn of the spinal cord and the dorsal raphe nuclei (obscuris and pallidus) in the brainstem (197,198). The latter neurons are either 5HT alone, sub P/5HT, or TRH/sub P/TRH. Sub P/5HT and 5HT alone neurons from the caudal raphe nuclei project to the entire gray matter of the spinal cord, while TRH/sub P/5HT neurons project primarilly to the ventral horn of the spinal cord in the ventro-lateral funiculus (199). Boutons apposed to motor neuron dendrites contain large (100 nm) dense core vesicles which contain sub P or TRH and small vesicles which contain 5HT (200). Released TRH is broken down by membrane-bound pyroglutamylpeptidase, which has different enzyme characteristics and cofactor dependence compared with the cytosolic pyroglutamylpeptidase, TRH deami-dase, or postproline endopeptidase (201). Like other neuropeptide transmitters, no uptake mechanism for released TRH has been demonstrable.

Actions of TRH. TRH iontophoretically applied alone to motor neurons may facilitate Glu- or Asp-induced discharges but does not directly cause motor neuron depolarization (148). The TRH effect, like the sub P and 5HT effects, is slow in onset and prolonged in duration. However, the TRH effect may be different from the effect that occurs with sub P or 5HT, which demonstrates only facillitation. Three additional effects seen with TRH, namely (a) inhibition of amino acid induced depolarization, (b) tachyphylaxis, and (c) TRH antagonism of 5HT facilitation of amino-acid-induced depolarization, require special atten-tion. TRH alone in some motor neurons can cause inhibition of Glu- or Asp-induced depolarization. In addition, motor neurons in the spinal cord and hypo-glossal nucleus also demonstrate a tachyphylaxis to iontophoretically applied TRH but not to 5HT. As discussed above, sub P and 5HT together are synergistic in producing an increased response to Glu- or Asp-induced depolarization when both are present, compared to either 5HT or sub P alone. Possible mechanisms for this synergism may include sub P induction of increased density of 5HT binding sites and inhibition of the 5HT autoreceptor that presynaptically inhibits 5HT release. However, unlike the simultaneous administration of sub P and 5HT, the simultaneous administration of TRH and 5HT together is antagonistic to Glu- or Asp-induced depolarization of motor neurons. The mechanism for this observation is unknown (183).

The effects of intravenously administered TRH on motor neuron field poten-tials ellicited by ventral root stimulation are different. In this situation, 5HT agonists and TRH or TRH analogs together may be additive if the animal is not spinalized but antagonistic if the animal is spinalized (183). One hypothesis is that TRH effects in this situation may be mediated through TRH-induced NE release providing motor neuron facilitation through another mechanism (202).

In addition to the above neurophysiological effects of TRH, there are also trophic effects of TRH and TRH analogs, including (a) TRH-induced neurite extension and ChAT elevation by neurons in culture (203), (b) TRH-induced delay of developmental death of neurons (204), and (c) TRH-potentiated recovery from nerve crush in vivo when pharmacological doses are administered (205,206).

Effect of Toxins or Injuries on TRH. Serotoninergic neurotoxins will deplete spinal cord ventral horn 5HT, sub P, and TRH but not histidyl-proline diketopiperazine (cyclo-histidyl-proline or cyclo-His-Pro, cHP) (207). Dorsal horn TRH is unaffected. Ventral horn TRH receptors are increased after serotoninergic neurotoxins (208) and micromolar amounts of sub P (209). Chronic prolonged TRH administration has variable effects (210). Serotonin synthesis inhibition with parachlorophenylalanine prevents the neonatal thyroidectomy-induced increase in spinal cord TRH (211). Spinal cord TRH and 5HT are increased above the site of spinal trauma (212). Neuronal degeneration induced by murine neurotropic retrovirus or genetically induced spinal muscular atrophy will result in increased spinal cord TRH demonstrable by radioimmunoassay (213,214).

Effect of ALS on TRH. In whole spinal cord segments there is no significant change in the spinal cord content of TRH, but cyclic His-Pro may be increased (215); however, in punch biopsy analysis of the ventral horn (Fig. 17) compared with intermediate horn gray matter, there is a significant reduction in TRH content (216,217). TRH content in brain is unchanged (218). TRH staining fibers in the ventral horn are relatively decreased in ALS patients (156). In addition, TRH receptors are significantly reduced (Fig. 17) in the ventral horn compared with the intermediate horn (64). TRH catabolism may be slightly increased in ALS spinal cords compared with controls but some specific enzymes are not increased (219–221). Chronic prolonged administration of TRH to ALS patients will induce TRH deamindase activity in the spinal cord, but not other regions (222). CSF levels of TRH (Fig. 18) are not decreased in ALS patients compared with controls, but cyclo His-Pro levels were increased in one study and not in another (215,223). Although there is controversy concerning whether the spinal cord content of TRH is decreased in ALS patients, the paradox is that TRH is not increased, as demonstrated in the animal models of motor neuron degeneration, including wobbler spinal muscular atrophy and murine neurotropic retrovirus-induced motor neuron disease. This suggests that a putative endogenous neuropeptide injury response mechanism is not activated in ALS. The possible reasons for this lack of response have not been fully elucidated (224).

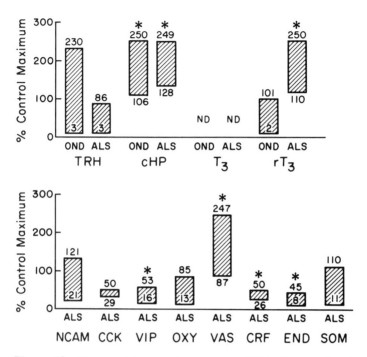

Figure 18 Neuropeptides and hormones in CSF. Thyrotropin-releasing hormone (TRH), cyclo-histidylproline (cHP), tri-iodo-thyronine (T3), reverse thyronine binding (rT3), (NCAM), cholecystokinin (CCK), vasoactive intestinal peptide (VIP), oxytocin (OXY), vasopressin (VAS), corticotrophin-releasing factor (CRF), beta-endorphin (END), and somatostatin (SOM) were measured by immunoassay in cerebrospinal fluid. Neuropeptide or hormone concentrations are presented as 95% confidence limits relative to the control maximum in other neurological disease (OND) and amyotrophic lateral sclerosis (ALS) patients as adapted from several studies [195,215,223,225,234,238, 242,253]. cHP is significantly ($p < 0.05$) increased in the CSF of both OND and ALS patients (223). Reverse thyronine binding is increased and thyronine content was not detectable (ND) in ALS patients (225). Vasopressin (VAS) is significantly increased (234) and vasoactive intestinal peptide (VIP), beta-endorphin (END), and corticotrophin-releasing factor (CRF) are significantly decreased in the cerebrospinal fluid of ALS patients (238,242,253).

CSF thyroxine [T_4] is identical in ALS and controls, while CSF thyronine [T_3] is not detectable by current radioimmunoassay in either group (Fig. 18). CSF reverse T_3, however, is present in increased amounts in ALS patients compared with controls (225). It is not clear how CSF reverse T_3 elevation relates to the decreased nuclear T_3 receptor in ALS precentral gyrus (226). Nuclear T_3 receptor is high up to the 16th week of gestation and decreases during developmental natural motor neuron death. The pathology of hypothyroidism, however, is similar to that seen in ALS, with attenuated dendrites and decreased number of dendritic spines (48,227). The observations of decreased nuclear T_3 receptors and dendritic atrophy in ALS should be integrated with the observation of increased NE in ALS. The usual effect of hypothyroidism on the CNS is to create a decreased neural sensitivity to NE (228). It is not clear whether the above findings are directly linked to the cause of motor neuron degeneration or are a consequence of motor neuron degeneration. Moreover, the relationship of nuclear T_3 receptors to peptidergic inputs to the motor neurons, namely axons that may contain TRH, is not at all known at the present time.

Hypothalamic and Other Peptides

Arginine Vasopressin (AVP) and Oxytocin (OXY)

AVP and OXY are nine-amino-acid nonapeptides. AVP is a nine-amino-acid peptide derived via cleavage from a precursor 166-amino-acid polyprotein, propressophysin, that also gives neurophysin II. OXY is a nine-amino-acid peptide produced in the same manner from the precursor 145-amino-acid polyprotein, prooxyphysin, that also gives neurophysin I (136). Leu-ENK is associated with AVP and met-ENK is associated with OXY immunoreactive neurons (229). AVP or OXY immunoreactive neurons in the parvocellular portion of the paraventricular nuclei in the hypothalamus project AVP or OXY immunoreactive fibers to the dorsal horn laminae I–II and lamina X. No AVP or OXY neurons are present in the spinal cord (74).

Actions of AVP and OXY. AVP and OXY variably alter firing rates of neurons (230). Salt loading will increase AVP mRNA expression throughout the CNS (231).

Effect of Toxins or Injuries on AVP and OXY. No information is available on dorsal and ventral horn changes in AVP or OXY following specific neurotoxins or injury.

Effect of ALS on AVP and OXY. No tissue studies of spinal cord AVP or OXY in ALS have been published (232). CSF AVP, but not CSF OXY, is decreased in one study (233) but increased in another study (234) of ALS patients (Fig. 18). The increased CSF AVP may correlate with the increased fast axonal transport demonstrated in the motor nerves of ALS patients because exogenously administered AVP may speed fast axonal transport (235).

Cholecystokinin (CCK)

The predominant form of this neuropeptide is as an eight-amino-acid octapeptide, but several other polypeptides ranging from 3 to 39 amino acids are derived from the 115-amino-acid preprocholecystokinin (136). CCK-positive neurons colocalized with sub P are present in the dorsal root ganglia and project fibers to the dorsal horn (137). CCK-positive oval neurons are present in laminae I–III of the dorsal horn, while CCK-positive multipolar neurons are present in laminae IV–V, VII, and X. CCK-positive neurons in the caudal raphe nuclei project in the lateral and dorsal funiculi to the intermediate horn or the ventral horn. CCK-positive neurons in the midbrain central gray matter also project to the intermediate and ventral horn (74).

Actions of CCK.   CCK is excitatory and potentiates large pyramidal cell discharge rates (236). CCK also has a trophic neurite-promoting effect on ventral horn cells in vitro (237).

Effect of Toxins or Injuries on CCK.   Capsaicin or dorsal rhizotomy will decrease dorsal horn CCK-positive fibers (163). Transection will result in accumulation of CCK in axons rostral to the lesion (74).

Effect of ALS on CCK.   CSF CCK (Fig. 18) is not altered in ALS patients (238).

Corticotrophin-Releasing Factor (CRF)

This 41-amino-acid peptide is present in cells in the hypothalamus and the dorsolateral pontine tegmentum (136). Numerous CRF immunoreactive fibers are present in the spinal cord and may be involved in autonomic functions such as the micturition reflex (239).

Actions of CRF.   CRF can be directly excitatory to large pyramidal cells (240). CRF will stimulate beta-endorphin secretion (241).

Effects of Toxins or Injuries on CRF.   Some toxins and injuries will result in a stress-related increase in CRF (239).

Effect of ALS on CRF.   CSF CRF is decreased in ALS patients compared with controls, parallelling the decreased CSF beta-endorphin noted below in ALS patients. However, the structural and physiological correlates of this observation have not been fully investigated (242).

Endorphin (END)

Beta-endorphin is a 31-amino-acid peptide that is one of many peptides derived by proteolytic cleavage from the 267-amino-acid precursor proopiomelanocortin polypeptide (136). This polypeptide is one of the opioid family precursor proteins that gives rise to beta-lipotropin from which beta-endorphin and gamma-lipotropin are cleaved, in addition to adrenocorticotropin hormone (ACTH), corticotropin-like intermediate lobe peptide (CLIP), and melanocyte-stimulating hormone (alpha-MSH) in different tissues, including pituitary gland, arcuate nucleus, and periarcuate regions of the medial basal hypothalamus and caudal medulla in the lower part of the nucleus tractus solitarius in a noradrenergic neuronal cell group. The arcuate nuclei beta-endorophin projections are to the periaqueductal region of the diencephalon. The anterior paraventricular nuclei of the hypothalamus and the locus ceruleus contain beta-endorphin and, with beta-endorphin-containing neurons in the nucleus solitarius, project to the pontine reticular formation and the caudal serotoninergic and peptidergic nuclei. POMC immunoreactivity is present in the dorsal horn, dorsolateral fasciculus (Lissauer's tract), and dorsal lamina X of spinal cord (243).

Actions of END. Iontophoretically applied beta-endorphin inhibits neuronal discharges in many CNS regions (244). Beta-endorphin also decreases ACh turnover (245). The beta-endorphin–induced reduction in DA release both in vitro and in vivo may explain the observed prolonged akinesia and muscular rigidity caused by intrathecal administration of this peptide (246,247). This akinesia caused by beta-endorphin occurs following the acute tremulousness characterized as "wet-dog" shakes, which is similar to the behavior seen in opioid withdrawal and TRH administration (248). Beta-endorphin actions are mediated via mu and delta opioid receptors (249). Antinociceptive effects of beta-endorphin are primarilly mediated through the delta opioid receptors (250).

Effect of Toxins or Injuries on END. Pain, electrical stimulation of the periaqueductal gray, and seizures will increase beta-endorphin release from CNS tissue with an increase in CSF beta endorphin (248,251). Motor nerve section increases beta-endorphin immunoreactivity at the neuromuscular junction (252).

Effect of ALS on END. CSF END is decreased in ALS patients (Fig. 18), but no tissue studies have been performed to determine the structural and physiological basis for this observation (253). The fact that beta-endorphin is decreased and that this may be mediator between the nucleus tractus solitarius and the caudal serotoninergic/peptidergic brainstem nuclei is made more interesting because of the fact that intraventricular administration of END will induce "wetdog" shakes similar to those seen with intravenous or intrathecal TRH administration (254). This suggests that END may also be a mediator of release of TRH from the brainstem peptidergic nuclei. Since spinal cord ventral horn TRH which is dependent on the brainstem caudal raphe nuclei is decreased in ALS, the concomitant decrease of a possible activator of this neuropeptide circuit is worthy of more investigation. In addition, cervical spinal cord arachnoid thickening and inflammation is seen in ALS. This observation may have a bearing on the decreased CSF END in ALS patients since CSF END is also decreased in primates with spinal arachnoiditis (255).

Somatostatin (SOM)

This cyclic peptide with an internal disulfide bond exists in several forms as a 14- or 28-amino-acid polypeptide derived from cleavage of the 116-amino-acid pre-prosomatostatin (136). Primarilly localized in the hypothalamus, this peptide inhibits growth hormone release from the anterior pituitary. SOM-positive fibers project to the spinal cord from neurons in the dorsal root ganglia. The amygdala contains SOM-positive neurons that project fibers ipsilaterally to lower brain-stem regions, including the cranial motor neuron nuclei (facial and hypoglossal) and the upper cervical spinal cord, particularly the ventral horn. In addition, there are SOM-positive neurons in the insular cortex that project to the spinal cord (74). SOM-positive neurons are found in lamina II of the dorsal horn with a higher concentration rostrally toward the medulla oblongta. SOM-positive nerve fibers in the spinal cord are small in diameter and unmyelinated, forming primarilly axodendritic synapses. Ventral horn SOM fibers derive primarily from SOM/5HT neurons in the raphe pallidus et obscurus, which project to the ventral horn with or without other peptides such as ENK, sub P, or TRH (256).

Actions of SOM.   SOM has variable effects when iontophoresed in vivo and in vitro. The direct effects of SOM are to cause slow membrane depolarization by blocking a resting potassium conductance and inhibit Glu-induced depolar-ization similarly to ENK (257, 258).

Effect of Toxins or Injuries on SOM.   Reserpine causes no change in dorsal or ventral horn SOM (177). Rhizotomy will decrease SOM ipsilaterally in the dorsal horn, as will capsaicin (259,260). Transection will decrease SOM in the spinal cord below the lesion (256). CSF SOM is increased in CNS varicella zoster and decreased in Alzheimer's disease (261,262).

Effect of ALS on SOM.   SOM immunoreactive fibers are relatively decreased in the ventral horn of the spinal cord in ALS patients (156). However, CSF SOM (Fig. 18) is unchanged in ALS patients (195). CSF neural cell adhesion molecule (NCAM) is also unchanged (238).

Vasoactive Intestinal Polypeptide (VIP) and Peptide Histidine Isoleucine (PHI)

VIP is a 28-amino-acid octocosapeptide that is derived from a large preVIP precursor (263). PHI is a 27-amino-acid polypeptide related to VIP that has an amino-terminal histidine and a carboxy-terminal isoleucine-amide (136). Its dis-tribution and function are similar to those of VIP. Historically, VIP and PHI below are classified with the glucagon-secretin family of neuropeptides. VIP-containing neurons are prominent interneurons in layers II–III of the cerebral cortex but do not project caudally (264). VIP-containing neurons are present in the dorsal root ganglia and project to the dorsal horn of the spinal cord where VIP-associated large (100 nm) granular vesicles are associated with axodendritic synapses (265–267). VIP-containing multipolar neurons with long dendrites in-trinsic to the spinal cord exist in lamina I and the lateral spinal nucleus of the dorsal horn of the spinal cord (74). VIP-containing fibers originate from the first group of neurons in lamina I and may project to laminae V and X. In addition,

VIP-containing oval neurons with short dendrites are present in lamina X near the central canal (268).

Actions of VIP and PHI. Systemically VIP is a vasodilator (136). In the CNS, VIP ionotophoretically applied to laminae I–VII will depolarize 75% of dorsal horn neurons and increase their firing rate (269). VIP and PHI may interact with NE to increase glycogenolysis in the CNS (270). VIP receptors are present on astrocytes (271), and the metabolic response to VIP is higher in cortical than spinal cord astrocytes (272). VIP administration increases cerebral glucose utilization measured by fluordeoxyglucose in specific brain regions (273). VIP is also a neurotrophic factor which promotes cholinergic neuron survival and is an astrocytic mitogen (274–276).

Effect of Toxins or Injuries on VIP and PHI. Capsaicin depletes VIP in the dorsal horn of neonates (277) but not adults (278). Neurectomy or nerve crush, distal to the dorsal root ganglion, will cause a significant increase in dorsal horn VIP and PHI (279,280). Dorsal rhizotomy, proximal to the dorsal root ganglion, will not cause an increase in the dorsal horn content of VIP or PHI (278,279). Transection of the spinal cord increases VIP in axons caudal to the lesion (281).

Effect of ALS on VIP and PHI. VIP is decreased in the CSF of ALS patients (Fig. 18), but tissue content studies by radiommunoassy have not been performed to determine the possible site in the CNS responsible for this decrease (238). The possible role of VIP as a missing neurotrophic factor for motor neurons in ALS has not been fully investigated (282). VIP and PHI are relatively increased in the sacral region of the spinal cord at the site where the autonomic motor neuron nuclei are spared in ALS (150,156). Moreover, the distinctive cortical gliosis that occurs in layers II–III in the premotor cerebral cortex of ALS patients (283) occurs in regions where VIP interneurons are common (270). Therefore, the role of VIP as a neurotrophic factor and as a glial mitogen in the pathogenesis of ALS requires further attention.

SECOND MESSENGERS—CYCLIC NUCLEOTIDES, CALMODULIN, PHOSPHOINOSITIDES

Evidence for Role of Second Messengers in Neurotransmitter Function

Second messengers may mediate, primarily intracellularly, some of the effects of neurotransmitters and hormones as well as certain metabolic processes. The establishment of the relationship between a neurotransmitter- or hormone-induced effect and a particular second messenger is supported by the following observations: (a) The presence of enzymes that synthesize the second messenger which are activated by some interaction with the neurotransmitter or hormone. (b) The presence of one or more ways to inactivate the effect of the second messenger by catabolism or extrusion from the cell. (c) The tissue or cellular content of the second messenger will be raised or lowered in response to the neurotransmitter or hormone. (d) Chemically stable analogs of the second messenger will recapitulate the effect of the neurotransmitter or hormone. (e) Inhibition of the catabolism or inactivation of the second messenger will potentiate or decrease the neurotransmitter- or hormone-induced effect. (f) The second messenger will activate specific protein kinases that phosphorylate specific protein sites in order to mediate the biochemical or electrical effect activated by the second messenger (284).

Within the CNS there are at least three major second messenger systems: (a) cyclic nucleotides (56), (b) calcium and calcium-binding proteins with effects separate from those that are mediated by cyclic nucleotides (285), and (c) polyphosphoinositides (286).

Cyclic Nucleotides

Both adenyl cyclase (AC) and guanyl cyclase (GC), which synthesize cyclic adenosine-3′,5′-monophosphate (cAMP) and cyclic guanosine-3′,5′-monophosphate (cGMP) are primarilly membrane-bound enzymes. AC is linked to the neurotransmitter or hormone effector receptor via an intermediatry G protein with a binding site for guanosine diphosphate (GDP). Activation of the receptor displaces GDP with guanosine triphosphate (GTP). The now activated G protein interacts with calcium bound to calmodulin to activate the adenyl cyclase which produces cAMP from adenosine triphosphate (ATP). G proteins may also inhibit AC activity. If the G protein is stimulatory, cAMP is produced and then diffuses or translocates to bind the regulatory subunit of the protein kinase linked to a particular AC. The kinase, now activated in this fashion, proceeds to phosphorylate its target protein, which, now activated, carries out is specific intracellular effect.

cAMP

Membrane-bound AC requires ATP to produce cAMP which is linked to several functions as noted below by:

1. Mediating, through cAMP, the effects of the following neurotransmitters
     Type I neurotransmitters
          AC stimulation by Glu, NMDA, cysteine sulfate, KA, quisqualate (287)
          AC inhibition by GABA (288)
     Type II neurotransmitters
          AC stimulation by DA through dopamine receptor, D1 (89)
          AC stimulation, including spinal cord, by NE through alpha receptor, alpha1 or alpha2 (289)

AC stimulation, including spinal cord, by E or NE equipotently, through beta receptor, beta1 (290)

AC stimulation, by E more potently that NE, through beta receptor, beta2 (87)

AC inhibition by ACh through muscarinic receptor, M2 (291)

AC inhibition by DA through dopamine receptor, D2 (292)

AC inhibition by NE through alpha receptor, alpha2 (86)

Type III neurotransmitters

AC stimulation by VIP in cortex, hypothalamus, striatum which is enhanced by $GABA_B$ receptor (293)

2. Regulating the biosynthesis of certain neurotransmitters

Type II neurotransmitters

AC stimulation of tyrosine hydroxylase by ACh (294)

3. Regulating microtubule function

AC stimulation of microtubule assembly (56)

AC is quite ubiquitous in many cell types and may affect both membrane-bound and cytosolic cAMP-dependent protein kinases. cAMP is present in many cell types and affects not only transmitter-mediated functions, but other general metabolic functions as well. Spinal cord AC is activated by alpha1, alpha2, and beta1 receptors (289,290). The release of cAMP from cells is proportional to the intracellular concentration, and now in vivo dialysis techniques can be used to measure cAMP kinetics in the active awake state (295).

cGMP

Both cytosolic and membrane-bound GC require guanosine triphosphate (GTP) to produce cGMP, which mediates the effects of the following neurotransmitters:

Type I neurotransmitters

GC stimulation by Glu in cerebellum without AC stimulation (296)

GC stimulation by GABA and Gly is slower than Glu-mediated stimulation (297)

Type II neurotransmitters

GC stimulation by ACh in some CNS regions is blocked by atropine (298)

GC stimulation by NE in cerebellum has same kinetics as Glu-induced GC stimulation (297)

GC in the spinal cord is not stimulated by NE (289,290)

GC in the cerebellum is not stimulated by ACh or histamine (297)

GC inhibition in the cerebellum by DA and 5HT (297)

Type III neurotransmitters

GC stimulation by TRH in cerebellum (299)

GC stimulation by TRH in spinal cord (300)

GC stimulation by atrial natiuretic peptide (301)

cGMP is present in neurons, glia, and probably endothelial cells that respond to prostaglandins and thromboxane by producing endoperoxides that may activate soluble GC.

Effect of Toxins and Injury on Cyclic Nucleotides

Injury, degeneration, toxins, electroshock, and decapitation can variably increase cAMP or cGMP in various CNS regions (302–306). AC response to NE in neurons postsynaptic to noradrengeric neurons is exaggerated by pretreatment with the neurotoxin 6-hydroxydopamine that causes degeneration of the noradrenergic neurons (90). AC response to DA is increased following spinal cord transection (307). Some cerebellar degenerations are associated with decreased CNS cGMP (308).

Effect of ALS on Cyclic Nucleotides

CNS tissue studies have not been performed in ALS. However, in both experimental animal models of motor neuron degeneration, wobbler spinal muscular atrophy and murine neurotropic retrovirus-induced motor neuron disease, CNS spinal cord content of cGMP is decreased (309,310). Systemically administered TRH will transiently and selectively increase spinal cord cGMP but not cAMP (300). The TRH-induced cGMP is not clinically beneficial (213,311).

Such studies as described above require special techniques to immediate process CNS tissue for proper evaluation of cyclic nucleotides. Human studies have relied on the relationship of extracellular cyclic nucleotides to intracellular content as measured directly in the CSF (110,295). Blockade of the transport of cyclic nucleotides from the CSF will follow proscribed kinetics allowing comparison of cyclic nucleotide accumulations in different patient groups or in the same patients after different drugs. These investigational techniques have demonstrated that baseline and postprobenecid CSF cGMP is significantly decreased in ALS patients (Fig. 12) compared with patients who have other neurological diseases (109,110). In two separate clinical trials, pthalazinol, a cAMP and cGMP phosphodiesterase inhibitor, increased selectively CSF cAMP, but not CSF cGMP, in treated ALS patients (110,312).

Calcium and Calcium-Binding Proteins

Calcium itself can serve as a second messenger by entry through a specific calcium channel in response to receptor-mediated (NMDA, etc.) or nonspecific depolarization. Calcium may act alone or through binding to calmodulin present in the membrane, vesicles, or cytoplasm. Calcium activates this 148-amino-acid, heat-stable protein with four calcium-binding sites to result in activation of specific protein kinases that are different from cAMP, cGMP, or phosphoinositide hydrolysis–activated protein kinases (56). Calcium-mediated changes require a specific ATP-dependent calcium uptake pump, specific binding proteins, and specific protein kinases, which allow alternate effects separate from the cyclical nucleotide or PI hydrolysis systems. Through calmodulin or other calcium-binding proteins, calcium may mediate the effects of the following neurotransmitters:

Type I neurotransmitters
> Glu-induced long-term potentiation in CA1 pyramidal cells by calcium mediated through calmodulin of calcium/calmodulin-dependent protein kinase II (313)

Type II neurotransmitters
> Release of NE, DA, or ACh from vesicles caused by calcium mediated through calmodulin (314)
>
> Phosphorylation of synapsin I following NE, DA, or 5HT release mediated by calcium through calmodulin (315)

Type III neurotransmitters
> VIP increase in hippocampal cAMP inhibited by calcium mediated through calmodulin (316)
>
> SOM-induced increase in calmodulin-dependent cyclic nucleotide phosphodiesterase (317)

Effect of Toxins or Injuries on Calcium/Calmodulin

Toxins or injuries that increase postsynaptic receptors will increase calcium/calmodulin-mediated changes in protein phosphorylation. Calmodulin antagonists can have enhancing or inhibiting effects on calcium-mediated neurotransmitter release, depending on the concentration of antagonists used and length of exposure to the antagonist.

Effect of ALS on Calcium/Calmodulin

Specific studies have not been reported in tissues of ALS patients compared with controls.

Polyphosphoinositides (PI)

Membrane-bound phosphoinositol-4,5-biphosphate (PIP2) is catabolized by membrane-bound phospholipase C when this enzyme is activated via a G protein–mediated event initiated by amino acid, biogenic amine, or neuropeptide binding to a specific receptor (318). PI hydrolysis yields diacylglycerol, which activates protein kinase C, and inositol triphosphate, which can mediate release of intracellular calcium. Protein kinase C leads to phosphorylation of specific cellular proteins that result in defined functions. Released intracellular calcium can mediate a number of postsynaptic transmitter and metabolic functions as described above. The reconstitution of the membrane PI required phosphoryl-ation of diacylglycerol mediated by ATP and formation of cytosine-diphos-phate-diacylglycerol following reaction with cytosine triphosphate. Inositol triphosphate is dephosporylated to inositol, which reacts with cytosine-diphos-phate-diacylglycerol to regenerate PI, which is rephosphorylated to form the membrane-bound phosphoinositol-4,5-biphosphate. PI hydrolysis is common to many tissues; however, in the CNS both neurons and astrocytes may demonstrate PI hydrolysis in response to several neurotransmitters. Within the CNS, how-ever, cerebral cortical and cerebellar astrocytic PI hydrolysis is stimulated by bradykinin, oxytocin, vasopressin, eledoisin, and neurokinin beta, whereas the spinal cord astrocytic PI hydrolysis is stimulated by bradykinin, substance P, eledoisin, and both neurokinin alpha and beta (319). The effects of PI hydrolysis are protean and include metabolic changes as well as mediating the effects of the following neurotransmitters:

Type I neurotransmitters
    PI hydrolysis mediated by Glu-stimulated receptor (320)
Type II neurotransmitters
    PI hydrolysis mediated by class A muscarinic agonists (carbachol or oxy-tremoline-M) (321)
    PI hydrolysis mediated by NE (322)
Type III neurotransmitters
    PI hydrolysis mediated directly by TRH in absence of other transmitters (323)
    PI hydrolysis mediated by CGRP linked to nicotinic ACh receptor synthesis and function (318)

Effect of Toxins or Injuries on PI Hydrolysis
Lithium inhibits PIP2 hydrolysis, which may explain one aspect of its pharma-cological function (324). Excitotoxic amino acid–induced lesions or cholinergic neurons in the nucleus basalis of Meynert will induce increased cortical ACh receptor-mediated PI hydrolysis (325). Neither electroshock, the serotoninergic toxin 5,7DHT, which decreases 5HT, nor the noradrenergic toxins DSP4 and reserpine, which deplete NE affect PI hydrolysis induced by NE (326, 327).

Effect of ALS on PI Hydrolysis
Specific studies have not been reported in tissues of ALS patients compared with controls.

FUTURE DIRECTIONS

This review has strived to provide the foundation for understanding some of the possible neurochemical changes that occur in ALS. In systematically reviewing specific neurotransmitter systems, the neuroanatomy of the neurons in the spinal cord and neurons projecting to the spinal cord were defined, the neurochemical processes for synthesis and degradation of the neurotransmitters were described, and the specific receptors and second-messenger systems, where known, were detailed. It is important to look at the neurochemical effects of specific neurotoxic and physical ablations to determine whether the observed changes in ALS bear any similarities or differences compared to known lesions. The known effects of injury, such as neurectomy, rhizotomy, transection, or blunt trauma, and the known effects of specific toxins were reviewed. The neurochemical data on CNS tissue in ALS suggest that there are some features that are similar to and some features that are not similar to known injuries and toxins. Future studies will have to identify the pathophysiological changes that are specific for ALS.

ACKNOWLEDGMENTS

This review owes much to the clear expositions of the pathophysiology of neurotransmitters described by McGeer et al., the pharmacology of spinal cord neurotransmitters edited by Davidoff, and the early work of Schoenen. The genesis of this review lay in several discussions with Roberto Guiloff (Westminster Hospital, London), Richard Smith (Center for Neurologic Study), Andreas Plaitakis (Mount Sinai School of Medicine), Michael Strong and Arthur Hudson (University of Western Ontario), and Theodore Munsat (Tufts University School of Medicine). Any errors are strictly my responsibility. The help of our ALS Clinic staff, especially Kathy Roelke, Nurse Clinician, in helping me keep to task, both clinical and research, is greatfully appreciated. The ALS Clinical Research Center Coordinator, Jennifer Cox, was extremely helpful in searching for references as well as preparing the text and figures. Much thanks is due my wife and children who put up with references throughout our house from cellar to attic as I tried to systematize the immense amount of data that had to be collated. This review was supported in part by grants from the Muscular Dystrophy Association for the MDA Midwest Regional ALS Research and Treatment Program as well as the Department of Veterans Affairs. Further support was provided by the Hamilton Roddis Foundation and donations in memory of Donald Dietz and Elaine Veith.

REFERENCES

1. Young AB, Penny JB, Dauth GW, Bromberg MB, Gilman S. Glutamate or aspartate as a possible neurotransmitter of cerebral corticofugal fibers in the monkey. Neurology 1983;33:1513–1516.
2. Eccles JC, Fatt P, Koketsu K. Cholinergic and inhibitory synapses in a pathway from motor-axon collaterals to motoneurons. J Physiol 1954;126:524–562.

3. Kuffler SW, Yoshikami D. The distribution of acetylcholine sensitivity at the postsynaptic membrane of vertebrate skeletal twitch muscles: Iontophoretic mapping in the micron range. J Physiol 1975;244:703–730.

4. Gibson SJ, Polak JM, Bloom SR, et al. Calcitonin gene-related peptide immunoreactivity in the spinal cord of man and eight other species. J Neurosci 1984;4: 3101–3111.

5. Takami K, Yriko K, Uchida S, Tohyama M, et al. Effect of calcitonin gene-related peptide on contraction of striated muscle in the mouse. Neurosci Lett 1985;60: 227–230.

6. Kirilovsky J, Duclert A, Fontaine B, Devillers-Thiery A, Osterlund M, Changeux JP. Acetylcholine receptor expression in the primary cultures of embryonic chick myotubes. II. Comparison between the effects of spinal cord cells and calcitonin gene-related peptide. Neuroscience 1989;32:289–296.

7. Ikuta F, Makifuchi T, Ichikawa T. Comparative studies of tract degeneration in ALS and other disorders. In: Tsubaki T, Toyokura Y, eds. Amyotrophic lateral sclerosis. Baltimore: Univrsity Park Press, 1979:177–200.

8. McGeer PL, Eccles JC, McGeer EG. Putative excitatory neurons: Glutamate and aspartate, Chapter 6. In: McGeer PL, Eccles JC, McGeer EG. Molecular neurobiology of the mammalian brain. 2nd ed. New York: Plenum Press, 1987:175–196.

9. Stone TW. Amino acids as neurotransmitters of corticofugal neurones in the rat: A comparison of glutamate and aspartate. Br J Pharmacol 1979;67:545–551.

10. Johnston GAR. The intraspinal distribution of some depressant amino acids. J Neurochem 1968;15:1013–1017.

11. Puil E. Actions and interactions of S-glutamate in the spinal cord. In: Davidoff RA, ed. Handbook of the spinal cord. Vols 2 and 3. Anatomy and physiology. Chapter 3. New York: Marcel Dekker, 1983:105–169.

12. Sonnhof U, Linder M, Grafe P, Krumnikl G. Postsynaptic actions of glutamate on somatic and dendritic membrane areas of the lumbar motoneurons of the frog. Pfluegers Arch 1975;355(Suppl):R86.

13. Potashner SJ, Tran PL. Decreased uptake and release of D-aspartate in the guinea pig spinal cord after partial cordotomy. J Neurochem 1985;44:1511–1519.

14. Potashner SJ, Dymczyk L. Amino acid levels in the guinea pig spinal gray matter after axotomy of primary and descending tracts. J Neurochem 1986;47:412–422.

15. Price DL, Stocks A, Griffin JW, Young A, Peck L. Glycine-specific synapses in rat spinal cord: identification by electron microscope autoradiography. J Cell Biol 1976;68:389–395.

16. Nistri A. Spinal cord pharmacology of GABA and chemically related amino acids. In: Davidoff RA, ed. Handbook of the spinal cord. Vol 1. Pharmacology. New York: Marcel Dekker, 1983:45–104.

17. Reubi JC. Comparative study of the release of glutamate and GABA, newly synthesized from glutamine, in various regions of CNS. Neuroscience 1980;5: 2145–2150.

18. Jansen KLR, Faull RLM, Dragunow M, Waldvogel H. Autoradiographic local-

ization of NMDA, quiasqualate and kainic acid receptors in human spinal cord. Neurosci Lett 1990;108:53–57.

19. Krnjevic K. Chemical nature of synaptic transmission in vertebrates. Physiol Rev 1974;54:418–540.

20. Nieoullon A, Dusdticier N. Glutamate uptake, glutamate decarboxylase and choline acetyltransferase in subcortical areas after sensorimotor cortical ablations in the cat. Brain Res Bull 1983;10:287–293.

21. McGeer PL, Eccles JC, McGeer EG. Inhibitory Amino Acid Neurotransmitters, Chapter 7. In: McGeer PL, Eccles J, McGeer EG. Molecular neurobiology of the mammalian brain. 2nd ed. New York: Plenum Press, 1987:197–234.

22. Young AB, MacDonald RL. Glycine as a spinal cord transmitter. In: Davidoff RA, ed. Handbook of the spinal cord. Vol 1. Pharmacology. New York: Marcel Dekker, 1983:1–44.

23. Krnjevic K, Puil E, Werman R. GABA and glycine action on spinal motoneurons. Can J Physiol Pharmacol 1977;55:658–669.

24. Holstege JC. Ultrastructural evidence for GABAergic brainstem projections to spinal motoneurons in the rat. J Neurosci 1991;11:159–167.

25. Lodge D, Johnston GAR, Stephenson AL. The uptake of GABA and beta-alanine in slices of cat and rat CNS tissue: Regional differences in susceptibility to inhibitors. J Neurochem 1976;27:1569–1570.

26. Barbeau A, Huxtable RJ, eds. Taurine and neurological disease. New York: Raven Press, 1978:298.

27. Schoenen J. Chemical neuroanatomy of the human spinal cord [French]. Rev Neurol 1988;144:630–642.

28. Kelly JS, Gottefeld Z, Schon FF. Reduction in GAD I activity from the dorsal lateral region of the deafferented rat spinal cord. Brain Res 1973;62:581–586.

29. Rizzoli AA. Distribution of glutamic acid, aspartic acid, gamma-aminobutyric acid and glycine in six areas of cat spinal cord after transection. Brain Res 1968;11: 11–18.

30. Perry TL, Hansen S, Jones K. Brain glutamate deficiency in amyotrophic lateral sclerosis. Neurology 1987;37:1845–1848.

31. Plaitakis A. Glutamate dysfunction and selective motor neuron degeneration in amyotrophic lateral sclerosis: A hypothesis. Ann Neurol 1990;28:308.

32. Plaitakis A, Constantakakis C, Smith J. The neuroexcitotoxic amino acids glutamate and aspartate are altered in the spinal cord and brain in amyotrophic lateral sclerosis. Ann Neurol 1988;24:446–449.

33. Constantakakis E, Plaitakis A. *N*-acetylasparate and acetylaspartylglutmate are altered in the spinal cord in amyotrophic lateral sclerosis. Ann Neurol 1988;24: 478.

34. Rothstein JD, Tsai G, Kuncl RW, et al. Abnormal excitatory amino acid metabolism in amyotrophic lateral sclerosis. Ann Neurol 1990;28:18–25.

35. Malessa S, Leigh N, Hornykiewicz O. Branched-chain amino acids in amyotrophic lateral sclerosis. Lancet 1988;2:681–692.

36. Hayashi H, Suga M, Satake M, Tsubaki T. Reduced glycine receptor in the spinal cord in amyotrophic lateral sclerosis. Ann Neurol 1981;9:292–294.

37. Whitehouse PJ, Wamsley JK, Zarbin MA, Price DL, Tourtellotte WW, Kuhar MJ. Amyotrophic lateral sclerosis: Alterations in neurotransmitter receptors. Ann Neurol 1983;14:8–16.

38. Whitehouse PJ, Wamsley JK, Zarbin MA, Price DL, Kuhar MJ. Neurotransmitter receptors in amyotrophic lateral sclerosis: Possible relationship to sparing of eye movements. Ann Neurol 1985;17:518.

39. De Belleroche J, Recordati A, Rose FC. Neurotransmitters and amino acids in motor neurone disease. In: Rose FC, ed. Research progress in motor neurone disease. Chapter 19. Pitman: London, 1984:276–282.

40. Meier DH, Schott KJ. Free amino acid pattern of cerebrospinal fluid in amyotrophic lateral sclerosis. Acta Neurol Scand 1988;77:50–53.

41. Patten BM, Harati Y, Acosta L. Free amino acid levels in amyotrophic lateral sclerosis. Ann Neurol 1978;3:305–309.

42. Perry TL, Krieger C, Hansen S, Eisen A. Amyotrophic lateral sclerosis: Amino acid levels in plasma and cerebrospinal fluid. Ann Neurol 1990;28:12–17.

43. Spink DC, Martin DL. Excitatory amino acids in amyotrophic lateral sclerosis. Ann Neurol 1991;29:110.

44. De Belleroche J, Recordati A, Rose CF. Elevated levels of amino acids in the CSF of motor neuron disease patients. Neurochem Pathol 1984;2:1–6.

45. Ziegler MG, Brooks BR, Lake CR. Norepinephrine and gamma-aminobutyric acid in amyotrophic lateral sclerosis. Neurology 1980;30:98–101.

46. Nothias F, Peschanski M. Homotypic fetal transplants into an experimental model of spinal cord neurodegeneration. J Comp Neurol 190;301:520–534.

47. Mattison MP, Guthrie PB, Kater SB. Intracellular messengers in the generation and degeneration of hppocampal neuroarchitecture. J Neurosci Res 1988;21:447–464.

48. Karpati G, Carpenter S, Dunham H. A hypothesis for the pathogenesis of amyotrophic lateral sclerosis. Rev Neurol 1988;144:672–675.

49. O'Brien RJ, Fischbach GD. Characterization of excitatory amino acid receptors expressed by embryonic chick motoneurons in vitro. J Neurosci 1986;6:3275–3283.

50. Oyanagi K, Ikuta F, Horikawa Y. Evidence for sequential degeneration of the neurons in the intermediate zone of the spinal cord in amyotrophic lateral sclerosis: A topographic and quantitative investigation. Acta Neuropathol 1989;77:343–349.

51. Sharif NA. Chemical and surgical lesions of the rat olfactory bulb: Changes in thyrotropin releasing hormone and other systems. J Neurochem 1988;50:388–394.

52. Beal MF, Swartz KJ, Finn SF, Mazurek MF, Kowall NW. Neurochemical characterization of excitotoxin lesions in the cerebral cortex. J Neurosci 1991;11:147–158.

53. Young AB. What's the excitement about excitatory amino acids in amyotrophic lateral sclerosis? Ann Neurol 1990;28:9–11.

54. Meldrum B, Garthwaite J. Excitatory amino acid neurotoxicity and neurodegenerative disease. Trends Pharmacol Sci 1990;11:379–387.

55. Schwarcz R, Whetsell WO, Mangano REM. Quinolinic acid: An endogenous

metabolite can produce axon sparing lesions in rat brain. Science 1983;219:316–318.

56. McGeer PL, Eccles J, McGeer EG. Principles of synaptic biochemistry. In: McGeer PL, Eccles J, McGeer EG. Molecular neurobiology of the mammalian brain. Chapter 5. New York: Plenum Press, 1987:151–173.

57. Zieglgansberger W, Reiter C. A cholinergic mechanism in the spinal cord of cats. Neuropharmacology 1974;13:519–527.

58. Krnjevic K. Acetylcholine and cyclic GMP. In: Hendon DJ, ed. Cholinergic mechanisms and psychopharmacology. Vol 24. Advances in behavioral biology. New York: Raven Press, 1977:261–266.

59. Weight FF, Salmoiraghi GC. Responses of spinal cord interneurons to acetylcholine, norepinephrine and serotonin administered by microelectrophoresis. J Pharmacol 1966;153:420–427.

60. Peng JH, McGeer PL, McGeer EG. Membrane-bound choline acetyltransferase from human brain: Purification and properties. Neurochem Res 1986;11:959–971.

61. Nagata Y, Okuya M, Watanabe R, Honda M. Regional distribution of cholinergic neurons in human spinal cord transections in the patients with and without motor neuron disease. Brain Res 1982;244:223–229.

62. McGeer PL, Eccles J, McGeer EG. Cholinergic neurons. In: McGeer PL, Eccles J, McGeer EG. Molecular neurobiology of the mammalian brain. 2nd ed. Chapter 8. New York: Plenum Press, 1987:235–263.

63. Ryall RW. Cholinergic transmission in the spinal cord. In: Davidoff RA, ed. Handbook of the spinal cord. Vol 1. Pharmacology. Chapter 5. New York: Marcel Dekker, 1983:203–239.

64. Manaker S, Caine SB, Winokur A. Alterations in receptors for thyrotropin-releasing hormone, serotonin and acetylcholine in amyotrophic lateral sclerosis. Neurology 1988;38:1464–1474.

65. Whitehouse PJ, Lynch D, Kuhar MJ. Effects of post-mortem delay and temperature on neurotransmitter receptor binding in a rat model of the human autopsy process. J Neurochem 1984;43:553–559.

66. Main AR. Structure and inhibitors of cholinesterase. In: Goldberg AM, Hamin I, eds. Biology of cholinergic function. New York: Raven Press, 1976:269–377.

67. Gwyn DG, Wolstencroft JH, Silver A. The effect of a hemisection on the distribution of acetylcholinesterase and choline acetyltransferase in the spinal cord of the cat. Brain Res 1972;47:289–301.

68. Nagata Y, Okuya M, Honda M. Regional distribution of choline acetyltransferase and acetylcholinesterase activity in spinal neurons of motor neuron disease patients. Neurosci Lett 1981;6(Suppl):571.

69. Hayashi H. Lactic dehydrogenase activities in single motoneurons in relations to amyotrophic lateral sclerosis. J Neurol Sci 1987;81:119–131.

70. Kato T. Cholinergic and GABA-ergic systems in ALS spinal motor neurons. In: Tsubaki T, Yase Y, eds. Amyotrophic lateral sclerosis. Amsterdam: Elsevier, 1988:125–130.

71. Poloni M, Partini C, Rocchelli B, Rindi G. Thiamine monophosphate in the CSF of patients with amyotrophic lateral sclerosis. Arch Neurol 1982;39:507–509.

72. Marshall KC. Catecholamines and their actions in the spinal cord. In: Davidoff RA, ed. Handbook of the spinal cord. Vol 1. Pharmacology. Chapter 7. New York: Marcel Dekker, 1983:275–328.

73. Westlund KN, Bowker RM, Ziegler MG, Coulter JD. Noradrenergic projections to the spinal cord of the rat. Brain Res 1983;263:15–31.

74. Tohyama M, Shiotani Y. Neuropeptides in spinal cord. Prog Brain Res 1986;66: 177–218.

75. Zivin JA, Reid JL, Saavedra JM, Kopin IJ. Quantitative localization of biogenic amines in the spinal cord. Brain Res 1975;99:293–301.

76. Lackovic Z, Jakupcevic M, Burnarevic A, Damjanov, Relja M, Kostovic I. Serotonin and norepinephrine in the spinal cord of man. Brain Res 1988;443:199– 203.

77. White SR, Neuman RS. Facilitation of spinal motoneurone excitability by 5-hydroxytryptamine and noradrenaline. Brain Res 1980;188:119–127.

78. Fung SJ, Barnes CD. Evidence of facilitatory coeruleospinal action in lumbar motoneurons of cats. Brain Res 1981;216:299–311.

79. McGeer PL, Eccles J, McGeer EG. Catecholamine neurons. In: McGeer PL, Eccles J, McGeer EG. Molecular neurobiology of the mammalian brain. Chapter 9. New York: Plenum Press, 1987:265–317.

80. Reid JL, Zivin JA, Foppen FH, Kopin IJ. Catecholamine neurotransmitters and synthetic enzymes in the spinal cord. Life Sci 1975;16:975–984.

81. Zivin JA, Reid JL, Tappaz ML, Kopin IJ. Quantitative localization of tyrosine hydroxylase, dopamine beta hydroxylase, phenyl-ethanolamine-N-methyl transferase, and glutamic acid decarboxylase in spinal cord. Brain Res 1976;105:151– 156.

82. Neff NH, Yang HT, Goridis C, Bialek D. The metabolism of indoleakylamines by type A and B monoamine oxidase of brain. In: Costa E, Gessa GL, Sandler M, eds., Serotonin—New vistas, Adv Biochem Psychopharmacol 1974;11:51–58.

83. Westlund KN, Denney RM, Kochersperger LM, Rose RM, Abell CW. Distinct monoamine oxidase A and B populations in primate brain. Science 1985;230: 181–183.

84. Li PP, Warsh JJ, Godse DD. Formation and clearance of norepinephrine glycol metabolites in mouse brain. J Neurochem 1984;43:1425–1433.

85. Langer SZ. Presynaptic regulation of the release of catecholamines. Pharmacol Rev 1980;32:337–362.

86. Bylund DB, U'Prichard DC. Characterization of alpha-1 and alpha-2 adrenergic receptors. Int Rev Neurobiol 1983;24:343–431.

87. Minneman KP, Hegstrand LR, Molinoff PB. Simultaneous determination of beta-1 and beta-2 adrenergic receptors in tissues containing both receptor subtypes. Mol Pharmacol 1979;16:34–46.

88. Schulz DW, Stanford EJ, Wyrick SW, Mailmand RS. Binding of 3H-SCH23390 in rat brain. Regional distribution and effects of assay conditions and GTP suggest interactions at a D-1-like dopamine receptor. J Neurochem 1985;45:1601–1611.

89. Kebabian JW, Calne DB. Multiple receptors for dopamine. Nature 1979;277: 223–234.

90. Jones DJ. Supersensitivity of the spinal cord cyclic AMP system following 6-hydroxydopamine. Eur J Pharmacol 1980;67:499–500.
91. Cadet JL, Karoum F. Central and peripheral effects of iminodipropionitrile on catecholamine metabolism in rats. Synapse 1988;2:23–27.
92. O'Kusky JR, Boyes BE, McGeer EG. Methylmercury-induced movement and postural disorders in developing rat: Regional analysis of brain catecholamines and indoleamines. Brain Res 1988;439:138–146.
93. De La Torre JC, Morassutti D, Merali Z, Fortin T, Richard M. Associated norepinephrine loss following clacium induced spinal paralysis. Brain Res 1988;442:297–304.
94. Nygren LG, Olson L. A new major projection from locus coeruleus: The main source of noradrenergic nerve terminals in the ventral and dorsal columns of the spinal cord. Brain Res 1977;132:85–93.
95. Commissiong JW, Hellstrom SO, Neff NH. A new projection from locus coeruleus to the spinal ventral columns: Histochemical and biochemical evidence. Brain Res 1978;148:207–213.
96. Colado MI, Arnedo A, Peraita E, Del Mio J. Unilateral dorsal rhizotomy decreases monoamine levels in the rat spinal cord. Neurosci Lett 1988;87:302–306.
97. Zivin JA, Doppman JL, Reid JL, et al. Biochemical and histochemical studies of biogenic amines in spinal cord trauma. Neurology 1976;26:99–107.
98. Brait K, Fahn S, Schwarz GA. Sporadic and familial parkinsonism and motor neuron disease. Neurology 1973;23:990–1002.
99. Gilbert JJ, Kish SJ, Chang LJ, Shannak K, Hornekiewicz O. Dementia, Parkinsonism and motor neuron disease: Neurochemical and neuropathological correlates. Ann Neurol 1988;24:688–691.
100. Hayashi H, Tsubaki T. Enzymatic analysis of individual anterior horn cells in amyotrophic lateral sclerosis and Duchenne muscular dystrophy. J Neurol Sci 1982;57:133–142.
101. Gillberg PG, Aquilonius SM, Askmark H. Autoradiographic distribution of high affinity nerve growth factor binding sites and of L-deprenyl binding sites in spinal cords of controls and of patients with amyotrophic lateral sclerosis. In: Rose FC, ed. New evidence in MND/ALS research. London: Smith-Gordon, 1991 (in press).
102. Brooks BR, Ziegler MG, Lake CR, Wood JH, Enna SJ, Engel WK. Cerebrospinal fluid norepinephrine and free gamma-aminobutyric acid in amyotrophic lateral sclerosis. Brain Res Bull 1980;5(suppl 2):765–768.
103. Brucke T, Graf M, Mamoli B, Riederer P. Biogenic amines, their metabolites and amino acids in cerebrospinal fluid of patients with amyotrophic lateral sclerosis. J Neurol 1985;232(Suppl):21.
104. Brooks BR, Turner J, Koch D. Baroreceptor-mediated and thyrotropin-releasing hormone-mediated catecholamine secretion in amyotrophic lateral sclerosis patients with bulbar involvement. Ann Neurol 1987;22:169.
105. Chase TN, Schnur JA, Brody JA et al. Parkinson-dementia and amyotrophic lateral sclerosis of Guam. Arch Neurol 1971;25:9–13.
106. Brody J, Chase TN, Gordon EK. Depressed monoamine catabolite levels in CSF of patients with Parkinson-dementia of Guam. N Engl J Med 1970;282:947–950.

107. Mendell JR, Chase TN, Engel WK. Amyotrophic lateral sclerosis: A study of central monoamine metabolism and therapeutic trial of levo-dopa. Arch Neurol 1972;25:320–325.

108. Forsgren L, Almay BGL, Haggendal J, Oreland L. Monoamine oxidase [MAO], 5-hydroxyindole acetic acid[5HIAA] and homovanillic acid [HVA] in motor neuron disease. Acta Neurol Scand 1987;75:22–27.

109. Ebert MH, Kartzinel R, Cowdry RW, Goodwin FK. Cerebrospinal fluid amine metabolites and the probenecid test. In: Wood JH, ed. Neurobiology of cerebrospinal fluid. Vol. 1. Chapter 8. New York: Plenum Press, 1980:97–112.

110. Brooks BR, Wood JH, Diaz M, et al. Extracellular cyclic nucleotide metabolism in the human central nervous system. In: Wood JH, ed. Neurobiology of cerebrospinal fluid. Vol 1. Chapter 9. New York: Plenum Press, 1980:113–139.

111. Garnett S, Chirakal R, Firnau G, Nahmias C, Hudson A. Recent developments in PET scanning related to amyotrophic lateral sclerosis and primary lateral sclerosis. In: Hudson JA, ed. Amyotrophic lateral sclerosis, concepts in pathogenesis and etiology. Toronto: Toronto Press, 1990:358–370.

112. Anderson EG, Holgerson LO. The distribution of 5-hydroxytryptamine and norepinephrine in cat spinal cord. J Neurochem 1966;13:479–485.

113. Oliveras JL, Bourgoin S, Hery F, Besson JM, Hamon M. The topographical distribution of serotonergic terminals in the spinal cord of the cat: Biochemical mapping by the combined use of microdissection and microassay procedures. Brain Res 1977;138:393–406.

114. Fone KCF, Bennett GW, Marsden CA. Regional distribution of substance P- and thyrotrophin releasing hormone-like immunoreactivity and indoleamines in the rabbit spinal cord. J Neurochem 1987;48:1027–1032.

115. Cooper CL, Marsden CA, Bennett GW. Measurement of catecholamines, indoleamines, thyrotrophin releasing hormone and substance P in rat and human spinal cord using a common extraction method. J Neurosci Meth 1987;22:31–39.

116. Skagerberg G, Bjorklund A. Topographic principles in the spinal projections of serotoninergic and non-serotonergic brainstem neurons in the rat. Neuroscience 1985;15:445–480.

117. Holstege JC, Kuypers HGJM. Brainstem projections to spinal motoneurons: An update. Neuroscience 1987;23:809–821.

118. Dahlstrom A, Fuxe K. Evidence for the existence of monamine neurons in the central nervous system. II. Experimentally induced changes in the intraneuronal amine levels of bulbospinal neuron systems. Acta Physiol Scand 1965;247(Suppl): 1–36.

119. Agajanian GK, McCall RB. Serotonergic synaptic input to facial motoneurons: Localization by electron microscopic autoradiography. Neuroscience 1980;5: 2155–2162.

120. Barasi S, Roberts MHT. The modification of lumbar motoneurone excitability by stimulation of a putative 5-hydroxytryptamine pathway. Br J Pharmacol 1974;52: 339–348.

121. Barasi S, Roberts MHT. The action of 5-hydroxytryptamine antagonists and precursors on bulbospinal facilitation of spinal reflexes. Brain Res 1973;52:385–388.

121a. Magnusson T. Effect of chronic transection on dopamine, noradrenaline and 5-hydroxytryptamine in the rat spinal cord. Naunyn-Schmiedeberg's Arch Pharmacol 1973;278:13–22.

122. VanderMaelen CP, Aghajanian GK. Intracellular studies showing modulation of facial motoneurone excitability by serotonin. Nature 1980;287:346–347.

123. McCall R, Aghajanian G. Serotonin facilitation of facial motoneuron excitation. Brain Res 1979;169:11–27.

124. McGeer PL, Eccles J, McGeer EG. Serotonin and other Brain indoles, chapter 10. In: McGeer PL, Eccles J, McGeer EG. Molecular neurobiology of the mammalian brain. New York: Plenum Press, 1987:319–317.

125. Anderson EG. The serotonin system of the spinal cord. In: Davidoff RA, ed. Handbook of the spinal cord. Vol. 1. Pharmacology. Chapter 6. New York: Marcel Dekker, 1983:241–274.

126. Kimelberg HK, Katz DM. High affinity uptake of serotonin into immunocytochemically identified astrocytes. Science 1985;228:889–890.

127. Blurton PA, Broadhurst AM, Cross JA, Ennis C, Wood MD, Wylie MG. Panuramine, a selective inhibitor of uptake of 5-hydroxytryptamine in the brain of the rat. Neuropharmacology 1984;23:1049–1052.

128. Peroutka SJ, Lebovitz RM, Snyder SH. Two distinct central serotonin receptors and different physiological functions. Science 1981;212:827–829.

129. Berge OG, Fasmer OB, Tveiten L, Hole K. Selective neurotoxic lesions of descending serotonergic and noradrenergic pathways in the rat. J Neurochem 1985;44:1156–1161.

130. Hadjiconstantinou M, Panula P, Lackovic Z, Neff NH. Spinal cord serotonin: A biochemical and immunohistochemical study following transection. Brain Res 1984;322:245–254.

131. Roberts MHT, Wright DM. The effects of chronic section of dorsal roots on the responsiveness of motoneurons to 5-hydroxytryptamine and a substance P analogue. Br J Pharmacol 1981;73:589–594.

132. Nelson DL, Herbet A, Bourgoin S, Glowinski J, Hamon M. Characteristics of central 5HT receptors and their adaptive changes following intracerebral 5,7-dihydroxytryptamine administration in the rat. Mol Pharmacol 1978;14:983–995.

133. Daval G, Verge D, Basbaum AI, Bourgoin S, Hamon M. Autoradiographic evidence of serotonin binding sites on primary afferent fibers in the dorsal horn of the spinal cord. Neurosci Lett 1987;83:71–76.

134. Pranzatelli MR, Dailey A, Markush S. The regulation of TRH and serotonin receptors: Chronic TRH and analog administration in the rat. J Receptor Res 1988;8:667–681.

135. Belendiuk K, Belendiuk GW, Freedman DX, Antel JP. Neurotransmitter abnormalities in patients with motor neuron disease. Arch Neurol 1981;38:415–417.

136. McGeer PL, Eccles J, McGeer EG. The prominent peptides, chapter 12. In: McGeer PL, Eccles J, McGeer EG. Molecular neurobiology of the mammalian brain. New York: Plenum Press, 1987:369–414.

137. Neale JH, Barker JL. Peptides: Diverse elements in spinal-sensory function. In:

Davidoff RA, ed. Handbook of the spinal cord. Vol 1. Pharmacology. Chapter 4. New York: Marcel Dekker, 1983:171–202.

138. Palkovits M. Topography of chemically identified neurons in the central nervous system. Neuroendocr Perspect 1984;1:1–69.

139. Fried G, Franck J, Brodin E. Differential distribution of 5-hydroxytryptamine and substance P in synaptosomal vesicles of rat ventral spinal cord. Neurosci Lett 1988;91:315–320.

140. Gilbert RFT, Emson PC, Hunt SP, et al. The effects of monoamine neurotoxins on peptides in the rat spinal cord. Neuroscience 1982;7:69–87.

141. Marti E, Gibson SJ, Polak JM, et al. Ontogeny of peptide- and amine-containing neurones in motor, sensory, and autonomic regions of rat and human spinal cord, dorsal root ganglia and rat skin. J Comp Neurol 1987;266:332–359.

142. Gibson SJ, Polak JM, Giaid A, et al. Calcitonin gene-related peptide messenger RNA is expressed in sensory neurones of the dorsal root ganglia and also in spinal motoneurones in man and rat. Neurosci Lett 1988;91:283–288.

143. Pittman QJ, Riphagen CL, Lederis K. Release of immunoassayable neurohypophyseal peptides from rat spinal cord, in vivo. Brain Res 1984;300:321–326.

144. Fried G, Franck J, Brodin E, et al. Evidence for differential storage of calictonin gene-related peptide, substance P and serotonin in synaptosomal vesicles of rat spinal cord. Brain Res 1989;499:315–24.

145. Hokfelt T, Johansson O, Goldstein M. Chemical anatomy of the brain. Science 1984;225:1326–1334.

146. Loy YP, Parish DC. Processing of neuropeptide precursors. In: Turner AJ, ed. Neuropeptides and their peptidases. Chapter 4. New York: VCH, 1987:65–84.

147. Sharif NA, Burt DR. Rat brain TRH receptors: kinetics, pharmacology, distribution and ionic effects. Regul Peptides 1983;7:399–411.

148. White SR. A comparison of the effects of serotonin, substance P and thyrotropin releasing hormone on excitability of rat spinal motoneurones in vivo. Brain Res 1985;335:63–70.

149. Bennett GW, Nathan PA, Wong KK, Marsden CA. Regional distribution of immunoreactive thyrotrophin releasing hormone and substance P and indoleamines in human spinal cord. J Neurochem 1986;46:1718–1724.

150. Benarroch EE, Aimone LD, Yaksh TL. Segmental analysis of neuropeptide concentrations in normal human spinal cord. Neurology 1990;40:137–144.8

151. Wimalaswansa SJ, Morris HR, Etienne A, Blench I, Panico M, MacIntyre I. Isolation, purification and characterization of beta-CGRP from human spinal cord. Biochem Biophys Res commun 1990;167:993–1000.

152. Hietanen M, Pelto-Huikko M, Rechardt L. Immunocytochemical study of the relations of acetylcholinesterase, enkephalin, substance P-, choline acetyltransferase- and calcitonin gene-related peptide immunoreactive structures in the ventral horn of rat spinal cord. Histochemistry 1990;93:473–477.

153. Newton BW, Unger J, Hamill RW. Calcitonin gene-related peptide and somatostatin immunoreactivities in the rat lumbar spinal cord: Sexually dimorphic aspects. Neuroscience 1990;37:471–489.

154. Pepper P, Miccych PE. The effect of castration on calitonin gene-related peptide in spinal motor neurons. Neuroendocrinology 1989;50:338–343.

155. Battaner F, Rodriquez del Castillo A, Guerra M, Mas M. Gonadal influences on spinal cord and brain monoamines in male rats. Brain Res 1987;425:391–394.

156. Gibson SJ, Polak JM, Katagiri T, et al. A comparison of the distribution of eight peptides in spinal cord from normal controls and cases of motor neurone disease with special reference to Onuf's nucleus. Brain Res 1988;474:255–278.

157. New HV, Mudge AW. Calcitonin gene-related peptide regulates muscle acetylcholine receptor synthesis. Nature 1986;232:809–811.

158. Ohhashi T, Jacobwitz DM. Effects of calcitonin gene-related peptide on neuromuscular transmission in the isolated diaphragm. Peptides 1988;9:613–617.

159. Oku R, Satoh M, Fujji N, Otaka A, Yajima H, Takagi H. Calcitonin gene-related peptide promotes mechanical nociception by potentiating release of substance P from the spinal dorsal horn in rats. Brain Res 1987;463:350–354.

160. Le Greves P, Nyberg F, Terenius L, Hokfelt T. Calcitonin gene-related peptide is a potent inhibitor of substance P degradation. Eur J Pharmacol 1985;115:309–311.

161. Miletic V, Tan H. Ionotophoretic application of calcitonin gene-related peptide produces a slow and prolonged excitation of neurons in the cat lumbar dorsal horn. Brain Res 1988;446:169–172.

162. Kangrga I, Randic M. Tachykinin and calcitonin gene-related peptide enhance release of endogenous glutamate and aspartate from the rat spinal dorsal horn slice. J Neurosci 1990;10:2026–2038.

163. Pohl M, Benoliel JJ, Bourgoin S, et al. Regional distribution of calcitonin gene-related peptide-substance P-, cholecystokinin-, met-enkephalin-, and dynorphin A(1–8)-like materials in the spinal cord and dorsal root ganglia of adult rats: Effects of dorsal rhizotomy and neonatal capsaicin. J Neurochem 1990;55:1122–1130.

164. Arvidsson U, Cullheim S, Ulfhake B, Hokfelt T, Terenius L. Altered levels of calcitonin gene-related peptide (CGRP)-like immunoreactivity of cat lumbar motoneurons after chronic spinal cord transection. Brain Res 1989;489:387–391.

165. Mannen T, Makoko I, Toyokura Y, Nagashima K. Preservation of a certain motoneurone group of the sacral cord in amyotrohic lateral sclerosis: Its clinical significance. J Neurol Neurosurg Psychiatry 1977;40:464–469.

166. Fisher LA, Kikkawa DO, Rivier JER, et al. Stimulation of noradrenergic sympathetic outflow by calcitonin gene-related peptide. Nature 1983;305:534–536.

167. Gibson SJ, Polak JM, Allen JM, Adrian TE, Kelly JS, Bloom SR. The distribution and origin of a novel brain peptide, neuropeptide Y, in the spinal cord of several mammals. J Comp Neurol 1984;227:78–91.

168. Gulbenkian S, Wharton J, Hacker GW, Varndell IM, Bloom SR, Polak JM. Co-localization of neuropeptide tyrosine(NPY) and its C-flanking peptide(C-PON). Peptides 1985;6:1237–1243.

169. Everitt BJ, Hokfelt T, Terenius L, Tatemoto K, Mutt V, Goldstein M. Differential co-existence of neuropeptide Y(NPY)-like immunoreactivity with catecholamines in the central nervous system of the rat. Neuroscience 1984;11:443–462.

170. Tiles P, Regenoid JT. Interaction between neuropeptide Y and noradrenaline on central catecholamine neurons. Nature 1990;344:62–63.

171. Petrusz P, Merchenthaler I, Maderdrut JL. Distribution of enkephalin-containing neurons in the central nervous system. In: Bjorklund A, Hokfelt T, eds. Handbook of chemical neuroanatomy. Vol 4. GABA and neuropeptides in the CNS. Part I. Chapter 6. Amsterdam: Elsevier 1985:273–326.

172. Hunt SP, Kelly JS, Emson PC, Kimmel JR, Miller R, Wu JY. An immunohistochemical study of neuronal populations containing neuropeptidergic or GABA within the superficial layers of the rat dorsal horn. Neuroscience 1981;6:1883–1898.

173. Hunt SP, Lovik TA. The distribution of 5HT, met-enkephalin and beta-lipotropin-like immunoreactivity in neuronal perikarya in the cat brain stem. Neurosci Lett 1982;30:139–145.

174. Zieglfansberger W, Tullock IF. The effects of methionine- and leucine-enkephalin on spinal neurons of the cat. Brain Res 1979;167:53–64.

175. Mudge AW, Leeman SE, Fischbach GD. Enkephalin inhibits release of substance P from sensory neurons in culture and decreases action potential duration. Proc Natl Acad Sci USA 1979;76:526–530.

176. Pohl M, Lombard MC, Bourgoin S, et al. Opioid control of the in vitro release of calcitonin gene-related peptide from primary afferent fibers projecting in the rat cervical cord. Neuropeptide 1989;14:151–159.

177. Gilbert RFT, Bennett GW, Marsden CA, Emson PC. The effects of 5-hydroxy-tryptamine-depleting drugs on peptides in the ventral spinal cord. Eur J Pharmacol 1981;76:203–210.

178. Ch'ng JLC, Christofides ND, Anand P, et al. Distribution of galanin in the central nervous system and the response of galanin-containing neuronal pathways to injury. Neuroscience 1985;16:343–354.

179. Fisone G, Wu CF, Consolo S, et al. Galanin inhibits acetylcholine release in the ventral hippocampus of the rat: histochemica, autoradiographic, in vivo and in vitro studies. Proc Natl Acad Sci USA 1987;84:7339–7343.

180. Nordstrom O, Melander T, Hokfelt T, Bartfai T, Goldstein M: Evidence for an inhibitory effect of the peptide galanin on dopamine release from the rat median eminence. Neurosci Lett 1987;73:21–36.

181. Villar MJ, Cortes R, Theodorsson E, et al. Neuropeptide expression in rat dorsal root ganglion cells and spinal cord after peripheral nerve injury with special reference to galanin. Neuroscience 1989;33:587–604.

182. Bowker RM, Westlund KN, Sullivan MC, Wilber JF, Coulter JD. Descending serotonergic, peptidergic and cholinergic pathways from the raphe nuclei: A multiple transmitter complex. Brain Res 1983;288:33–48.

183. White SR, Crane GK, Jackson DA. Thyrotropin-releasing hormone (TRH): Effects on spinal cord neuronal excitability. Ann NY Acad Sci 1989;553:337–350.

184. Takahashi T, Otsuka M. Regional distribution of substance P in the spinal cord and nerve roots of the cat and the effect of dorsal root section. Brain Res 1975;87:1–11.

185. Naftchi NE, Abrahams SJ, St Paul HM, Lowman EW, Schlosser W. Localization of substance P in spinal cord of paraplegic cats. Brain Res 1978;153:507–513.

186. Mantyh P, Hunt SP. The autoradiographic localization of substance P receptors in the rat and bovine spinal cord and the rat and cat spinal trigeminal nucleus pars caudalis and the effects of neontal capsaicin. Brain Res 1985;332:315–324.

187. Wright Dm, Roberts MHT. Supersensitivity to a substance P analogue following dorsal root section. Life Sci 1978;22:19–24.

188. Helke CJ, Charlton CG, Wiley RG. Studies on the cellular localization of spinal cord substance P receptors. Neuroscience 1986;19:523–533.

189. Schoenen J. Chemical neuroanatomy of the human spinal cord: Applications to disease including amyotrophic lateral sclerosis [French]. Rev Neurol 1988;144: 664–671.

190. Patten BM, Croft S. Spinal cord substance P in amyotrophic lateral sclerosis. In: Rose FC, ed. Research progress in motor neuron disease. Bath: Pitman, 1984: 283–289.

191. Gillberg PG, Aquilonuis SM, Eckmas SA, Lundqvist G, Winblad B. Choline acetyltransferase and substance P-like immunoreactivity in the human spinal cord: Changes in amyotrophic lateral sclerosis. Brain Res 1982;250:394–397.

192. Otsuka M, Kanazawa I, Sugita H, Toyokura Y. Substance P in the spinal cord and serum of amyotrophic lateral sclerosis. In: Tsubaki T, Toyokura Y, eds. Amyotrophic lateral sclerosis. Baltimore: University Park Press, 1978:405–411.

193. Dietl MM, Sanchez M, Probst A, Palacios JM. Substance P receptors in the human spinal cord: decrease in amyotrophic lateral sclerosis. Brain Res 1989;483: 39–49.

194. Nutt JG, Mroz EA, Leeman SE, Williams AC, Engel WK, Chase TN. Substance P in human cerebrospinal fluid: Reductions in peripheral neuropathy and autonomic dysfunction. Neurology 1980;30:1280–1285.

195. Cramer H, Rosler N, Rissler K, Gagnieu MC, Renaud B. Cerebrospinal fluid immunoreactive substance P and somatostatin in neurological patients with peripheral and spinal cord disease. Neuropeptides 1988;12:119–124.

196. Lechan RM, Segerson TP. ProTRH gene expression and precursor peptides in rat brain: Observations by hybridization analysis and immunocytochemistry. Ann NY Acad Sci 1989;553:29–59.

197. Coffield JA, Miletic V, Zimmerman E, Hoffert MJ, Brooks BR. Demonstration of thyrotropin-releasing hormone immunoreactivity in neurons of the mouse spinal dorsal horn. J Neurosci 1986;6:1194–1197.

198. Hokfelt T, Tsuruo Y, Ulfhake B, et al. Distribution of TRH-like immunoreactivity with special reference to coexistence with other neuroactive compounds. Ann NY Acad Sci 1989;553:76–105.

199. Bowker RM, Westlund KN, Sullivan MC, Wilber JF, Coulter JD. Transmitter of the raphe-spinal complex: Immunocytochemical studies. Peptides 1982;3: 291–298.

200. Ulfake B, Arvidsson U, Cullheim S, et al. An ultrastructural study of 5-hydroxytryptamine, thyrotropin-releasing hormone and substance P-immunoreactive axonal boutons in the motor nucleus of spinal cord segments L7-S1 in the adult cat. Neuroscience 1987;23:917–929.

201. Griffiths EC, Kelly JA, Ashcroft A, Ward DJ, Robson B. Comparative metabolism

and conformation of TRH and its analogues. Ann NY Acad Sci 1989;553:217–231.

202. Paakkari I, Siren AL, Nurminen ML, Svartstrom-Fraser M. Injection of thyrotropin releasing hormone into the locus coeruleus increases blood pressure. Eur Heart J 1987;8(Suppl B):147–151.

203. Askanas V, Engel WK, Eagleson K, Micaglio G. Influence of TRH and TRH analogues RGH-2202 ad DN-1417 on cultured ventral spinal cord neurons. Ann NY Acad Sci 1989;553:325–336.

204. Banda RW, Means ED, Fitzgerald M. Thyrotropin releasing hormone decreases neuronal loss induced by axotomy in infant rats. Neurology 1987;37(Suppl 1):285.

205. Van den Bergh P, Kelly JJ, Adelman L, Munsat TL, Jackson IMD, Lechan R. Effect of spinal cord TRH deficiency on lower motor neuron function in the rat. Muscle Nerve 1987;10:397–405.

206. Van den Bergh P, Kelly JJ, Adelman L, Munsat TL, Jackson IMD, Lechan R. Spinal cord TRH deficiency is associated with incomplete recovery of denervated muscle in the rat. Neurology 1988;38:452–459.

207. Lechan RM, Jackson IMD. Thyrotropin releasing hormone but not histidyl proline diketopeperazine is depleted from rat spinal cord following 5,7-dihyroxytryptamine. Brain Res 1983;326:152–155.

208. Sharif NK, Towle AC, Burt DR, Mueller RA, Breese GR. Co-transmitters: differential effects of serotonin (5-HT) depleting drugs on levels of 5-HT and TRH and their receptors in rat brain and spinal cord. Brain Res 1989;480:365–371.

209. Sharif NA, Burt DR. Micromolar substance P reduces spinal receptor binding for thyrotropin releasing hormone-possible relevance to neuropeptide coexistence. Neurosci Lett 1983;43:245–251.

210. Prasad C, Spahn SA. Chronic thyrotropin releasing hormone decreases the affinity and increases the number of its own receptor in the spinal cord. Neurosci Lett 1989;103:309–313.

211. Lighton C, Marsden CA, Bennett GW. The efffsects of 5,7-dihydroxytryptamine and parachlorophenylalanine on thyrotropin releasing hormone in regions of the brain and spinal cord of the rat. Neuropharmacology 1984;23:55–60.

212. Faden AI, Hill TG, Kubek MJ. Changes in TRH immunoreactivity in spinal cord after experimental spinal injury. Neuropeptides 1985;7:11–18.

213. Kozachuk WE, Mitsumoto H, Salanga VD, Beck GJ, Wilber JF. Thyrotropin releasing hormone (TRH) in murine motor neuron disease (the wobbler mouse). J Neurol Sci 1987;78:253–260.

214. Zimmermann EM, Coffield JA, Miletic V, Brooks BR. Changes in substance P (Sub P)-, 5-hydroxytryptamine (5-HT)- and thryotropin releasing hormone (TRH)-like immunoreactivity (LI) in spinal cord during murine neurotropic retrovirus induced motor neuron degeneration. Neurology 1985;35(Suppl 1):157–158.

215. Jackson IM, Adelson LS, Munsat TL, Forte S, Lechan R. Amyotrophic lateral sclerosis: Thyrotropin releasing hormone and histidyl proline diketopiperazine in the spinal cord and cerebrospinal fluid. Neurology 1986;1218–1223.

216. Mitsuma T, Nogumou T, Adachi K, Mukoyama M, Ando K. Concentrations of

immunoreactive thyrotropin releasing hormone in spinal cord of patients with amyotrophic lateral sclerosis. Am J Med Sci 1984;287:34–36.

217. Banda RW, Kubek MJ, Means ED. Decreased content of thyrotropin releasing hormone(TRH) in cervical ventral horn of patients with amyotrophic lateral sclerosis (ALS). Neurology 1986;36(Suppl 1):139.

218. Mitsuma T, Adachi K, Muroyama M, Ando K. Concentration of thyrotropin releasing hormone in the brain of patients with amyotrohic lateral sclerosis. J Neurol Sci 1986;76:277–281.

219. Brooks BR, Turner J, Schwartz T. Spinal cord thyrotropin releasing hormone (TRH) catabolism in animal and human motor neuron disease. Soc Neurosci Abstr 1986;12(Part 1):82.

220. Brooks BR, Turner J, Schwartz T, Tourtellotte WW. Human spinal cord thyrotropin releasing hormone (TRH) metabolism: Increased TRH catabolism with histidylproline(His-Pro-OH) and proline formation in amyotrohic lateral sclerosis. Neurology 1987;37(Suppl 1):163.

221. Court JA, McDermott JR, Gibson AM, et al. Raised thyrotropin releasing hormone pyroglutamylamino peptidase, and proline endopeptidase are present in the spinal cord of wobbler mouse but not in human motor neurone disease. J Neurochem 1987;49:1084–1090.

222. Turner J, Schwartz T, Tourtellotte WW, Brooks BR. Increased deamindation of thyrotropin releasing hormone (TRH) in spinal cord of TRH-treated amyotrophic lateral sclerosis (ALS) patients. Neurology 1988;38(Suppl 1):326.

223. Engel WK, Wilber JF, Van den Bergh P, Siddique T. CSF thyrotropin releasing hormone (TRH) and histidine-proline diketopeperazine (cyclo-HisPro, cHP) in neuromuscular diseases and during TRH infusion. Neurology 1983;34(Suppl 1): 210.

224. Brooks BR. A summary of the current position of TRH in ALS therapy. Ann NY Acad Sci 1989;553:431–461.

225. Malin JP, Kodding R, Fuhrmann H, von zur Muhlan A. T4, T3 and rT3 levels in serum and cerebrospinal fluid of patients with amyotrophic lateral sclerosis. J Neurol 1989;236:57–59.

226. Yoshio Y, Irie H, Akai K. Assay of nuclear triiodothyronine receptors in the precentral gyrus in patients with amyotrophic lateral sclerosis [Japanese]. Rinsho Shinkeigaku 1990;30:45–49.

227. Nozaki M. Changes in free amino acids in the central nervous system of hypo- and hyper-thryoid rats [Japanese]. Rinsho Shinkaigaku 1989;29:713–719.

228. Whybrow P, Prange A. A hypothesis of thyroid-catecholamine-receptor interaction. Arch Gen Psychiatry 1981;38:106–113.

229. Martin R, Geis R, Holl R, Schafer M, Voigt KH. Co-existence of unrelated peptides in oxytocin and vasopressin terminals of rat neurohypophyses: immunoreactive methionine-enkephalin-, leucin-enkephalin- and cholecystokinin-like substances. Neuroscience 1983;8:213–227.

230. Dreifuss JJ. Vasopressin an oxytocin as neuromediators. Arch Intern Physiol Biochem 1989;97:A1–A14.

231. Pretel S, Piekut DT. Mediation of changes in paraventricular vasopressin and

oxytocin mRNA content to the medullary vagal complex and spinal cord of the rat. J Chem Neuroanat 1989;2:327–334.

232. Jenkins JS, Ang VTY, Hawthorn J, Rossor MN, Iverson LL. Vasopressin, oxytocin and neurophysins in the human brain and spinal cord. Brain Res 1984;291: 111–117.

233. Olsson JE, Forsling ML, Lindvall B, Akerlund M. The cerebrospinal fluid vasopressin in Parkinson's disease, dementia and other degenerative disorders. J Neurol 1985;232(Suppl):176.

234. Seckl JR, Lightman SL, Guiloff RJ. Elevated cerebrospinal fluid vasopressin in moror neuron disease. J Neurol Neurosurg Psychiatry 1987;50:795–797.

235. Breuer AC, Atkinson MB. Fast axonal transport alterations in amyotrophic lateral sclerosis (ALS) and in parathyroid hormone (PTH) treated axons. Cell Motil Cytoskeleton 1988;10:321–330.

236. Dockray GJ. Cholecystokinin, chapter 34. In: Krieger DT, Brownstein MJ, Martin JB, eds. Brain peptides. New York: Wiley, 1983:851–869.

237. Iwasaki Y, Kinoshita M, Ikeda K, Shiojima T. Trophic effects of cholecystokinin and calcitronin gene-related peptide on ventral spinal cord in culture. Int J Neurosci 1989;48:285–289.

238. Werdelin L, Gjerris A, Boysen G, Fahrenkrug J, Jorgensen OS, Rehfeld JF. Neuropeptides and neural cell adhesion molecule (NCAM) in CSF from patients with ALS. Acta Neurol Scand 1989;79:177–181.

239. Kalin NH. Behavioral and endocrine studies of corticotropin-releasing hormone in primates. In: De Souza EB, Nemeroff CB, eds. Corticotropin-releasing factor: Basic and clinical studies of a neuropeptide. Chapter 19. Boca Raton, FL: CRC Press, 1990:275–290.

240. Vale WW, Rivier C, Spiess J, Rivier J. Corticotropin releasing factor. In: Krieger DT, Brownstein MJ, Martin JB, eds. Brain peptides. Chapter 38. New York: Wiley. 1983;961–980.

241. Vale W, Spiess J, Rivier C, Rivier J. Characterization of a 41-residue ovine hypothalaminic peptide that stimulates secretion of corticotropin and beta-endorphin. Science 1981;213:1394–1397.

242. Klimek A, Cieslak D, Szulc-Kuberska J, Stepien H. Reduced lumbar cerbrospinal fluid corticotropin releasing factor (CRF) levels in amyotrophic lateral sclerosis. Acta Neurol Scand 1986;74:72–74.

243. Gianoulakis C, Angelogianni P. Characterization of beta-endorphin peptides in the spinal cord of the rat. Peptides 1989;10:1048–1054.

244. Nicoll RA, Siggins GR, Ling N, Bloom FE, Guillemin R. Neuronal actions of endorophins and enkephalins among brain regions: A comparative microiontophoretic study. Proc Natl Acad Sci USA 1977;74:2584–2588.

245. Moroni F, Cheney DL, Costa E. The turnover rate of acetylcholine in brain nuclei of rats injected intraventricularly and intraseptally with alpha and beta endorphin. Neuropharmacology 1978;171:191–198.

246. Berney S, Hornkiewicz O. The effect of beta-endorphin and met-enkephalin on striatal dopamine metabolism and catalepsy: Comparison with morphine. Commun Psychopharmaol 1977;1:597–604.

247. Loh HH, Brase DA, Sampath-Khanna S, Mar JB, Way EL, Li CH. Beta-endorphin in vitro inhibition of striatal dopamine release. Nature 1976;264:567–568.

248. Bloom FE, Segal DS. Endorphins in cerebrospinal fluid. In: Wood, JH, ed. Neurobiology of cerebrospinal fluid. Vol 1. Chapter 45. New York: Plenum Press, 1980:651–664.

249. Besse D, Lombard MC, Zajac JM, Roques BP, Besson JM. Pre- and post-synaptic distribution of mu, delta and kappa opioid receptors in the superficial layers of the cervical dorsal horn of the rat spinal cord. Brain Res 1990;52:15–22.

250. Suh HH, Tseng LF. Delta, but not mu-opioid receptors in the spinal cord are involved in antinociception induced by beta-endorphin given intracerebroventricularly in mice. J Pharmacol Exp Ther 253:981–986.

251. Iadarola MJ, Brady LS, Draisc G, Dubner R. Enhancement of dynorphin gene expression in spinal cord following experimental inflammation stimulus specificity, behavioral parameters and opioid receptor binding. Pain 1988;35:313–326.

252. Hughes S, Smith ME. Pro-opiomelanocaortin-derived peptides in transected and contralateral motor nerves of the rat. J Chem Neuroanat 1989;2:227–237.

253. Klimek A, Szulc-Kuberska J, Stepien H. Beta-endorphin level in cerebrospinal fluid of ALS patients. J Neurol Sci 1990;88(Suppl):218.

254. Fone KCF, Johnson JV, Dix P, Bennett GW, Marsden CA. Repeated intrathecal TRH analogue injections, but not 5,7 DHT treatment, induces tolerance to wet-dog shake behavior and increases ventral horn ChAT activity. Ann NY Acad Sci 1989;553:598–601.

255. Lipman BT, Haughton VM. Diminished cerebrospinal fluid beta-endorphin concentration in monkeys with arachnoiditis. Invest Radiol 1988;23:190–192.

256. Chiba T, Masuko S. Coexistence of varying combinations of neuropeptides with 5-hydroxytryptamine in neurons of the raphe pallidus et obscurus projecting to the spinal cord. Neurosci Res 1989;7:13–23.

257. Macdonald RL. Neuropharmacology of spinal cord and dorsal root ganglion neurons in primary dissociated cell culture. In: Davidoff RA, ed. Handbook of the spinal cord. Vol 1. Pharmacology. Chapter 9. New York: Marcel Dekker, 1983: 381–408.

258. Sah DW. Neurotransmitter modulation of calcium current in rat spinal cord neurons. J Neurosci 1990;10:136–141.

259. Tuchscherer MM, Seybold VS. A quantitative study of the coexistence of peptides in varicosities within the superficial lamine of the dorsal horn of the rat spinal cord. J Neurosci 1989;9;195–205.

260. Jancso G, Hokfelt T, Lundberg JM, et al. Immunohistochemical studies on the effect of capsaicin on spinal and medullary peptide and monoamine neurons using antisera to substance P, gastrin-CCK, somatostatin, VIP, enkephalin, neurotensin and 5-hydroxytryptamine. J Neurocytol 1981;10:963–980.

261. Unger J, Weindl A, Ochs G, Struppler A. CSF somatostatin is elevated in patients with postzoster merualgia. Neurology 1988;38:1423–1427.

262. Reinikainen KJ, Reikkinene PJ, Jolkkonen J, Kosma VM, Soininen H. Decreased somatostatin-like immunoreactivity in cerebral cortex and cerebrospinal fluid in Alzheimer's disease. Brain Res 1987;402:103–108.

263. Linder S, Barkheim T, Norberg A, et al. Structure and expression of the gene encoding the vasoactive intestinal peptide precursor. Proc Natl Acad Sci USA 1987;84:605–609.
264. Abrams GM, Nilaver G, Zimmerman EA. VIP-containing neurons. In: Bjorklund A, Hokfelt T, eds. Handbook of chemical neuroanatomy. Vol 4. GABA and neuropeptides in the CNS. Part I. Chapter 7. Amsterdam: Elsevier, 1985:335–354.
265. Yaksh TL, Michener SR, Bailey JE, et al. Survey of distribution of substance P, vasoactive intestinal polypeptide, cholecystokinin, neurotensi, ret-enkephalin, bombesin and PHI in the spinal cord of cat, dog, sloth and monkey. Peptides 1988;9:357–372.
266. Chung K, Briner RP, Carlton SM, Westlund KN. Immunohistochemical localization of seven different peptides in the human spinal cord. J Comp Neurol 1989;280:
267. Du F, Dubois P. Distribution of substance P and vasoactive intestinal polypeptide neurons in the chicken spinal cord, with note on postnatal development. J Comp Neurol 1988;278:253–264.
268. LaMotte CC. Vasoactive intestinal polypeptide cerebrospinal fluid-contacting neurons of the monkey and cat spinal central canal. J Comp Neurol 1987;258:527–541.
269. Jeftinija S, Murase K, Nedelijkov V, Randic M. Vasoactive intestinal polypeptide excites mamalian dorsal horn neurons in vivo and in vitro. Brain Res 1982;243:158–164.
270. Magistretti PJ. VIP-containing neurons in the cerebral cortex: Cellular actions and interactions with the noradrenergic system. In: Ritchie JM, Keynes RD, Bolis L, eds., Ion channels in neural membranes. New York: Alan R Liss, 1986:323–331.
271. Hosli L, Hosli E, Heuss L, Rojas J. Electrophysiological evidence for receptors for vasoactive intestinal peptide and angiotensin II on astrocytes of cultured rat central nervous system. Neurosci Lett 1989;102:217–222.
272. Cholewinski AJ, Wilkin GP. Astrocytes from forebrain, cerbellum, and spinal cord differ in their response to vasoactive intestinal peptide. J Neurochem 1988;51:1626–1633.
273. McCulloch J, Kelly PAT, Uddman R, Edvinsson L. Functional role of vasoactive intestinal polypeptide in the caudate nucleus: A 2-deoxy(14C)glucose investigation. Proc Natl Acad Sci USA 1983;80:1472–1476.
274. Brenneman DE, Nicol T, Warren D, Bowers LM. Vasoactive intestinal peptide: A neurotrophic releasing agent and an astroglial mitogen. J Neurosci Res 1990;25:386–394.
275. Brenneman DE, Foster GA. Structural specificity of peptides influencing neuronal survival during development. Peptides 1987;8:687–694.
276. Wang FZ, Nelson PG, Fitzgerald SC, Hersh LB, Neale EA. Cholinergic function in cultures of mouse spinal cord neurons. J Neurosci Res 1990;25:312–323.
277. Gibson SJ, Polak JM, Anand P, et al. The distribution of origin of VIP in the spinal cord of six mammalian species. Peptides 1984;5:201–207.
278. Yaksh T, Abay EO, Go VL. Studies on the localization and release of cholecys-

tokinin and vasoactive intestinal polypeptide in the rat and cat spinal cord. Brain Res 1982;242:279–290.

279. McGregor GP, Gibson SJ, Sabate IM, et al. Effect of peripheral nerve crush on spinal cord neuropeptides in the rat: Increased VIP and PHI in the dorsal horn. Neuroscience 1984;13:207–216.

280. Shehab SAS, Atkinson ME. Vasoactive intestinal polypeptide increases in areas of the dorsal horn of the spinal cord from which other neuropeptides are depleted following peripheral axotomy. Exp Brain Res 1986;62:422–430.

281. Fuji K, Senba E, Tohyama M, Fujji S, Ueda Y, Wu JW. Distribution, ontogeny and fiber connections of cholecystokinin-8, vasoactive intestinal polypeptide and gamma-aminobutyric acid containing neuron systems in the rat spinal cord: An immunohistochemical analysis. Neuroscience 1985;14:881–896.

282. Iwasaki Y, Kinoshita M, Ikeda K, Shionjima T. Neurotrophic effect of vasoactive intestinal polypeptide (VIP) on the ventral spinal cord of rat embryo. Acta Neurol scad 1990;81:87.

283. Kamo H, Haebara H, Akiguchi I, Kameyama M, Kimura H, McGeer PL. A distinctive distribution of reactive astroglia in the precentral cortex in amyotrophic lateral sclerosis. Acta Neuropathol 1987;74:33–38.

284. Northup JK. Regulation of cyclic nucleotides in the nervous system. In: Siegel G, Agranoff B, Albers RW, Molinoff P, eds. Basic neurochemistry, molecular, cellular and medical aspects. 4th ed. Chapter 17. New York: Raven Press, 1989: 349–363.

285. Nestler EJ, Greengard P. Protein phosphorylation in the nervous system. New York: Wiley, 1984.

286. Kaczmarek LK, Levitan IB, eds. Neuromodulation: The biochemical control of neuronal excitability. Oxford: Oxford University Press, 1986.

287. Baba A, Nishiuchi Y, Uemura A, Tatsuno T, Iwata H. Inhibition by forskolin of excitatory amino acid-induced accumulation of cyclic AMP in guinea pig. J Neurochem 1988;51:237–242.

288. Wojcik WJ, Neff NH. Gamma-aminobutyric acid B receptors are negatively coupled to adenylate cyclase in brain and in the cerebellum these receptors may be associated with granule cells. Mol Pharmacol 1984;25:24–28.

289. Jones DJ, McKenna LF. Norepinephrine-stimulated cyclic AMP formation in rat spinal cord. J Neurochem 1980;34:467–469.

290. Jones DJ, McKenna LF. Cyclic AMP formation in rat spinal cord tissue slices. Neuropharmacology 1980;19:669–674.

291. Brown JH, Brown SL. Agonists differentiate muscarinic receptors that inhibit cyclic AMP formation from those that stimulate phosphoinositide metabolism. J Biol Chem 1984;259:3777–3781.

292. Kebabian JW, Steiner AL, Greengard P. Pharmacological and biochemical evidence for the existence of two categories of dopamine receptor. Can J Neurol Sci 1984;11:114–117.

293. Watling KJ, Bristow DR. GABAB receptor-mediated enchancement of vasoactive intestinal peptide stimulated cyclic AMP production in slices of rat cerebral cortex. J Neurochem 1986;46:1756–1762.

294. Tachikawa E, Tank AW, Yanagihara N, Mosimann W, Weiner N. Phosphorylation of tyrosine hydroxylase on at least three sites in rat phenochromocytoma PC12 cells treated with 56 mM potassium: Determination of the sites on tyrosin hydroxylase phosphorylated by cyclic AMP-dependent protein kinases. Mol Pharmacol 1986;30:4760485.

295. Stone EA, John SM. In vivo measurement of extracellular cyclic AMP in the brain: Use in studies of beta-adenoceptor function in anonanesthetized rats. J Neurochem 1990;55:1942–1949.

296. Garthwaite J, Garthwaite G. Cellular origina of cyclic GMP responses to excitatory amino acid receptor agonists in rat cerebellum in vitro. J Neurochem 1987;48: 29–39.

297. Ferrendelli JA. Role of cyclic GMP in the function of the central nervous system. In: Weiss B, ed. Cyclic nucleotides in disease. Baltimore: University Park Press, 1975:377–390.

298. Ferrendelli JA, Steiner AL, McDougal DB, Kipnis DM. The effect of oxotremorine and atropine on cGMP and CAMP levels in mouse cerebral cortex and cerebellum. Biochem Biophys Res Commun 1970;41:1061–1067.

299. Mailman RB, Frye GD, Mueller RA, Breese GR. Change in brain quanosine-3'.5'-monophosphate (cGMP) content by thyrotropin releasing hormone. J Pharmacol Exp Ther 1979;208:169–175.

300. Brooks BR, Priester E, Lust WD. Behavioral and neurochemical effects of acute and chronic administration of thyrotropin releasing hormone (TRH) in NIH:N mice. Neurology 1984;34(Suppl 1):239.

301. Friedl A, Harmening C, Hamprecht B. Atrial natriuretic hormones raise the level of cyclic GMP in neural cell lines. J Neurochem 1986;46:1522–1527.

302. Naftchi NE, Kirschner AK, Demenyu M, Viau AT. Alterations in norepinephrine, serotonin, cAMP, and transsynaptic induction of tyrosine hydroxylase after spinal cord transection in the rat. Neurochem Res 1981;6:1205–1216.

303. Ghetti B, Truex L, Sawyer B, Strand S, Schmidt M. Exaggerated cyclic AMP accumulation and glial cell reaction in the cerebellum during Purkinje cell degeneration in pcd mutant mice. J Neurosci Res 1981;6:789–801.

304. Brodie ME, Aldridge WN. Elevated cerebellar cyclic GMP levels during the deltamethrin-induced motor syndrome. Neurobehav Toxicol Teratol 1982;4:109–113.

305. Lust WD, Kupferberg JH, Yonekawa WD, Penry JK, Passonneau JV, Wheaton AB. Changes in brain metabolites induced by convulsants or electroshock: Effects of anticonvulsant drugs. Mol Pharmacol 1978;14:347–356.

306. Lust WD, Feussner GK, Passonneau JV, McCandless DW. Distribution of cyclic nucleotides in layers of cerebellum after decapitation. J Cyclic Nucleotide Res 1981;7:333–337.

307. Gentleman S, Parenti M, Commissiong JS, Neff NH. Dopamine-activated adenylate cyclase of spinal cord: supersensitivity following transection of the cord. Brain Res 1979;210:271–275.

308. Mao C, Guidotti A, Landis S. Cyclic GMP: Reduction of cerebellar concentrations in "nervous" mutant mice. Brain Res 1975;90:335–339.

309. Brooks BR, Lust WD, Andrews JM, Engel WK. Decreased cyclic GMP in murine (wobbler) spontaneous motor neuron degeneration. Arch Neurol 1978;35:590–591.

310. Brooks BR, Feussner GK, Lust WD. Spinal cord metabolic changes in murine retrovirus induced neuron disease. Brain Res Bull 1983;11:681–686.

311. Sandmire DA, Turner JG, Priester E, Brooks BR. Non-equilibrium uptake kinetics of 125-I thyrotropin-releasing hormone (TRH) into spinal cord and brain following intravenous, intraperitoneal, or subcutaneous administration in NIH:N mice. Neurology 1985;35(Suppl 1):93.

312. Kaneko Y, Suzuki S, Hayakawa T, Yashima Y, Kumashiro H. Non-typical matters occurring in motor neuron disease and cyclic nucleotide metabolism. Fukushima J Med Sci 1983;29:113–123.

313. Malenka RC, Kauer JA, Perkel DJ, et al. An essential role for postsynaptic calmodulin and protein kinase activity in long term potentiation. Nature 1989;340:554–557.

314. De Lorenzo RJ. Calmodulin modulations of the calcium signal in synaptic transmission. In: Bradford HF, ed. Neurotransmitter interactions and compartmentalization. New York: Raven Press, 1982:101–120.

315. Imai S, Onozuika M. Clearer demonstration of calcium/calmodulin-dependent events in synaptosomes by use of the differential effects of two calmodulin antagonists, *N*-(aminohexyl)-5-chloro-1-naphthalenesulfonamide and *N*-(6-aminonohexyl)-1-naphthalenesulfonamide. Comp Biochem Physiol (C) 1988;91:535–540.

316. Ahlijanian MK, Cooper DM. Distinct interactions between Ca2+/calmodulin and neurotransmitter stimulation of adenylate cyclase in striatum and hippocampus. Cell Mol Neurobiol 1988;8:459–469.

317. Rendon MC, Toro MJ, Mellado M, Montoya E. Somatostatin stimulates phosphodiesterase in rat anterior pituitary and brain and GH4Cl cells. Second-Messengers-Phosphoproteins 1988;12:75–81.

318. Agranoff BW. Phosphoinositides, Chapter 16. In: Siegel GJ, Agranoff B, Albers RW, Polinoff P, eds. Basic neurochemistry: Molecular, cellular and medical aspects. 4th ed. New York: Raven Press, 1989:333–347.

319. Cholewinski AJ, Hanley MR, Wilkin GP. A phosphoinositide-linked peptide response in astrocytes: Evidence for regional heterogeneity. Neurochem Res 1988;13:389–394.

320. Nicoletti F, Meek JL, Iadarola MJ, Chuang DM, Roth BL, Costa E. Coupling of inositol phospholipid metabolism with excitatory amino acid recognition sites in rat hippocampus. J Neurochem 1986;46:40–46.

321. Gongora JL, Sierra A, Marisca S, Aceves J. Physostigmine stimulates phosphoinositide breakdown in the rat neostriatum. Eur J Pharmacol 1988;155:49–55.

322. Nicoletti F, Canonico PL, Favit A, Nicoletti G, Albanese V. Receptor-mediated stimulation of inositol phospholipid hydrolysis in human brain. Eur J Pharmacol 1989;160:299–301.

323. Imai A, Gershengorn MC. Phosphatidylinositol 4,5-biphosphate turnover is tran-

sient while phophatidylinositol turnover is persistent in thyrotropin releasing hor-
mone-stimulated rat pituitary cells. Proc Natl Acad Sci USA 1986;83:5840–8544.

324. Lenox RH, Hendley D, Ellis J. Desensitization of muscarinic receptor-coupled
phosphoinositide hydrolysis in rat hippocampus: Comparisons with the alpha 1-
adrenergic response. J Neurochem 1988;50:558–564.

325. Reed LJ, de Belleroche J. Induction of ornithine decarboxylase in cerebral cortex
by excitatoxin lesion of nucleus basalis: Association with postsynaptic responsiveness and *N*-methyl-D-aspartate receptor activation. J Neurochem 1990;55:780–
787.

326. Fowler CJ, Thorell G, Sundstrom E, Archer T. Norepinephrine-stimulated inositol
phospholipid breakdown in the rat cerebral cortex following serotoninergic lesion.
J Neural Transm 1988;73:205–215.

327. Blendy JA, Stockmeier CA, Kellar KJ. Electroconvulsive shock and resperpine
increase alpha 1-adrenergic binding sites but not norepinephrine-stimulated phosphoinositide hydrolysis in rat brain. Eur J Pharmacol 1988;156:267–270.

28

Protease Cascade Dysregulation and Synaptic Degeneration in Amyotrophic Lateral Sclerosis

Barry W. Festoff

*Veterans Affairs Medical Center, Kansas City, Missouri,
and University of Kansas Medical Center, Kansas City, Kansas*

INTRODUCTION

The neuromuscular junction has traditionally been a model for the study of cell-cell interaction in the nervous system. The interaction of the motor neuron's presynaptic axonal twigs with the subsynaptic portion of the muscle fiber surface at this peripheral cholinergic synapse is influenced by humoral factors as well as by specific adhesive components of the extracellular matrix. Neuromuscular synapse formation is initiated with the outgrowth of a neurite destined to be the axon of the motor neuron. This initial ramification begins a complex cascade of steps, which include the directed extension of this axonal process through an inhospitable extracellular milieu, the recognition of an appropriate site(s) on the muscle fiber's surface, and the localized deposit, removal, and subsequent redeposition of components of the muscle fiber's basal lamina. Eventually, in the neonatal period, a stabilization or linkage of macromolecules of the motor neuron and muscle fiber with the synaptic basal lamina occurs during the process known as elimination of polyneuronal innervation (1). This process, and its underlying mechanisms, may allow for plasticity or remodeling over the life of the organism. The very nature of these cascade events suggests that the well-studied biochemical events associated with regulated extracellular proteolysis underlying thrombogenesis and fibrinolysis may participate in this process (2).

Activation of extracellular protease activity at the neuromuscular junction was proposed 10 years ago (3) as a common pathogenetic mechanism in amyotrophic

Table 1 Comparison of ALS Etiological Theories and
Protease Activation

Theory	Activates neutral proteases
Deficiency	Unknown
Environmental	
Lead	Yes
Mercury	Yes
Manganese	Unknown
Calcium	Yes
Aluminum	Yes
Metabolic	
Glucose/insulin	Yes
Pancreatic	Yes
Catecholamine	Unknown
Free amino acids	Yes
Aging (abiotrophy)	Yes
Viral	Yes
Cancer	Yes
Circulating toxic factor	Possibly (i.e., plasminogen)

lateral sclerosis (ALS). Such an hypothesis fits with the concept of "dying back" as it relates to ALS (4,5). Dying back still remains an attractive model for continued motor unit destruction in ALS despite one contrary report (6). Furthermore, the unexplained feature of the neuropathology of ALS, the apparent differential susceptibility of individual motor neurons even in areas of severe motor neuronal loss (7–9), is also consistent with a dying-back process coexisting with regenerative sprouting and reinnervation. Dysregulation of protease activity in the central nervous system, coupled with the loss of peripheral target organ and retrograde transsynaptic degeneration, could account for the corticospinal tract involvement in addition to the motor unit disturbance in ALS. In this regard, if we compare the various theories of etiology with known increases in neutral protease activity, we can generate a listing such as Table 1. The intention of this review is to bring this hypothesis concerning a protease:inhibitor imbalance underlying ALS with current concepts of the roles of these molecules in the development as well as the degeneration of the nervous system.

Our laboratory has been actively testing the hypothesis that synapse formation, more specifically neuromuscular junction formation, may be based on molecular mechanisms similar to clot formation and retraction. Recently, the Maratea Conference (see 10) took place and the participants explored theoretical considerations and empirical observations that implicated serine proteases of the fibrinolytic cascade in muscle and neural cells both in culture and in vivo. As it may relate to ALS, some of this information has been presented elsewhere (see 11–14).

BACKGROUND

Neuromuscular Junction Acetylcholinesterase Localization and Release

The junctional acetylcholinesterase (AChE) terminates the action of acetycholine (ACh) at the synapse, and most of this fraction is attached to or lies within the basal lamina. Although much remains in the basal lamina after injury, denervation, or x-irradiation of frog muscle (see 15,16), less remains in mammalian muscle. This end-plate AChE is extremely sensitive to extracellular proteases, the AChE activity released into the bathing medium in organ culture (17–19), without affecting neuromuscular transmission. Maintenance of the basal lamina localization of this fraction of extracellular AChE depends on innervation (16). Much of this extracellular-bound AChE is the asymmetrical, collagen-tailed form known as A_{12} AChE. It is this collagenous "tail" of asymmetrical A_{12} AChE that is exquisitely sensitive to proteolysis, not the globular catalytic subunits of the "head" region (20–22). Our studies demonstrating very rapid decline of asymmetrical AChE in synaptic regions following short stump axotomy (17) represented one of the earliest changes in muscle following denervation. They demonstrated a neurotrophic influence of the nerve to localize A_{12} AChE to the synaptic basal lamina (18,19). Subsequent studies indicated that exogenous protease inhibitors protected AChE localization after denervation (23,24). An extract of peripheral nerve had similar properties to exogenous protease inhibitors by protecting A_{12} AChE localization to end-plates in organ culture (24). These experiments led to studies of endogenous protease regulation after denervation and the balance between proteases and inhibitors in muscle.

We had earlier suggested that end-plate instability in ALS patients might result in release of AChE into the blood (see 8), just as synaptic AChE was released into organ culture bathing medium. This was consistent with studies by others in chicken dystrophy (neural) and immaturity (25,26). Neurotrophic regulation of the extracellular localization of AChE at the junction, its susceptibility to proteases, and the dramatic reduction following denervation all supported this concept. To test this further, we assayed "true" plasma AChE in control and ALS patients. In humans circulating AChE is quite low, compared with pseudocholinesterase or even with erythrocyte AChE. We found a twofold elevation in plasma AChE in ALS patients compared to controls (27), subsequently confirmed by others (28). This demonstrated that release of AChE from some bound site may account for this increase in ALS patients. Protease-susceptible sites on the basal lamina seem reasonable to explain these results. These data were also consistent with reports indicating that junctional pathology existed in ALS patients' muscle (29).

Basal Lamina of Skeletal Muscle and NMJ

The 80–100-nm-thick basal lamina ensheathes the adult skeletal muscle fiber, continues through, and contributes the synaptic matrix material at the junction. This synaptic basal lamina has many important roles in the formation, function, and maintenance of the end-plate (see 16): the binding of A_{12} acetylcholinesterase via specific sites; the adhesion of nerve to muscle; ''induction'' or maintenance of ACh receptor clustering in the postsynaptic membrane; regulation of nerve terminal differentiation or regenerating axons during muscle reinnervation; and the precise reinnervation at original synaptic regions of muscle following denervation. The maintenance function of the junctional basal lamina likely has special importance to ALS research.

Three classes of matrix components are known to exist in the muscle basal lamina: global, synapse-excluded and synapse-specific (see 16). In the latter group are included, in addition to asymmetrical AChE, heparan sulfate proteoglycan, agrin (see below), and S-laminin. Specific biochemical relationships exist between AChE and other basal lamina components. For instance, certain basal lamina glycoproteins interact with sugar-site-specific plant lectins, such as concanavalin A, that prevent solubilization of AChE from electric organ membranes and precipitate A_{12} AChE in vitro (30). Labeled eel AChE (31), as does rat AChE (32), sediments with dense, carbohydrate-containing membrane particles. One such carbohydrate, the glycosaminoglycan chondroitin sulfate, caused low-ionic-strength aggregation of eel AChE (33). In addition, heparin was shown to both bind to as well as solubilize asymmetrical AChE from basal lamina–binding sites (34).

We initiated studies of extracellular matrix synthesis in clonal muscle cells in an effort to explore the relationship of AChE to basal lamina components (35–37). In recent studies of proteoglycan synthesis by primary chick (38) and clonal mouse (39) muscle cells in culture, we found that synthesis of a large Mr chondroitin sulfate proteoglycan depended on stage of myogenic development. A smaller Mr heparan sulfate proteoglycan also showed this developmental regulation in the primary cultures (39). These cultures demonstrate clusters of AChRs quite readily, a fact used to develop a bioassay to purify the AChR-aggregating molecule, agrin (40), and show developmental regulation of AChE isoforms (18,19). A large chondroitin sulfate proteoglycan similar to that detected in cultured muscle cells has been identified as a terminal anchorage protein (TAP-1) at neuromuscular synapses (41).

Possible explanations for why the clonal cells did not show developmental regulation of the large proteoglycan might be degradation of the core protein or some genetic deficiency in the transformed state. In this regard, these clonal cells contain significant levels of proteases, and a plasminogen activator was the major secreted protease found (42). Primary chick cultures have extremely low levels of plasminogen activators (PAs) and must be infected by Rous sarcoma virus for PA activity to be demonstrated (43,44). The PA induced has prominent effects on AChRs in these chick cells, in particular, acceleration of receptor internalization and degradation (43). Furthermore, as mentioned, clonal cells demonstrate constitutively high-specific-activity PA, their major secreted neutral protease (42), without viral infection. The locally produced plasmin accelerates internalization of AChRs, thus allowing more rapid intralysosomal degradation (45), but also reducing the numbers of receptors on the muscle membrane and, thereby, inhibiting cluster formation (44). Clonal cells cannot be used to demonstrate spontaneous clustering of AChRs. This may relate to unopposed surface proteolysis since we have found colocalization of patches of protease nexin I, a protease inhibitor, with AChR clusters in mature primary cultures but not in clonal cells (46). Of interest to the relationship between AChR aggregation or clustering and protease inhibition was the mention at the Winter Brain Conference meeting in 1990 that agrin, the chondroitin sulfate–associated AChR-aggregating factor, possessed protease inhibitory activity.

Extracellular Proteases: Plasminogen Activators, Collagenase, and Kallikreins

Plasminogen activators (PAs) are serine proteases that are specific and selective, converting plasminogen to plasmin (47). They are found in plasma, urine (urokinase), various tissues, and transformed or "activated" cells in culture. Two types of PAs are known in mammalian species, tissue-type PA (tPA) and urokinase-like PA (uPA). PAs have been associated with processes of tissue remodeling, invasive potential of malignant cells, or migratory behavior of others (47–49). Plasminogen is present in abundant quantities in plasma (0.1 mg/ml) and many cells are capable of synthesizing and releasing specific PAs; plasmin itself, once active, has broad proteolytic specificity (47).

Mammalian collagenase is a Ca^{2+}-activated neutral protease that cleaves helical regions of reticular, fibrillar collagen such as types I and III. Type IV collagenases and "gelatinases" also exist. Activation of collagenase is known to occur by specific plasmin proteolytic cleavage and under the control of urokinase (50).

Kallikreins are serine proteases that either circulate (plasma kallikrein) or are present in, but can also be released from, tissues (glandular or tissue kallikrein).

Table 2 Chronology of Protease Regulation in Neuromuscular System

Release of lysosomal enzymes at end-plate by nerve stimulation	(53,54)
Decrease in lysosomal enzymes with end of polyneuronal innervation	(1)
ACh causes release of lysosomal enzymes in developing muscle	(1)
Cultured muscle secretes PA after Rous sarcoma virus infection	(43,44)
PA:plasmin affects ACh receptors on Rous-infected chick muscle	(45)
Denervation causes early release of A12 AChE from basal lamina	(17)
Hypothesis of neutral proteases in synaptic disorders such as ALS	(2)
Finding of protease nexin in clonal mouse muscle cells	(13)
PA:plasmin involves in muscle basal lamina degradation in culture	(35)
PA major secreted neutral protease of cultured muscle	(42)
PA:plasmin speeds internalization of ACh receptors in muscle	(45)
uPA followed by tPA activated early in denervated muscle	(58)
uPA:plasmin degrades matrix components in situ with denervation	(14)
PNI localizes to end-plate along with ACh receptors	(46)
uPA and tPA decline rapidly as polyneural innervation is eliminated	(59)
PMI prevents uPA-driven myotube basal lamina degradation	(101)
Muscle uPA not tPA rapidly regulated by nerve	(60)

These are separate molecules by a variety of criteria (51). Of interest to neurobiology and any discussion of ALS is that tissue kallikrein is a major enzyme in salivary secretions, along with the PAs and the growth factors, NGF and EGF. By sequence studies, sufficient homology exists between NGF and the EGF-binding protein to consider these molecules in the glandular kallikrein subclass (52).

Neutral Proteases and the End-Plate Basal Lamina

The normal turnover of synaptic AChE, as well as that of other matrix-associated glycoproteins, may involve one or more of these enzymes. That proteases release basal lamina–bound AChE experimentally from the end-plate has already been discussed. In addition, a number of studies have shown release of these enzymes by nerve stimulation (53,54), by disease processes, and following experimental manipulation. Their involvement has been proposed to account for the elimination of polyneuronal innervation seen frequently in neonatal mammals (1). An inexhaustive list of these are presented in Table 2.

Early studies indicated that lysosomal proteases increased in skeletal muscle following denervation (55), with the earliest increase 48 hr after nerve section (56). Initial attempts to define a topographic representation for muscle collagenase were unrewarding (Festoff et al., unpublished). We did not assay whether a type IV "collagenase," similar to the serine protease elastase, isolated from neutrophils, was more critical in basal lamina protein turnover. This enzyme may be associated with junctional basal lamina destruction in ALS. We did find, however, ample evidence for participation of the PA:plasmin system (11–14,35–37). Since this system, like most members of the serine protease family, involves zymogen precursors in cascades of activity, a mechanism for tissue remodeling that can be controlled locally is possible. This type of balanced system is more likely to be involved in the changes in the neuromuscular system.

Our own studies demonstrated that PAs were the major secreted neutral proteases in clonal muscle cultures (42). Both tPA and uPA were produced and secreted (57). In innervated, adult muscle, low levels of PAs are present but denervation rapidly increases these enzymes, especially uPA, which increased hours after nerve section and reached levels 8- to 10-fold above controls 7 days later (58). In developing muscle, postnatal regulation of uPA and tPA was found, and both enzymes decreased dramatically during the period of elimination of polyneuronal innervation 2–3 weeks after birth (59). uPA, but not tPA, is under tight neural regulation since levels return almost to control values after reinnervation when crush, rather than axotomy, is used (60). The messenger RNA encoding urokinase (uPA) is in high concentration in adult muscle but is not completely translated, the translation being under some, as yet undefined, negative translational control signal from the nerve (61). What role this untranslated mRNA for uPA has in the pathogenesis of ALS is currently under study in our laboratory.

Proteolytic/Collagenolytic Activity in Skin of ALS Patients

The previous finding that skin of patients with ALS and other denervating disorders possessed increased proteolytic or collagenolytic activity may be the link between the neurotrophic control of muscle basal lamina protein turnover/degradation by uPA:plasmin and other proteases with enhanced protease activity in other ALS tissues. Fullmer and his associates detected alteration in collagen fibrils in skin of Guamanian ALS patients (62), postulating that the alteration was the result of enhanced catalytic activity of collagen and *predicted* the presence of an activated collagenase, or other protease. They extended this finding to sporadic ALS and to other denervating and degenerative neurological conditions (63). More recent studies by Toyokura and Mannen and colleagues have confirmed these observations and found them to be specific for ALS (64,65). Thus, they represent a potentially important clue to this enigmatic and fatal disease. We assayed collagenase activity in dissociated skin biopsies of Guamanian ALS patients and found no increase in fibroblast collagenase activity. However, after 1 week in organ culture, collagenase activity increased, suggesting that interaction of components in the tissue was required to uncover latent enzyme (66). This also suggested that activation of latent collagenase in ALS patients' skin by some "factor," perhaps the plasminogen activator:plasmin (50), accounted for these results.

In addition to hypothesizing the participation of neutral extracellular proteases in the degradation of extracellular matrix (ECM) components, the original hypothesis (2) also introduced the concept of a protease inhibitor produced by one or more of the cell types present at the neuromuscular junction. This has subsequently been tested and resulted in the demonstration of localized concentration of a specific protease inhibitor, protease nexin I (PNI), at adult murine junctions (see below).

INHIBITORS OF SERINE PROTEASES

With all the steps and mechanisms mentioned above to *augment* proteolysis, how then is it possible to control widespread extracellular proteolysis? Control is exerted over plasma proteases by circulating antiprotease or protease inhibitors (PIs), proteins capable of inhibiting plasmin, collagenase, and other proteases, and which include alpha$_2$-macroglobulin, alpha$_1$-antitrypsin, C$_1$-inactivator, and others (67). Many of these are members of the serpin superfamily (68), others belong to the Kunitz family of inhibitors (67). The balance of this system depends partly on the PI concentration in plasma and partly on the local concentration of proteases synthesized and released. A preliminary study sought to determine the levels of α_2-macroglobulin (α_2-mac), a major circulating PI in plasma in ALS patients (69). ALS patients had significantly lower levels of α_2-mac. However, in a subsequent unstratified study, this reduction in α_2-mac was not confirmed by others (70), whereas reduction in antithrombin III (ATIII), a serpin homologous to protease nexin I (71,72), was found. Extension of the study of circulating serpins into (a) grouping by subtype, (b) comparison with other neuromuscular diseases, and (c) possible use of such analyses as prognostic indicators and baseline for therapeutic trials is warranted. Several experiments have already been performed to determine whether ALS patients' sera contain the same or different capacity as normal sera to inhibit extracellular proteolytic (tryptic) activity in a rather simple assay. They indicated that ungrouped ALS patients' sera was less effective than normal sera in inhibiting trypsin (69), but further studies in this area are indicated.

Kunitz-Type Inhibitors ("Kunins")

This group of polypeptides and glycoproteins represents the oldest-known and best-studied of the serine protease inhibitors. Members of this class include the bovine pancreatic trypsin inhibitor (Kunitz inhibitor; aprotinin or Trasylol) as well as the inter-α-trypsin inhibitor (IαI) and the lipoprotein-associated coagulation inhibitor (LACI; see 73). The class also includes the Kunitz protease inhibitor (KPI)-domain-containing forms of the β-amyloid precursor protein

(βAPP_{751} and βAPP_{770}; see 74,75). "Kunins" may be single, double, or tri-headed. Of interest to the concept of synapse formation involving a balance between one or more of the serine proteases and the peptide/polypeptide serine proteinase inhibitors is the close association of kunins with glycosaminoglycans, especially heparan sulfate and chondroitin sulfate (see above), as well as the disulfide links based on their intra- and interchain cysteines. In unpublished studies, we have also localized protease nexin II (75–77), the soluble forms of the β-amyloid precursor (βAPP_{751} and βAPP_{770}) to human and rodent end-plates. From studies of IαI and the βAPPs, the kunins, apparently unlike the serpins, have been embedded in larger precursors and are specifically cleaved to yield the functional inhibitor (73).

Serpins, a Growing Family of Serine Protease Inhibitors

These include circulating and cellular inhibitors and structurally homologous molecules for which a serine protease inhibiting function has not, as yet, been found (68). Members in the former subgroup are α_1-protease inhibitor ($\alpha_1 PI$), or α_1-antitrypsin, and α_1-antichymotrypsin ($\alpha_1 ACT$). The serpins without known inhibitory activity include angiotensinogen and ovalbumin.

Protease nexin I (PNI) is a cell-associated member of the serpin superfamily of serine protease inhibitors (71,72,78,). It is a heparin-activatable thrombin inhibitor with reported molecular masses (M_r) of 38–54 kDa. The variability in M_r is presumably due to differences in glycosylation. In addition to inhibiting thrombin at rates faster than any other mammalian inhibitor (in the presence of heparin, $1 \times 10^9 \, mol^{-1} \, sec^{-1}$), PNI is also a "respectable" inhibitor of uro-kinase (uPA) and tissue (tPA) plasminogen activators, although a much less potent inhibitor of plasmin and trypsin, and it does not inhibit chymotrypsin. Like other serpins, PNI is "single-headed" and forms 1:1 molar complexes with serine proteinases. Most serpins have a primary, physiological target protease and for PNI it is likely to be thrombin, but this may vary during development. Although originally found in human foreskin fibroblasts, PNI is synthesized by a number of anchorage-dependent, extravascular mammalian cells. Impor-tant to its possible role in cholinergic neuromuscular synapse formation is the fact that PNI binds to and is localized to the basal lamina (92). This finding has prompted Cunningham and colleagues to postulate that cell surfaces can regulate the amount and type (i.e., target protease) of inhibitory activity by PNI (79,80).

Plasminogen activator inhibitors 1, 2, and 3 (PAI-1,2,3) are more specific cellular serpins than PNI and have little or no inhibitory specificity toward serine proteases other than the PAs (81,82). PAI-1 is the major regulator of the extrinsic pathway of fibrinolysis. It is present in plasma, and in great amounts in platelets, and is bound, in a latent form, to the basal lamina. Other PAIs have been isolated and purified (83).

Protease nexin II (PNII), another serine protease inhibitor, was first detected by its ability to "link" up with the epidermal growth factor (EGF)-binding protein (84) and γ subunit of nerve growth factor (NGF; 100), itself a serine protease homologous with tissue kallikrein (52). Once isolated and purified, it was found to be an effective inhibitor of chymotrypsin (84). Recent exciting work has demonstrated that the sequence of PNII is identical to the β-amyloid precursor protein (βAPP_{751}) isolated from senile amyloid plaques from Alzheimer's disease (AD) patients' brains (75–77). However, a controversy currently exists as to whether PNII is a serpin or, perhaps, a kunin (see above), based on its ability to form 1:1 molar ratio complexes with EGF-binding protein or chymotrypsin that are resistant to boiling SDS (76,77,84).

SERPINS IN THE NERVOUS SYSTEM

Serpins in the central nervous system (CNS) were first evaluated by Monard and his co-workers, who isolated a polypeptide initially from rat C6 glioma conditioned medium that promoted neurite outgrowth from mouse neuroblastoma cells cultured in the absence of NGF (85). The isolated and purified molecule was shown to be a protease and fibrinolytic inhibitor and, subsequently, to be virtually identical to protease nexin I (86). When the cDNAs for the glioma factor (86), subsequently termed the glial derived nexin (GDN), and human fibroblast PNI were compared, GDN differed from PNI by only three amino acids (87,88). Peripheral tissues, fibroblasts, and muscle (Festoff et al., unpublished data) produce two forms, termed alpha and beta, which are in a 2:1 ratio, while CNS cells produce only, or primarily, the β form. No differences in terms of activity, spectrum of proteases inhibited, or heparin binding have been found in the two forms (88).

Neurite outgrowth promotion was the bioassay used by Monard's group to define, isolate, and, ultimately, clone the GDN (85,86,89). This effect has been attributed to PNI's inhibition of a thrombin-like enzyme (90). This has been confirmed for PNI's equipotent promotion of neurite outgrowth, while the thrombin present in the culture medium was found to be inhibitory in the outgrowth bioassay (90). Recently, Monard's group, using the polymerase chain reaction (PCR), has detected the mRNA encoding for prothrombin in rat brain (91).

Neuronal survival has been stated by Monard to be unaffected by GDN (85,86,92). In previous experiments with day 8 chick embryo mixed spinal cord cultures, it was found that an extract of adult chicken ischiatic (sciatic) nerve, after transferrin was removed by affinity chromatography, markedly enhanced neuronal survival, as well as neurite outgrowth (93). Preliminary characterization of this extract showed that antithrombin and anti-urokinase-like PA (uPA) activity was present in a heparin-agarose affinity elution peak. This peak has recently been shown to contain PNI (Festoff et al., unpublished). Similarly, studies have been performed showing that PNI enhanced survival of cortical neurons in culture, and that endogenous PNI is released from cortical glial cells under the influence of vasoactive intestinal polypeptide (94). No reports of neuronal survival enhancement have been reported for the PAIs. Thus, PNI and/or other serpins may also have neuronal survival properties, along with their effects on neurite outgrowth, further suggesting their roles as trophic factors in the nervous system.

Distribution of serpins in the CNS has recently been reported by Monard and his colleagues, who have shown that GDN is enriched in the olfactory system: bulb, tract, and lobe (95). This finding is of considerable interest and importance since the olfactory system undergoes almost continuous degeneration and regeneration in the adult mammalian nervous system. In addition, in Alzheimer's disease (AD) several groups of investigators have recently focused attention on the olfactory system as a region susceptible to aluminum intoxication and where amyloid plaques are found in high concentration (96,97). PNI has also recently been shown to be present in amyloid plaques in AD brain (98). The relationship between these neuropathological changes in AD and ALS is underscored by recent findings of immature, noncongophilic plaques in brains of Guamanian victims of ALS/Parkinsonism-dementia complex (ALS/PDC).

SERPINS IN THE PERIPHERAL NERVOUS SYSTEM (PNS)

The original hypothesis regarding ALS and the end-plate predicted that the normal balance and regulation of protease activity at the synapse must involve participation of one or more inhibitors (3). This prediction coincided chronologically with the demonstration of the first cellular serine protease inhibitor, protease nexin (71), now called PNI (87,88). As remarked above, we found that a partially purified factor in chicken sciatic nerve distinct from transferrin ("sciatin," "neurotrophic factor"), promoted neurite outgrowth and survival of motor neurons in chick spinal cord cell cultures (93). This factor is a fibrinolytic inhibitor homologous to PNI (Festoff et al., in preparation). Recently, Monard and colleagues showed a rapid increase in mRNA encoding for GDN/PNI in the distal stump of a crushed rat sciatic nerve (99). In crush injury of mouse sciatic nerve, PNI mRNA also increases in the distal stump (Festoff et al., in preparation) over the same time course as that of uPA increase in the denervated muscle (60).

Critical in their selectivity as inhibitors, and probably accounting for GDN/PNI's neurotrophic ability to promote neurite outgrowth (89,90), are the reactive centers of the serpins (Table 3). As shown in the table, there is an overrepre-

Table 3 Partial Reactive Center of Serpin Inhibitors

	Sequence	P2	P1	P1′	P2′	P3′
Rodent						
	cos3E-46	Phe	Arg-	Ser-	Arg-	Arg
	subC	Pro-	Leu-	Ser-	Ala-	Lys
	subD	Leu-	Arg-	Cys-	***-	Gly
	2A1	Gln-	Cys-	Cys-	Gln-	Gly
	2A2	Gly-	Cys-	Cys-	Ala-	Val
	subE	Phe-	Met-	Ser-	Ala-	Lys
	3E2	Phe-	Gln-	Ser-	Ser-	Lys
	Mouse α1-PI	Pro-	Tyr-	Ser-	Met-	Pro
	Contrapsin	Gly-	Arg-	Lys-	Ala-	Ile
Human						
	α1-PI	Pro-	Met-	Ser-	Ile-	Pro
	PCI	Phe-	Arg-	Ser-	Ala-	Arg
	α1-ACT	Leu-	Leu-	Ser-	Ala-	Leu
	ATIII	Gly-	Arg-	Ser-	Leu-	Asn
	HCII	Pro-	Leu-	Ser-	Thr-	Gln
	PAI-1	Ala-	Arg-	Met-	Ala-	Pro
	PAI-2	Gly-	Arg-	Thr-	Gly-	His
	PNI	Ala-	Arg-	Ser-	Ser-	Pro
	I-αI	Cys-	Arg-	Ala-	Phe-	Ile
	APP	Cys-	Arg-	Ala-	Met-	Ile

sentation of arginine in the P1 position, the serpin reactive center (68). *Arg-serpins* have a greater capacity to inhibit serine proteases that cleave after an arginine residue. These include thrombin, trypsin, kallikrein, and the PAs. The amyloid precursor protein (βAPP), thought to be a serpin and recently identified as protease nexin II (PNII; 76,77), also has an Arg at the P1 center and has now been found in high concentration in the α granules of human platelets (100). We found that muscle cells produce significant quantities of PNI (46), which at picomolar concentrations, totally inhibited uPA:plasmin-mediated muscle ECM degradation (101). βAPP/PNII has also been localized to skeletal muscle (102) and we have identified both PNI and PNII at synaptic sites in human muscle (12,14,46, unpublished), where they are ideally located for inhibition of excessive serine protease activity and to promote terminal anchorage at the synapse, probably in association with the terminal anchorage protein, TAP-1 (41) and/or cell adhesion molecules such as N-CAM (103) with which PNI, and possibly PNII, might interact.

The junctional concentration of PNI is significant for several reasons. First, although several antigens have been localized to the synaptic basal lamina in

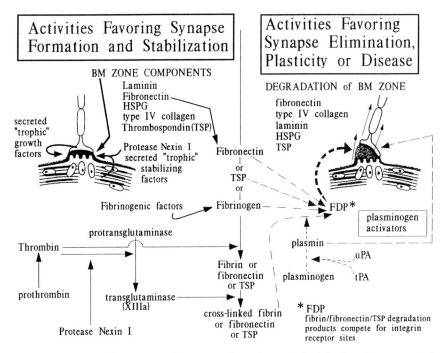

| Activities Favoring Synapse Formation and Stabilization | Activities Favoring Synapse Elimination, Plasticity or Disease |

Figure 1 Model of neuromuscular synapse formation and plasticity based on concept of thrombogenic and fibrinolytic cascades operating with ECM components and RGDS receptors (integrins). Balance of serine proteases (secreted "trophic" factors of nerve) and inhibitors (serpins, such as protease nexin I, secreted "trophic" stabilizing factors of target muscle fiber) essential for this mode. [From Festoff et al. (12).]

muscle, as mentioned above only A_{12} AChE, a form of heparan sulfate proteoglycan, agrin and S-laminin are concentrated at the junction. Second, forms of heparan sulfate proteoglycan shown to be associated with both the high concentration of membrane ACh receptors and A_{12} AChE are present at the junction and appear to undergo nerve-induced remodeling in culture (see 104). PNI binds to heparin in solution and a component(s) of the basal lamina, most likely heparan sulfate. Third, several proteins are known to be selectively expressed by nuclei under the end-plate area, the so-called subsynaptic nuclei. PNI localization to this region suggests that it, too, may be selectively expressed by these nuclei, likely to be strongly influenced by specific signals emanating from the nerve (99). Finally, the recent discovery that agrin possesses protease inhibitory activity suggests that one aspect of PNI's colocalization with AChR clusters may relate to its fibrinolytic/proteolytic function.

THROMBOGENIC AND FIBRINOLYTIC CASCADE MODELS OF SYNAPSE FORMATION AND PLASTICITY

Based on the foregoing information, we have proposed a model for synapse formation at the neuromuscular junction, which is testable for central synapses as well. In Figure 1, the principal features of the model are diagrammatically represented. Here seemingly opposing forces, or activities, favoring synapse formation (left-hand side) or synapse plasticity (as might occur in programmed elimination of polyneuronal synapses) or disintegration (as might occur in synaptic disorders, such as ALS) are presented on the right-hand side.

Prominent components of the basal lamina (i.e, fibronectin, laminin, type IV collagen, and heparan sulfate proteoglycan) are displayed along with thrombospondin, a platelet α-granule glycoprotein found to be a constituent of a number of basement membranes, including muscle. Thrombospondin has recently been shown to be uniquely increased in ALS muscle (105). In addition, PNI is depicted as one of several secreted trophic stabilizing factors from muscle that interact with one or more secreted trophic growth factors from the nerve. Another may be PNII/βAPP, recently localized at the junction (unpublished results). One or more PAs, secreted by axonal growth cones, may fall into the trophic growth factor category. In forming a synapse, the focus is on adhesion and stabilization. At the level of the membrane are the matrix components receptors, the integrins (106), which allow for the multifunctional glycoproteins of the basal lamina to interact with both nerve terminal and postsynaptic membranes. These elements are shown overlying several zymogen components of the thrombogenic cascade. Activation of prothrombin to active serine protease, in turn activating protransglutaminase to Factor XIIa, capable of cross-linking fibronectin, thrombospondin, or other multifunctional basal lamina glycoproteins to effectively stabilize the nascent neuromuscular junction, is shown as well.

SERINE PROTEASES, SERPINS, AND ALS

An important aspect for testing this hypothesis as it relates to ALS would be to determine whether a diathesis exists in ALS patients for generalized increases in specific serine proteases that cleave after arginines and are involved in tissue remodeling such as the PAs and kallikreins. Sensitive assays are now available to detect activity and antigen content of these enzymes in biological fluids of ALS patients compared to aged-matched normal and disease controls. Although numerous attempts have been made to identify consistent systemic abnormalities, a biological marker for ALS does not currently exist. Our preliminary data on PAs in plasma (see 11) show exceedingly high levels of uPA in several ALS patients. Pilot data on tissue kallikrein in ALS patients' urine and CSF suggest, but do not prove, that such a diathesis exists (Festoff and Chao, unpublished). By confirming the uPA results (11) and determining tissue kallikrein activity in ALS plasma, this will be important in demonstrating that such a diathesis, indeed, exists for elevated serine protease activity. Such a propensity for elevated serine protease activity may be exaggerated in the tissues typically affected in ALS, i.e., skeletal muscle and spinal cord. Also important would be obtaining a biochemical marker that could be used to correlate with disease progression. Such a marker might be extremely useful in measuring response to experimental therapeutic agents.

A major goal of future work in this laboratory is to determine whether serine protease dysregulation is involved in ALS. To accomplish this, we are assaying for content and activity of the major serine proteases and their inhibitors (serpins), many of which are acute-phase proteins. In addition, estimating the acute-phase protein-inducing cytokine, interleukin-6 (IL-6), in plasma of ALS patients compared to aged-matched normal and disease controls is underway. A number of previous reports suggested that ALS was an inflammatory or infectious condition (see 107). This has recently been reevaluated and ALS has been considered an "unconventional autoimmune disease," since it lacks the generally accepted hallmarks of autoimmune diseases (107).

Acute phase proteins are produced primarily by the liver and induced by B-cell stimulatory factor, shown to be identical to hepatocyte-stimulatory factor and interferon β_2. This T-cell-independent B-cell response molecule is now known as IL-6 (108). The major circulating serpins are included in the acute-phase proteins (Table 4); in particular, α_1-antitrypsin (α_1-protease inhibitor; α_1PI) and α_1-antichymotrypsin (α_1ACT) are dramatically increased. Although a recent study (109) did not show an increase in IL-6 in Alzheimer's disease, no studies of IL-6 or acute-phase proteins have been reported in ALS. If statistically significant differences can be detected in ALS patients' sera, it would lend support for systemic alteration in the response to exogenous factors.

EPILOGUE—PROTEASE:INHIBITOR IMBALANCE AND THE PATHOGENESIS OF ALS

The last 25 years have witnessed 15 or more international symposia documenting the progress in our understanding of this enigmatic disease, described in the medical literature almost 150 years ago (110,111). Most of these symposia have focused on research approaches to the etiology of ALS (see 112–115). Past approaches to etiopathogenesis have concentrated on uncovering *the single cause* of ALS. Despite expenditure of considerable human and consumable resources, the etiology of ALS is not yet known, in contrast to other, more recently appearing diseases, such as the acquired immunodeficiency syndrome (AIDS). Is ALS a true nosological entity (a "disease") or a syndrome (stereotyped signs

Table 4 Acute-Phase Proteins Induced by Interleukin-6

	Increase				
Species	10–100-fold	2–10-fold	≤ 2-fold	No change	Decrease
Human	C-reactive protein Serum amyloid A	α_1-Proteinase inhibitor α_1-Acid glycoprotein α_1-Antichy-motrypsin Fibrinogen Haptoglobin	Ceruloplasmin C3 of complement α_2-Antiplasmin C_1-inactivator	α_2-Macro-globulin Hemopexin Serum amyloid P Prothrombin	Inter-α-trypsin inhibitor Transferrin α_1-Lipopro-tein Prealbumin Albumin
Rat	α_2-Macro-globulin α_1-Acid glyco-protein	Fibrinogen Haptoglobulin Cysteine proteinase inhibitor	α_1-Proteinase inhibitor Ceruloplasmin Prekallikrein Hemopexin C-reactive protein	α_1-Macro-globulin Antithrombin III Serum amyloid P Prothrombin	α_1-Inhibitor 3 Transferrin Prealbumin Albumin

and symptoms, different causes; 116–118)? Is the nomenclature correct for this disorder and all "motor neuron diseases"? The literature reveals that conditions considered as "ALS" for purposes of therapeutic trials or testing of etiological hypotheses may not actually have been ALS (119). The International Classification of Disease (ICD) in its most recent edition (9th revision) continues to "lump" the major forms of sporadic motor neuron disorders (120).

Significance of Pathogenetic Approach

Inadequate clinical diagnosis, casting doubt on the conditions being treated experimentally, as well as on the underlying hypotheses, abound in the ALS literature (119). Various historical theories of the etiology of "ALS" (112–115) may still be viable, at least for the patients described in those specific studies. For a theory to be valid, it must be applicable to all forms of "ALS"; otherwise it risks being considered anecdotal. As an alternative approach, this laboratory has pursued a common pathogenesis for classical ALS, perhaps having the possibility of several, diverse etiologies. Why might this be important? For current and future ALS victims, testing a common pathogenesis theory might be more rapidly confirmed or refuted by other investigators. If confirmed, candidate therapies might move quickly from research bench to clinic. Second, with increased interest in ALS clinical trial testing (see 121,122) and genetic linkage

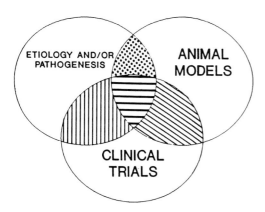

Figure 2   Three-ring sign of research in ALS/MND.

studies for familial ALS (123,124), pathogenesis studies can be further tested in animal model experiments. These areas of current ALS research—etiopathogenesis, clinical trials, and animal studies—may be visualized using a Venn diagram, as shown in Figure 2. Third, a pathogenetic approach would be *complementary* to studies on causation. This becomes particularly important in renewed studies of the changing epidemiology of the ALS/Parkinsonism/dementia complex (ALS/PDC) of Micronesia (Guam/Marianas type), along with studies of neurotoxic metals and excitatory amino acids in sporadic ALS and genetic linkage studies in familial ALS.

SUMMARY

A pathogenetic model based on dysregulation of serine proteases and their inhibitors has been presented for ALS. If it is to be seriously considered, alterations in the activity and amounts of critical proteases and/or their serpin inhibitors must be demonstrated in affected, and accessible, tissues. Assay for plasminogen-dependent and independent proteases in muscle and skin biopsy samples of ALS patients and disease controls can be done, in efforts to confirm pilot data. From our own results and those of others there is ample evidence for participation of the muscle PA:plasmin system in simple denervation. Previous studies have shown increases in other proteases in ALS patients' muscle (125). In addition, the principal posttranslational regulators of serine protease activity, cellular serpins such as PNI, PAI-1, and PNII, are synthesized by muscle and concentrated at synapses, possibly to provide the balance previously predicted (3,14). Such studies would provide the evidence in ALS muscle tissue for the disturbed delicate balance that results in synaptic disorganization which, if continued unabated, would result in neuronal exhaustion and death.

ACKNOWLEDGMENTS

Partial support for some of the studies described was provided by the Muscular Dystrophy Association, the ALS Association, the I.N.S.E.R.M., the NSF, the American Health Assistance Foundation, and the Medical Research Service of the Department of Veterans Affairs (DVA). Dr. Festoff is a Medical Investigator Awardee of the DVA, and gratefully acknowledges the participation of Drs. Jasti Rao, Daniel Hantaï, and Rajendra Reddy along with Alan Rayford, Cecilia Maben, and Riichiro Suzuki in some of the studies, as well as Joyce Capps in preparation of the manuscript.

REFERENCES

1. O'Brien RAD, Östberg Vrbová G. Observations on the elimination of polyneuronal inervation and the developing mammalian skeletal muscle. J Cell Physiol 1978;282:571–582.
2. Lijnen HR, Collen D. Regulation and control of the fibrinolytic system. In Festoff BW, ed. Serine proteases and serpins in the nervous system: Roles in development and malignant and degenerative disease. New York: Plenum Press, 1990:9–19.
3. Festoff BW. Role of neuromuscular junction macromolecules in the pathogenesis of amyotrophic lateral sclerosis. Med Hypothesis 1980;6:121–131.
4. Cavenaugh JB. The significance of the "dying back" process in experimental and human neurological disease. Int Rev Exp Pathol 1964;3:219–267.
5. Mott FW. Brain 1895;18:21–36.
6. Bradley WG, Kelemen J, Adelman LS, et al. The absence of dying-back in the phrenic nerve in amyotrophic lateral sclerosis (ALS). Neurology 1980;30:409a.
7. Iwata M, Hirano A. Sparing of the Onufrowicz nucleus in sacral anterior horn lesions. A Neurol Med (Tokyo) 1979;11:569–594.
8. Hirano A. In pursuit of the early pathological alterations in ALS. In: Tsubaki T, Toyokara Y, eds. Proc. International Symposium on Amyotrophic Lateral Sclerosis Tokyo: University of Tokyo Press, 1979:193–198.
9. Hirano A. Amyotrophic lateral sclerosis. In: Zimmerman HM, ed. Progress in neuropathology. New York: Grune & Stratton, 1973:181–215.
10. Festoff BW, ed. Serine proteases and serpins in the nervous system: Roles in development and malignant and degenerative disease. New York: Plenum Press, 1990:356 pp.
11. Hantaï C, Soria J, Soria C, et al. Plasminogen activators in development, injury and pathology of the neuromuscular system. In: Festoff BW, ed. Serine proteases and serpins in the nervous system: Roles in development and malignant and degenerative disease. New York: Plenum Press, 1990:219–228.
12. Festoff BW, Rao JS, Reddy BR, Hantaï D. A cascade approach to synapse formation based on thrombogenic and fibrinolytic models. In: Festoff BW, ed. Serine proteases and serpins in the nervous system: Roles in development and malignant and degenerative disease. New York: Plenum Press, 1990:245–252.

13. Festoff BW, Hantaï D. Plasminogen activators and inhibitors: Specific roles in neuromuscular regeneration. Prog Brain Res 1987;71:423–431.

14. Hantaï D, Rao JS, Festoff BW. Serine proteases and serpins: Their possible roles in the motor system. Rev Neurol 1988;144:680–687.

15. McMahan UJ, Sanes JR, Marshall LM. Cholinesterase is associated with the basal lamina at the neuromuscular junction. Nature 1978;271:172–174.

16. Sanes JR. Extracellular matrix molecules that influence neural development. Annu Rev Neurosci 1989;12:491–516.

17. Fernandez HL, Duell MJ, Festoff BW. Neurotrophic regulation of 16S acetylcholinesterase at the neuromuscular junction. J Neurobiol 1979;10:442–454.

18. Festoff BW. Release of acetylcholinesterase in amyotrophic lateral sclerosis. In: Rowland LP, ed. Pathogenesis of human motor neuron diseases. New York: Raven Press, 1982:503–516.

19. Beach RL, Popiela H, Festoff BW. Trophic factors and neuromuscular function: Implications for ALS. In: Rose FC, ed. Research progress in motor neuron diseases. London: Pitman, 1984:228–248.

20. Sketelj J, Brzin M. Attachment of acetylcholinesterase to structures of the motor end-plate. Histochemistry 1979;61:239–248.

21. Hall ZW, Kelly RB. Enzymatic detachment of endplate acetylcholinesterase from muscle, Nature (New Biol) 1971;232:62–63.

22. Dudai Y, Silman IJ. The effects of solubilization procedures on the release and molecular state of acetylcholinesterase from electric organ tissue. Neurochemistry 1974;23:1177–1187.

23. Fernandez HL, Duell MJ. Protease inhibitors reduce effects of denervation on muscle end-plate acetylcholinesterase. J Neurochemistry 1984;4:1166–1171.

24. Fernandez HL, Patterson MR, Duel MJ. Neurotrophic control of 16S acetylcholinesterase from mammalian skeletal muscle in organ culture. Neurobiology 1980;11:557–570.

25. Wilson BW, Montgomery WA, Asmundson RV. Cholinesterase activity and inherited muscular dystrophy of the chicken. Proc Soc Exp Biol 1968;129:199–206.

26. Wilson BW, Kaplan MC, Merhoff WC, Mori SS. Innervation and the regulation of acetylcholinesterase activity during the development of normal dystrophic chick muscle. J Exp Zool 1970;174:39–54.

27. Festoff BW, Fernandez HL. Plasma and red cell acetylcholinesterase in amyotrophic lateral sclerosis. Muscle Nerve 1981;4:41–47.

28. Rasool CG, Chad D, Bradley WG, Connolly B, Baruah BK. Acetylcholinesterase and ATPases in motor neuron degenerative diseases. Muscle Nerve 1983;430–435.

29. Bjornskov F, Norris FH, Jr., Mowe-Kuby J. Quantitative axon terminal and endplate morphology in amyotrophic lateral sclerosis. Arch Neurol 1985;41:527–530.

30. Bon S, Rieger F. Interactions between lectins and electric eel acetylcholinesterase. FEBS Lett 1975;53:282–286.

31. Lweburga-Mukuasa JS, Lappi S, Taylor D. Molecular forms of acetylcholinesterase from *Torpedo californica*: Their relationship to synaptic membranes. Biochemistry 1976;15:1425–1434.

32. Festoff BW, Engel WK. In vitro analysis of the general properties and junctional receptor characteristics of skeletal muscle membranes: Isolation, purification and partial characterization of sarcolemmal fragments. Proc Natl Acad Sci USA 1974;71:2435–2439.

33. Bon S, Cartaud J, Massoulié J. The dependence of acetylcholinesterase aggregation at low ionic strength upon a polyanionic component. Eur J Biochem 1978;85: 1–14.

34. Brandan E, Inestrosa NC. Binding of the asymmetric forms of acetylcholinesterase to heparin. Biochem J 1984;221:415–422.

35. Beach RL, Burton WV, Hendricks WJ, Festoff BW. Extracellular matrix synthesis by skeletal muscle in culture: proteins and effect of enzyme degradation. J Biol Chem 1982;257:11437–11442.

36. Beach RL, Rao JS, Festoff BW. Production of extracellular matrix by cultured muscle cells: Characterization of media collagens of myoblasts. Biochem J 1985;225:619–627.

37. Rao JS, Beach RL, Festoff BW. Extracellular matrix synthesis in muscle cell cultures: Quantitative and qualitative studies during myogenesis. Biochem Biophys Res Commun 1985;130:440–446.

38. Miller R, Rao JS, Festoff BW. Proteoglycan synthesis by primary chick skeletal muscle during in vitro myogenesis. J Cell Physiol 1987;133:257–266.

39. Miller R, Rao JS, Burton WJ, Festoff BW. Proteoglycan synthesis by clonal skeletal muscle cells during in vitro myogenesis: Differences detected in the types and patterns from primary cultures. Int J Dev Neurosci 1991;9:259–267.

40. Godfrey EW, Nitkin RM, Wallace WG, Rubin LL, McMahan UL. Components of Torpedo electric organ and muscle that cause aggregation of acetylcholine receptors on cultured muscle cells. J Cell Biol 1984;99:615–627.

41. Carlson S, Wight TN. Nerve terminal anchorage protein (TAP-1) is a chondroitin sulfate proteoglycan: biochemical and election microscopic characterization. J Cell Biol 1987;105:3075–3086.

42. Festoff BW, Patterson MR, Romstedt K. Plasminogen activator: The major secreted neutral protease of cultured skeletal muscle cells. J Cell Physiol 1982;110: 190–195.

43. Miskin R, Eaton TG, Reich E. Plasminogen activator in chick embryo muscle cells: Induction of enzyme by RSV, PMA and retinoic acid. Cell 1978;15:1301–1312.

44. Hatzfeld J, Miskin R, Reich E. Acetylcholine receptor: Effects of proteolysis on receptor metabolism. J Cell Biol 1982;92:176–182.

45. Romstedt K, Beach RL, Festoff BW. Studies of acetylcholine receptor in clonal muscle cells: Role of plasmin and effects of protease inhibitors. Muscle Nerve 1983;6:283–290.

46. Festoff BW, Hantaï D, Rao JS. Plasminogen activators and inhibitors in the neuromuscular system. III. Protease nexin I, a neurite-outgrowth promoting serine protease inhibitor (serpin) synthesized by muscle, co-localizes with acetylcholine receptors at neuromuscular synapses. J Cell Physiol 1991;147:76–86.

47. Danø K, Andreasen PA, Grøndahl-Hansen J, Kirstensen P, Nielsen IS, Skriver L.

Plasminogen activators, tissue degradation, and cancer. Adv Cancer Res 1985;44: 139–266.

48. Blasi F, Vassali JD, Danø K. Urokinase-type plasminogen activator: Proenzyme, receptor, and inhibitors. J Cell Biol 1987;104:801–804.

49. Grøndahl-Hansen J, Agerlin N, Munkholm-Larsen P, et al. Sensitivity and specific enzyme-linked immunosorbent assay for urokinase-type plasminogen activator and its application to plasma from patients with breast cancer. J Lab Clin Med 1988;111:42–51.

50. Werb A, Aggeler J. Proteases induce secretion of collagenase and plasminogen activator by fibroblasts. Proc Natl Acad Sci USA 1978;75:1839–1843.

51. MacDonald RJ, Margolis HS, Erdos EG. Molecular biology of tissue kallikrein. Biochem J 1988;253:313–321.

52. Bradshaw RA, Dunbar JC, Isaakson PJ, et al. In: Ford JR, Maized Al, eds. Mediators of cell growth and differentiation. New York: Raven Press, 1985:87–101.

53. Poberai M, Sávay G. Time course of proteolytic enzyme alterations in the motor end-plates after stimulation. Acta Histochem (Jena) 1976;57:44–48.

54. Poberai M, Sávay G, Csillik B. Function-dependent proteinase activity in the neuromuscular synapse. Neurobiology 1972;2:1–7.

55. Gutmann E, Melichna JA, Herbrychová A, et al. Different changes in contractile and histochemical properties of reinnervated and regenerated slow soleus muscles of guinea pigs. Pflüegers Arch 1976;364:191–194.

56. McLaughlin J, Abood LG, Bosmann HB. Early elevations of glycosidase, acid phosphatase and acid proteolytic enzyme activity in denervated skeletal muscle. Exp Neurol 1974;42:541–550.

57. Festoff BW, Rao JS, Maben C, Hantaï D. Plasminogen activators and their inhibitors in the neuromuscular system: I. Developmental regulation of plasminogen activator isoforms during in vitro myogenesis in two cell lines, J Cell Physiol 1990;144:262–271.

58. Festoff BW, Hantaï D, Soria J, Thomaïdis A, Soria C. Plasminogen activator in mammalian skeletal muscle: characteristics of effect of denervation or urokinase-like and tissue activator. J Cell Biol 187;103:1415–1421.

59. Hantaï D, Rao JS, Kahler CB, Festoff BW. Decrease in plasminogen activator correlates with synapse elimination during neonatal development of mouse skeletal muscle. Proc Natl Acad Sci USA 1989;86:362–366.

60. Hantaï D, Rao JS, Festoff BW. Rapid neural regulation of muscle urokinase-like plasminogen activator as defined by nerve crush. Proc Natl Acad Sci USA 1990;87:2926–2930.

61. Botteri FM, Der Putten H, Rajput B, Ballmer-Hofer K, Nagamine Y. Induction of the urokinase-type plasminogen activator gene by cytoskeleton-disrupting agents. In: Festoff BW, ed. Serine proteases and serpins in the nervous system: Roles in development and malignant and degenerative disease. New York: Plenum Press, 1990:105–114.

62. Fullmer HM, Seidler HD, Krooth RS, et al., A cutaneous disorder of connective

tissue in amyotrophic lateral sclerosis. A histochemical study. Neurology 1960;10: 717.

63. Fullmer HM, Lazarus G, Stam AC, Gibson WA. In: Norris FH, Kurland LT, eds. Motor neuron diseases. New York, London: Grune & Stratton, 1969:242–248.

64. Ono S, Mannen T, Toyokura YJ. Differential diagnosis between amyotrophic lateral sclerosis and spinal muscular atrophy by skin involvement. J Neurol Sci 1989;91:301–310.

65. Ono S, Hashimoto K, Shimizu T, Mannen T, Toyokura YJ. Amyotrophic lateral sclerosis: electrophoretic study of amorphous material of skin. J Neurol Sci 1989;92:159–167.

66. Beach RL, Rao JS, Festoff BW, et al. Collagenase activity in skin fibroblasts of patients with amyotrophic lateral sclerosis. J Neurol Sci 1987;72:49–60.

67. Laskowski M Jr, Kato I. Protein inhibition of proteinases. Annu Rev Biochem 1980;49:593–626.

68. Carrell RW, Boswell DR. Serpins: the superfamily of plasma serine proteinase inhibitors. In: Barret A, Salvesen G, eds. Proteinase inhibitors. Amsterdam: Elsevier, 1987:403–420.

69. Festoff BW. α_2-macroglobulin and plasma anti-protease activity (APA) in amyotrophic lateral sclerosis. Ann NY Acad Sci 1984;421:369–376.

70. Adachi N, Shoji SJ. Studies of protease inhibitors in sera of patients with amyotrophic lateral sclerosis. J Neurol Sci 1989;89:165–168.

71. Baker JB, Low DA, Simmer RL, Cunningham DD. Protease nexin: A cellular component that links thrombin and plasminogen activator and mediates their binding to cells. Cell 1980;21:37–45.

72. Baker JB, Knauer DJ, Cunningham DD. Protease nexin: secreted protease inhibitors that regulate protease actions at and near the cell surface. In: Conn PM, ed. The receptors. Vol 3. New York: Academic Press, 1986:153–172.

73. Enghild JJ, Thørgersen IB, Pizzo SV, Salvesen G. Polypeptide chain structure of inter-α-trypsin inhibitor and pre-α-trypsin inhibitor: Evidence for chain assembly by glycan and comparison with other ''kunin''-containing proteins. In: Festoff BW, ed. Serine proteases and serpins in the nervous system: Roles in development and malignant and degenerative disease. New York: Plenum Press, 1990:79–91.

74. Tanzi R. A serine protease inhibitor domain encoded with the Alzheimer's disease-associated amyloid β-protein precursor gene. In: Festoff BW, ed. Serine proteases and serpins in the nervous system: Roles in development and malignant and degenerative disease. New York: Plenum Press, 1990:313–319.

75. Selkoe, DJ. Deciphering Alzheimer's disease: The amyloid precursor protein yields new clues. Science 1990;248:1058–1060.

76. Oltersdorf T, Fritz LC, Schenk DB, Lieberburg J, Johnson-Wood KL, Beattie EC, Ward PJ, Blacher RW, Dovey HF, Sinha S. The secreted form of the Alzheimer's amyloid precursor protein with the Kunitz domain is protease nexin II. Nature 1989;341:144–147.

77. Van Nostrand WE, Wagner SL, Suzuki M, Choi BM, Farrow JS, Geddes JW, Cotman CW, Cunningham DD. Protease nexin II, a potent antichymotrypsin, shows identity to amyloid β-protein precursor. Nature 1989;341:546–569.

78. Knauer D, Thompson JT, Cunningham DD. Protease nexins: Cell secreted components that mediate the binding, internalization and degradation of regulatory serine proteases. J Cell Physiol 1983;117:385–396.
79. Farrell DH, Cunningham DD. Glycosaminoglycans on fibroblasts accelerate thrombin inhibition by protease nexin I. Biochem J 1988;245:543–550.
80. Cunningham, DD, Farrell DH, Wagner SL. Regulation of protease nexin I activity and target protease specificity by the extracellular matrix. In: Festoff BW, ed. Serine proteases and serpins in the nervous system: Roles in development and malignant and degenerative disease. New York: Plenum Press, 1990:93–101.
81. Loskutoff DJ, Edgington TS. Synthesis of a fibrinolytic activator and inhibitor by endothelial cells. J Biol Chem 1982;256:4142–4145.
82. Holmberg L, Lecander I, Persson B, Astedt B. An inhibitor from placenta specifically binds urokinase and inhibitor plasminogen activator released from ovarian carcinoma in tissue culture. Biochim Biophys Acta 1978;544:128–137.
83. Stump DC, Theinpont M, Collen D. Purification and characterization of a novel inhibitor of urokinase from human urine quantitation and preliminary characterization. J Biol Chem 1986;261:12759–12766.
84. Van Nostrand WE, Cunningham DD. Purification of protease nexin II from human fibroblasts. J Biol Chem 1987;262:8508–8514.
85. Monard D, Stockel K, Goodman R, et al. Distinction between nerve growth factor and glial factor. Nature 1975;258:444.
86. Gloor S, Odink K, Guenther J, Nick H, Monard D. A glial-derived neurite promoting factor with protease inhibitory activity belongs to the protease nexins. Cell 1986;47:687–693.
87. McGrogan MP, Kennedy J, Li MP, Hsu C, Scott RW, Simonsen C, Baker JB. Molecular cloning and expression of two forms of human protease nexin I. Biotechnology 1988;6:172–177.
88. McGrogan MP, Kennedy J, Golini F, Ashton N, Dunn F, Bell K, Tate E, Scott RW, Simonsen CC. Structure of the human protease nexin gene and expression of recombinant forms of PNI. In: Festoff BW, ed. Serine proteases and serpins in the nervous system: Roles in development and malignant and degenerative disease. New York: Plenum Press, 1990:147–161.
89. Monard D, Niday E, Limat A, et al. Inhibition of protease activity can lead to neurite extension in neuroblastoma cells. Prog Brain Res 1983;58:359.
90. Gurwitz D, Cunningham DD. Thrombin modulates and reverses neuroblastoma neurite outgrowth. Proc Natl Acad Sci USA 1988;85:3440–3445.
91. Dihanich M, Kaser M, Reinhard E, Cunningham DD, Monard D. Prothrombin mRNA is expressed by cells of the nervous system. Neuron 1991;6:575–581.
92. Monard D, Reinhard E, Meier R, Sommer J, Farmer L, Rovelli G, Ortmann R. Steps in establishing a biological relevance for glia-derived nexin. In: Festoff BW, ed. Serine proteases and serpins in the nervous system: Roles in development and malignant and degenerative disease. New York: Plenum Press, 1990:275–282.
93. Popiela H, Porter T, Beach RL, Festoff BW. Peripheral nerve extract promotes long-term survival and neurite outgrowth in cultured spinal cord neurons. Cell Mol Neurobiol 1984;4:67–77.

94. Festoff BW, Rao JS, Brenneman DE. Vasoactive intestinal polypeptide (VIP) is a secretagogue for protease nexin I (PNI) from astrocytes. Neurosci Abstr 1990; 16:909.
95. Reinhard E, Meier R, Halfter W, et al. Detection of glia-derived nexin in the olfactory system of the rat. Neuron 1988; 1:387.
96. Perl DP, Good PF. Uptake of aluminum into central nervous system along nasal-olfactory pathways. Lancet 1987;2:1028.
97. Perl DP, Good PF. The association of aluminum, Alzheimer's disease and neurofibrillary tangles. J Neurol Transm 1987;24(Suppl):205–211.
98. Rosenblatt DE, Geula C, Mesulam HH. Protease nexin immunostaining in Alzheimer's disease. Ann Neurol 1989;26:628–63.
99. Meier R, Spreyer P, Ortmann R, Harel A, Monard D. Induction of glial-derived nexin after lesion of a peripheral nerve. Nature 1989;342:548–550.
100. Van Nostrand WE, Schmaier AH, Farrow JS, Cunningham DD. Protease nexin-II (amyloid β-protein precursor): A platelet α-granule protein. Science 1990;248: 745–748.
101. Rao JS, Kahler CB, Baker JB, Festoff BW. Protease nexin I, a serpin, inhibits plasminogen dependent degradation of muscle extracellular matrix. Muscle Nerve 1989;12:640–646.
102. Zimmerman K, Herget T, Salbaum J, et al. Localization of the putative precursor of Alzheimer's disease-specific amyloid at nuclear envelopes of adult human muscle. EMBO J 1988;7:367–372.
103. Cashman NR, Covault J, Wollman RL, Sanes JR. Neural cell adhesion molecule in normal, denervated, and myopathic human muscle. Ann Neurol 1987;21:481–489.
104. Anderson MJ. Nerve-induced remodelling of muscle basal lamina during synaptogenesis. J Cell Biol 1986;102:863–877.
105. Rao JS, Hantaï D, Reddy BR, Festoff BW. Thrombospondin, not other matrix glycoproteins, is uniquely increased in muscle basement membrane of amyotrophic lateral sclerosis patients. Arch Neurol (in press).
106. Ruoshlahti R, Pierschbacher MD. New perspectives in cell adhesion: RGD and integrins. Science 1987;238:491–496.
107. Drachman DB, Kuncl RR. Amyotrophic lateral sclerosis: An unconventional autoimmune disease? Ann Neurol 1989;26:269–274.
108. Heinrich PC, Castell JV, Andus T. Interleukin-6 and the acute phase response. Biochemistry 1990;265:621–636.
109. Duijn CM, van Hoffman A, Nagelkerkan L. Neurosci Lett 1990;108:350–354.
110. Aran FA. Recherches sur une maladie non encore décrite du systéme musculaire (atrophic musculaire progressive). Arch Med 1850;24:5–35.
111. Charcot JM, Joffrey A. Deux cas d'atrophie musculaire progressive avec lésions de la substance grise et des faiseceaux antérolatéraux de la moëlle épinière. Arch Physiol 1869;2:354(629,744).
112. Andrews JM, Johnson RT, Brazier MAB, eds. Amyotrophic lateral sclerosis: Recent research trends. New York: Academic Press, 1976.

113. Mulder DW, ed. The diagnosis and treatment of amyotrophic lateral sclerosis. Boston: Houghton Mifflin, 1980.

114. Cosi V, Kato AC, Parlette W, Pinelli P, Polani M, eds. Amyotrophic lateral sclerosis: Therapeutic, psychological and research aspects. Vol 209. New York: Plenum Press, 1987.

115. Rowland LP, ed. Amyotrophic lateral sclerosis and other motor neuron diseases. New York: Raven Press, 1991.

116. Munsat TL, Bradley WG. Amyotrophic lateral sclerosis. In: Tyler HR, Dawson PM, eds. Current neurology. Boston: Houghton Mifflin, 1979:79–103.

117. Tanden R, Bradley WG. Amyotrophic lateral sclerosis. Part 1. Clinical features, pathology and ethical issues in management. Ann Neurol 1985; 18:271–280.

118. Tanden R, Bradley WG. Amyotrophic lateral sclerosis. Part 2. Clinical features, pathology and ethical issues in management. Ann Neurol 1985; 18:419–431.

119. Festoff BW, Crigger NJ. Therapeutic trials in amyotrophic lateral sclerosis: A review. In: Mulder DM, ed. The diagnosis and treatment of amyotrophic lateral sclerosis. Boston: Houghton Mifflin, 1980:337–366.

120. International Classification of Disease. 9th rev. 1979.

121. Brooks BR, DePaul R, Tan Y-D, Sanjak M, Sufit RL, Robbins R. Motor neuron disease. In: Schoenberg BS, Porter R, eds. Controlled clinical trials in neurology. New York: Marcel Dekker, 1990:249–281.

122. Brooks BR, Beaulieu D, Erickson, et al. Pilot studies and clinical therapeutic trials in amyotrophic lateral sclerosis. Muscle Nerve 1986; 9(Suppl 5):90.

123. Siddique T, Pericak-Vance, Brooks BR, Roos RP, et al. Linkage analysis in familial amyotrophic lateral sclerosis. Neurology 1989;39:919–925.

124. Siddique T, Figlewicz D, Perieak-Vance MA, Haones JL, et al. Assignment of a gene causing familial amyotrophic sclerosis to chromosome 21 and evidence for genetic heterogeneity. N Engl J Med 1991;324:1381–1384.

125. Antel LP, Chelmicka-Schorr E, Sportiello M, et al. Muscle acid protease activity in amyotrophic lateral sclerosis. Correlation with clinical and pathologic features. Neurology 1982; 8:901–903.

29

Genetic Linkage Studies in Hereditary Amyotrophic Lateral Sclerosis

Denise A. Figlewicz and Guy A. Rouleau

Montreal General Hospital and Centre for Research in Neuroscience,
McGill University
Montreal, Quebec, Canada

James F. Gusella

Massachusetts General Hospital, Charlestown, Massachusetts, and
Harvard Medical School
Boston, Massachusetts

INTRODUCTION

Amyotrophic lateral sclerosis (ALS) is a disease of unknown cause. Pathologically, the disease is characterized by the highly selective death of large motor neurons in the cerebral cortex and anterior horn. Despite extensive analysis, the pathophysiology and underlying biochemical defect(s) leading to this cell death remain(s) a mystery. Many plausible hypotheses have been proposed, which may in fact account for the development of the disease in some percentage of cases. However, specific therapies will not be found until the common or primary events underlying the death of motor neurons become clear. Although ALS is an adult-onset disease, there is no way at the moment of determining at which age or even stage of nervous system development the disease process actually begins. A cause for ALS has eluded conventional investigation by approaches that help to shed light on diseases of other tissues. For these reasons, we have opted to use a new approach to discover the pathophysiology of ALS—genetic linkage mapping.

Historically, genetic linkage studies of certain human traits had begun as early as the 1920s. However, linkage for any human trait only became feasible when Botstein and associates (1) proposed that sufficient variations occur in the nucleotide sequence of homologous regions of human chromosomes to provide polymorphic markers throughout the genome. They hypothesized that these markers would serve as a genetic map to which additional anonymous markers and actual genetic traits could be linked. This approach implied that it is not necessary to isolate a given gene in order to map it. Therefore, mapping of hereditary diseases of unknown etiology should be possible given sufficient heritable and easily detectable DNA markers.

The feasibility of this approach was demonstrated in 1983, when Gusella and co-workers were able to map Huntington's disease—a hereditary neurodegenerative disorder somewhat akin to ALS—to the telomere of the short arm of chromosome 4 by linkage to just such a polymorphic anonymous marker (2).

Since then, the genetic linkage approach has been used to localize the disease gene(s) for a number of neurological disorders, including Charcot-Marie-Tooth type I, chr. 17p (3); neurofibromatosis type 1 (NF1), chr. 17q (4,5); neurofibromatosis type 2 (NF2), chr. 22q (6); Friedreich's ataxia, chr. 9q (7); and, most recently, childhood-onset spinal muscular atrophy, chr. 5q (8).

The ultimate goal of genetic linkage mapping is to identify the disease gene. Within the last few years, this goal has been attained for many diseases, three of which are common hereditary disorders—cystic fibrosis, Duchenne muscular dystrophy, and NF1 (9–13).

The familial form of ALS accounts for only approximately 10% of the cases of ALS. However, clinical and epidemiological analyses of sporadic versus familial forms of ALS suggest few differences between the two forms (14–20). Thus, successful mapping of the familial form of ALS could provide information about the primary biochemical defect, which might prove applicable to sporadic cases as well.

TOOLS OF LINKAGE MAPPING

Linkage mapping is based on the simple principle that the closer two genes are to each other, the more likely it is that they will segregate together during meiosis. Genes on different chromosomes will segregate randomly. In fact, even genes on the same chromosome may, if widely separated, not be inherited in a linked manner. Crossover and exchange of homologous regions of paired chromatids occurs during gametogenesis. It is estimated that at least one such crossover event occurs for every chromosome per meiosis. Thus, the farther apart two genes are on a given chromosome, the greater the likelihood that they will be separated by a crossover event and not passed on to the offspring together. The likelihood of such a crossover, or recombination, between any two loci defines genetic distance. The unit of this genetic map distance is the centiMorgan (cM). For two fixed loci spaced close enough on a chromosome so that one would expect at most one crossover in the interval, the genetic distance in cM is equivalent to the chance of recombination between two loci. When the distance between two loci is sufficiently large, one must consider the chance of multiple crossovers occuring in this interval. The Haldane function allows for the more precise estimation of genetic distance, correcting for this possibility. In addition, the occurence of one crossover event tends to inhibit the formation of other crossovers in the immediate vicinity. This phenomenon, interference, has been taken into account in two more sophisticated mapping functions: the Kosambi function, correcting for positive interference, and the Felsenstein function, correcting for variable interference. [See Ott (21) for detailed discussion.] At a sufficiently great genetic distance, there will be 50% chance of recombination between two loci on the same chromsome (i.e., random segregation), as is seen between any two loci on separate chromsomes. The human genome is 3300 cM in "genetic size" and contains approximately 3×10^9 base pairs (bp). Thus, on the average, 1 cM genetic distance is equivalent to 1×10^6 bp physical distance. However, this rough measure can vary considerably.

Humans have 46 chromosomes divided into 22 pairs of autosomes and one pair of sex chromosomes. All genetic loci on the 22 autosomes thus exist as pairs, one copy on each homologue. Different versions of any one locus are referred to as alleles. Examples of different alleles for some genetic traits are enzyme isoforms, ABO blood groups, HLA markers, and color blindness. In the case of a hereditary disease, one (or more) mutant allele(s) is (are) responsible for the phenotype, i.e., the disease. Linkage mapping in a hereditary disease is simply an attempt to find a polymorphic genetic locus (i.e., a locus for which two or more alleles are somehow identifiable = a genetic marker) that is so close to the disease locus that the two loci can be seen to segregate together when traced through a given family tree.

A successful linkage study depends on: (a) appropriate polymorphic genetic markers (discussed below) and (b) DNA samples from the members of a family or families with the hereditary disorder in question (discussed in the next section).

Certain observations can narrow the search for linkage to a given hereditary disorder. For example, sex-linked disorders are on the X chromosome. Deletions or translocations demonstrated by chromosomal karyotyping may also provide a clue, as was the case in NF1, as to the localization of a disease trait. However, in ALS, as in many hereditary disorders, our only clue is that the disease is not sex-linked. [In fact, most reports of familial ALS indicate an autosomal dominant mode of transmission (17–20,22,23); there has been one report of an autosomal recessive variant (24).] Therefore, all 22 autosomes must be searched.

How does one find enough polymorphic markers to test their segregation against the disease trait? Until 10 years ago, the only polymorphic markers known were those based on recognizable differences in protein products (viz., isozymes, etc., as mentioned above) or in a phenotypic trait (such as color blindness). Then in 1980, Botstein et al. (1) identified an even better source of polymorphic markers, which could be found in genomic DNA itself. It has been estimated, on the average, that a single base pair difference between two homologous regions of DNA occurs once every 500 bp. Such variations in sequence, or polymorphisms, will fall in coding as well as noncoding regions of the genome, the majority of which have no phenotypic expression. How, then, can they serve as identifiable markers? Differences in the base pair sequence, even a single base pair substitution, will be recognized when the change alters the site of recognition of a restriction enzyme. These bacterial enzymes recognize with high fidelity and cleave with great efficiency a very specific sequence of 4-, 6-, or 8-bases. Thus, two homologous regions of DNA, one bearing a restriction site and one missing this site as a result of a base pair alteration, will yield different-sized restriction fragments when the DNA is digested by the appropriate enzyme. DNA fragments are separated on the basis of size by agarose gel electrophoresis. DNA from the gel is denatured to single strands and transferred to a nylon membrane ("Southern blotting"). A probe, typically 0.5–10.0 kB in size, containing the region of the particular polymorphic restriction site, is labeled with ^{32}P, also denatured to single strands, and allowed to hybridize against the filter. Radioactive bands of different size will identify the two alleles resulting from the single base pair change. Typically, DNA samples from a given family are electrophoresed in adjacent lanes. By this means, one can rapidly verify the Mendelian inheritance of the polymorphism in question, determine nonpaternity for a given offspring, and tabulate the results for computer analyses (see Fig. 1) (25). The simplest kind of polymorphic marker is commonly called a restriction fragment length polymorphism (RFLP). The linkage map of the entire human genome, proposed by Botstein et al. (1), suggested that a minimum of 150 such markers, evenly spaced 20 cM apart, should allow the mapping of any genetic trait. However, since it would prove unrealistic to expect to locate perfectly spaced polymorphic markers, a minimum of 200 such markers, well spaced throughout the genome, would be a realistic set to use for linkage mapping. By the late 1980s, a linkage map based on 403 polymorphic markers, linked to 95% of the human genome (Donis-Keller) (26) and a 255-locus map with linkage groups on 2/3 of the chromsomes (White) (27) were made available. As of their most recent meeting, Human Gene Mapping Workshop 10, information is now available for more than 5100 mapped gene markers (28).

RFLP markers described above most often provide two allelic possibilities. Assuming that the two alleles are present in the human population in a 1:1 ratio (often not the case), then any given individual has a 50% chance of being homozygous at this locus (two copies of the same allele) and 50% chance of being heterozygous (one copy of each allele). The usefulness, or "informativeness," of a polymorphic marker for linkage mapping is based on the probability that a given individual is a heterozygote, thereby allowing identification (marking) of the parental chromosomes. Statistically, the usefulness of a marker

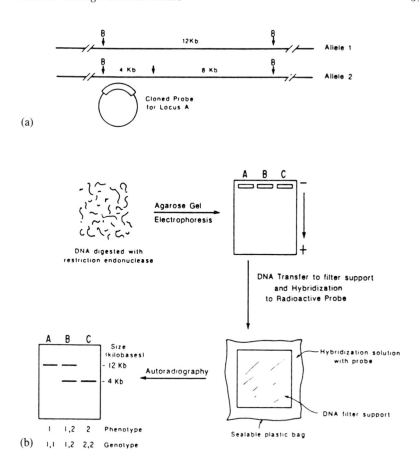

Figure 1 (a) Map of enzyme B sites at hypothetical locus A. A hypothetical restriction fragment length polymorphism is revealed at an arbitrary locus (A) by digestion with endonuclase B. Alleles 1 and 2 differ by the presence of an additional restriction enzyme site in the latter that reduces from 12 kilobases to 4 kilobases the size of fragment detected by a probe for the locus cloned in a plasmid vector. (b) Detection of RFLP with probe for locus A. This flowchart depicts the steps taken to determine the phenotype and corresponding genotype at locus A in genomic DNA of three individuals using hybridization to the cloned probe from A. The resultant autoradiograph indicates that the three individuals each have a different phenotype, corresponding to one homozygote for 1 allele, one heterozygote, and one homozygote for the 2 allele. (Reproduced from Ref. 25, with permission from Annual Reviews, Inc.)

is reflected in the polymorphism information content (PIC). [For detailed presentation of this subject, see Botstein et al. (1).] A polymorphic marker with more than two allelic possibilities will likely be more informative than a simple two-allele RFLP simply because the chance of any given individual in the population being a heterozygote at the marker locus will increase.

Another variation in genomic DNA sequence based on the insertion or deletion of small, repetitive blocks of DNA was first reported in yeast and *Drosophila*. When this was explored in the human genome, it was discovered that changes in spacing of restriction enzyme sites due to the insertion or deletion of such repeating units were very frequent and so constitute an important source of highly informative polymorphic markers. Many of these markers, known as variable number of tandem repeats (VNTRs), are now available or being developed (27). (See Fig. 2.) In contrast to RFLPs, eight or more different alleles can be found for some VNTR markers. In principle, the high PIC of VNTR makes them significantly more useful than two-allele polymorphisms for mapping. In practice, however, the processing of information from a VNTR probe, for a very large family with many branches and many deceased individuals, can be very difficult.

Another source of polymorphic markers is candidate genes. In ALS, for example, interesting candidate genes that have been tested for linkage to the disease trait include beta-tubulin, nerve growth factor, Tau heat shock proteins, and heavy neurofilament. This approach can be used for mapping of any disease trait. Since it is estimated that a variation in DNA sequence occurs approximately every 500 bp, and the genomic span of a gene is typically 5–10,000 bp, one would expect to be able to identify at least one polymorphism in a given candidate gene. This can be done quite simply by screening panels of 5–10 unrelated individuals' DNA (i.e., 10–20 alleles of any locus) which have been digested with various restriction enzymes. Useful enzymes include: MspI; TaqI; PstI; HindIII; BamHI; EcoRI; EcoRV; SacI; Bg1II; and RsaI. Tight linkage to a candidate gene, with no recombination between the two loci, would provide presumptive evidence that mutation in the candidate results in the disease itself. The advantage of this approach is that positional cloning strategies are not needed. At the very least, a polymorphic candidate gene that has been mapped can provide exclusion data, i.e., delineate a region of the genome where the diesease gene is not.

More recently, polymorphisms have been detected using the polymerase chain reaction (PCR) (29). PCR allows amplification of small regions of DNA; oligomers synthesized from the $3'$ and $5'$ ends of the region to be amplified are incubated with template (genomic DNA, cosmid DNA, etc.) and DNA polymerase from the bacterium *Thermus aquaticus*. By cyclically varying the temperature, n cycles of PCR will produce 2^n copies of the region between the oligomers. Variations in genomic DNA, on a scale of 10–200 bp, based on small

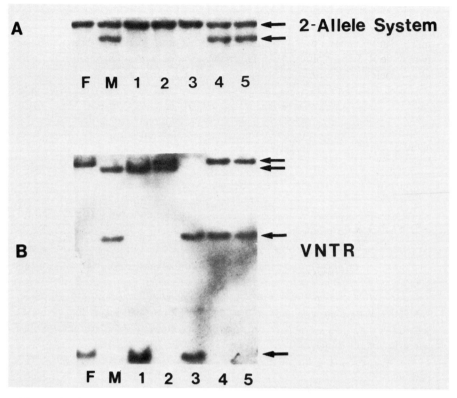

Figure 2 Comparison of the segregation of two polymorphic markers in a nuclear family; F = father; M = mother; 1–5 = children. One can notice that three out of seven individuals are heterozygotes for the probe with the two-allele polymorphism while seven out of seven individuals are heterozygotes for the VNTR probe.

insertion/deletions or changes in restriction sites can be identified this way. A limitation to this method is that the sequence of the DNA in the region to be amplified must be known. However, this may prove to be a useful way to expand the locus (i.e., increase the informativeness) of a marker that has proved interesting or reveal a polymorphic locus in a candidate gene.

A new source of polymorphisms is GT/CA repeats. These are VNTR polymorphisms where the repeated sequence is a dinucleotide, CA. Regions of GT repeats are believed to be found throughout the human genome; it is estimated that there are 50–100,000 interspersed $(CA)n$ blocks. The number of repeats in any one stretch can also be highly variable, with the range of n being 15–30. [See Weber and May (30) for detailed discussion.] As with VNTRs, these vari-

Table 1 LOD-Scores Obtained from Two-Point
Liped Analysis

Recombination fraction	Locus 0 FALS versus locus 3	Locus 0 FALS versus locus 11
0.35	−0.04028	0.06167
0.30	−0.07470	0.11452
0.25	−0.12363	0.18235
0.20	−0.19234	0.26201
0.15	−0.29098	0.34983
0.10	−0.44254	0.44242
0.05	−0.72073	0.53704
0.00	−99.99000	0.63169

ations have been shown to be inherited in a Mendelian fashion. Polymorphisms based on GT repeats need to be resolved using sequencing gels, as the difference between two alleles may be as small as 2 bp. However, several hundred individuals may be analyzed using one sequencing gel. GT repeats can probably provide needed polymorphisms or increase the informativeness for any locus of interest.

We are currently using all these approaches in our linkage analysis of ALS families.

Once allelic information for a given marker locus has been tabulated for the members of a family, linkage or exclusion (= nonlinkage) is determined statistically and expressed as a LOD score.

First we will discuss the LOD score in terms of the simplest analysis: two-point analysis. The segregation of the alleles of the marker locus and the segregation of the alleles of the disease locus (i.e., affected versus normal, in the simplest situation) are compared. Two likelihoods are calculated. The first is the likelihood of obtaining this segregation pattern if the two loci are linked, allowing for a certain percentage of recombination (i.e., distance in centiMorgans) between the two loci. The second is the likelihood that this pattern of alleles would have arisen as the result of completely random segregation (i.e., nonlinkage). The ratio of these two probabilities tells us how much more likely the data are to have arisen under one premise (linkage) than the other (nonlinkage). The $\log_{10}$ of this odds ratio is the LOD score. Table 1 shows two-point analysis testing markers at two particular loci.

In human genetics, a LOD score of 3.0 is accepted as the threshold for linkage. This odds ratio, 10^3 or 1000:1 in favor of the data arising as a result of linkage is offset by the likelihood of nonlinkage (roughly 50:1) for any two random loci in the human genome [that is to say, a priori, the chance of any two randomly chosen loci being on different arms of different chromosomes. See Lander (31) for elaboration of this point.] Thus, a LOD score of 3 corresponds to about 20:1 odds in favor of linkage (95% confidence interval). Therefore, one time in 20, a LOD score of 3 will be misleading. On the other hand, a LOD score of -2.0 or less is accepted as exclusion of the marker locus from linkage to the disease trait. Very informative families and/or very informative probes can provide exclusion data to a distance of 10 or more cM on either side of the marker locus.

Calculation of LOD scores, once done by hand, is now achieved by computer programs, such as LIPED (32) and LINKAGE (33,34). In addition, in the past 5 years, strategies have been devised to allow analysis of more difficult or complicated linkage situations. For example, multipoint analysis (LINKAGE program), where cosegregation of several loci within the same chromosomal region are analyzed simultaneously, provides a substantial improvement of the efficiency of linkage analysis and allows more precise placement of the loci involved on the genetic map (33,35). This is done by varying the position of one locus in relation to a set of loci whose relative positions are known on the genetic map and ascertaining which locus order is the most probable. This strategy proved useful in assigning the disease locus in NF1, for example. In this case, two-point linkage analysis resulted in a LOD score of 4.37; after multipoint analysis using three marker loci, the LOD score almost doubled (4). This technique was also used for more precise localization of the Huntington's disease gene (36).

New approaches to analysis are being developed, such as simultaneous search (37). This is a useful strategy when many families are being tested for linkage and it is suspected that the disease may result from a mutation at one of two or more loci (heterogeneity). In this situation, one can ascertain the likelihood of linkage to either of a pair of marker loci. Simultaneous search may be a necessary strategy for analysis of linkage results in familial ALS. Another approach, homozygosity mapping, is a strategy for linkage mapping of autosomal recessive disease traits, taking advantage of regions of homozygosity found in genomic DNA from offspring of first- and second-cousin marriages in inbred populations (38).

For more theoretical discussion of these approaches, see Lathrop et al. (35), Lander and Botstein (39), and Lander (31).

ALS FAMILIES

Clearly, the tools needed for linkage mapping are at hand, and they are constantly improving. The other critical resource needed for a successful linkage analysis is family material.

Table 2 Familial ALS Epidemiology

	Number families	Number family members	Total number collected	Total affecteds collected	Sex ratio M:F	Mean age at onset (years)	Mean survival (years)
FALS-AD	87	2697	472	67	1.5	50 ± 12 (*n* = 181)	2.6 ± 1.7 (*n* = 143)
FALS-ATYP	5	276	37	15	0.44	46 ± 10 (*n* = 36)	11.0 ± 6 (*n* = 16)
FALS-UNI	13	219	41	10	0.58	52 ± 14 (*n* = 19)	2.1 ± 1.4 (*n* = 12)
FALS total	105	3192	550	92	1.15	50 ± 12 (*n* = 236)	3.4 ± 3.5 (*n* = 171)

We have identified more than 100 families with ALS (see Table 2). The first two subgroups display clear autosomal dominant inheritance with multiple affecteds in multiple generations. They correspond quite closely to two of the three types described by Horton et al. (20). Familial ALS-autosomal dominant (FALS-AD), representing by far the majority of the families, strongly resembles sporadic ALS in terms of onset age, survival, and M:F ratio. An atypical subgroup of familial ALS (FALS-ATYP) differs somewhat from the sporadic ALS population, having a preponderance of lower motor neuron symptoms and average survival >10 years. The unigenerational (FALS-UNI) group includes multiple affected individuals in the same family, but all from the same generation. Families chosen by us for linkage analysis come only from the FALS-AD subgroup.

The ideal resource for a linkage study of a dominantly inherited trait would be: (a) a single very large family (to avoid the complication of heterogeneity); (b) disease survival long enough to enable one to obtain DNA samples from affected individuals in several generations; and (c) a disease trait showing high penetrance. (Penetrance reflects the frequency with which the disease phenotype is expressed in an individual with the disease genotype.) A family such as described above is the Venezuelan pedigree that was used to establish linkage in Huntington's disease. The use of a single large family helps to minimize the possibility that one is searching for linkage to more than one locus (i.e., genetic heterogeneity). However, in the absence of genetic heterogeneity, it is valid to add the LOD scores obtained from several smaller families for a given marker locus. Such an approach was successful in establishing linkage in NF1 and Friedreich's ataxia, for example. For a hereditary disorder with autosomal dominant inheritance, representing a unique locus in the genome, it is estimated that 12–15 families with two or three affecteds in each family are needed to obtain a

LOD score of 3.0 if markers are screened every 30 cM and only two-point analysis is used (39).

In a recent paper, Lander described the process of linkage mapping of a simple Mendelian trait as straightforward and quite likely to be successful. However, characteristics can make the trait less favorable for linkage mapping. These problems include (31):

Incomplete penetrance: where a fraction of individuals carrying the disease gene never express the phenotype.

Phenocopies: a similar disease may be the result of nongenetic causes.

Genetic heterogeneity: in which a mutation at any one of two or more loci can produce a similar disease (phenotype).

Genetic interactions: the disease phenotype is the result of interactions among more than one genetic locus.

Rarity: either families with the disease, or multiple affected individuals in a given family may be very difficult to obtain.

Unfortunately, in terms of these problems, ALS may prove to be one of the most difficult diseases for linkage analysis.

Penetrance

For a trait with autosomal dominant inheritance, one would expect 50% of the offspring of an affected individual to also be affected. However, one must take into consideration the age when the phenotype first appears. The average age of onset for affecteds from our FALS collection is 50 ($\pm$ 12 years), meaning that one can expect a certain number of carriers with the FALS trait to die of other causes before showing symptoms. In addition, we have encountered several examples of obligate carriers (see Fig. 3, Pedigrees AIII16, BII9, and BIII6), where someone has transmitted the disease without ever developing symptoms. To further complicate the picture, penetrance can be quite variable from family to family (23) (see Fig. 3, Pedigrees A–D). Taking all the variables into account, we calculate penetrance in our total family collection to be about 80%. When a dominant trait shows complete penetrance, unaffected siblings prove to be as informative as affected individuals—that is, in both cases, phenotype reflects genotype. In situations of reduced penetrance, as seen in our ALS pedigrees, the information contributed by unaffected individuals is decreased. For example, with 80% penetrance, an unaffected individual contributes roughly one-third the information of an affected (31). Since we have a large family collection, we were able to construct an age-of-onset curve and calculate the likelihood of succumbing to ALS, if one carries the trait, in each decade from 20 years to 70 years old. Using these age-of-onset classes, we can maximize the information obtainable from the unaffecteds.

(A)

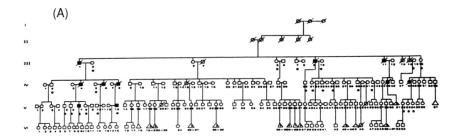

(B)

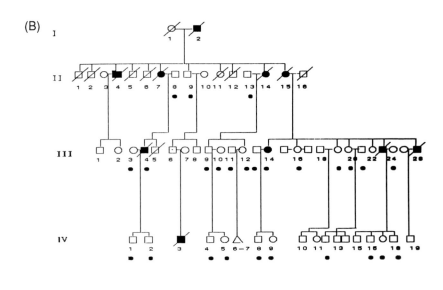

(C)

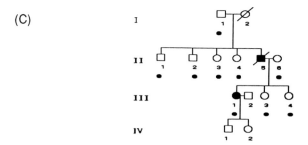

Figure 3 Familial ALS pedigrees. (A–D) Autosomal dominant inheritance, with varying penetrance. (E) Unigenerational. (F) Autosomal recessive.

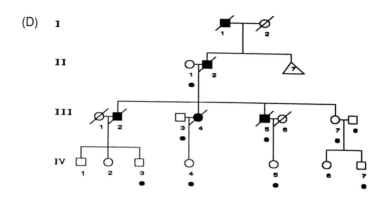

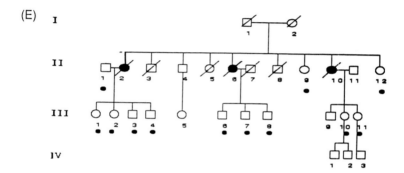

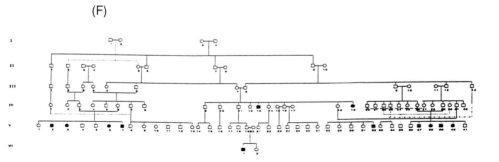

Phenocopies

Although our hereditary ALS population represents only 10% of the total patient population, the odds are small that the motoneuron disease of an affected individual in one of the families has a nongenetic etiology. On the other hand, in our group of unigenerational families, we cannot claim parent-to-child transmission and must consider the possibility of some other, perhaps environmentally related, cause for this "clustering" (see Fig. 3, Pedigree E).

Genetic Heterogeneity

It is possible that different genes may, when mutated, lead to FALS (22). Therefore, we cannot tell whether the gene affected in different families is the same or different. While it is true that, on clinical grounds, we are able to divide our families with autosomal dominant transmission into two subgroups, it must be kept in mind that variable clinical severity has been documented for a number of diseases known to be linked to only one genetic locus. This is the case with NF1, cystic fibrosis, and X-linked muscular dystrophy. On the other hand, diseases that are phenotypically very similar have been linked to different loci in different families. Examples of this are Charcot-Marie-Tooth and manic-depressive illness.

Since two-point analysis of LOD scores is calculated separately for each family, genetic heterogeneity, if it exists for familial ALS, can be detected. If linkage to more than one locus is suspected, the simultaneous search strategy can be employed.

Rarity

ALS is estimated to affect 1/20,000 individuals in the population. Worldwide epidemiology does not seem to indicate much variation from this incidence, with the exception of the high-incidence foci of ALS-Parkinsonism-dementia on Guam and the Kii Peninsula of Japan. Approximately 10% of ALS cases (i.e., 1/200,000) are hereditary in nature. Based on these statistics, we have estimated that, together with our colleagues at Duke and Columbia Universities, we have possibly identified most of the ALS families in North America. Thus, we do not expect the family resources available to us to improve much, except that with time, some individuals currently showing no symptoms may develop the disease, increasing the informativeness of a given pedigree. The median survival after onset for affected individuals in the FALS-AD subgroup is 2 years. This means that it is virtually impossible to obtain affected individuals from multiple generations, at least within a few years of identifying and collecting blood from the family. It also means that it is rather difficult to find multiple living affected siblings.

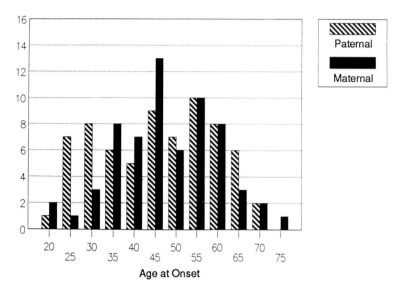

Figure 4 Protective effect of maternal inheritance of the ALS trait (autosomal dominant families, only). A later age at onset for those inheriting the trait from their mother is statistically significant for individuals whose age at onset is less than 50.

Table 3 LOD Scores Achievable Using 10 FALS Kindreds Assuming 85% Penetrance

FALS pedigree	Marker allele frequency		
	0.9[a] 0.1	0.5[a] 0.5	0.1[a] 0.9
1	1.49	2.08	3.35
3	1.60	1.84	2.13
4	1.29	1.29	1.29
7	1.91	2.10	2.18
8	1.40	1.40	1.40
9	0.42	0.50	0.54
11	2.09	2.38	2.62
15	3.11	4.30	5.84
20	2.56	2.76	3.22
30	1.64	1.85	2.28
Total	17.51	20.50	24.85

[a]Denotes allele segregating with the defect.

Inheritance

We have calculated the effect of maternal versus paternal inheritance on age of onset of affected offspring and found that maternal inheritance does seem to confer a protective effect, delaying the age of onset by several years in the affecteds whose age of onset was younger than 50 (see Fig. 4).

Before embarking on a genetic study such as this, the usefulness of any family for linkage can be rapidly assessed by running the LIPED program using dummy RFLPs, in a simple two-allele, two-point analysis. Estimated LOD scores obtained in this way can give an indication of the potential usefulness of any given pedigree. Table 3 illustrates the results of one such estimation.

HOMOZYGOSITY MAPPING

The recent identification of many families with a clearly autosomal recessive form of motor neuron disease allows the application of new mapping strategies. This recessive FALS has been best described in some highly inbred families in Tunisia. One such family has been made available to us by Drs. F. Hentati and M. BenHamida (see Fig. 3, Pedigree 3F).

Genetic linkage in this family will be sought using the strategy of homozygosity mapping, as described by Lander and Botstein (38). In families where a recessive disease trait is the result of inbreeding, one can expect the region of the genome flanking the disease locus to also be homozygous by descent. This region could be quite large, many centiMorgans in length. Statistical analyses demonstrate that using markers of only 50% heterozygosity, spaced every 15 cM in the genome, linkage can be achieved using only 15 affected individuals (children of first-cousin marriages).

The clinical phenotype of recessive ALS is similar, though not identical, to that of FALS-AD. Therefore, recessive ALS may, but probably does not, represent a mutation of the FALS-AD gene(s). In any event, recessive ALS genetic studies are an important alternative approach to identify genes responsible for motor neuron death.

LINKAGE RESULTS

While linkage to familial ALS has not yet been established, tentative linkage is being investigated to loci on chromosome 21q. Weak positive LOD scores have also been found for loci on chromosomes 11p and 22q. There have been some preliminary reports of results (40–42).

Genetic linkage is very powerful for the exclusion of linkage, particularly of candidate genes. Recombination occurring between a disease gene and a candidate gene (or a polymorphism detected by this candidate gene) strongly implies

Table 4 Collaborative Familial ALS Study Group

M. BenHamida	Tunis, TUNISIA
T. Bird	Seattle, WA
E. P. Bosch	Iowa City, IA
R. Campbell	London, Ont., CANADA
D. Chad	Worcester, MA
J. Daube	Rochester, MN
J. de Belleroche	London, UK
B. W. Festoff	Kansas City, KS
J. P. Fryns	Leuven, BELGIUM
J. Glasberg	Detroit, MI
M. R. Glasberg	Detroit, MI
J. Halperin	Stony Brook, NY
F. Hentati	Tunis, TUNISIA
A. J. Hudson	London, Ont., CANADA
H. Husquinet	Liège, BELGIUM
W. Johnson	New York, NY
B. Jubelt	Chicago, IL
A. King	London, UK
H. Lipe	Seattle, WA
K. Matthews	Iowa City, IA
D. W. Mulder	Rochester, MN
T. L. Munsat	Boston, MA
G. Nicholson	Sydney, AUSTRALIA
M. Pericak-Vance	Durham, NC
F. C. Rose	London, UK
A. Roses	Durham, NC
A. Server	Cambridge, MA
T. Siddique	Chicago, IL
R. L. Sullivan	Portland, ME
L. Thomson	Madison, WI
E. Toms	Providence, RI
P. Van den Bergh	Leuven, BELGIUM
R. Van den Bergh	Leuven, BELGIUM
D. Williams	Rochester, MN
A. Windebank	Rochester, MN
M. Zeidman	Durham, NC

that the candidate gene is not primarily responsible for the observed phenotype. As discussed previously, genetic distance of 1 cM roughly corresponds to 10^6 bases, a region larger than most genes. Exclusion, by linkage, of a region 2 cM on either side of a candidate gene virtually excludes it from involvement in the disease. A composite of results obtained by the authors and results obtained by Siddique et al. (Duke University) have excluded the linkage of familial ALS to some interesting candidate markers: beta-nerve growth factor, spectrin, fibroblast growth factor, beta-tubulin, nerve growth factor receptor, insulin receptor, glutamate dehydrogenase, estrogen receptor, and epidermal growth factor receptor.

CONCLUSION

Linkage studies in the familial forms of ALS are currently well underway. Many obstacles make this a long, difficult task. Nonetheless, the linkage strategy is important for the simple reason that it will eventually work. It is encouraging to realize that since the earliest descriptions of application of molecular genetic techiques to neurological disease (43,44), many of these methods and strategies have been successful. In addition, new approaches to more difficult aspects of the methodology continue to be developed (29,30,45–49). Thus, the greatest hurdle for genetic studies of familial ALS remains the nature of the family material itself. Once linkage has been established, it will become possible to apply strategies to clone the familial ALS gene(s) and subsequently analyze the mutant gene product(s). We believe that insight thus obtained will provide an enormous contribution to understanding of the etiology of ALS—not only the familial forms, but the sporadic form as well.

ACKNOWLEDGMENTS

The authors thank their many collaborators in the ALS linkage effort, in particular Drs. R. H. Brown and J. Haines, Boston; Drs. R. Horvitz and A. Server, Cambridge, Massachusetts; and Dr. T. Siddique, Durham, North Carolina (see also Table 4). They also acknowledge the support of the Pierre L. De-Bourghknecht Foundation; Cambridge NeuroScience Research, Inc.; the ALS Society of Canada; the ALS Association (USA); the Muscular Dystrophy Association of America; and the Muscular Dystrophy Association of Canada.

REFERENCES

1. Botstein D, White RL, Skolnick M, Davis R. Construction of a genetic linkage map in man using restriction fragment length polymorphisms. Am J Hum Genet 1980;32: 314–331.

2. Gusella JF, Wexler NS, Conneally PM, et al. A polymorphic DNA marker genetically linked to Huntington's disease. Nature 1983;306:234–238.

3. Bird TD, Ott J, Giblett ER. Evidence for linkage of Charcot-Marie-Tooth neuropathy to the Duffy locus on chromosome 1. Am J Hum Genet 1982;34:388–394.

4. Barker D, Wright E, Nguyen K, et al. Gene for von Recklinghausen Neurofibromatosis is in the pericentromeric region of chromosome 17. Science 1987;236: 1100–1102.

5. Seizinger BR, Rouleau GA, Ozelius LJ, et al. Genetic linkage of von Recklinghausen Neurofibromatosis to the nerve growth factor receptor gene. Cell 1987;49: 589–594.

6. Rouleau GA, Wertelecki W, Haines JL, et al. Genetic linkage of a bilateral acoustic neurofibromatosis to a DNA marker on chromsome 22. Nature 1987;329:246–248.

7. Chamberlain S, Shaw J, Rowland A, et al. Mapping of mutation causing Friedreich's ataxia to human chromosome 9. Nature 1988;334:248–250.

8. Brzustowicz LM, Lehner T, Castilla LH, et al. Genetic mapping of chronic childhood-onset spinal muscular atrophy to chromosome 5q11.2–13.3. Nature 1990;344: 540–541.

9. Monaco A, Neve R, Colletti-Feener C, Bertelson C, Kurnit D, Kunkel L. Isolation of candidate cDNAs for portions of the Duchenne muscular dystrophy gene. Nature 1986;323:646–650.

10. Koenig M, Hoffman EP, Bertelson CJ, Monaco AP, Freener C, Kunkel L. Complete cloning of the Duchenne muscular dystrophy cDNA and preliminary genomic organization of the DMD gene in normal and affected individuals. Cell 1987;50: 509–517.

11. Rommens JM, Ianuzzi MC, Kerem B, et al. Identification of the cystic fibrosis gene: Chromosome walking and jumping. Science 1989;245:1059–1065.

12. Riordan JR, Rommens JM, Kerem B, et al. Identification of the cystic fibrosis gene: Cloning and characterization of complementary DNA. Science 1989;245:1066–1073.

13. Cawthon RM, Weiss R, Xu G, et al. A major segment of the Neurofibromatosis Type 1 gene: cDNA sequence, genomic structure and point mutations. Cell 1990;62:193–201.

14. Gubbay SS, Kahana E, Zilber N, Cooper G, Pintov S, Leibowitz Y. Amyotrophic lateral sclerosis. A study of its presentation and prognosis. J Neurol 1985;232: 295–300.

15. Buckley J, Warlow C, Smith P, Hilton-Jones D, Irvine S, Tew JR. Motor-neuron disease in England and Wales, 1959–1979. J Neurol Neurosurg Psychiatry 1983;46: 197–205.

16. Forsgren L, Almay BG, Holmgren G, Wahl S. Epidemiology of motor-neuron disease in northern Sweden. Acta Neurol Scand. 1983;68:20–29.

17. Kurland LT, Mulder DW. Epidemiologic investigations of amyotrophic lateral sclerosis. 2. Familial aggregations indicative of dominant inheritance. Neurology 1955;5:182–268.

18. Li TM, Alberman E, Swash M. Comparison of sporadic and familial disease

amongst 580 cases of motor neuron disease. J Neurol Neurosurg Psychiatry 1988;51:778–784.

19. Mulder DW, Kurland LT, Offord KP, Beard CM. Familial adult motor neuron disease: Amyotrophic lateral sclerosis. Neurology 1986;36:511–517.

20. Horton WA, Eldridge R, Brody JA. Familial motor neuron disease. Evidence for at least three different types. Neurology 1976;26:460–465.

21. Ott J. Analysis of human genetic linkage. Baltimore: Johns Hopkins University Press, 1985.

22. Chio A, Brignolio F, Meineri P, Schiffer D. Phenotypic and genotypic heterogeneity of dominantly inherited amyotrophic lateral sclerosis. Acta Neurol Scand 1987;75:277–282.

23. Williams DB, Floate DA, Leicester J. Familial motor neuron disease: Differing penetrance in large pedigrees. J Neurol Sci 1988;86:215–230.

24. Schmitt HP, Emser W, Heimes E. Familial occurence of ALS, Parkinsonism, and dementia. Ann Neurol 1984;16:642–648.

25. Gusella JF. DNA polymorphism and human disease. Annu Rev Biochem 1986;55: 831–854.

26. Donis-Keller H, Green P, Helms C, et al. A genetic linkage map of the human genome. Cell 1987;51:319–337.

27. White R, Lalouel JM, Sets of linked genetic markers for human chromosomes. Annu Rev Genet 1988;22:259–279.

28. Cytogenetics and cell genetics. Vol 51. No. 1–4. Human gene mapping 10. Basel: S. Karger, AG, 1989.

29. Skolnick MH, Wallace RB. Simultaneous analysis of multiple polymorphic loci using amplified sequence polymorphisms. Genomics 1988;2:273–279.

30. Weber JL, May PE. Abundant class of human DNA polymorphisms which can be typed using the polymerase chain reaction. Am J Hum Genet 1989;44:388–396.

31. Lander E. Mapping complex traits in human genetics. In: Davies K, ed. Human genetic disease: A practical approach. Oxford: IRL Press, 1989.

32. Ott J. Estimation of the recombination fraction in human pedigrees: efficient computation of the likelihood for human linkage studies. Am J Hum Genet 1974;26: 588–597.

33. Lathrop GM, Lalouel JM, Julier C, Ott J. Strategies for multi locus linkage analysis in humans. Proc Natl Acad Sci USA 1984;81:3443–3446.

34. Lathrop GM, Lalouel JM. Easy calculation of LOD scores and genetic risks on small computers. Am J Hum Genet 1984;36:460–465.

35. Lathrop GM, Lalouel JM, Julier C, Ott J. Multilocus linkage analysis in humans: Detection of linkage and estimation of recombination. Am J Hum Genet 1985;37: 482–498.

36. Gilliam TC, Tanzi RE, Haines JL, et al. Localization of the Huntington's disease gene to a small segment of chromosome 4 flanked by D4S10 and the telomere. Cell 1987;50:565–571.

37. Lander E, Botstein D. Strategies for studying heterogeneous genetic traits in humans using a linkage map of restriction length polymorphisms. Proc Natl Acad Sci USA 1986;83:7353–7357.

38. Lander E, Botstein D. Homozygosity mapping: A way to map human recessive traits with the DNA of inbred children. Science 1987;236:1567–1570.
39. Lander E, Botstein D. Mapping complex genetic traits in humans: new methods using a complete RFLP linkage map. Cold Spring Harbor Symp Quant Biol 1986;51:49–62.
40. Figlewicz DA, Rouleau GA, Haines JL, Horvitz R, Brown RH Jr. Genetic linkage studies in familial amyotrophic lateral sclerosis (ALS). 18th Annual Society for Neuroscience Abstr. 1988;14:273.2.
41. Siddique T, Pericak-Vance MA, Brooks BR, et al. Linkage analysis in familial amyotrophic lateral sclerosis. Neurology 1989;39:919–925.
42. Siddique T, Pericak-Vance MA, Roos RP, et al. Chromosome 21 markers in familial amyotrophic lateral sclerosis. Neurology 1990;40(Suppl 1):315.
43. Roses AD, Pericak-Vance MA, Yamaoka LH, et al. Recombinant DNA strategies in genetic neurological diseases. Muscle Nerve 1983;6:339–355.
44. Gusella JF, Tanzi RE, Anderson MA, et al. DNA markers for nervous system diseases. Science 1984;225:1320–1326.
45. Carle GF, Frank M, Olson MV. Electrophoretic separation of large DNA molecules by periodic inversion of the electric field. Science 1986;232:65–68.
46. Michaels F, Burmeister M, Lehrach H. Derivation of clones close to met by preparative field inversion electrophoresis. Science 1987;236:1305–1308.
47. Poustka A, Pohl TM, Barlow DP, Frischauf AM, Lehrach H. Construction and use of human chromosome jumping libraries from NotI-digested DNA. Nature 1987;325:353–355.
48. Collins FS, Drumm ML, Cole JL, Lockwood WK, VandeWoude GF, Iannuzzi MC. Construction of a general human chromosome jumping library, with application to cystic fibrosis. Science 1987;235:1046–1049.
49. Estivill X, Farrall M, Scambler PJ, et al. A candidate for the cystic fibrosis locus isolated by selection for methylation-free islands. Nature 1987;326:840–845.

30

Gene Expression in Motor Neurons

Kenneth E. M. Hastings

Montreal Neurological Institute and McGill University
Montreal, Quebec, Canada

INTRODUCTION

Motor neurons are the subject of a voluminous literature extending over many years and including many classic neuroscience investigations. However, our understanding of the molecular biology of motor neurons, particularly of those aspects which might be unique to this class of neurons, is very limited. The impetus to further such understanding comes from a desire to comprehend the development, structure, and function of this important component of the nervous system and also from the knowledge that certain devastating diseases, including amyotrophic lateral sclerosis (ALS), have motor neurons as a particular target (1–3). The existence of motor neuron diseases is an indication of special biological properties, but the diseases themselves do not provide direct insight into the nature of these special motor neuron characteristics. Obviously, it would be of great medical importance to know which aspects of motor neuron biology make them particularly vulnerable to these diseases. Moreover, such motor-neuron-specific characteristics may also be of great relevance to understanding the normal biology of motor neurons.

Many aspects of cell biology depend on gene expression. The set of proteins synthesized by a cell reflects the gene set active in that cell and the rate of synthesis of each protein is a quantitative reflection of gene activity. The generation of diverse cell types during development is largely based on mechanisms of differential expression of cell-type-specific genes. In addition, even fully differentiated adult cells are capable of quantitative and qualitative changes in gene expression in response to changing physiological conditions. Each of these aspects of gene expression and regulation—qualitative and quantitative, developmental and physiological—must be important in the normal biology of motor neurons. Moreover, one or more of these aspects may also be important in motor neuron diseases, whether these clearly involve gene defects, as in familial ALS (4) and the hereditary spinal muscular atrophies (5), or whether gene involvement is less clear, as in sporadic ALS. In this chapter I review and discuss various aspects of gene expression in motor neurons, under the following general headings: quantitative aspects related to the very large cell size of motor neurons, characterization of the genes expressed in motor neurons, with a particular focus on possible motor neuron-specific genes, and gene regulatory phenomena related to the development, differentiation, and physiology of motor neurons. Several recent reviews have considered gene expression in the brain, or in the nervous system as a whole (6–9), but the particular subject of gene expression in motor neurons has not been considered before.

QUANTITATIVE ASPECTS RELATED TO LARGE CELL-BODY AND AXON SIZE

Motor neurons are very large cells, and this has implications for quantitative aspects of gene expression, i.e., the synthesis and accumulation of RNA and protein molecules. Motor neurons (and other similarly large neurons) are the largest somatic cells in vertebrates thought to be supported by the transcriptional activity of a single diploid nucleus. Among somatic cells, only skeletal muscle cells are larger, and these are syncytial cells containing hundreds or thousands of nuclei. Invertebrates produce giant cells, including giant neurons (and giant axons), which can be much larger than the largest vertebrate neurons or axons. However, these giant cells are sustained by the transcriptional activity of many individual nuclei, as in the giant motor axon of the squid, which is produced by the fusion of hundreds of individual axons of unremarkable size (10), or of single, but manyfold polyploid, nuclei, as in the R2 and L6 neurons of the marine mollusc *Aplysia*, whose nuclei contain 10^5 times the diploid DNA value (11,12). Neither of these mechanisms for giantism is utilized in vertebrates. High polyploidy is unknown in vertebrate tissue cells, including neurons, although evidence has been presented both for (13) and against (14, 15) low (up to eightfold) polyploidy in large neurons, including motor neurons and Purkinje cells (see Ref. 16 for review). Therefore, it is conceivable that vertebrate motor neurons may be near an upper size limit for a diploid cell.

What is the maximum amount of biosynthetically active cytoplasm that can be supported by a single diploid nucleus? In general, the factors that limit cell growth are unknown, but it is reasonable to consider as a possible limit the production and maintenance of ribosomes. The highest rate of production of ribosomes known for a mammalian cell is 4–5000 per minute, seen in exponentially growing fibroblasts in culture (see Ref. 17 for review), although rates about fourfold higher could occur if the theoretical maximum gene transcription rate calculated by Kafatos (18) (48 transcripts per minute) is applied to the case of a cell having 400 copies of the ribosomal cistron, as do diploid G1 human cells (see Ref. 19). The possibility that large neurons may, like oocytes of many organisms, specifically amplify their ribosomal genes (19) has been considered and ruled out, at least in the case of Purkinje cells (20). In all likelihood, motor neurons also produce their ribosomes from diploid or near-diploid numbers of ribosomal genes. No somatic tissue cell in the adult is known to produce ribosomes at as high a rate as rapidly dividing fibroblasts in culture. Hepatocytes produce 1100–1400 per minute per cell, although this is increased to 3700 per minute during liver regeneration (17). Brain cells produce ribosomes at a much slower rate, 220–260 per minute per cell (21).

Ribosome accumulation is determined by synthesis and turnover, which, in a cell in steady state, are exactly balanced. Relatively few adult tissue cells have been characterized in terms of ribosome turnover. Ribosomes turn over with a half-life of 3–5 days in liver (reviewed in Ref. 17) and adrenal gland (22), but more slowly (6–15-day half-life) in brain (21,23). The ribosome half-life of motor neurons is unknown. However, it is intriguing to note that given the number of ribosomes present in a motor neuron cell body (an average of 9×10^7)* and using as a hypothetical rate of production the highest known rate for a vertebrate diploid somatic cell (4–5000 per minute) (17), then the ribosome half-life necessary to maintain a steady state is 8.9 days. This is within the range estimated for brain (6–15 days) (21,23). Therefore, it is a realistic possibility that the cell bodies of motor neurons and other large neurons[†] could be near the limit of biosynthetically active cytoplasm that can be supported by a single diploid nucleus. They may be at or close to the limit if ribosome half-lives much

---

* Calculated on the basis of an RNA content of 500 pg/cell, an approximate average for human spinal cord motor neurons [25,26; early data on rabbit, human, and lower vertebrate anterior horn cells reviewed in Ref. 24; see also 25,26 for additional data on humans, and Ref. 27, which shows a higher RNA content [1350 pg] for bovine motor neurons], and assuming that this RNA is 70–75% ribosomal RNA with most of the rest being transfer RNA (28).

† This is particularly true for larger motor neurons (27,29), the large cells of Dieter's nucleus in the medulla oblongata (30), and large dorsal root ganglion neurons (31), all of which contain 1–2 ng of RNA, and for the Mauthner neuron of lower vertebrates, whose cell body contains 2 ng of RNA (32).

longer than about 10 days are not practical in a synthetically active cell in steady state.*

If it is true that motor neurons are near the limit of diploid cell ribosome accumulation, then they would likely also be near the limit of diploid cell protein synthesis capacity. The absolute rate of protein synthesis has not been measured in motor neurons or in any other neuron type, so estimates must be based on comparison with other tissues. Cell types that are classic examples of high-level protein synthesis in vertebrates, hepatocytes, pancreatic acinar cells (which secrete digestive enzymes), and tubular gland cells of chicken oviduct (which secrete ovalbumin and other egg-white proteins) have fractional daily synthesis rates in the range of 30–80%; i.e., they synthesize each day an amount of protein equal to 30–80% of their steady-state protein content (Table 1). Higher fractional daily synthesis rates are known for cells in culture, some of which have cell (and, presumably, protein) doubling times as short as 10 hr (36). In a nongrowing adult tissue cell the corresponding fractional daily synthesis rate would be about 250%. Applying this rather high figure to the case of an average-sized (30 pl) motor neuron cell body containing 6 ng of protein suggests a maximum likely synthesis rate of about 15 ng protein per day.

It is interesting to compare this calculated maximal synthesis rate with the demand represented by axonal transport/maintenance. Assuming that slow axonal transport (on the scale of ~ 1 mm/day) represents the rate of continuous de novo synthesis of the major axoplasmic proteins and their passage from the neuronal cell body into the axon (46), then this would demand the daily synthesis of approximately 1 axon-mm equivalent of protein. (For alternative views on axonal protein synthesis, see Refs. 47,48.) In the case of motor neurons with axons of 8–10 μm diameter (average for human lumbar alpha motor neurons, see Ref. 49), this would amount to approximately 12–16 ng/day (assuming 20% protein by weight, as is the case for cell bodies and other typical tissues, although this could be a severalfold overestimate; see Ref. 45). Fast transport (46) would represent an additional protein synthetic demand. These considerations indicate that axonal transport/maintenance must require a large fraction of the protein synthetic activity of motor neuron cell bodies. This suggests that perhaps evolutionary drive to maximize axon caliber has led to the generation of maximal or near-maximal cell body size in vertebrate motor neurons.[†]

---

* Virtually complete ribosome stability occurs under some conditions [exponentially growing cells in culture (33,34) and oocytes (35)] but is unknown in synthetically active cells in steady state (i.e., adult tissue cells). Moreover, the biological significance of ribosome turnover is unknown, i.e., is it merely a means to maintain steady state in the face of imperfect control over production rates? Or is it a mechanism for maintaining a "fresh" ribosome population for efficient protein synthesis?

[†]Although axons of approximately 10 μm diameter are, in general, the greatest caliber axons in vertebrate organisms, there is one cell type, the Mauthner cell of fish and amphibians, whose axon

Table 1 Protein Synthesis Rates in Various Cell Types

Cell type	Cell volume (pl)	RNA content (pg)	Protein content (pg)	Fractional daily protein synthesis (%)
Rodent pancreatic acinar cell	4.2[a]	39[a]	850[a]	30–70[b]
Rodent hepatocyte	3.7[c]	37[c]	670[c]	66[d]
Chicken oviduct magnum tubular gland cell	1.2[e]	16[f]	240[e]	50–80[f]
Mammalian spinal motor neuron cell-body	30[g]	500[h]	6000[i]	See text

[a]Based on data in Ref. 37.
[b]Based on data in Refs. 37 and 38.
[c]Based on data in Ref. 39.
[d]Ref. 40.
[e]Based on data in Ref. 41.
[f]Based on data in Ref. 42.
[g]Based on Refs. 25, 26, 29, 43, 44. This is an average estimate for fixed spinal alpha motor neurons in humans and cats; sizes range up to severalfold higher than this average value.
[h]See text footnote.
[i]Assuming 30 pl volume and 20% protein by wet weight, the typical tissue protein content; see also Refs. 30,44,45.

Although this discussion has been focused on the ribosomal genes, similar comments apply to protein-coding genes. In these cases also, transcript (mRNA) accumulation is determined by the balance between production and degradation. To understand the impact of large cell size, consider any particular "housekeeping" mRNA species present at similar concentrations in hepatocytes and in motor neurons. Since motor neuron cell bodies are 8 times the volume of hepatocytes (Table 1), it follows that either the cell nucleus of the motor neuron must produce the mRNA at a rate 8 times higher than the hepatocyte nucleus, or the half-life of the mRNA must be 8 times longer in motor neurons than in hepato-

---

has a significantly greater diameter (approximately 30 μm, Refs. 50,51). The Mauthner neuron cell body volume and RNA content are also severalfold higher than the average for motor neurons (see Refs. 24,32). Although some higher vertebrate neurons overlap the Mauthner cell in terms of size and approach it in terms of RNA content (24), the diameter of the Mauthner axon is uniquely large. Whether this reflects the operation of synthetic or transport mechanisms peculiar to this cell type is presently unknown.

cytes. This kind of demand may push some protein-coding genes close to the biological limits of transcription or of useful mRNA half-life in motor neurons.

The importance of these size-related considerations for ALS and other motor neuron disease is that they may suggest a particular vulnerability of motor neurons. If these cells are operating near a biological limit of RNA and protein synthesis under normal conditions, then they may be more susceptible to various insults than are cells which operate well within the maximum limits and which therefore may have a considerable reserve capacity. Another size-related issue concerns responsiveness to changing environmental conditions. Large cells may be relatively sluggish in terms of environmentally induced gene expression, e.g., heat shock (52), or interferon (53) gene expression, since following maximal transcriptional activation, smaller cells would be able to accumulate the induced mRNAs to any given cytoplasmic concentration in a shorter period of time. There is suggestive evidence that cell size may be an important factor in ALS susceptibility. Analysis of motor neuron cell-body sizes in ALS suggests (but cannot prove) that smaller motor neurons (presumably gamma fusimotor neurons; see below) are relatively spared (54). Moreover, large sensory neurons in dorsal root ganglia can also be affected in ALS (54), although sensory deficit is not usually clinically prominent. The involvement of pyramidal cells of the cerebral cortex (Betz cells; 1,3) is also consistent with the possibility of size-related susceptibility. It would be of interest to know whether other large neurons, including Dieter's cells in the lateral vestibular nucleus and cerebellar Purkinje cells, may also be affected.

Cellular RNA concentrations have been studied in ALS spinal motor neurons and have been found to be 30–40% lower than control values (25,26; see also 26a). Other neurons (nucleus dorsalis) in ALS patients do not show reduced RNA levels relative to controls (26). The lower RNA concentration and content in ALS motor neurons presumably reflects lower ribosome levels (28), which could result from either a decreased rate of production or an increased rate of turnover in comparison with normal motor neurons. It has been suggested that the lower RNA levels of ALS motor neurons may be related to cytological changes in motor neuron nuclear chromatin (26a) and/or to a DNA repair deficit that is detectable in ALS skin fibroblasts (2,55). The reduction in ribosome levels in ALS motor neurons would be expected to result in a significant reduction in protein synthetic capacity of the cells, which could, according to our earlier calculations, render the cells incapable of normal axonal transport/maintenance (see also Ref. 2, pp. 425–426). However, it is not clear that this should lead to cell death, nor is it known whether the reduction in ribosomes represents a primary ALS pathology, or whether it is a secondary effect observed in cells that may already be moribund due to a dysfunction that has no direct relationship to overall RNA accumulation. The plausibility of a primary RNA accumulation defect is indicated by the experimental induction in cats of a motor neuron disease–like condition by treatment of the animals with actinomycin D, an inhibitor of RNA synthesis (work of Koenig and colleagues, cited in Ref. 26a); however, this does not prove that an RNA defect is primary in human ALS.

Only one specific mRNA, that encoding one of the neurofilament subunits, NF-L, has been quantitatively assessed (by in situ hybridization) in ALS spinal motor neurons. NF-L mRNA was found to be of equal concentration in ALS and control motor neurons (56). This need not imply that NF-L protein synthesis proceeds at normal rates, given that ribosome levels are reduced in ALS motor neurons. Whether all or the generality of mRNA species are at normal levels in ALS motor neurons remains to be established. If so, this could suggest that the reduction in RNA levels is a specific effect for ribosomal RNA and does not affect mRNA production and accumulation.

GENES EXPRESSED IN MOTOR NEURONS

Gene Products Identified in Motor Neurons

Gene expression in motor neurons has been extensively investigated by histochemical and immunohistochemical methods. However, with few exceptions (see below) the protein/peptide/enzyme/antigen visualized in motor neurons using these procedures is one that is already known from other sources. Therefore this approach has provided little information about motor-neuron-specific genes. It is nonetheless of interest in terms of establishing the overall profile of gene expression in motor neurons. In the following paragraphs the proteins/peptides/ enzymes/antigens that have been demonstrated in motor neurons are collected in terms of general cell functions.

Cytoskeletal proteins: actin (57), fodrin (58), neurofilament 200K, 150K, and 68K (57), peripherin (59), tubulin (alpha and beta) (57), tau microtubule-associated protein (57).

Neuroendocrine vesicle-related proteins: caligulin (60), cholinergic vesicle marker proteoglycan (61), chromogranin A (60,62), clathrin (58), SV2 (60), synapsin I (60), synaptophysin (p38) (60).

Neuropeptides/neurotransmitter enzymes: calcitonin gene–related peptide (CGRP) (63–67), galinin (66,67), neuropeptide Y (66), somatostatin (66,68), vasoactive intestinal peptide (69), acetylcholinesterase (60,70), choline acetyltransferase (71).

Receptors: androgen receptor (72), dopamine receptor (73), glycine receptor (74), muscarinic acetylcholine receptor (73,74), nerve growth factor (NGF) receptor (75).

Metabolic enzymes: acetylCoA synthetase (76), ATP-citrate lyase (76), carnitine acetyltransferase (76), citrate synthetase (76), creatine kinase (57), cytochrome oxidase (77), glucose-6-phosphate dehydrogenase (78,79), glutamate dehydrogenase (78,79), glutamate-oxaloacetate transaminase (78,79), gluta-mate-pyruvate transaminase (24), glycogen phosphorylase (80,81), hexokinase (78,79), isocitrate dehydrogenase (78,79), lactate dehydrogenase (80,81), malate dehydrogenase (78,79), monoamine oxidase (82), NADH diaphorase (80,81), NADPH diaphorase (80), neuron-specific enolase (57), phosphoglucoi-somerase (79), 6-phosphogluconate dehydrogenase (78,79), pyruvate dehydro-genase (76), succinate dehydrogenase (80,81,83), UDP-glucose glycogen trans-ferase (84).

Hydrolytic enzymes: acid phosphatase (81,82,85), acid proteinase (cathepsin D) (85), alkaline phosphatase (86), arylsulfatase (70,85), enkephalinase (87), beta-galactosidase (79,88), galactosylceramidase (70), GM$_1$-ganglioside-beta-galactosidase (70), beta-glucosidase (88), beta-glucuronidase (70,79), beta-gly-cosidase (82,85), hexosaminidase (70,85), 5'-nucleotidase (82,89), phospholi-pase A$_2$ (70), ribonuclease (acid) (70), ribonuclease (alkaline) (70).

Miscellaneous: agrin (90), calmodulin (58), choline phosphotransferase (70), phosphocholine acyltransferase (70), neural cell adhesion molecule (N-CAM; 91,92).

Induced during axonal regeneration: growth-associated protein 24 (GAP-24) (93), growth-associated protein 43 (GAP43) (93,94), major histocompatability (class I) antigen (95), gamma-interferon (95).

Known only as antigens: SC1 (96), MO-1 (97,159), Tor 23 (98), Cat-201 (99), Cat-301 (99).

Several comments can be made about this list. First, other proteins are un-doubtedly present [presumably about 10,000 species if motor neurons, like most cell types, express about 10,000 different mRNA species (100)], but have not been specifically identified or shown to be synthesized in motor neurons. In addition to a host of general housekeeping proteins, e.g., ribosomal proteins, other proteins that are expected to be present include the Na$^+$, K$^+$, and Ca^{2+} channels involved in carrying axonal action potentials and initiating neurosecre-tory activity and receptors for neurotransmitter glutamate and possibly also nor-epinephrine, serotonin, and GABA (see Ref. 101).

A second aspect of the list is that some of the entries are proteins which may not be detectably expressed in some or even all normal adult motor neurons. Several products are expressed in limited subsets of adult motor neurons (e.g., galinin in some cranial, but not in spinal, motor neurons; Ref. 67), or in em-bryonic, but not in adult motor neurons (66,68,96), or in some species but not others (e.g., VIP in *Torpedo* electromotor neurons but not in mammalian motor neurons; Refs. 60,69), or depending on the nature of the afferent input (102). In addition, several proteins are not expressed in adult motor neurons or are ex-pressed at extremely low levels, but are strongly induced during axonal regen-eration (93–95, see also 70,75,103). This variability and plasticity presumably reflects the fact that motor neurons are capable of considerable gene regulatory behavior that is sensitive to physiological and/or developmental conditions.

Motor-Neuron-Specific Genes

In terms of functional and morphological criteria, motor neurons are a well-defined neuronal cell type. Is this distinct phenotype associated with the expression of cell-type-characteristic proteins? Are there motor-neuron-specific proteins and genes? In the above list of proteins/peptides/enzymes/antigens known to be expressed in motor neurons, only one product—the MO-1 antigen (159)—is potentially a motor-neuron-specific molecule. Otherwise, the list would appear to be a partial recipe that could perhaps be valid for any cholinergic neuron. Several products that are not motor-neuron-specific appear to be more abundant in motor neurons than in other cholinergic neurons, although whether this is a qualitative or a quantitative difference is not clear (see below). Other experimental approaches than the histochemical/immunohistochemical ones have also identified candidate motor-neuron-specific proteins (see below) but these have not yet been characterized. Before reviewing studies bearing on the issue of motor-neuron-specific gene expression, I can state the general conclusion that, although several intriguing candidates have been put forward, no well-characterized molecule is presently known to have a motor-neuron-specific distribution.

Four general approaches have been used in the search for motor neuron-specific gene products; (a) generation of shotgun monoclonal antibody libraries, which might include antibodies recognizing motor-neuron-specific epitopes, (b) direct biochemical and gel electrophoretic analysis of proteins extracted from isolated motor neurons, (c) analysis of labeled proteins undergoing axonal transport in motor axons, and (d) analysis of electric organ of electric fish, which is a hyperdeveloped neuromuscular junction rich in both pre- and postsynaptic proteins.

Monoclonal Antibody Approaches

In this approach it is supposed that motor-neuron-specific epitopes exist. In possible support of this notion is the recent finding that guinea pigs immunized with bulk-isolated bovine motor neurons may develop a motor neuron disease that is presumably antibody-mediated (104). The technical difficulty of motor neuron isolation is such that no attempts to characterize anti–motor-neuron antibodies generated in response to immunization with isolated motor neurons have been reported. Instead, investigators have taken the approach of using heterogeneous immunogens which contain motor neuron material (e.g., spinal cord), preparing a battery of monoclonal hybridomas, and screening each monoclonal antibody by immunohistochemical reaction with motor neurons in spinal cord histological sections. A monoclonal antibody, MO-1, raised against embryonic rat ventral hemicord was found to react exclusively with motor neurons (97,159). The MO-1 antigen is therefore the first (and only) motor-neuron-specific macromolecule, and its full characterization is eagerly awaited. In a similar study using feline (99) spinal cord gray matter, two monoclonal antibodies, Cat-201 and Cat-301, were found to react with motor neurons, although there was also extensive reaction with many other neuronal cell types. In a study using avian material, several monoclonal antibodies generated against embryonic spinal cord membranes were found to react with embryonic/fetal motor neurons, although in this study also, none was motor-neuron-specific (96). Monoclonal antibodies have also been raised by immunization with synaptic vesicles isolated from *Torpedo* electric organ. One of these, Tor 23, recognizes a cell surface epitope present on a specific subclass of mammalian neurons including, but not limited to, motor neurons (98).

General Analysis of Extracted Proteins

Perhaps the most direct experimental approach to the study of motor-neuron-specific gene expression is to isolate and directly analyze motor neuron proteins and mRNAs. Several motor neuron isolation procedures have been reported (27,105,106). To date, there is one report on comparative analysis of motor neuron proteins and none on analysis of motor neuron mRNA. In the study of motor neuron proteins Weil and McIlwain (107) isolated bovine spinal motor neuron perikarya (cell bodies and proximal dendrites) and analyzed the soluble proteins (extracted by homogenization in 50 mM phosphate buffer) by two-dimensional gel electrophoresis. They carried out a quantitative comparison of the motor-neuron-soluble protein pattern with that of ventral gray matter, which includes motor neurons as well as other neuronal cell types. The overall patterns were similar, but 6 of the 50 most abundant proteins were found to be much more abundant (17 times, or more) in the motor neuron prep than in the ventral gray matter prep. These proteins, which were not identified, therefore appear to be much more abundant in motor neurons than in other neurons of the ventral gray matter and should be considered as candidate motor-neuron-specific proteins. However, it has not been directly confirmed that any of these proteins is in fact synthesized in motor neurons, nor has their possible expression in neuronal cell bodies in other regions of the nervous system been investigated.

Weil and McIlwain also analyzed proteins similarly extracted from dorsal and ventral spinal roots and considered these proteins to be derived largely from either sensory or motor axons, respectively. The protein patterns were qualitatively identical, and quantitative analysis of the 50 most abundant proteins showed no consistent differences between the dorsal and ventral root preparations (107). Therefore, the extractable proteins of sensory and motor axons represent largely or entirely identical populations.

Axonal Transport of Labeled Proteins

Other information relating to motor neuron proteins comes from studies based on axonal transport. Following central nervous system injection of radiolabeled amino acids, proteins synthesized in motor neuron cell bodies become labeled and their subsequent transport to distal axonal segments in motor nerve trunks can be analyzed by polyacrylamide gel electrophoresis and autoradiography. A comparative study of slowly transported axonal proteins showed no major differences between sensory and spinal motor neurons (57); minor proteins were not analyzed. Comparative studies of fast-transported components also show extremely similar profiles in sensory and motor nerves. No significant differences were noted in one-dimensional gel analysis in rat (108), and in a two-dimensional analysis in the frog (109), the approximately 45 most heavily labeled proteins were found to be the same in sensory and motor nerves. At most four minor spots may have been motor neuron (ventral root)-specific in the latter study, but because they were near the limits of detection, their undetectability in sensory nerve could simply be due to the presence of severalfold lower levels.

Comparative studies involving other axon types revealed overall similarities, but also specific molecular differences. Optic nerve contains a slowly transported, 52-kDa protein not observed in sensory and motor nerves (57,58), and preganglionic parasympathetic axons of the vagus nerve contain a fast-transported protein of 50 kDa that is not present in hypoglossal motor axons (110). Because these cytotypic differences concern proteins that are absent from motor neuron axons, they do not suggest candidates for motor-neuron-specific gene products.

Thus general studies of accumulated and transported protein species indicate that sensory and motor axons are extremely similar, with no definite, reproducible differences having been noted. Given that a significant fraction of motor neuron protein synthesis must be concerned with axonal proteins (see above), the similarity of accumulated and transported protein species in sensory and motor axons implies a great similarity of major mRNA species in these two cell types. This is remarkable given the embryonic origins of these two cell neuronal cell types (motor neurons from neural tube and sensory neurons from neural crest; Ref. 111).

Although major axonal proteins do not appear to include any motor-neuron-specific species, the analysis of Weil and McIlwain (107) suggests that as many as 10% of abundant perikaryal protein species may be motor-neuron-specific. The six proteins they identified as being much more abundant in purified motor neurons than in ventral gray matter have not been characterized. However, they remain of great interest as possible motor-neuron-specific gene products, especially because they are quantitatively major proteins.

Proteins from Electric Organ

An additional experimental approach to motor neuron proteins is through analysis of electric organ of electric fish, which is a rich source of pre- and postsynaptic components. Protein extracts of electric organ have not been subjected to general protein analysis with a view to discovering motor-neuron-specific proteins. However, one protein discovered initially from this source has been shown to be expressed in motor neurons. This protein, agrin (90), was first identified as an activity promoting the aggregation of acetylcholine receptors on cultured muscle cells. The production of antiagrin antibodies permitted the demonstration that motor neurons contain agrin. Indeed, within spinal cord sections agrin antibodies selectively stained motor neurons, indicating that agrin was particularly prominent in motor neurons (90). However, vascular and/or perivascular cells also are strongly stained with antiagrin antibodies, indicating that this is not strictly a neuronal protein. Moreover, quantitative analysis of extracts of brain regions not containing prominently staining cells indicated that antibody-neutralizable agrin activity is present, presumably at concentrations too low to provide definite immunohistochemical staining (90). Thus, although agrin does not appear to be a motor-neuron-specific protein, or even a neuron-specific protein, among spinal cord cells it seems to be expressed at much higher levels in motor neurons than in any other neuronal cell type.

Summary

No well-characterized protein or gene is known to be specifically and uniquely expressed in motor neurons. The MO-1 antigen is the only molecule that has been histochemically identified as showing a motor-neuron-specific expression pattern. However, other than the fact that the MO-1 antigen is sensitive to trypsin and therefore is, or contains, a polypeptide (97), we know nothing about its structure or function. The six motor-neuron-enriched proteins identified by Weil and McIlwain (107) are strong candidates for motor-neuron-specific proteins, but at the moment we know nothing of their structure or function, nor do specific molecular probes exist for these proteins or the genes and mRNAs that encode them.

It is worthwhile noting that several products that are definitely not motor-neuron-specific appear to be expressed at higher levels in motor neurons than in other spinal cord cells. Among these the most notable are agrin (90) and peripherin (59), although chromogranin A and CGRP also show this phenomenon (60,63,112). It may be that expression of these genes is widespread or even ubiquitous among neurons, but is quantitatively correlated with some feature that is particularly well developed in motor neurons, e.g., large size, large axon diameter, numerous terminals, and so forth. In a semiquantitative analysis of only spinal ventral gray matter, this could result in a misleading impression of motor neuron specificity. Such products, although expressed at particularly high levels in motor neurons, do not correspond to the notion of cell-type-specific gene expression reflecting unique developmental gene regulatory mechanisms. This type of gene regulation would be expected to be associated with unconditional cell-type-specific gene expression, of the kind that might provide stable cell-type-specific molecular markers and might be of particular significance in defining and specifying the fundamental motor neuron phenotype.

Finally, it should be noted that although the great majority of gene products listed earlier are also known to be expressed in cell types other than motor neurons and are therefore apparently not motor-neuron-specific, it has not been rigorously established in any case that the particular product expressed in motor neurons corresponds precisely to the product expressed in other cell types. That is, it remains possible that motor-neuron-specific isoforms of any or all of these products may exist, produced by mechanisms of alternative RNA splicing (113) or by the use of separate but related genes (gene families).

GENE REGULATION IN MOTOR NEURONS

Gene regulatory mechanisms presumably play numerous important roles in motor neuron biology. In the following sections gene regulation in motor neurons is discussed in relation to (a) neuronal gene activation during the embryonic formation of motor neurons, (b) axonal regeneration, (c) transsynaptic signaling, and (d) motor neuron functional heterogeneity.

Neuronal Differentiation

Embryonic neuroectodermal cells give rise both to glia and to neurons. The undifferentiated precursor cells contain vimentin intermediate filaments, but during the formation of definitive neuronal cells, cell-type-specific intermediate filaments, neurofilaments, appear (114,115). Therefore, the activation of neurofilament gene expression is a key point in the development of a neuronal cell type. In the spinal cord, the first cells to express immunohistochemically detectable neurofilament protein are presumptive motor neurons, which are therefore the first spinal cord cells in which neuronal differentiation occurs (66,116–118). This occurs in the rat at E11–E13. Choline acetyl transferase is also first detectable in rat motor neurons at E13 (119). The early establishment of neurons from precursor cells may involve the coordinated activation of a battery of neuronal genes. The mechanisms that control the tissue-specific expression of neurofilament genes, and other neuron-specific genes, and their activation during neuronal differentiation have not been elucidated. Transgenic mouse studies are underway that should permit the mapping of *cis*-regulatory elements that direct the neuronal-specific expression of the human NFL-L gene, and such studies should lead to the identification of neuron-specific transcription factors active during motor neuron differentiation (120,121).

During development of the rat spinal cord, CGRP, galinin, and somatostatin are first detected in motor neurons several days later than the first appearance of neurofilament (66). It is possible that the delay of neuropeptide expression with respect to neurofilament expression may reflect serial stages of gene activation during neuronal development (although other explanations based on the elaborate posttranslational processing involved in neuropeptide accumulation could also account for the delay). Some neuronal gene products are first expressed much later in development; the MO-1 antigen (97) is not readily detectable on motor neurons until the end of the first week after birth. In other neuronal types, although apparently not in motor neurons (115,118), the neurofilament 200-kDa subunit (NF-H) gene is not actively expressed until after birth (122,123), long after the activation of NF-M (150 kDa) and NF-L (68 kDa) neurofilament subunit expression.

In addition to late-appearing products, there are products expressed in embryonic motor neurons which are expressed only at very low levels, if at all, in adult motor neurons. For example, neuropeptide expression is more diverse and more widespread in embryonic as opposed to adult motor neurons (66,68). Whether the maturation-associated restriction of neuropeptide expression reflects a developmentally programmed loss of cells or a reduction in neuropeptide expression within individual cells has not been clarified. In other cases, transient expression in embryonic neurons seems clearly established, e.g., the cell-surface antigen recognized by the monoclonal antibody SC-1 (96) and the growth-associated proteins whose synthesis is reactivated in adult motor neurons during axonal regeneration (see below). These features suggest that the gene expression profile of adult motor neurons is based on multiple gene regulatory systems involving serial stages of gene activation and repression, presumably related to distinct and important stages in motor neuron development.

Axonal Regeneration

In mature, fully developed neurons, gene expression and cell biology can be considerably perturbed by axotomy. The overall response of the neuron is to regenerate the missing distal axon by establishing a growth cone at or near the severed end and extending a thin axonal process at a rate on the order of 1 mm/day (124–126). This can lead to reestablishment of synaptic contact with the target tissue and, in time, to the reformation of an axon of appropriate caliber (often much larger than the regenerating axonal process) and complete recovery of original neuronal properties. During the regeneration period, the neurons differ in several respects from normal adult neurons, including in the size and the overall histological appearance of the cell body, and also in the synthesis of growth-associated proteins and other proteins not actively synthesized in normal adult neurons.

During axonal regeneration in rabbit hypoglossal motor neurons (45) and frog spinal cord motor neurons (127), there is an increase in cell-body size and RNA (ribosome) content up to levels greater than twice as high as control, nonaxotomized neurons. These increases peak over a long course, 30–50 days following axotomy, and return to normal by 70–80 days following reinnervation. Both these classes of motor neuron have rather small cell sizes compared with the average mammalian spinal cord motor neuron used in the earlier calculations of ribosome production and stability. It would be of great interest to know whether larger mammalian spinal motor neurons, which have as much as, or more than, double the RNA content of hypoglossal neurons or frog spinal motor neurons, and which the calculations suggest could be near a limit of ribosome production and accumulation, could also double their volumes and ribosome contents during regeneration. Several observations (see Ref. 126, p. 53) suggest that the volume changes, at least, may be less pronounced in mammalian spinal motor neurons than in hypoglossal motor neurons. The increased RNA accumulation seen in regenerating neurons undoubtedly represents largely ribosomal RNA (124,126). Whether the increase represents increased synthesis or increased stability is an important question which has not been resolved; numerous studies (reviewed in Refs. 124,125) have shown greater incorporation of radioactivity from labeled RNA precursors into regenerating motor neurons, but in fact, it has never been established whether this phenomenon reflects an increased rate of RNA synthesis or an increased nucleotide pool specific activity.

Regenerating motor neurons generally, but not invariably (127), show the typical cytological reaction to axotomy termed chromatolysis, i.e., dispersal of the Nissl substance, or rough endoplasmic reticulum (126). It is not clear whether this change affects the amount, or only the distribution, of the rough endoplasmic reticulum. Some studies (reviewed in Ref. 126) suggest that the ratio of free to membrane-bound ribosomes is increased in chromatolysis. Such a change in ribosome distribution could reflect changes in the cellular mRNA population, since the attachment of ribosomes to the endoplasmic reticulum depends on the nature of nascent polypeptide being synthesized, and hence on the mRNA being translated (128). A reduction in the proportion of cellular ribosomes bound to the endoplasmic reticulum could reflect a reduction in the fraction of the mRNA population that encodes membrane/secretory proteins. Specific changes in the mRNA population undoubtedly occur (see below). However, the relative levels of mRNAs for membrane/secretory proteins have not been systematically evaluated. Moreover, some of the known changes do not fit the expected pattern; e.g., neurofilament (presumably translated on free polysomes) synthesis is decreased (103) and CGRP (presumably translated on membrane bound polysomes) accumulation is increased (129). The cause and significance of chromatolysis remain unknown.

In terms of specific gene expression, evidence has been presented for an increased synthesis of the growth-associated proteins (125), actin and tubulin (103), nerve growth factor receptor (75), and for increased accumulation of CGRP (129), interferon (95), histocompatability antigen (95), enzymes of hexose monophosphate shunt (glucose-6-phosphate dehydrogenase and 6-phosphogluconate dehydrogenase, 130), and acid phosphatase (reviewed in Ref. 126, p. 92). Decreased expression has been noted for neurofilament (103), proteins related to cholinergic neurotransmitter function (131), and glycogen phosphorylase (84). The signals initiating the gene expression responses to axotomy have not been characterized (124). It is also not known if or how the various changes observed are coordinated. It is possible that each gene may be responding to different stimuli and conditions. For example, although both actin and tubulin genes show enhanced expression following axotomy of facial motor neurons, they display different time courses of response and also differ in their reaction to successful versus unsuccessful regeneration (103). It therefore seems possible that multiple gene regulatory mechanisms may be involved in the gene expression changes seen during axonal regeneration.

Transsynaptic Gene Regulation

Transsynaptic gene regulation, i.e., the regulation of genes in postsynaptic cells by mechanisms depending on synaptic activity, has been documented in several neurobiological contexts. Transsynaptic regulation affects genes encoding neurotransmitter receptors [e.g., nicotinic acetylcholine receptor in muscle (132,133)], enzymes involved in neurotransmitter synthesis [e.g., tyrosine hydroxylase in postganglionic sympathetic neurons (134)], transcription factors (135), and proteins that may function in long-term synaptic modulation (136). Possible transsynaptic gene regulation in motor neurons has not been extensively studied, although expression of CGRP has been shown to be influenced by both descending and dorsal root inputs (102). Given the variety and density of synaptic input into motor neurons, there is abundant opportunity for transsynaptic gene regulatory mechanisms, and it is likely that further study will reveal more examples of this type of regulation.

Motor Neuron Heterogeneity

Motor neurons are functionally heterogeneous. In higher vertebrates one can distinguish between the gamma motor neurons that innervate the muscle spindle organs (fusimotor neurons) and the alpha motor neurons (skeletomotor neurons) that innervate the force-generating muscle fibers that make up the bulk of a muscle (49,137,138). Among the alpha skeletomotor neurons, one can recognize several distinct motor unit types each of which is associated with skeletal muscle fibers of either the slow (type I) or the fast (type IIA and type IIB) fiber types (137,138).

The gamma (fusimotor) axons in a motor nerve are much smaller than the alpha (skeletomotor) axons and a similar relationship likely applies to the cell bodies (49,137). Among the skeletomotor axons, slow motor unit axons conduct more slowly than fast motor unit axons, presumably reflecting a slightly smaller caliber (137). Cell body sizes are similarly related; slow motor neurons tend to be somewhat smaller than fast motor neurons, although there is a wide overlap (137). Characteristic fast/slow differences also exist in the maximum firing rate and in the EPSPs generated by comparable synaptic inputs (see Ref. 137 for review). In addition, slow units are used much more often than fast units (139), and hence, slow motor neurons are more active than fast motor neurons. Gamma (fusimotor) neurons are also relatively active (140). Histochemical analysis indicates that gamma motor neurons, and other smaller spinal cord neurons, are richer in oxidative enzymes than are the larger, alpha skeletomotor neurons (80,83,84). Subsequent studies have also suggested that among the alpha motor neuron class, slow motor neurons are richer in oxidative enzymes than are fast motor neurons (141).

It is unclear to what extent the differences among the various classes of motor neuron are based on differences in gene expression. This is likely to be the case at least for the quantitative differences in levels of oxidative enzymes. Any or all of the electrophysiological differences could involve regulation of genes encoding, for example, neurotransmitter receptors and ion channels, although possible posttranslational or other regulatory mechanisms could also account for the functional differences observed. Differences in gene expression among motor neuron classes could reflect either developmentally preprogrammed differences inherent in the cells or plasticity within a single fundamental cell type in response to differing physiological and environmental conditions. Such factors might include the kinds of synaptic input and the frequencies of use (transsynaptic regulation) and the nature and number of axon terminals, which may influence gene expression in cell bodies in the spinal cord by effects on the materials retrogradely transported from the terminals to the cell bodies. Regarding the possibility of axonal retrograde regulation, there is evidence to indicate that a mechanism based on information originating at the neuromuscular junction could play a role in establishing the difference in maximal firing rates of fast and slow motor neurons (142).

CURRENT AND FUTURE RESEARCH DIRECTIONS

A major goal of molecular biological analysis of motor neuron gene expression in the short- and intermediate-term future will likely remain the identification and characterization of motor-neuron-specific genes and gene products. At present, a monoclonal antibody reacting with a motor-neuron-specific antigen has been isolated (159), and several protein spots separated on two-dimensional gels represent likely candidate motor-neuron-specific proteins (107). I outline below possible future research directions that could lead to further characterization of these apparent examples of motor-neuron-specific gene expression, and to the identification of additional examples of motor-neuron-specific genes/gene products.

Anti–spinal cord monoclonal antibodies showing motor-neuron-specific immunohistochemical reaction, such as MO-1 (159), or others developed in future studies, may be amenable to Western blot analysis (143) of the antigen. This procedure can reveal the apparent molecular weight of the antigen and, in conjunction with the use of glycosidases and proteases, can establish whether the epitope recognized is a carbohydrate moiety, or part of a polypeptide chain. In the latter case it would be possible to use the antibody for immunological screening of an expression vector [e.g., lambda gt11 (144)] cDNA library representing spinal cord mRNA. This could lead to the isolation of cloned cDNA copies of the mRNA species encoding the motor-neuron-specific protein, and such cDNA clones would be useful in several applications (see below).

One possible approach to the further characterization of candidate motor-neuron-specific proteins such as those identified by Weil and McIlwain (107) is through protein microsequencing of the protein spots recovered from gels (145). On the basis of partial amino acid sequence information, specific oligonucleotides corresponding to the deduced protein-coding mRNA sequence can be synthesized and used as hybridization probes to screen a spinal cord cDNA clone library or as primers for polymerase chain reaction (PCR) amplification (see, e.g., Ref. 146). These approaches can lead directly to the isolation of cloned cDNA copies of mRNAs encoding the candidate motor-neuron- specific proteins.

The availability of motor neuron isolation procedures (27,105,106) also opens the possibility of isolating motor neuron mRNA and preparing (a) a motor neuron cDNA library and (b) hybridization probes representing the motor neuron mRNA population. Although overall mRNA and cDNA yields may be low, such difficulties could perhaps be overcome by exploiting some of the possibilities of PCR amplification (147). With a motor neuron cDNA library and a probe representing the motor neuron mRNA population, one would be in a position to employ differential hybridization screening of the library in order to identify cloned sequences present in motor neuron mRNA but not in mRNA from other neuronal sources. This could also lead directly to the isolation of cDNA clones of motor-neuron-specific mRNAs. In a related approach, Dickson et al. (148) reported the preparation of a cDNA library of embryonic chick spinal cord and the isolation of cDNA clones corresponding to mRNAs which were neuronal-specific (i.e., not expressed in optic nerve) and which showed distinct developmental expression patterns. (Whether any of these mRNAs are expressed in motor neurons was not determined.)

In order to avoid difficulties of purity and limited yield encountered in the physical isolation of any particular neuronal type, neurobiologists in recent years have attempted to produce immortal derivatives of primary neuronal cells as cell culture models. Two general immortalization approaches have been used: (a) infection with oncogene-expressing viruses (149,150), and (b) hybrid cell formation with an immortal tumor cell line, e.g., neuroblastoma (151–153). Immortalized cells can be used in a variety of research applications, including identification of cell-type-specific proteins and genes. For example, a putative motor neuron × neuroblastoma hybrid cell line has been used in immunological and cDNA cloning studies in order to identify proteins and mRNAs expressed in the hybrid cell, but not in the neuroblastoma parental cell line. Molecular probes for several hybrid-specific molecules, including surface antigens (154) and mRNA species (155), have been produced, and the possible motor-neuron-specificexpression of these molecules in situ can now be investigated. This represents a possible general approach to the identification of motor-neuron-specific genes/ gene products.

The isolation of cDNA clones of motor-neuron-specific mRNAs could lead to further studies of great interest. For example, DNA sequencing would reveal the amino acid sequence of the corresponding motor-neuron-specific protein, and upon comparison with known classes of cellular proteins, this could result in considerable insight into the possible cellular role of the newly identified protein. Such insight into the possible cellular functions of motor-neuron-specific proteins may lead to further understanding of motor-neuron-specific properties, including their susceptibility to motor neuron disease. Another important use of cDNA clones of motor-neuron-specific mRNAs concerns the possibility that the genetic motor neuron diseases (familial ALS and the genetic spinal muscular atrophies) could represent mutations in motor-neuron-specific genes. Once cDNA probes are available for motor-neuron-specific genes, the possibility that the corresponding gene is the one responsible for any genetic motor neuron disease can be assessed by gene polymorphism analysis in affected pedigrees (156–158). Tight linkage between the disease locus and the motor-neuron-specificgene locus, or characteristic Southern blot abnormalities in affected individuals, would be good evidence for the involvement of that particular gene in the disease. Identification of candidate genes by this procedure is unrelated to the more general approach of isolating linked marker DNA segments by restriction fragment length polymorphism linkage analysis using anonymous DNA probes. The latter approach, since it does not make any assumptions regarding the nature of the defective gene, is more certain of eventual success, i.e., identifying a piece of DNA near the defective gene (160). On the other hand, the former approach may give a fortunate result that would bypass not only the work of establishing a linked marker, but also the very difficult subsequent steps of ''walking'' along the chromosome from the linked marker to the disease locus itself.

Motor-neuron-specific cDNA clones or antibodies may also be of great utility in motor neuron research by providing objective and qualitative molecular markers of the motor neuron phenotype. Such markers would be useful for the identification of motor neurons in the absence of normal morphological clues, as in pathological and experimental conditions, including cell culture.

ACKNOWLEDGMENTS

I thank Stirling Carpenter, Neil Cashman, Ronald Chase, Heather Durham, and Jean-Pierre Julien for valuable discussions.

REFERENCES

1. Tandan R, Bradley WG. Amyotrophic lateral sclerosis. Part I. Clinical features, pathology, and ethical issues in management. Ann Neurol 1985;18:271–280.
2. Tandan R, Bradley WG. Amyotrophic lateral sclerosis. Part 2. Etiopathogenesis. Ann Neurol 1985;18:419–431.
3. Banker BQ. The pathology of the motor neuron disorders. In: Engel AG, Banker BQ, eds. Mycology. Vol 2. New York: McGraw-Hill, 1986:2031–2067.
4. Horton WA, Eldridge R, Brody JA. Familial motor neuron disease: Evidence for at least three different types. Neurology 1976;26:460–465.
5. Gomez MR. Motor neuron diseases in children. In: Engel AG, Banker BQ, eds. Mycology. Vol 2. New York: McGraw-Hill, 1986:1993–2012.
6. Sutcliffe JG. mRNA in the mammalian central nervous system. Annu Rev Neurosci 1988;11:157–198.
7. Hahn WE, Owens GP. Genes expressed in the brain: Evolutionary and developmental considerations. In: Rosenberg RN, Harding AE, eds. The molecular biology of neurological disease. Toronto: Butterworth, 1988:22–34.
8. Chikaraishi DM. Characteristics of brain messenger RNAs. In: Easter SS, Barald KF, Carlson BM, eds. From message to mind. Sunderland, MA: Sinauer, 1988:52–65.
9. Milner RJ, Bloom FE, Sutcliffe JG. Brain-specific genes: Strategies and issues. Curr Topics Dev Biol 1987;21:117–150.
10. Young JZ. The giant nerve fibers and epistellar body of cephalopods. Q J Microsc Soc 1936;78:367–386.
11. Coggeshall RE, Yaksta BA, Swartz FJ. A cytomorphometric analysis of the DNA of the nucleus of the giant cell, R2, in Aplysia. Chromosoma 1970;32:205–212.
12. Lasek RJ, Dower WJ. *Aplysia californica*: Analysis of nuclear DNA in individual nuclei of giant neurons. Science 1971;172:278–280.
13. Herman CJ, Lapham LW. Neuronal polyploidy and nuclear volumes in the cat central nervous system. Brain Res 1969;15:35–48.

14. Fujita S. DNA constancy in neurons of the human cerebellum and spinal cord as revealed by Fuelgen cytophotometry and cytofluorometry. J Comp Neurol 1974;155:195–202.
15. McIlwain DL, Capps-Covey P. The nuclear DNA content of large ventral spinal neurons. J Neurochem 1976;27:109–112.
16. Giuditta A. Role of DNA in brain activity. In: Lajtha A, ed. Handbook of neurochemistry Vol 5. New York: Plenum Press, 1983:251–276.
17. Hadjiolov AA. The nucleolus and ribosome biogenesis. Cell Biol Monogr 1985;12.
18. Kafatos FC. The cocoonase zymogen cells of silk moths: A model of terminal cell differentiation for specific protein synthesis. Curr Topics Dev Biol 1972;7:125–192.
19. Long EO, Dawid IB. Repeated genes in eukaryotes. Annu Rev Biochem 1980;49:727–764.
20. Brodsky VY, Marshak TL, Karavanov AA, Zatsepina OV, Nosikov VV, Korochkin LI, Braga EA. Cell differentiation as assayed by the topography and number of ribosomal genes. Cell Differ 1988;24:201–207.
21. Stoykova AS, Dudov KP, Dabeva MD, Hadjiolov AA. Different rates of synthesis and turnover of ribosomal RNA in rat brain and liver. J Neurochem 1983;41:942–949.
22. Boyadjiev SI, Hadjiolov AA. Fractionation and biosynthesis of ribonucleic acids of the rat adrenals. Biochim Biophys Acta 1968;161:341–351.
23. Retz KC, Steele WJ. Ribosome turnover in rat brain and liver. Life Sci 1980;27:2601–2604.
24. Brand MM, Lehrer GM. The biochemistry of single nerve cell bodies. In: Lajtha A, ed. Handbook of neurochemistry. Vol 5A. New York: Plenum Press, 1971:337–371.
25. Davidson TJ, Hartmann HA, Johnson MD. RNA content and volume of motor neurons in amyotrophic lateral sclerosis. I. The cervical swelling. J Neuropathol Exp Neurol 1981;40:32–36.
26. Davidson TJ, Hartman HA. RNA content and volume of motor neurons in amyotrophic lateral sclerosis. II. The lumbar intumescence and nucleus dorsalis. J Neuropathol Exp Neurol 1981;40:187–192.
27a. Mann DMA, Yates PO. Motor neurone disease: The nature of the pathogenic mechanism. J Neurol Neurosurg Psychiatry 1974;37:1036–1046.
27. Capps-Covey P, McIlwain DL. Bulk isolation of large ventral spinal neurons. J Neurochem 1975;25:517–521.
28. Hartmann HA, Davidson TJ. Neuronal RNA in motor neuron disease. In Rowland LP, ed. Human motor neuron diseases. New York: Raven Press, 1982:89–103.
29. Edstrom JE. The content and concentration of ribonucleic acid in motor anterior horn cells from the rabbit. J Neurochem 1956;1:159–165.
30. Hyden H, Pigon A. A cytophysiological study of the functional relationship between oligodendroglial cells and nerve cells of Deiter's nucleus. J Neurochem 1960;6:57–72.

31. Edstrom J-E, Pigon A. Relation between surface, ribonucleic acid content and nuclear volume in encapsulated spinal ganglion cells. J Neurochem 1958;3:95–99.

32. Edstrom J-E, Eichner D, Edstrom A. The ribonucleic acid of axons and myelin sheaths from Mauthner neurons. Biochim Biophys Acta 1962;61:178–184.

33. Weber MJ. Ribosomal RNA turnover in contact inhibited cells. Nature New Biol 1972;235:58–61.

34. Bowman LH, Emerson CP. Post-transcriptional regulation of ribosome accumulation during myoblast differentiation. Cell 1977;10:587–596.

35. Davidson EH. Gene activity in early development. 2nd ed. New York: Academic Press, 1976:365.

36. Buckley PA, Konigsberg IR. Myogenic fusion and the duration of the mitotic gap. Dev Biol 1974;37:193–212.

37. Junqueira LCU, Rothschild HA, Fajer A. Protein production by the rat pancreas. Exp Cell Res 1957;12:338–341.

38. Kramer MF, Poort C. Unstimulated secretion of protein from rat exocrine pancreas cells. J Cell Biol 1972;52:147–158.

39. Scornik OA. In vivo rate of translation by ribosomes of normal and regenerating liver. J Biol Chem 1974;249:3876–3883.

40. Scornik OA. Role of protein degradation in the regulation of cellular protein content and amino acid pools. Fed Proc 1984;43:1283–1288.

41. Palmiter RD. Rate of ovalbumin messenger ribonucleic acid synthesis in the oviduct of estrogen-primed chicks. J Biol Chem 1973;248:8260–8270.

42. Palmiter RD. Quantitation of parameters that determine the rate of ovalbumin synthesis. Cell 1975;4:189–197.

43. Schade JP, Van Harreveld A. Volume distributions of moto- and interneurons in the peroneus-tibialis neuron pool of the cat. J Comp Neurol 1961;117:387–398.

44. Hyden H. Cytophysiological aspects of the nucleic acids and proteins of nervous tissue. In: Elliot KAC, Page IH, Quastel JH, eds. Neurochemistry. The chemistry of brain and nerve. Springfield, IL: Charles C Thomas 1962:331–375.

45. Brattgaard S-O, Edstrom J-E, Hyden H. The chemical changes in regenerating neurons. J Neurochem 1957;1:316–325.

46. Lasek RJ, Garner JA, Brady ST. Axonal transport of the cytoplasmic matrix. J Cell Biol 1984;99:212s–221s.

47. Koenig E. Local synthesis of axonal protein. In: Lajtha A, ed. Handbook of neurochemistry. 2nd ed. Vol 7. New York: Plenum Press, 1984:315–340.

48. von Bernardi R, Alvarez J. Is the supply of axoplasmic proteins a burden for the cell body? Morphometry of sensory neurons and amino acid incorporation into their cell bodies. Brain Res 1989;478:301–308.

49. Dyck PJ. Diseases of peripheral nerves. In: Engel AG, Banker BQ, eds. Myology Vol 2. New York: McGraw-Hill, 1986:2069–2108.

50. Zottoli SJ. Comparative morphology of the Mauthner cell in fish and amphibians. In: Faber DS, Korn H, eds. Neurobiology of the Mauthner cell. New York: Raven Press, 1978:13–45.

51. Celio MR. Die Schmidt-lantermann'schen Einkerbungen der Myelinscheide des

Mauthner-axons: orte Longitudinalen Myelinwachstums? Brain Res 1976;108: 221–235.

52. Lindquist S. The heat shock response. Annu Rev Biochem 1986;55:1151–1191.
53. Pestka S, Langer JA, Zoon KC, Samuel CE. Interferons and their actions. Annu Rev Biochem 1987;56:467–496.
54. Kawamura Y, Dyck PJ, Shimono M, Okazaki H, Tateishi J, Doi H. Morphometric comparison of the vulnerability of peripheral motor and sensory neurons in amyotrophic lateral sclerosis. J Neuropathol Exp Neurol 1981;40:667–675.
55. Tandan R, Robison SH, Munzer JS, Bradley WG. Deficient DNA repair in amyotrophic lateral sclerosis. J Neurol Sci 1987;79:189–203.
56. Clark AW, Tran PM, Parhad IM, Krekoski CA, Julien J-P. Neuronal gene expression in amyotrophic lateral sclerosis. Mol Brain Res 1990;7:75–83.
57. Oblinger MM, Brady ST, McQuarrie IG, Lasek RJ. Cytotypic differences in the protein composition of the axonally transported cytoskeleton in mammalian neurons. J Neurosci 1987;7:453–462.
58. McQuarrie IG, Brady ST, Lasek RJ. Diversity in the axonal transport of structural proteins: major differences between optic and spinal axons in the rat. J Neurosci 1986;6:1593–1605.
59. Leonard DGB, Gorham JD, Cole P, Greene LA, Ziff EB. A nerve growth factor-regulated messenger RNA encodes a new intermediate filament protein. J Cell Biol 1988;106:181–193.
60. Booj S, Goldstein M, Fischer-Colbrie R, Dahlstrom A. Calcitonin gene-related peptide and chromogranin A: Presence and intra-axonal transport in lumbar motor neurons in the rat, a comparison with synaptic vesicle antigens in immunohistochemical studies. Neuroscience 1989;30:479–501.
61. Walker JH, Obrocki J, Zimmermann CW. Identification of a proteoglycan antigen characteristic of cholinergic synaptic vesicles. J Neurochem 1983;41:209–216.
62. Volknandt W, Schober M, Fisher-Colbrie R, Zimmerman H, Winkler H. Cholinergic terminals in the rat diaphragm are chromogranin A immunoreactive. Neurosci Lett 1987;81:241–244.
63. Gibson SJ, Polak JM, Bloom SR, Sabate IM, Mulderry PM, Ghatei MA, McGregor GP, Morrison JFB, Kelly JS, Evans RM, Rosenfeld MC. Calcitonin gene-related peptide immunoreactivity in the spinal cord of man and eight other species. J Neurosci 1984;12:3101–3111.
64. Kawai Y, Takami K, Shiosaka S, Emson PC, Hillyard CJ, Girgis S, MacIntyre I, Tohyama M. Topographic localization of calcitonin gene-related peptide in the rat brain: An immunohistochemical analysis. Neuroscience 1985;15:747–763.
65. Fontaine B, Klarsfeld A, Hokfelt T, Changeux JP. Calcitonin gene–related peptide, a peptide present in spinal cord motoneurons, increases the number of acetylcholine receptors in primary cultures of chick embryo myotubes. Neurosci Lett 1986;71:59–65.
66. Marti E, Gibson SJ, Polak JM, Facer P, Springall DR, Van Aswegan G, Aitchison M, Koltzenburg M. Ontogeny of peptide- and amine-containing neurones in motor, sensory, and autonomic regions of rat and human spinal cord, dorsal root ganglia, and rat skin. J Comp Neurol 1987;266:332–359.

67. Moore RY. Cranial motor neurons contain either galinin- or calcitonin gene–related peptidelike immunoreactivity. J Comp Neurol 1989;282:512–522.

68. Villar MJ, Huchet M, Hokfelt T, Changeux JP, Fahrenkrug J, Brown JC. Existence and coexistence of calcitonin gene–related peptide, vasoactive intestinal polypeptide, and somatostatin like immunoreactivities in spinal cord motor neurons of developing embryos and posthatch chicks. Neurosci Lett 1988;86:114–118.

69. Agoston DV, Conlon JM. Presence of VIP-like immunoreactivity in the cholinergic electromotor system of *Torpedo marmorata*. J Neurochem 1986;47:445–453.

70. Alberghina M, Giuffrida Stella AM. Changes in phospholipid-metabolizing and lysosomal enzymes in hypoglossal nucleus and ventral horn motoneurons during regeneration of craniospinal nerves. J Neurochem 1988;51:15–20.

71. Armstrong DM, Saper CB, Levey AI, Wainer BH, Terry RD. Distribution of cholinergic neurons in rat brain: Demonstrated by the immunocytochemical localization of choline acetyltransferase. J Comp Neurol 1983;216:53–68.

72. Sar M, Stumpf WE. Androgen concentration in motor neurons of cranial nerves and spinal cord. Science 1977;197:77–79.

73. Ganguly DK, Das M. Effects of oxotremorine demonstrate presynaptic muscarinic and dopaminergic receptors on motor nerve terminals. Nature 1979;278:645–646.

74. Whitehouse PJ, Wamsley JK, Zarbin MA, Price DL, Toutellotte WW, Kuhar MJ. Amyotrophic lateral sclerosis: Alterations in neurotransmitter receptors. Ann Neurol 1983;14:8–16.

75. Ernfors P, Henschen A, Olson L, Persson H. Expression of nerve growth factor receptor mRNA is developmentally regulated and increased after axotomy in rat spinal cord motoneurons. Neuron 1989;2:1605–1613.

76. Hayashi H, Kato T. Acetyl-CoA synthesizing enzyme activities in single nerve cell bodies in rabbits. J Neurochem 1978;31:861–869.

77. Wong-Riley MT, Kageyama GH. Localization of cytochrome oxidase in the mammalian spinal cord and dorsal root ganglia, with quantitative analysis of ventral horn cells in monkeys. J Comp Neurol 1986;245:41–61.

78. Lowry OH. In: Richter D, ed. Metabolism of the nervous system. New York: Pergamon Press, 1957:323–328.

79. Robins E. In: Symposium on the histochemistry of the nervous system. J Histochem Cytochem 1960;8:431–436.

80. Campa JF, Engel WK. Histochemistry of motor neurons and interneurons in the cat lumbar spinal cord. Neurology 1970;20:559–568.

81. Sickles DW, McLendon RE. Metabolic variation among rat lumbosacral alpha-motoneurons. Histochemistry 1983;79:205–217.

82. Robinson N. Histochemistry of human cervical posterior root ganglion cells and a comparison with anterior horn cells. J Anat 1969;104:55–64.

83. Chalmers GR, Edgerton VR. Single motoneuron succinate dehydrogenase activity. J Histochem Cytochem 1989;37:1107–1114.

84. Campa JF, Engel WK. Histochemical and functional correlations in anterior horn neurons of the cat spinal cord. Science 1971;171:198–199.

85. Hirsch HE, Parks ME. The quantitative histochemistry of acid proteinase in the nervous system: localization in neurons. J Neurochem 1973;21:453–458.
86. Lowry OH. In: Waelsch H, ed. Progress in neurobiology: Ultrastructure and cellular chemistry of neural tissue. New York: Hoeber-Harper, 1957:69–82.
87. Back SA, Gorenstein C. Fluorescent histochemical localization of neutral endopeptidase-24.11 (enkephalinase) in the rat spinal cord. J Comp Neurol 1989; 280:436–450.
88. Robins E, Hirsch HE. Glycosidases in the nervous system. II. Localization of beta-galactosidase, beta-glucuronidase, and beta-glucosidase in individual nerve cell bodies. J Biol Chem 1968;243:4253–4257.
89. Nandy K, Bourne GH. Adenosine triphosphatase and 5'-nucleotidase in spinal cord. Arch Neurol 1964;11:547–553.
90. Magill-Solc C, McMahan UJ. Motor neurons contain agrin-like molecules. J Cell Biol 1988;107:1825–1833.
91. Rieger F, Grumet M, Edelman GM. N-CAM at the vertebrate neuromuscular junction. J Cell Biol 1985;101:285–293.
92. Tosney KW, Watanabe M, Landmesser L, Rutishauser U. The distribution of N-CAM in the chick hindlimb during axon outgrowth and synaptogenesis. Dev Biol 1986;114:437–452.
93. Redshaw JD, Bisby MA. Proteins of fast axonal transport in the regenerating hypoglossal nerve of the rat. Can J Physiol Pharmacol 1984;62:1387–1393.
94. Skene JHP, Willard M. Axonally transported proteins associated with axon growth in rabbit central and peripheral nervous systems. J Cell Biol 1981;89:96–103.
95. Olsson T, Kristensson K, Ljungdahl A, Maehlen J, Holmdahl R, Klareskog L. Gamma-interferon-like immunoreactivity in axotomized rat motor neurons. J Neurosci 1989;9:3870–3875.
96. Tanaka H, Obata K. Developmental changes in unique cell surface antigens of chick embryo spinal motoneurons and ganglion cells. Dev Biol 1984;106:26–37.
97. Urakami H, Chiu AY. A monoclonal antibody distinguishes somatic motor neurons from other neuronal populations in the rat nervous system. Soc Neurosci Abstr 1989;15:67.
98. Kushner PD. A library of monoclonal antibodies to Torpedo cholinergic synaptosomes. J Neurochem 1984;43:775–785.
99. McKay RDG, Hockfield SJ. Monoclonal antibodies distinguish antigenically discrete neuronal types in the vertebrate central nervous system. Proc Natl Acad Sci USA 1982;79:6747–6751.
100. Hastie ND, Bishop JO. The expression of three abundance classes of mRNA in mouse tissues. Cell 1976;9:761–774.
101. Ryall RW. Neuropharmacology: Types of chemical transmission and drug interactions. In: Austin GM, ed., The spinal cord. New York: Igaku-Shoin, 1983: 106–118.
102. Arvidsson U, Cullheim S, Ulfhake B, Hokfelt T, Terenius L. Altered levels of calcitonin gene-related peptide (CGRP)-like immunoreactivity of cat lumbar motoneurons after chronic spinal cord transection. Brain Res 1989;489:387–391.

103. Tetzlaff W, Bisby MA, Kreutzberg GW. Changes in cytoskeletal proteins in the rat facial nucleus following axotomy. J Neurosci 1988;8:3181–3189.

104. Engelhardt JI, Appel SH, Killian JM. Experimental autoimmune motoneuron disease. Ann Neurol 1989;26:368–376.

105. Engelhardt J, Joo F, Pakaski M, Kasa P. An improved method for the bulk isolation of spinal motoneurons. J Neurosci Methods 1985;15:219–227.

106. Dohrmann U, Edgar D, Sendtner M, Thoenen H. Muscle-derived factors that support survival and promote fiber outgrowth from embryonic chick spinal motor neurons in culture. Dev Biol 1986;118:209–221.

107. Weil DE, McIlwain DL. Distribution of soluble proteins within spinal motoneurons: a quantitative two-dimensional electrophoretic analysis. J Neurochem 1981;36:242–250.

108. Bisby MA. Similar polypeptide compositions of fast-transported proteins in rat motor and sensory axons. J Neurobiol 1977;8:303–314.

109. Stone GC, Wilson DL. Qualitative analysis of proteins rapidly transported in ventral horn motoneurons and bidirectionally from dorsal root ganglia. J Neurobiol 1979;10:1–12.

110. Black MM, Lasek RJ. A difference between the proteins conveyed in the fast component of axonal transport in guinea pig hypoglossal and vagus motor neurons. J Neurobiol 1978;9:433–443.

111. Jacobson M. Developmental neurobiology. New York: Plenum Press, 1978.

112. Gibson SJ, Polak JM, Giaid A, Hamid QA, Kar S, Jones PM, Denny P, Legon S, Amara SG, Craig RK, Bloom SR, Penketh RJA, Rodek C, Ibrahim NBN, Dawson A. Calcitonin gene–related peptide messenger RNA is expressed in sensory neurones of the dorsal root ganglia and also in spinal motoneurones in man and rat. Neurosci Lett 1988;91:283–288.

113. Breitbart RE, Andreadis A, Nadal-Ginard B. Alternative splicing: A ubiquitous mechanism for the generation of multiple protein isoforms from single genes. Annu Rev Biochem 1987;56:4.

114. Tapscott SJ, Bennet GS, Toyama Y, Kleinbart F, Holtzer H. Intermediate filament proteins in the developing chick spinal cord. Dev Biol 1981;86:40–54.

115. Bennett GS. Changes in intermediate filament composition during neurogenesis. Curr Topics Dev Biol 1987;21:151–183.

116. Raju T, Bignami A, Dahl D. In vivo and in vitro differentiation of neurones and astrocytes in the rat embryo. Dev Biol 1981;85:344–357.

117. Ayer LeLievre CS, Dahl D, Bjorklund H, Sieger A. Neurofilament immunoreactivity in developing rat autonomic and sensory ganglia. Int J Dev Neurosci 1985;3:385–399.

118. Cochard P, Paulin D. Initial expression of neurofilaments and vimentin in the central and peripheral nervous system of the mouse embryo in vivo. J Neurosci 1984;4:2080–2094.

119. Phelps PE, Barber RP, Brennan LA, Maines VM, Salvaterra PM, Vaughn JE. Embryonic development of four different subsets of cholinergic neurons in rat cervical spinal cord. J Comp Neurol 1990;291:9–26.

120. Julien J-P, Tretjakoff I, Beaudet L, Peterson AC. Expression and assembly of a

human neurofilament protein in transgenic mice provide a novel neuronal marking system. Genes Dev 1987;1:1085–1095.

121. Julien J-P, Beaudet L, Tretjakoff I, Peterson AC. Neurofilament gene expression in transgenic mice. J Physiol (Paris) 1990;84:50–52.

122. Shaw G, Weber K. Differential expression of neurofilament triplet proteins in brain development. Nature 1982;298:277–279.

123. Julien J-P, Meyer D, Flavell D, Hurst J, Grosveld F. Cloning and developmental expression of the murine neurofilament gene family. Mol Brain Res 1986;1:243–250.

124. Austin L. Molecular aspects of nerve regeneration. In: Lajtha A, ed. Handbook of Neurochemistry. Vol 9. New York: Plenum Press, 1985:1–29.

125. Skene JHP. Axonal growth-associated proteins. Annu Rev Neurosci 1989;12:127–156.

126. Lieberman AR. The axon reaction: A review of the principal features of perikaryal responses to axon injury. Int Rev Neurobiol 1971;14:49–124.

127. Edstrom J-E. Ribonucleic acid changes in the motoneurons of the frog during axon regeneration. J Neurochem 1959;5:43–49.

128. Walter P, Gilmore R, Blobel G. Protein translocation across the endoplasmic reticulum. Cell 1984;38:5–8.

129. Streit WJ, Dumoulin FL, Raivich G, Kreutzberg GW. Calcitonin gene–related peptide increases in rat facial motoneurons after peripheral nerve transection. Neurosci Lett 1989;101:143–148.

130. Tetzlaff W, Kreutzberg GW. Enzyme changes in the facial nucleus following a conditioning lesion. Exp Neurol 1984;85:547–564.

131. Hoover DB, Hancock JC. Effect of facial nerve transection on acetylcholinesterase, choline acetyltransferase, and [^{3}H]quinuclidinyl benzilate binding in rat facial nuclei. Neuroscience 1985;15:481–487.

132. Merlie JP, Isenberg KE, Russel SD, Sanes JR. Denervation supersensitivity in skeletal muscle: Analysis with a cloned cDNA probe. J Cell Biol 1984;99:332–335.

133. Merlie JP, Kornhauser JM. Neural regulation of gene expression by an acetylcholine receptor promoter in muscle of transgenic mice. Neuron 1989;2:1295–1300.

134. Black IB, Chikairishi DM, Lewis EJ. Trans-synaptic increase in RNA coding for tyrosine hydroxylase in a rat sympathetic ganglion. Brain Res 1985;339:151–153.

135. Cole AJ, Saffen DW, Baraban JM, Worley PF. Rapid increase of an immediate early gene messenger RNA in hippocampal neurons by synaptic NMDA receptor activation. Nature 1989;340:474–476.

136. Castellucci VF, Kennedy TE, Kandel ER, Goelet P. A quantitative analysis of 2-D gels identifies proteins in which labeling is increased following long-term sensitization in *Aplysia*. Neuron 1988;1:321–328.

137. Burke RE. Motor units: Anatomy, physiology and functional organization. In: Brooks VB, ed. Handbook of physiology. Section 1. The nervous system. Vol 2. Motor systems. Washington, DC: American Physiological Society, 1981:345–422.

138. Burke RE. Physiology of motor units. In: Engel AG, Banker BQ, eds. Myology. New York: McGraw-Hill, 1986:419–443.

139. Hennig R, Lomo T. Firing patterns of motor units in normal rats. Nature 1985;314: 164–166.

140. Murthy KSK. Vertebrate fusimotor neurones and their influences on motor behavior. Prog Neurobiol 1978;11:249–307.

141. Sickles DW, Oblak TG. Metabolic variation among alpha-motoneurons innervating different muscle-fiber types. I. Oxidative enzyme activity. J Neurophysiol 1984;51:529–537.

142. Czeh G, Gallego R, Kudo N, Kuno M. Evidence for the maintenance of motoneurone properties by muscle activity. J Physiol (Lond) 1978;281:239–252.

143. Towbin H, Staehlin T, Gordon J. Electrophoretic transfer of proteins from polyacrylamide gels to nitrocellulose sheets: procedure and some applications. Proc Natl Acad Sci USA 1979;76:4350–4354.

144. Young R, Davis R. Efficient isolation of genes by using antibody probes. Proc Natl Acad Sci USA 1983;80:1194–1198.

145. Aebersold RH, Leavitt J, Saavedra RA, Hood LE, Kent SB. Internal amino acid sequence analysis of proteins separated by one- or two-dimensional gel electrophoresis after in situ protease digestion on nitrocellulose. Proc Natl Acad Sci USA 1987;84:6970–6974.

146. Gonzalez GA, Yamamoto KK, Fischer WH, Karr D, Menzel P, Biggs W, Vale WW, Montminy MR. A cluster of phosphorylation sites on the cyclic AMP-regulated nuclear factor CREB predicted by its sequence. Nature 1989;337:749–752.

147. Erlich HA, ed. PCR technology: Principals and applications for DNA amplification. New York: Stockton Press, 1989.

148. Dickson JG, Prentice HM, Kenimer JG, Walsh FS. Isolation of cDNAs corresponding to neuron-specific and developmentally regulated mRNAs from chick embryo spinal cord. J Neurochem 1986;46:787–794.

149. Fredriksen K, Jat PS, Valtz N, Levy D, McKay R. Immortalization of precursor cells from the mammalian CNS. Neuron 1988;1:439–448.

150. Cepko CL. Immortalization of neural cells via retrovirus-mediated oncogene transduction. Annu Rev Neurosci 1989;12:47–65.

151. Greene LA, Rein G. Dopaminergic properties of a somatic cell hybrid line of mouse neuroblastoma × sympathetic ganglion cells. J Neurochem 1977;29:141–150.

152. Platika D, Boulos MH, Baizer L, Fishman MC. Neuronal traits of clonal cell lines derived by fusion of dorsal root ganglia neurons with neuroblastoma cells. Proc Natl Acad Sci USA 1985;82:3499–3503.

153. Hammond DN, Wainer BH, Tsonsgard JH, Heller A. Neuronal properties of clonal hybrid cell lines derived from central cholinergic neurons. Science 1986;234:1237–1240.

154. Shaw IT, Boulet S, Wong E, Cashman NR. Unique immunologic determinants of neuroblastoma-spinal cord (NSC) hybrid cells. Neurology 1990;40 (suppl 1); 273.

155. Pasternak S, Cashman NR, Hastings KEM. Motor neuron-specific genes: A hybrid cell cDNA cloning strategy. Soc Neurosci Abstr 1989;15:958.
156. Botstein D, White RL, Skolnock M, Davis RW. Construction of a genetic linkage map in man using restriction fragment length polymorphisms. Am J Hum Genet 1980;32:314–331.
157. Housman D, Gusella J. Molecular genetic approaches to neural degenerative disorders. In: Schmitt FO, Bird SJ, Bloom FE, eds. Molecular genetic neuroscience. New York: Raven Press, 1982:415–422.
158. Harding AE, Rosenberg RN. Molecular genetics and neurological disease: basic principles and methods. In: Rosenberg RN, Harding AE, eds. The molecular biology of neurological disease. Toronto: Butterworth, 1988:1–21.
159. Urakami H, Chiu AY. A monoclonal antibody that recognizes somatic motor neurons in the mature rat nervous system. J Neurosci 1990;10:620–630.
160. Melki J, Abdelhak S, Sheth P, Bachelot MF, Burlet P, Marcadet A, Aicardi J, Barois A, Carriere JP, Fardeau M, Fontan D, Ponsot G, Billette T, Angelini C, Barbosa C, Ferriere G, Lanzi G, Ottolini A, Babron MC, Cohen D, Hanauer A, Clerget-Darpoux F, Lathrop M, Munnich A, Frezal J. Gene for chronic spinal muscular atrophies maps to chromosome 5q. Nature 1990;344:767–768.

31

Research Directions in Amyotrophic Lateral Sclerosis: Problems and Prospects

Robert H. Brown, Jr.

Massachusetts General Hospital
Boston, Massachusetts

H. Robert Horvitz

Massachusetts Institute of Technology and Howard Hughes Medical Institute
Cambridge, Massachusetts

INTRODUCTION

As this volume documents, while numerous possible etiologies for amyotrophic lateral sclerosis (ALS) have been proposed and are being actively explored, the cause of this devastating disease remains unknown. Any adequate hypothesis must explain the following features of the illness: the highly selective deaths of motor neurons, particularly those within the spinal cord; the existence of both familial and sporadic forms of the disease; midlife onset; survival of only a few years; greater incidence among men than women; and a uniform prevalence worldwide, with the notable exception of the foci of endemic ALS in the Western Pacific basin.

In considering strategies for research concerning ALS, it is instructive to ask why investigations of this disease have been so unyielding. In our view, five major factors are relevant. (a) Relatively little is known about the basic cellular biology of the motor neuron. Embedded within the spinal cord and column, the motor neuron is highly inaccessible to in vivo study. As a consequence, we have only a limited understanding of the physiology of this cell type and in particular of the pathophysiological changes that occur during the course of the illness. For example, it is unclear how long prior to the clinical manifestations of ALS motor

This manuscript is dedicated to the memory of Oscar Horvitz, who died of ALS on Aug. 1, 1989.

neurons are first functionally compromised and first begin to die. Nor is it known how the pathology of these cells changes as the disease progresses. In addition, in vitro studies of motor neuron biology have been limited. (b) Little is known about the basic biology of cell death. Motor neuron degeneration in ALS is only one of numerous examples of cell death in biology. The major clinical features not only of the approximately 30 known neurodegenerative diseases, but also of stroke and certain types of trauma, are caused by cell death. In addition, cell death is a normal aspect of both development and tissue homeostasis. Yet our understanding of the cellular and molecular processes that lead to cell death in any biological system is rudimentary. (c) Other than the fact that both autosomal dominant and autosomal recessive forms of ALS exist, nothing is known about the genetics of ALS. Whereas the methods of molecular genetics have been applied with vigor to a variety of other neuromuscular disorders—the most successful example being Duchenne's muscular dystrophy (1)—comparable efforts to study familial ALS have just begun. (d) Good animal models for ALS have only recently been identified and have not yet been analyzed in detail. (e) No even marginally effective therapy for ALS has been discovered, which means that neither the classical method of pharmaceutical development—the synthesis and testing of a wide range of related molecules—nor a more systematic approach, based on knowledge of the mechanisms of action of a given agent, can be attempted.

We discuss below current research directions in each of these five areas. We do not intend this discussion to be comprehensive, but rather wish to express our view of the progress and promise in specific areas of biology relevant to ALS. We hope that the types of studies we discuss, as well as other types of investigations described throughout this book, will lead rapidly and effectively to the understanding, prevention, and cure of ALS.

THE MOTOR NEURON

Basic Motor Neuron Biology

Fundamental investigations into the cellular biology of the motor neuron seem highly likely to provide invaluable insight into possible causes of ALS and strategies for the treatment of this disease. For example, it is known that a substantial fraction of motor neurons dies during normal embryogenesis (reviewed in Ref. 2) and that these deaths can be modulated by factors derived both from muscle (3,4) (the target of the motor neurons) and from glial cells (5). It is possible that the mechanism that causes motor neuron death during normal embryogenesis is also responsible for motor neuron death in ALS, so that an understanding of motor neuron development will be directly relevant to the problem of motor neuron degeneration in ALS. Even if this is not the case, it is possible that the factors that protect motor neurons from dying embryonically might also protect motor neurons from dying in ALS patients. At least one candidate muscle-derived motor neuron trophic factor has been identified; this factor rescues motor neurons from death both in vitro and in vivo and has been partially purified and characterized (6,7). Other neurotrophic factors that promote the survival of cholinergic motor neurons, such as cholinergic neurotrophic factor (CNTF), have also been isolated and characterized molecularly (8). Such growth factors offer approaches both to an understanding of motor neuron death and to the development of agonists that might be effective pharmaceutical agents.

Factors necessary for sustaining the viability of mature, differentiated motor neurons or for promoting the ability of these cells to regenerate after injury are less well characterized. Terminally differentiated motor neurons have some capacity for regeneration, as distal motor neuron terminals can be induced to sprout (9). However, the limits to this form of neuronal plasticity and the factors that trigger and regulate it are unknown. Although the molecules that control neurogenesis during development might also act during motor neuron maintenance or regeneration, it seems equally plausible that distinct sets of molecules function in these various processes. The identification of factors that sustain mature motor neurons and/or promote their regeneration would be a promising step toward an understanding, and perhaps inhibition, of mechanisms that cause mature motor neurons to die.

Any molecule unique to motor neurons, or at least relatively important to motor neuron function, might also prove relevant to ALS. For example, androgen receptors have been reported to be localized to motor neurons, based on the observation that radiolabeled dihydrotestosterone is concentrated in motor neurons of the cranial nerves and spinal cord (10). Furthermore, this localization displays a specificity that corresponds to regions affected in ALS patients. This finding is consistent with the hypothesis that a defect in androgen function could be responsible for ALS and is intriguing given the higher incidence of ALS among men than among women.

More generally, the systematic identification of molecules that are relatively specific to motor neurons could provide a significant step toward explaining the specificity of motor neuron dysfunction in ALS. In addition, motor-neuron-specific molecules would constitute useful markers for studies of motor neuron biology. Both antibodies that recognize motor-neuron-specific antigens and cDNAs isolated by differential screening procedures and that correspond to motor-neuron-specific mRNAs are currently being sought (11).

Nonetheless, it should be noted that the specific involvement of motor neurons in ALS need not reflect defects in molecules that are specific to motor neurons. For example, it is known that enzyme deficiencies can have devastating and apparently specific consequences on motor neurons. Thus, in infantile acid maltase deficiency, the inaccessibility of glycogen leads to the death of motor neurons in the spinal cords of newborns, resulting in Pompe's disease, a malignant paralytic disorder that mimics the primary infantile motor neuron disorder Werdnig-Hoffman disease (12). Interestingly, a milder form of dysfunction of the same enzyme produces in adults a chronic progressive myopathy with less prominent motor neuron impairment and dysfunction in other tissues (13). Thus, deficiencies in this enzyme can lead to an apparently motor-neuron-specific disorder despite the fact that this enzyme clearly functions more broadly than in motor neurons. A similar example is provided by hexosaminidase deficiency, which can produce an adult-onset progressive motor neuropathy that mimics spinal muscular atrophy (14–16). In addition, a truly unique feature of motor neuron biology (such as size, shape, or soma or axonal localization, etc.) could be a consequence of the actions of many factors responsible for motor neuron development and function, no one of which is specific to motor neurons.

Motor Neuron Toxicology

The possibility that the demise of motor neurons in ALS might result from exposure to extrinsic toxins has been considered for decades. For example, lead toxicity is known to produce a motor neuropathy and in some cases myelopathic features (17). Nevertheless, in most cases of ALS studied, elevated lead levels have not been observed (Refs. 18,19, although see Ref. 20 for an alternative view). Another metal known to be toxic to motor neurons is aluminum, which is highly abundant in Western society and relatively uninvestigated with respect to neurological disorders other than dialysis dementia and Alzheimer's disease. Gajdusek and Salazar (21), Perl et al. (22), and Yase (23,24) have proposed that aluminum might be important in the high-incidence foci of ALS in Guam, Papua, New Guinea, and elsewhere in the Western Pacific. Garruto and colleagues (25) recently demonstrated that chronic, low-level toxicity from dietary (oral) aluminum can produce neurofibrillary pathology in motor neurons in primates.

Endogenous toxins have also been suggested as a possible cause of ALS. It has been proposed that intrinsic excitatory neurotransmitters might be responsible for neuronal cell death in a variety of neurological disorders, possibly by inducing excessive levels of intracellular calcium (26). More specifically, it has been reported that fasting plasma levels of the excitotoxic amino acid glutamate are elevated in ALS patients (27,28). A further possible relevance of excitotoxicity to motor neuron disease has been suggested by studies of the disorder lathyrism, which is indigenous to parts of India and is characterized by a progressive, disabling spasticity that reflects a degeneration of the anterior and lateral columns of regions of the spinal cord. Lathyrism has been shown by Spencer et al. (29)

to be a consequence of ingestion of the excitotoxin BOAA (beta-*N*-oxalylamino-L-alanine), a glutamate analog found in the legume *Lathyrus sativus*. Spencer et al. (30) also raised the possibility that endemic motor neuron disease in the Western Pacific might follow from the ingestion of the toxin BMAA (beta-*N*-methylamino-L-alanine), a component of the cycad nut. Primates fed large quantities of BMAA have been reported to develop behavioral and pathological changes referrable to motor neurons (predominantly, but not exclusively, in the spinal cord) and to large neurons in the extrapyramidal and frontal cortical regions. While the level of BMAA likely to be consumed by ingesting the cycad appears to be substantially lower than that fed to the primates in these studies (31), these findings are nonetheless provocative and bear further investigation.

The excitotoxin glutamate interacts with at least three classes of neuronal receptors, the best characterized of which is the *N*-methyl-D-aspartate (NMDA) receptor (26). NMDA antagonists protect against neuronal cell death in a variety of model systems (26). The identification and further characterization of NMDA antagonists, or of other agents that prevent excitotoxin-induced neuronal cell death, offer a promising approach to the development of pharmaceuticals that might be useful in the treatment of ALS.

Other substances toxic to motor neurons also warrant consideration. For example, antibodies directed against critical components of motor neurons (see below) might also be viewed as motor-neuron-specific toxins. Certain medicines also seem to be particularly toxic to motor neurons; for example, intrathecal or retrogradely transported Adriamycin produces major motor neuron pathology, presumably by intercalating into motor neuron DNA (32).

Motor Neuron Immunopathology

As recently reviewed by Appel et al. (33) and Drachman and Kuncl (34), there is considerable current interest in the possibility that some forms of motor neuron disease might be autoimmune. The clearest example is probably provided by cases of selective lower motor neuron disease in patients with monoclonal gammopathies (35). In some affected individuals, there is evidence of high titers of both monoclonal and polyclonal antibodies to specific antigens, such as GM1 ganglioside (36). Moreover, some of these patients have responded dramatically to aggressive anti-immune therapy (37). These findings are seminal, as they have established a reversible autoimmune pathogenesis for some forms of human motor neuron disease and raise the possibility that other forms of motor neuron disease might be similarly treatable. Although various studies have indicated that most forms of combined upper and lower motor neuron disease do not respond to conventional immunotherapy (38), further studies of immunosuppression of ALS are currently underway.

Potentially useful animal models for autoimmune-induced motor neuron disease have recently been developed. For example, guinea pigs immunized with bovine motor neurons develop a lower motor neuron disorder associated with high titers of anti–motor neuron antibodies and the presence of guinea pig immunoglobulin within the motor neurons of the affected animals (39). This latter observation suggests that immunoglobulins may be ingested by the motor neuron distally and transported to the soma, which raises the possibility that internalized antibodies can cause motor neuron degeneration. Different types of immunoglobulins might be routed through different intracellular compartments of the motor neuron and thereby have access to different intracellular organelles and antigens (40,41). Experimental autoimmune distal motor neuron dysfunction has also been induced by immunizing animals with other constituents of motor neurons, such as choline acetyltransferase (42).

Such autoimmune models for motor neuron disease are potentially important. First, they should allow identification of the target antigens that initiate the immune response and that are implicated in motor neuron pathology in these experimental disorders. Although these antigens might or might not be of direct relevance to ALS, they should certainly be useful in studies of basic motor neuron biology. Second, these experimental models should allow analysis of components of the immune system that lead to motor neuron dysfunction, including both the affector and effector immune mechanisms as well as the immunogenetic background of the affected strains. Finally, these models should not only facilitate studies of immunotherapy of autoimmune motor neuron disease, but, more generally, might also allow tests of strategies for enhancing function during the course of motor neuron involution from any cause.

CELL DEATH

The major pathological feature of ALS is motor neuron cell death. As noted above, cell death occurs not only in neurological disease, but also in normal development and tissue homeostasis (43–45). Studies of both normal and abnormal cell deaths that occur in organisms as diverse as mammals, insects, and nematodes have suggested that many of the distinct primary events that initiate the process of cell death act by triggering one of only a few general mechanisms that cause cells to die (e.g., Ref. 46). If so, an understanding of cell death processes gained from any of these experimental systems might help reveal the cell death processes that cause motor neuron degeneration in ALS patients.

Relatively little is understood about the basic biology of cell death. Abnormally high levels of excitatory neuronal input, growth factor deprivation, hormone stimulation or deprivation, as well as cell intrinsic events have all been shown to initiate cell death processes. Excessive levels of calcium have been implicated in a large variety of cell deaths and might prove to be a general step in the cell death process (26,43,45,47,48). Interestingly, many cell deaths are active processes on the parts of dying cells, requiring the de novo expression of new genes within cells that will die. For example, the inhibition of RNA or protein synthesis within cells otherwise destined to die prevents cell death in a broad variety of experimental systems, including vertebrate motor neurons that die in response to nerve growth factor deprivation (49), insect interneurons that die during normal development (50), glucocorticoid-treated thymocytes (51), and cells in the mammalian prostate gland that die in response to androgen deprivation (52). Similarly, the cell deaths that occur during normal nematode development or in various nematode genetic neurodegenerative disorders require the expression of specific "killer" genes within cells that will die (53–55). These observations suggest that the cell death process in ALS patients might well require the activation within motor neurons of specific genes that cause these cells to die. It seems plausible that these genes will prove to be both functionally and structurally similar to genes that cause the deaths of other cell types in humans and even to genes that cause cell deaths in other organisms. By inhibiting the activities of such genes, it may be possible to prevent the process of cell death. Thus, the identification of genes and molecules that function in cell death offers a promising approach to the understanding of the cell death process in ALS and to the development of therapeutic agents that could interfere with this process.

GENETICS OF ALS

Many forms of human motor neuron disease are inherited. Examples include familial ALS, which afflicts both upper and lower motor neurons; familial spastic paraparesis, which afflicts only upper motor neurons; and the spinal muscular atrophies, which afflict only lower motor neurons. Familial ALS has been estimated to account for 5–20% of all ALS (56). This ratio necessarily reflects a minimal value, and it is possible that a genetic basis for or a genetic predisposition toward ALS is responsible for a significantly greater fraction of cases. Most familial ALS displays simple Mendelian autosomal dominant inheritance. Familial ALS seems to be indistinguishable from sporadic ALS by clinical symptoms, age of onset, and duration (56,57). Some pathological findings, e.g., degeneration of posterior columns, seem to be more common in familial than sporadic ALS, but are nonetheless evident in both disorders (58). Overall, the similarities between familial and sporadic ALS suggest similar pathogenic mechanisms, although the disease process might be triggered in different ways. Thus, an understanding of the mutant gene(s) responsible for familial ALS promises to be relevant not only to familial ALS, but to sporadic ALS as well.

Current methodologies in human molecular genetics offer the prospect for the mapping and molecular cloning of the disease gene(s) responsible for familial

ALS. This approach has been enormously successful in identifying the general genetic map positions of numerous human genetic disorders (59,60). Knowledge of the map position of a disease gene allows genetic testing and hence genetic counseling. The techniques of molecular genetics have also led to the isolation of a number of disease genes, such as those for Duchenne's muscular dystrophy (61) and cystic fibrosis (62). With the gene in hand, one can identify and characterize in detail both the gene and its protein product. Knowledge of the structure and function of a familial ALS disease gene would offer the possibility of developing therapeutic agents that prevent the effects of that gene.

Studies of familial ALS are inherently more difficult than studies of other adult-onset neuromuscular diseases, primarily because the short survival period of afflicted individuals precludes the ready availability of blood samples from many patients within a single pedigree. Nonetheless, such studies, which we believe are extremely promising, have been begun; DNA samples have been obtained from affected individuals in approximately 250 families (57,63). Chromosomes from affected individuals are being examined cytologically, with the hope of identifying a chromosome aberration that will reveal the site of the familial ALS gene, much as was done to localize the gene responsible for Duchenne's muscular dystrophy (64). In addition, genetic linkage analysis is being performed. These linkage studies have the short-term goal of defining the general position of the gene on the genetic map as well as the longer-term goal of isolating the gene itself. These familial ALS pedigrees are also being used to test candidate genes (genes that one suspects might be responsible for familial ALS) for linkage to the disease. Genes that function within motor neurons, genes that function in cell death processes (possibly identified by homology with such genes from other organisms; see above), and genes that encode receptors for putative excitotoxins are examples of candidate genes worthy of examination. The advantages of using a candidate gene for these linkage studies are twofold. First, a successful candidate gene would display absolute linkage, which increases the likelihood of finding linkage with the relatively limited pedigrees available for familial ALS. Second, a successful candidate gene could result in direct identification of the disease gene, rather than of a linked DNA polymorphism that would still require extensive subsequent studies prior to isolation of the disease locus.

A more powerful and novel method for human genetic linkage studies has been proposed (65). This method, called "homozygosity mapping," is applicable only to diseases that display recessive inheritance and can be effectively used to study diseases expressed by unrelated inbred children. Although most familial ALS displays autosomal dominant transmission, a recessive form of familial ALS has been identified in Tunisia, where there is considerable consanguinity in marriages (66). This Tunisian disorder involves both upper and lower motor neurons. It differs from the dominant forms of familial ALS as well as from sporadic ALS in that it is juvenile-onset and of prolonged duration. The neuro-pathology of this disorder has not been described. Despite the differences in onset and duration, the clinical presentation of this recessive disease at any point in the course of the illness is strikingly similar to that of typical ALS, which suggests that the two disorders may be similar in pathogenesis as well. If so, the relative ease with which the genetics of the Tunisian disorder can be pursued offers the hope of rapid progress in this area.

ANIMAL MODELS FOR MOTOR NEURON DISEASE

In addition to the guinea pig model for autoimmune motor neuron disease dis-cussed above, a number of other intriguing mammalian models for motor neuron diseases have been described. *Mnd* mutant mice show late-onset degeneration of both upper and lower motor neurons (67). Furthermore, these mice share many pathological features with ALS patients, including increased ubiquitin levels, altered neurofilament distribution, and thyrotropin-releasing-hormone abnormal-ities. Thus, the *Mnd* mouse seems an extremely promising model for ALS. By contrast, the wobbler mutant mouse and the Brittany mutant spaniel are affected in only lower motor neurons and might be reasonable models for the spinal muscular atrophies (reviewed in Ref. 68). The disorder in the *Mnd* mouse is transmitted as an autosomal dominant trait, while the other two disorders are recessive. These genetic animal models could be advantageous in a variety of ways. First, they offer an approach to the isolation of genes responsible for ALS-like disorders; these genes would certainly be candidate genes for human ALS and could be used as discussed above. Second, these animal models offer the opportunity for pathological and physiological studies that are difficult or impossible to perform with ALS patients. Third, these models could be used for testing possible therapies, including gene therapies. It should be noted that even though these models all involve a primary genetic etiology, they nonetheless may well share cellular and molecular processes not only with familial, but also with sporadic ALS.

Other types of animal models could also be very informative. For example, when the gene for familial ALS is cloned, transgenic mice could be generated using this gene or its murine equivalent. Such a model might closely mimic the molecular and possibly the cellular defects seen in the human disease. Inverte-brate models might also be useful, in part because of their much greater ease of manipulation and analysis. For example, it has been proposed that genetic neu-rodegenerative disorders of the nematode *Caenorhabditis elegans* might be ap-propriate models for the analysis of, and perhaps even for the development of therapeutic agents for the treatment of, ALS (69,70). Two distinct classes of *C. elegans* neurodegenerative disorders have been described. First, mutations in the genes *deg-1* (neuronal *deg*eneration) and *mec-4* (*mec*hanosensory abnormal) lead to the late-onset degeneration of a small number of specific neuron types, and this degenerative phenotype displays a dominant inheritance pattern. Based on studies of these genes, it seems plausible that familial ALS could be caused by a mutant, cytotoxic form of a membrane protein that normally is expressed by and functions within motor neurons. This mutant protein might result in the abnormal activation of a receptor or of a second-messenger system or in the more frequent or prolonged opening of a membrane channel. Sporadic ALS could involve a similar mechanism, with an exogenous agent responsible for triggering the same physiological process.

The *C. elegans* gene *egl-1* (*egg*-laying abnormal) provides an alternative model for ALS (70,71). As noted above, in many organisms, including both nematodes and humans, cell death is a normal feature of development. In *C. elegans* mutants that carry dominant mutations in the gene *egl-1*, a specific class of motor neurons expresses the genes responsible for naturally occurring or "programmed" cell death, and these neurons die. By analogy, ALS could involve the inappropriate expression of genes that normally function in the programmed cell deaths that occur during human development.

CLINICAL STUDIES

It seems reasonable to expect that additional clinical studies of ALS will enhance our understanding of this disease. To the extent that it is feasible, efforts to characterize the motor neuron early during the course of ALS should be considered. Thus, one might perform cortical motor stimulation studies to quantify the degree of involvement of the corticospinal tracts as a function of the severity of the clinical symptoms. More speculatively, one might obtain spinal cord biopsies from selected patients, with the goal of defining the earliest histopathology of the motor neurons. Such findings would bear directly on the consideration of which of the model systems for cell death might be most relevant, as, for example, certain cell death processes begin with cell shrinking while others begin with cell swelling (46). Additional studies using pathological material from ALS patients would also be informative. For example, one might examine the expression in ALS autopsy or biopsy material of molecules identified in motor neurons and postulated to be involved in the process of motor neuron death in ALS (e.g., ubiquitin and phosphorylated neurofilament proteins; Refs. 72,73).

Excitotoxin receptor antagonists, calcium channel blockers, and neuronal growth factors all should be tested for efficacy in the treatment of ALS. In addition, it is arguable that clinical studies of ALS should include trials of drugs even remotely suspected to be of possible benefit. Such drug trials should be rigorously designed and controlled, so their outcomes can be interpreted in a meaningful way. In addition, such trials optimally should test specific hypotheses and thus be potentially informative not only with respect to the pharmacotherapy of ALS, but also with respect to the etiology of the disease. Given the devastating nature of ALS and our current complete inability to combat this disorder, this empirical and classical approach to medicine should continue to complement the more basic investigative approaches to the understanding, prevention, and cure of ALS discussed above.

ACKNOWLEDGMENTS

Studies of ALS in the authors' laboratories have been supported by funds from the Muscular Dystrophy Association, the ALS Association, the Pierre L. de Bourgknecht ALS Foundation, and the Cecil B. Day Foundation (to R.H.B.) and from the Howard Hughes Medical Institute and Cambridge NeuroScience, Inc. (to H.R.H.). H.R.H. is an Investigator of the Howard Hughes Medical Institute.

REFERENCES

1. Brown RH, Jr., Hoffman EP. Molecular biology of Duchenne muscular dystrophy. Trends Neurosci 1988;11:480–484.
2. Hamburger V, Oppenheim RW. Naturally occurring neuronal death in vertebrates. Neurosci Commentaries 1982;1:39–65.
3. Giller EL, Neale JH, Bullock PN, Schrier BK, Nelson PG. Choline acetyltransferase activity of spinal cord cell cultures increased by co-culture with muscle and by muscle-conditioned medium. J Cell Biol 1977;74:16–29.
4. Schnaar RL, Schaffner AE. Separation of cell types from embryonic chicken and rat spinal cord: Characterization of motoneuron-enriched fractions. J Neurosci 1981;1: 204–214.
5. Dohrmann U, Edgar D, Thoenen H. Distinct neurotrophic factors from skeletal muscles and the central nervous system interact synergistically to support the survival of cultured embryonic spinal motor neurons. Dev Biol 1987;124:145–152.
6. McManaman JL, Crawford FG, Stewart SS, Appel SH. Purification of a skeletal muscle polypeptide which stimulates choline acetyltransferase activity in cultured spinal cord neurons. J Biol Chem 1988;263:5890–5897.
7. Oppenheim RW, Haverkamp LJ, Prevette D, McManaman JL, Appel SH. Reduction of naturally occurring motoneuron death in vivo by a target-derived neurotrophic factor. Science 1988;240:919–922.
8. Stockli KA, Lottspeich F, Sendtner M, Masiakowski P, Carroll P, Gotz R, Lindholm D, Thoenen H. Molecular cloning, expression and regional distribution of rat ciliary neurotrophic factor. Nature 1989;342:920–923.
9. Brown MC, Holland RL, Hopkins WG. Motor nerve sprouting. Annu Rev Neurosci 1981;4:17–42.
10. Sar M, Stumpf WE. Androgen concentration in motorneurons of cranial neurons and spinal cord. Science 1977;197:77–79.
11. Shaw IT, Boulet S, Wong E, Cashman NR. Unique immunologic determinants of neuroblastoma–spinal cord (NSC) hybrid cells. Neurology 1990;40:273A.

12. Adams RD, Victor M. Principles of neurology. 3rd ed. New York: McGraw-Hill, 1985:1061.
13. Engel AG. Acid maltase deficiency. In: Engel AG, Banker BQ, eds. Myology. Chapter 55. New York: McGraw-Hill, 1986:1629–1651.
14. Kolodny EH, Raghavan SS. GM2-gangliosidosis: Hexosaminidase mutations not of the Tay-Sachs type produce unusual clinical variants. Trends Neurosci 1983;6: 16–20.
15. Navon R, Argov Z, Frisch A. Hexosaminidase A deficiency in adults. Am J Med Genet 1986;24:179–196.
16. Karni A, Navon R, Sadeh M. Hexosaminidase A deficiency manifesting as spinal muscular atrophy of late onset. Ann Neurol 1988;24:451–453.
17. Conradi S, Ronnevi L-O, Norris FH. Motor neuron disease and toxic metals 1982. In: Rowland LP, ed. Advances in neurology: Human motor neuron diseases. Vol 36. New York: Raven Press, 1982:201–231.
18. House AO, Abbot RJ, Davidson DLW, Ferguson JT, Lenman JAR. Penicillamine of lead concentrations in CSF and blood in patients with motor neuron disease. Br Med J 1978;2:1684.
19. Manton WJ, Cook JD. Lead content of cerebrospinal fluid and other tissue in amyotrophic lateral sclerosis (ALS). Neurology 1979;29:611–612.
20. Conradi S, Ronnevi L-O, Nise G, Vesterberg O. Abnormal distribution of lead in amyotrophic lateral sclerosis. Reestimation of lead in the cerebrospinal fluid. J Neurol Sci 1980;48:413–418.
21. Gajdusek DC, Salazar AM. Amyotrophic lateral sclerosis and parkinsonian syndromes in high incidence among the Auyu and Jakai people of West New Guinea. Neurology 1982;32:107–126.
22. Perl DP, Gajdusek DC, Garruto RM, Yanagihara RT, Gibbs CJ. Intraneuronal aluminum accumulation in amyotrophic lateral sclerosis and Parkinsonism-dementia of Guam. Science 1982;217:1053–1055.
23. Yase Y. A.L.S. in the Kii Peninsula: One possible etiological hypothesis. In: Tsubaki T, Toyokura Y, eds. Amyotrophic lateral sclerosis. Baltimore: University Park Press, 1979:307–318.
24. Yase Y. The pathogenetic role of metals in motor neuron disease—The participation of aluminum. Adv Exp Med Biol 1987;209:89–96.
25. Garruto RM, Shankar SK, Yanagihara R, Salazar AM, Amyx HL, Gajdusek DC. Low-calcium, high-aluminum diet-induced motor neuron pathology in cynomolgus monkeys. Acta Neuropathol 1989;78:210–219.
26. Choi DW. Glutamate neurotoxicity and diseases of the nervous system. Neuron 1988;1:623–634.
27. Plaitakis A, Caroscio JT. Abnormal glutamate metabolism in ALS. Ann Neurol 1985;18:271–280.
28. Plaitakis A, Caroscio JT. Abnormal glutamate metabolism in amyotrophic lateral sclerosis. Ann Neurol 1987;22:575–579.
29. Spencer PS, Ludolph A, Dwivedi MP, Roy DN, Hugon J, Schaumburg HH. Lathyrism: Evidence for the role of the neuroexcitatory amino acid BOAA. Lancet 1986;2:1066–1067.

30. Spencer PS, Nunn PB, Hugon J, Ludolph AC, Ross SM, Roy DN, Robertson RC. Guam amyotrophic lateral sclerosis–Parkinsonism-dementia linked to a plant excitant neurotoxin. Science 1987;237:517–522.

31. Duncan MW, Steele JC, Kopin IJ, Markey SP. 2-Amino-3-(methylamino)-propanoic acid (BMAA) in cycad flour: An unlikely cause of amyotrophic lateral sclerosis and parkinsonism-dementia of Guam. Neurology 1990;40:767–772.

32. England JD, Asbury AK, Rhee KE, Summer AJ. Lethal retrograde axoplasmic transport of doxorubicin (Adriamycin) to motorneurons. A toxic motor neuropathy. Brain 1988;111:915–926.

33. Appel SH, Stockton-Appel V, Stewart SS, Kerman RH. Amyotrophic lateral sclerosis: Associated clinical disorders and immunological evaluations. Arch Neurol 1986;43:234–238.

34. Drachman DB, Kuncl RW. Amyotrophic lateral sclerosis: An unconventional autoimmune disease? Ann Neurol 1989;26:269–274.

35. Latov N, Hayes AP, Sherman WH. Peripheral neuropathy and anti-MAG antibodies. Crit Rev Neurobiol 1988;3:301–332.

36. Pestronk A, Adams RN, Clawson L, Cornblath D, Kuncl RW, Griffin D, Drachman DB. Serum antibodies to GM1 ganglioside in amyotrophic lateral sclerosis. Neurology 1988;38:1457–1461.

37. Pestronk A, Cornblath DR, Ilyas AA, Baba H, Quarles RH, Griffin JW, Alderson K, Adams RN. A treatable multifocal motor neuropathy with antibodies to GM1 ganglioside. Ann Neurol 1988;24:73–78.

38. Brown RH, Hauser SL, Harrington H, Weiner HL. Failure of immunosuppression with a ten- to 14-day course of high-dose intravenous cyclophosphamide to alter the progression of amyotrophic lateral sclerosis. Arch Neurol 1986;43:383–384.

39. Englelhardt JI, Appel SH, Killian JM. Experimental autoimmune disease. Ann Neurol 1989;26:368–376.

40. Fabian RH, Petroff G. Intraneuronal IgG in the central nervous system: Uptake by retrograde axonal transport. Neurology 1987;37:1780–1784.

41. Fabian RH. Uptake of plasma IgG by central nervous system motor neurons: Comparison of anti-neuronal and normal IgG. Neurology 1988;38:1775–1780.

42. Chao L-P, Kan K-SK, Angelini C, Keesey J. Autoimmune neuromuscular disease induced by a preparation of choline acetyltransferase. Exp Neurol 1982;75:23–35.

43. Bowen I, Lockshin R, eds. Cell death in biology and pathology. New York: Chapman and Hall, 1981.

44. Cowan WM, Fawcett J, O'Leary D, Stanfield B. Regressive events in neurogenesis. Science 1984;225:1258–1265.

45. Potten C. Perspectives on mammalian cell death. Oxford: Oxford University Press, 1987.

46. Walker N, Harmon B, Gobe G, Kerr J. Patterns of cell death. Meth Achiev Exp Pathol 1988;13:18–54.

47. Cohen J, Duke R. Glucocorticoid activation of a calcium-dependent endonuclease in thymocyte nuclei leads to cell death. J Immunol 1984;132:38–42.

48. Conner J, Sawczuk I, Benson M, Tomashevsky P, O'Toole K, Olsson C, Buttyan

R. Calcium channel antagonists delay regression of androgen-dependent tissues and suppress gene activity associated with cell death. Prostate 1987;13:119–130.

49. Martin D, Schmidt R, DiStefano P, Lowry O, Carter J, Johnson E. Inhibitors of protein synthesis and RNA synthesis prevent neuronal cell death caused by nerve growth factor deprivation. J Cell Biol 1988;106:829–843.

50. Fahrbach S, Truman J. Mechanisms for programmed cell death in the nervous system of a moth. In: Selective neuronal death, Ciba Foundation Symposium no. 126. Chichester: Wiley, 1987:65–81.

51. Cohen J, Duke R. Glucocorticoid activation of a calcium-dependent endonuclease in thymocyte nuclei leads to cell death. J Immunol 1984;132:38–42.

52. Stanisic T, Sadlowski R, Lee C, Grayhack J. Partial inhibition of castration induced ventral prostate regression with acinomycin D and cyclohexamide. Invest Urol 1978;16:19–22.

53. Herman R. Mosaic analysis of two genes that affect nervous system structure in *Caenorhabditis elegans*. Genetics 1987;116:377–388.

54. Chalfie M, Au M. Genetic control of differentiation of *Caenorhabditis elegans* touch receptor neurons. Science 1989;243:1027–1033.

55. Yuan J, Horvitz HR. The *Caenorhabditis elegans* genes *ced-3* and *ced-4* act cell autonomously to cause programmed cell death. Dev Biol 1990;138:33–41.

56. Mulder DW, Kurland LT, Offord KP, Beard CM. Familial adult motor neuron disease: Amyotrophic lateral sclerosis. Neurology 1986;36:511–517.

57. Brown R Jr, Horvitz HR, Rouleau G, McKenna-Yaskek D, Beard C, Sapp P, Haines J, Gusella J, Figlewicz D. Progress report: Investigation of gene linkage in familial amyotrophic lateral sclerosis. In: Rowland LP, ed. Amyotrophic lateral sclerosis. New York: Raven Press.

58. Rowland LP. Human motor neuron diseases. In: Advances in neurology 36. New York: Raven Press: 1981.

59. Gusella JF. DNA polymorphism and human disease. Annu Rev Biochem 1986;55: 831–854.

60. Conneally PM, Rivas ML. Linkage analysis in man. Adv Hum Genet 1980;10: 209–266.

61. Koenig M, Hoffman EP, Bertelson CJ, Monaco AP, Feener C, Kunkel LM. Complete cloning of the Duchenne muscular dystrophy (DMD) cDNA and preliminary genomic organization of the DMD gene in normal and affected individuals. Cell 1987;50:507–517.

62. Rommens JM, Iannuzzi MC, Kerem B-S, et al. Identification of the cystic fibrosis gene: Chromosome walking and jumping. Science 1989;245:1059–1065.

63. Siddique T, Pericak-Vance M, Brooks B, Roos R, Hung W-Y, Antel J, Munsat T, Phillips K, Warner K, Speer M, Bias W, Siddique N, Roses A. Linkage analysis in familial amyotrophic lateral sclerosis. Neurology 1989;39:919–925.

64. Francke U, Ochs HD, de Martinville B. Minor Xp21 chromosome deletion in a male associated with expression of Duchenne muscular dystrophy, chronic granulomatous disease, retinitis pigmentosa and McLeod's syndrome. Am J Hum Genet 1985;37:250–267.

About the Editor

RICHARD ALAN SMITH is Director of the Center for Neurologic Study in San Diego, California, and he also serves on the senior medical staff of Scripps Memorial Hospital in La Jolla. He is the author or coauthor of numerous articles, book chapters, and proceedings papers, which focus on research and clinical aspects of presently incurable neurological disorders, including amyotrophic lateral sclerosis and multiple sclerosis, and is the editor of one book, *Interferon Treatment of Neurologic Disorders* (Marcel Dekker, Inc.). In 1968 the San Francisco Neurologic Society honored Dr. Smith with its Henry Newman Award for his studies on the management of ALS—a subject that has interested him throughout his career. Dr. Smith has pursued laboratory studies dealing with a possible viral or cytoskeletal origin of ALS. This evolved into a more general interest in the experimental treatment of neurological diseases, first with interferons and more recently with growth factors and NMDA receptor blockers. An associate member of the American Academy of Neurology, he is a member of the American Association for the Advancement of Science. He is a scientific advisor to the International Motor Neuron Disease Association and NeuroTherapeutics Corporation. Dr. Smith received the M.D. degree (1965) from the University of Miami School of Medicine and completed his internship (1965-1966) at Jackson Memorial Hospital in Miami, Florida, and residency in neurology (1966-1969) at Stanford University Hospital in Palo Alto, California.